Teaching Atlas of Chest Imaging

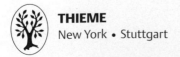

THIEME
New York • Stuttgart

Teaching Atlas of Chest Imaging

Mark S. Parker, M.D.
Associate Professor
Department of Radiology
Thoracic Imaging Section
Medical College of Virginia Hospitals–VCU Health System
Richmond, Virginia

Melissa L. Rosado-de-Christenson, M.D., F.A.C.R.
Clinical Professor
Department of Radiology
The Ohio State University College of Medicine
Columbus, Ohio
Adjunct Professor
Department of Radiology and Nuclear Medicine
Uniformed Services University of the Health Sciences
Bethesda, Maryland

Gerald F. Abbott, M.D.
Associate Professor
Brown Medical School
Director of Chest Radiology
Rhode Island Hospital
Providence, Rhode Island

Thieme Medical Publishers, Inc.
333 Seventh Ave.
New York, NY 10001

Editor: Timothy Hiscock
Vice President, Production and Electronic Publishing: Anne T. Vinnicombe
Production Editor: Print Matters, Inc.
Sales Manager: Ross Lumpkin
Chief Financial Officer: Peter van Woerden
President: Brian D. Scanlan
Compositor: Compset
Printer: Edwards Brothers

Library of Congress Cataloging-in-Publication Data

Parker, Mark S.
Teaching atlas of chest imaging / Mark S. Parker, Melissa L. Rosado-de-Christenson, Gerald F. Abbott.
    p. ; cm.
    Includes bibliographical references and index.
    ISBN 1-58890-230-7 — ISBN 3-13-139021-2
        1. Chest—Radiography—Atlases. 2. Diagnosis, Radioscopic—Atlases. 3. Chest—Diseases—Diagnosis—Atlases.
    [DNLM: 1. Diagnostic Imaging—Atlases. 2. Diagnostic Imaging—Case Reports. 3. Thoracic Diseases—diagnosis—Atlases. 4. Thoracic Diseases—diagnosis—Case Reports. 5. Radiography, Thoracic—Atlases. 6. Radiography, Thoracic—Case Reports. WF 17 P242t 2005] I. Rosado de Christenson, Melissa L. II. Abbott, Gerald F. III. Title.
    RC941.P285 2005
    617.5′407572—dc22

                                                                                    2005050647

Important note: Medical knowledge is ever-changing. As new research and clinical experience broaden our knowledge, changes in treatment and drug therapy may be required. The authors and editors of the material herein have consulted sources believed to be reliable in their efforts to provide information that is complete and in accord with the standards accepted at the time of publication. However, in view of the possibility of human error by the authors, editors, or publisher of the work herein or changes in medical knowledge, neither the authors, editors, or publisher, nor any other party who has been involved in the preparation of this work, warrants that the information contained herein is in every respect accurate or complete, and they are not responsible for any errors or omissions or for the results obtained from use of such information. Readers are encouraged to confirm the information contained herein with other sources. For example, readers are advised to check the product information sheet included in the package of each drug they plan to administer to be certain that the information contained in this publication is accurate and that changes have not been made in the recommended dose or in the contraindications for administration. This recommendation is of particular importance in connection with new or infrequently used drugs.

Some of the product names, patents, and registered designs referred to in this book are in fact registered trademarks or proprietary names even though specific reference to this fact is not always made in the text. Therefore, the appearance of a name without designation as proprietary is not to be construed as a representation by the publisher that it is in the public domain.

Printed in the United States of America
5 4 3 2 1
TMP ISBN 1-58890-230-7

GTV ISBN 3-13-139021-2

DEDICATION

To my heavenly Father, for the many blessings He has afforded me in life.
To my parents, for the encouragement and opportunities they provided.
To my wife Cindy, son Steven, and daughter Casey for their love, support, and countless sacrificed hours of family time.
To my best friends and colleagues, Melissa and Gerry, for their friendship, relentless dedication, and hard work.

Mark S. Parker, M.D.

To my husband, Paul J. Christenson, M.D., and my children, Heather, Jennifer, and Jon, for their love, support, and encouragement. To the countless radiology residents it has been my privilege to teach over the course of my career. Your curiosity, enthusiasm, and case contributions greatly enhance my academic life.

Melissa L. Rosado de Christenson, M.D., F.A.C.R.

To my family, friends, and colleagues for their patience, support, and encouragement.

Gerald F. Abbott, M.D.

CONTENTS

ANOMALIES OF THE PULMONARY ARTERIES AND VEINS

CARDIAC ANOMALIES

SECTION III
Airways Disease

SECTION IV
Atelectasis
MECHANISMS

DIRECT SIGNS OF ATELECTASIS

INDIRECT SIGNS OF ATELECTASIS

PATTERNS OF LOBAR COLLAPSE

SECTION V
Pulmonary Infections and Aspiration Pneumonia

SECTION VI
Neoplastic Diseases

SECTION VII
Trauma
THORACIC AORTA AND GREAT VESSEL INJURIES

LUNG INJURY

PLEURAL MANIFESTATIONS OF TRAUMA

AIRWAY INJURIES

DIAPHRAGMATIC INJURIES

THORACIC SKELETAL INJURIES

BAROTRAUMA

SECTION VIII
Life Support Tubes, Lines, and Monitoring Devices
ENDOTRACHEAL TUBES: TRACHEOSTOMY DEVICES

CENTRAL VENOUS CATHETERS

SECTION XIII
Pleura, Chest Wall, and Diaphragm

FOREWORD

Radiologists involved in education face a series of new and unique challenges. Our knowledge of the process of adult learning continues to evolve, and it is clear that some of the traditional tools that have been used in the past, including the standard textbook and traditional lectures, are probably not the best teaching instruments. In the field of radiology, there is increasing evidence that radiologists at all levels, including residents in training, learn better from practical case-based material. The current requirements for maintenance of certification emphasize a lifelong learning process and the need for self-assessment.

The *Teaching Atlas of Chest Imaging* fulfills many of the requirements for adult learning in the field of radiology. It is an eminently readable text that provides content related to the important categories of chest disease through a series of well-illustrated case-based material.

The book opens with an image gallery that illustrates normal anatomy on all imaging modalities pertinent to chest imaging. Each disease entity and subsequent sections or chapters open with a representative case. Each case is typically illustrated with four images, complete with image captions, diagnosis, and differential diagnosis. In addition, there is a comprehensive discussion of each disease entity, including background information, etiology, and clinical findings, as well as bulleted descriptions of pathology, imaging findings, treatment, and prognosis. Especially helpful features include bulleted "pearls" pertinent to each disease, where appropriate, and bulleted "pitfalls" pertinent to each disease. There are additional figures included with each case, demonstrating additional imaging manifestations of the disease being discussed and in some cases illustrations of related diseases. There is an excellent up-to-date list of suggested readings at the end of each case discussion.

The quality of the imaging figures is excellent, and a computer graphic artist has produced pertinent illustrations for many sections of this book.

Practicing radiologists, those involved in the process of maintaining certification, as well as residents and fellows in chest radiology and pulmonary medicine will all find this case-based textbook extremely useful. The approach is comprehensive, and 192 cases are included, covering the entire spectrum of chest disease.

I have known all of the authors for quite some time. As expected, the text reflects their experience at the Armed Forces Institute of Pathology. The content is rigorous and comprehensive and the case material is excellent. This text should be on the bookshelf of all physicians interested in chest disease.

Theresa C. McLoud, M.D.

PREFACE

Chest imaging remains one of the most complex subspecialties of diagnostic radiology. Advances in the use of imaging for the evaluation of airway disease, cardiovascular disease, diffuse lung disease, pulmonary thromboembolism, and thoracic trauma, as well as an increasing role of imaging in the critical care setting, and in lung cancer screening, introduce additional complexity to the study and understanding of thoracic imaging. Successful delivery of thoracic imaging services is further jeopardized by the marked shortage of thoracic radiologists and residents pursuing thoracic imaging fellowship training. Radiology residents need to be exposed to a large volume of thoracic imaging cases in order to master image interpretation, generate appropriate differential diagnoses, and play a valuable role in patient management. General radiologists and body imagers often find themselves in the uncomfortable position of covering the "chest service" and interpreting complex studies, without adequate resources. This book, *Teaching Atlas of Chest Imaging*, was developed to meet these needs. We also hope thoracic radiologists and pulmonary physicians will find this book a useful resource.

We encourage all our readers to review this atlas from cover to cover and study the common and uncommon manifestations of frequently encountered thoracic diseases. We recognize that a strong foundation in normal anatomy is essential to the understanding of chest diseases and their various imaging manifestations. Thus, the atlas begins with an overview of normal chest radiography, computed tomography, and magnetic resonance imaging anatomy. The remainder of the atlas is formulated as a case-based review of numerous congenital, traumatic, and acquired thoracic conditions. Each case is supported by a brief discussion of the etiology, pathology, imaging findings, treatment, and prognosis of the disease process illustrated in a concise bulleted format. These discussions are based on up-to-date reviews of the current literature as well as classic or landmark articles. Additional images illustrate other manifestations of a given entity or entities to be considered. Major teaching points ("Pearls") are provided for most cases to emphasize those features that may strongly support a specific diagnosis. Suggested readings are provided for those who desire additional or more in-depth information.

Mark S. Parker, M.D.
Melissa L. Rosado de Christenson, M.D.
Gerald F. Abbott, M.D.

ACKNOWLEDGMENTS

The authors wish to thank Rob Walker of Walker Illustration for his outstanding efforts in creating the graphic illustrations for this project and Heather K. Christenson for the immense research assistance she provided.

CONTRIBUTORS

Michael Atalay, M.D., Ph.D.
Assistant Professor,
  Diagnostic Imaging
Brown Medical School
Rhode Island Hospital
Providence, Rhode Island

Cynthia K. Brooks, M.D.
Department of Diagnostic Radiology
Medical College of Virginia
  Hospitals–VCU Health System
Richmond, Virginia

William R. Corse, D.O.
Director of MRI Imaging
Doylestown Hospital
Doylestown, Pennsylvania

John J. Cronan, M.D.
Professor, Diagnostic Imaging
Brown Medical School
Radiologist-in-Chief
Rhode Island Hospital
Providence, Rhode Island

Jeremy J. Erasmus, M.D.
Professor
Department of Radiology
University of Texas
M.D. Anderson Cancer Center
Houston, Texas

Harold L. Floyd, M.D.
Associate Professor
Department of Radiology
Thoracic Imaging Section
Medical College of Virginia
  Hospitals–VCU Health System
Richmond, Virginia

Aletta A. Frazier, M.D.
Department of Radiologic Pathology
Armed Forces Institute of Pathology
Washington, DC
Clinical Associate Professor
Department of Radiology
University of Maryland School of Medicine
Baltimore, Maryland

Jud W. Gurney, M.D., F.A.C.R.
Professor
Department of Radiology
University of Nebraska Medical Center
Omaha, Nebraska

Daniel A. Henry, M.D.
Associate Professor
Department of Radiology
Director Thoracic/Chest Radiology
Medical College of Virginia
  Hospitals–VCU Health System
Richmond, Virginia

Kenneth C. Hite, M.D.
Department of Radiology
Medical College of Virginia
  Hospitals–VCU Health System
Richmond, Virginia

Wanda M. Kirejczyk, M.D.
Department of Radiology
New Britain General Hospital
New Britain, Connecticut

Michael J. Landay, M.D.
Professor
Department of Radiology
University of Texas Southwestern
  Medical Center
Dallas, Texas

Maysiang Lesar, M.D.
Department of Radiology
National Naval Medical Center
Bethesda, Maryland

Gael J. Lonergan, M.D.
Department of Pediatric Radiology
Children's Hospital of Austin
Austin, Texas
Associate Professor
Departments of Radiology and Pediatrics
Uniformed Services University of the Health
    Sciences
Bethesda, Maryland

Martha B. Mainiero, M.D.
Assistant Professor
Department of Diagnostic Imaging
Brown Medical School
Rhode Island Hospital
Providence, Rhode Island

H. Page McAdams, M.D.
Professor
Department of Radiology
Duke University School of Medicine
Durham, North Carolina

Theresa C. McLoud, M.D.
Associate Radiologist-in-Chief
Director of Education
Professor of Radiology
Harvard Medical School
Boston, Massachussetts

Lakshmana Das Narla, M.D.
Professor
Department of Radiology, Pediatrics
Medical College of Virginia Hospitals–VCU
    Health System
Richmond, Virginia

D. Laurie Persson
Department of Radiology
Photographic Section and
    Radiographic Design
Virginia Commonwealth University
    School of Medicine
Richmond, Virginia

Rakesh D. Shah, M.D., F.C.C.P.
Assistant Professor
Department of Radiology
New York School of Medicine
Chief of Thoracic Radiology
North Shore University Hospital
Manhasset, New York

Rosita M. Shah, M.D.
Clinical Associate Professor
Department of Diagnostic Radiology
Hospital of the University
    of Pennsylvania
Philadelphia, Pennsylvania

Stephanie E. Spottswood, M.D.
Associate Professor
Department of Radiology
Children's Hospital of the
    King's Daughters
Norfolk, Virginia

Diane C. Strollo, M.D., F.C.C.P.
Clinical Associate Professor
Department of Radiology
University of Pittsburgh
    School of Medicine
Pittsburgh, Pennsylvania

Malcolm K. Sydnor, Jr., M.D.
Assistant Professor
Department of Radiology
Medical College of Virginia Hospitals–VCU
    Health System
Richmond, Virginia

Rob Walker, B.F.A.
Rob Walker Illustration
Providence, Rhode Island

Helen T. Winer-Muram, M.D.
Department of Radiology
Indiana University School of Medicine
Indianapolis, Indiana

Jill D. Wruble, D.O.
Mandel and Blaum, D.S.P.C.
Hartford, Connecticut

Teaching Atlas of Chest Imaging

SECTION I
Normal Thoracic Anatomy

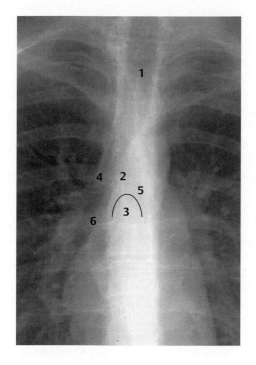

Figure I-1 Coned-down PA chest radiograph demonstrates the normal trachea and main bronchi. (Courtesy of Michael J. Landay, M.D., University of Texas Southwestern Medical Center at Dallas, Dallas, Texas.)

1. Trachea
2. Carina
3. Carinal angle
4. Right mainstem bronchus
5. Left mainstem bronchus
6. Bronchus intermedius

Airways

Trachea and Main Bronchi (Fig. I-1)

The trachea is a midline structure ranging from 6 to 9 cm in length. The anterior and lateral walls are composed of cartilaginous rings; the posterior wall is membranous. The tracheal diameter varies with the patient's sex:

Coronal diameter 13–25 mm; sagittal diameter 13–27 mm (men)
Coronal diameter 10–21 mm; sagittal diameter 10–23 mm (women)

The airway divides into the right and left main bronchi at the carina. Before 12 years of age, the right and left main bronchi follow a relatively vertical course. In adolescence and adulthood, the right main bronchus assumes a more vertical course than the left, which lies more horizontal. The carinal angle ranges between 40 and 75 degrees in adults.

Lobar and Segmental Bronchi (Figs. I-2 and I-3)

RIGHT LUNG

The *right upper lobe bronchus* arises from the lateral wall of the main bronchus and divides into three branches, supplying the apical, anterior, and posterior segments. The *bronchus intermedius* continues distally from the right upper lobe bronchus take-off, is about 3 to 4 cm long, and bifurcates into the

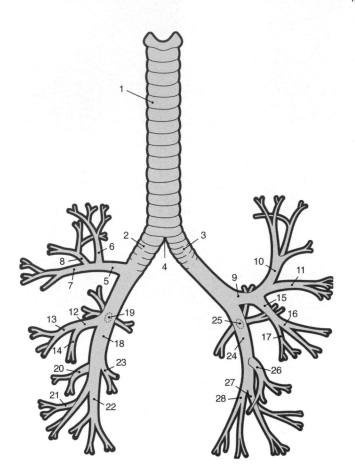

Figure I-2 Lobar and segmental bronchial anatomy (artistic illustration).

1.   Trachea
2.   Right main bronchus
3.   Left main bronchus
4.   Carina
5.   Right upper lobe bronchus
6.   Apical segmental bronchus; right upper lobe
7.   Anterior segmental bronchus; right upper lobe
8.   Posterior segmental bronchus; right upper lobe
9.   Left upper lobe bronchus
10. Apical-posterior segmental bronchus; left upper lobe
11. Anterior segmental bronchus; left upper lobe
12. Right middle lobe bronchus
13. Lateral segmental bronchus; right middle lobe
14. Medial segmental bronchus; right middle lobe
15. Lingular bronchus
16. Superior lingular bronchus
17. Inferior lingular bronchus
18. Right lower lobe bronchus
19. Superior segmental bronchus; right lower lobe
20. Anterior basal segmental bronchus; right lower lobe
21. Lateral basal segmental bronchus; right lower lobe
22. Posterior basal segmental bronchus; right lower lobe
23. Medial basal segmental bronchus right lower lobe
24. Left lower lobe bronchus
25. Superior segmental bronchus; left lower lobe
26. Anteromedial basal segmental bronchus; left lower lobe
27. Lateral basal segmental bronchus; left lower lobe
28. Posterior basal segmental bronchus; left lower lobe

middle and lower lobe bronchi. The *middle lobe bronchus* arises from the anterolateral wall of the bronchus intermedius opposite the origin of the lower lobe superior segmental bronchus and bifurcates into medial and lateral segments. The *lower lobe* has five segmental branches. The superior segment is the first branch and arises from the posterior wall of the lower lobe bronchus just beyond its origin. The four basal branches sequentially arise, lateral to medial, from the lower lobe bronchus in the following order: anterior, lateral, posterior, and medial.

LEFT LUNG

The *left upper lobe bronchus* arises from the left main bronchus and either bifurcates or trifurcates. The upper division is the main left upper lobe bronchus and divides into the combined apical-posterior segment and the anterior segment. The lower division is the lingular bronchus, which originates anterior to the take-off of the superior segmental bronchus to the lower lobe and bifurcates into superior and inferior branches. The lower lobe has four segmental divisions: the superior segment and three basal segments—anteromedial, lateral, and posterior. The latter arise sequentially in a manner similar to the basal divisions of the right lower lobe.

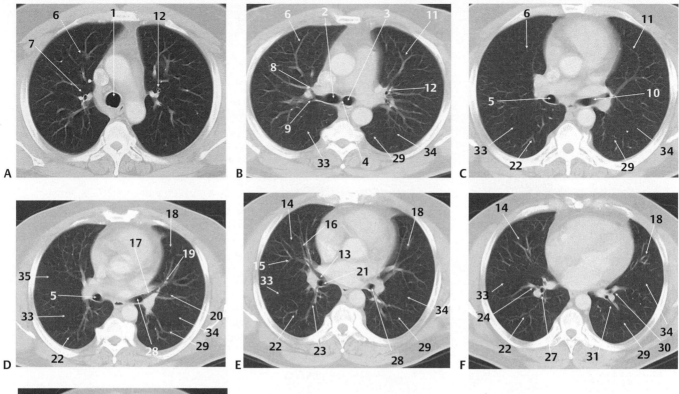

Figure I-3 (A–G) Contrast-enhanced chest CT (lung windows) demonstrates normal lobar and segmental bronchial anatomy.

1. Trachea
2. Right main bronchus
3. Left main bronchus
4. Carina
5. Bronchus intermedius
6. Right upper lobe
7. Apical segmental bronchus; right upper lobe
8. Anterior segmental bronchus; right upper lobe
9. Posterior segmental bronchus; right upper lobe
10. Left upper lobe bronchus
11. Left upper lobe
12. Apical-posterior segmental bronchus; left upper lobe
13. Right middle lobe bronchus
14. Right middle lobe
15. Lateral segmental bronchus; right middle lobe
16. Medial segmental bronchus; right middle lobe
17. Lingular bronchus
18. Lingula
19. Superior lingular bronchus
20. Inferior lingular bronchus
21. Right lower lobe bronchus
22. Right lower lobe
23. Superior segmental bronchus; right lower lobe
24. Anterior basal segmental bronchus; right lower lobe
25. Lateral basal segmental bronchus; right lower lobe
26. Posterior basal segmental bronchus; right lower lobe
27. Medial basal segmental bronchus; right lower lobe
28. Left lower lobe bronchus
29. Left lower lobe
30. Anteromedial basal segmental bronchus; left lower lobe
31. Lateral basal segmental bronchus; left lower lobe
32. Posterior basal segmental bronchus; left lower lobe
33. Right major fissure
34. Left major fissure
35. Minor fissure

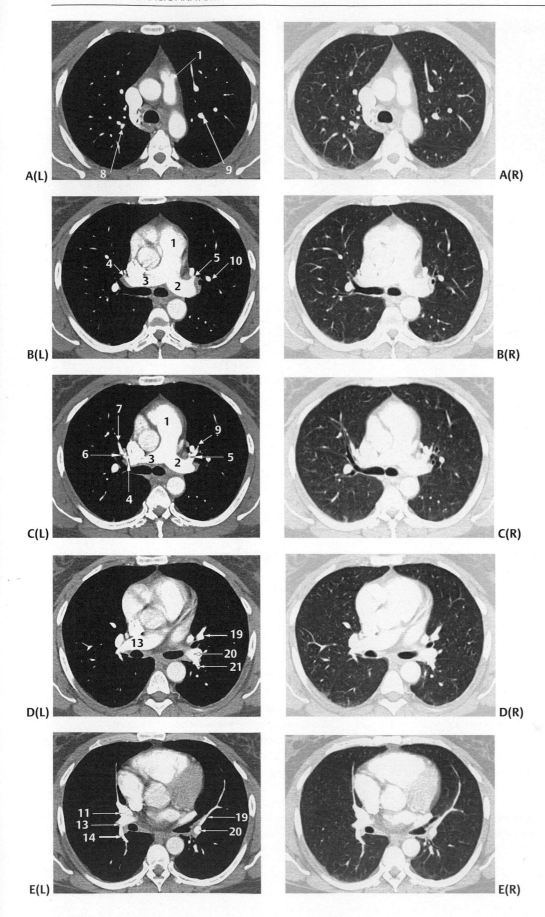

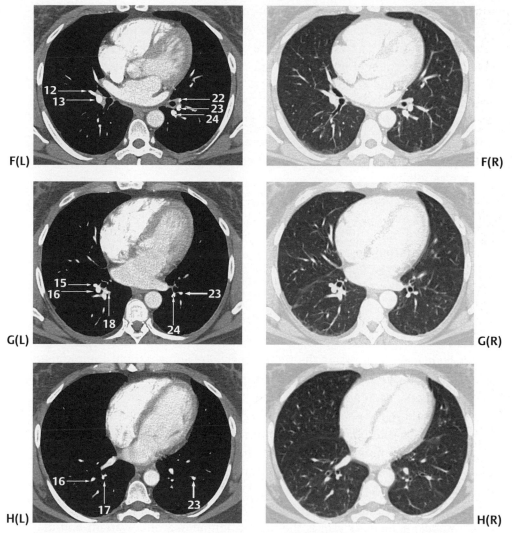

Figure I-4 (A–H) Contrast-enhanced chest CT (mediastinal windows and accompanying lung windows) demonstrates the normal main pulmonary artery and its segmental divisions.

1. Main pulmonary artery
2. Left main pulmonary artery
3. Right main pulmonary artery
4. Truncus anterior
5. Left upper lobe pulmonary artery
6. Right upper lobe pulmonary artery
7. Anterior segmental artery; right upper lobe
8. Posterior segmental artery; right upper lobe
9. Anterior segmental artery; left upper lobe
10. Posterior segmental artery; left upper lobe
11. Right middle lobe artery
12. Lateral segmental artery; right middle lobe
13. Right interlobar (descending) pulmonary artery
14. Superior segmental artery; right lower lobe
15. Anterior basal segmental artery; right lower lobe
16. Lateral basal segmental artery; right lower lobe
17. Posterior basal segmental artery; right lower lobe
18. Medial basal segmental artery; right lower lobe
19. Lingular artery
20. Left interlobar (descending) pulmonary artery
21. Superior segmental artery; left lower lobe
22. Anterior basal segmental artery; left lower lobe
23. Lateral basal segmental artery; left lower lobe
24. Posterior basal segmental artery; left lower lobe

Pulmonary Vessels

Main Pulmonary Artery and Segmental Branches (Fig. I-4)

The pulmonary valve gives rise to the main pulmonary artery, which courses superiorly and to the left. Before exiting the pericardium, the main pulmonary artery bifurcates into a long right, and a shorter left, main pulmonary artery. The *right main pulmonary artery* courses behind the ascending aorta. Behind the superior vena cava, and in front of the right main bronchus (eparterial), it divides into the truncus anterior, which supplies the upper lobe, and the interlobar branch, which supplies the lower lobe. The *interlobar artery* divides into segmental arteries that supply the middle and lower lobes and that parallel each of the segmental bronchi. The *left main pulmonary artery* courses over the left main bronchus (hyparterial) and continues as a vertical interlobar artery that gives off segmental branches to both the left upper and lower lobes. The interlobar pulmonary artery lies directly behind the lower lobe bronchus. Similarly, the arteries parallel each of the segmental bronchi. The normal diameter of the right interlobar pulmonary artery measured at the bronchus intermedius on frontal chest radiography is 16 mm in males and 15 mm in females. The normal diameters of the pulmonary arteries on CT are as follows:

Main pulmonary artery: 28.6 mm (rounded off to 29 mm)
Left main pulmonary artery: 28 mm
Right main pulmonary artery: 24 mm
Ratio of pulmonary artery to bronchus size:
1.3–1.4:1 distal to the take-off of the upper lobe bronchi
Peripheral bronchovascular bundles 1:1

Pulmonary Veins

Normally, the *right superior pulmonary vein* drains the right upper lobe and the right middle lobe, and descends medially into the superior aspect of the left atrium. The *left superior pulmonary vein* drains the left upper lobe and lingula, descends medially into the mediastinum, and drains into the superior portion of the left atrium. Both the *right* and *left inferior pulmonary veins* drain their respective lower lobes, and follow a medial and oblique course into the posterior-lateral left atrium. The ostia of the *inferior pulmonary veins* are more posterior and medial relative to the *superior pulmonary veins*. The *superior pulmonary veins* tend to have a longer trunk and are larger (mean 21.6 mm +/− 7.5 [SD] mm) than the *inferior pulmonary veins* (mean 14.0 mm +/− 6.2 [SD] mm). There is no significant difference in the average diameters of the *right and left inferior pulmonary vein* ostia (mean 18.0 +/− 3.7 mm). An *accessory right middle pulmonary vein* is the most common anatomic variant and may be identified in up to 16% of CT pulmonary vein examinations. In such cases, the *middle lobe vein* passes underneath the middle lobe bronchus and drains into the left atrium at the base of the superior pulmonary venous confluence. The *right middle pulmonary vein* has an ostial diameter much smaller than that of other pulmonary veins (mean 9.9 +/− 1.9 mm). Another anatomic variant, a *common left pulmonary vein trunk*, is characterized by an ostial diameter greater than those of the other pulmonary veins (32.5 +/− 0.5 mm).

Hila (Fig. I-5)

The hilum (root) of the lung contains bronchi, pulmonary and systemic arteries, pulmonary and systemic veins, lymphatic vessels, lymph nodes, and autonomic nerves. The hila are divided into upper and lower zones. The *upper zone of the right hilum* contains the superior pulmonary vein, the truncus anterior, short portion of the right upper lobe bronchus, anterior segmental artery, and bronchus (visualized *en face*). The *upper zone of the left hilum* contains the distal left main pulmonary artery and the superior pulmonary vein. The *lower zone of the right hilum* contains the right interlobar (descending) pulmonary artery, which lies medial to the bronchus intermedius. The inferior pulmonary vein is horizontally oriented and lies posterior and inferior to the hilum. The *lower zone of the left hilum* contains the distal interlobar (descending) pulmonary artery, the inferior pulmonary vein, and lingular and lower lobe bronchi.

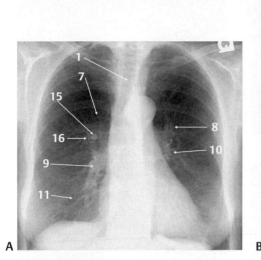
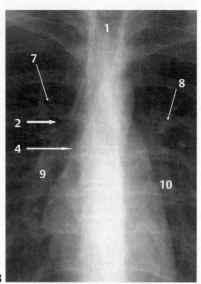
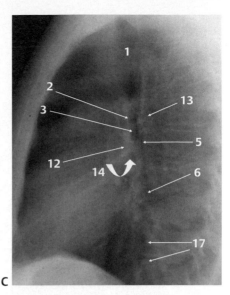

Figure I-5 PA **(A)**, coned down PA **(B)**, and coned down lateral **(C)** chest radiographs demonstrates the normal pulmonary hila and their anatomic relationships. (Images I-5A and I-5B courtesy of Michael J. Landay, M.D., University of Texas Southwestern Medical Center at Dallas; Dallas, Texas.)

1. Trachea
2. Right upper lobe bronchus
3. Left upper lobe bronchus
4. Bronchus intermedius
5. Posterior wall of the bronchus intermedius
6. Lower lobe bronchus
7. Right superior pulmonary vein
8. Left superior pulmonary vein
9. Right interlobar pulmonary artery
10. Left interlobar pulmonary artery
11. Right inferior pulmonary vein
12. Right pulmonary artery
13. Left pulmonary artery
14. Inferior hilar window (curved arrow)
15. Right upper lobe anterior segmental artery
16. Right upper lobe anterior segmental bronchus
17. Confluence of pulmonary veins

NORMAL HILAR RELATIONSHIPS ON FRONTAL CHEST RADIOGRAPHS (FIG. I-5A,B)

In 97% of individuals, the proximal left pulmonary artery is higher than the right interlobar pulmonary artery. In 3% of individuals, the proximal left pulmonary artery and the right interlobar pulmonary artery lie at the same horizontal level. The right pulmonary artery is never higher than the left in normal individuals.

NORMAL HILAR RELATIONSHIPS ON LATERAL CHEST RADIOGRAPHS (FIG. I-5C)

The tracheal air column is always conspicuous and should end in a well-defined rounded radiolucency that represents the proximal left upper lobe bronchus seen *en face*. The *right pulmonary artery* is seen as a spherical opacity anterior to the left upper lobe bronchus. The *left pulmonary artery* is more tubular and arches over the left main or left upper lobe bronchus (hyparterial). The right upper lobe bronchus is seen as a lucent circle approximately 1.0 cm higher than the left upper lobe bronchus. The posterior wall of the bronchus intermedius can be seen as a thin, vertically oriented white stripe, no more than 3 mm thick, between the right and left upper lobe bronchi. It separates the lumen of the bronchus intermedius from the aerated right lung and the azygoesophageal recess. The *inferior hilar window* is a radiolucent area immediately beneath the left upper lobe bronchus. An opacity in this areas suggests a hilar or subcarinal mass.

NORMAL HILAR ANATOMY ON CT AND MRI (FIGS. I-6 TO I-9)

The hila are optimally imaged with thin collimated and contrast-enhanced CT. Although intravenous contrast is not necessary in all cases, it simplifies interpretation, improves diagnostic accuracy and confidence, and provides insight into the potential vascular nature of various structures. Magnetic resonance

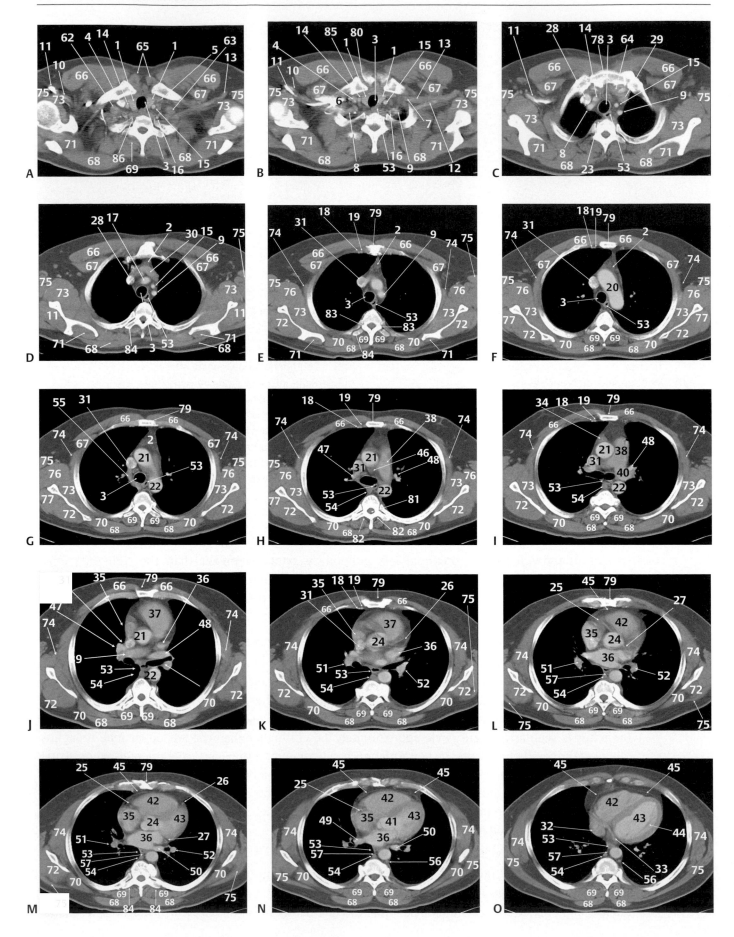

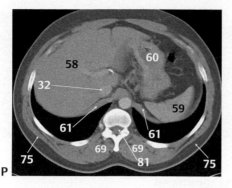

Figure I-6 (A–P) Sequential contrast-enhanced chest CT images from the thoracic inlet to the diaphragm illustrate normal hilar and mediastinal anatomy.

1. Thyroid gland
2. Involuting thymic tissue
3. Trachea
4. Right jugular vein
5. Left jugular vein
6. Right subclavian vein
7. Left subclavian vein
8. Right subclavian artery
9. Left subclavian artery
10. Right axillary artery
11. Right axillary vein
12. Left axillary artery
13. Left axillary vein
14. Right carotid artery
15. Left carotid artery
16. Left vertebral artery
17. Brachiocephalic artery
18. Internal mammary arteries
19. Internal mammary veins
20. Transverse aorta
21. Ascending aorta
22. Proximal descending thoracic aorta
23. Right superior intercostal vein
24. Aortic root
25. Right coronary artery
26. Left anterior descending coronary artery
27. Circumflex coronary artery
28. Right brachiocephalic vein
29. Left brachiocephalic vein
30. Crossing brachiocephalic vein
31. Superior vena cava
32. Inferior vena cava
33. Coronary sinus
34. Right atrial appendage
35. Right atrium
36. Left atrium
37. Right ventricular outflow tract
38. Main pulmonary artery
39. Right pulmonary artery
40. Left pulmonary artery
41. Left ventricular outflow tract
42. Right ventricle
43. Left ventricle
44. Papillary muscle
45. Pericardium
46. Transverse pericardial recess
47. Right superior pulmonary vein
48. Left superior pulmonary vein
49. Right inferior pulmonary vein
50. Left inferior pulmonary vein
51. Right interlobar pulmonary artery
52. Left interlobar pulmonary artery
53. Esophagus
54. Azygos vein
55. Azygos arch
56. Hemiazygos vein
57. Thoracic duct
58. Liver
59. Spleen
60. Stomach
61. Crux of diaphragm
62. Right anterior scalene muscle
63. Left anterior scalene muscle
64. Sternothyroid-sternohyoid muscles
65. Sternocleidomastoid muscles
66. Pectoralis major muscle
67. Pectoralis minor muscle
68. Trapezius muscle
69. Erector spinae muscle
70. Rhomboid muscle
71. Supraspinatus muscle
72. Infraspinatus muscle
73. Subscapularis muscle
74. Serratus anterior muscle
75. Latissimus dorsi muscle
76. Teres major muscle
77. Teres minor muscle
78. Manubrium
79. Sternum
80. Sternoclavicular joint
81. Spinal cord
82. Lamina
83. Pedicle
84. Transverse process
85. Clavicle
86. Head of the first rib

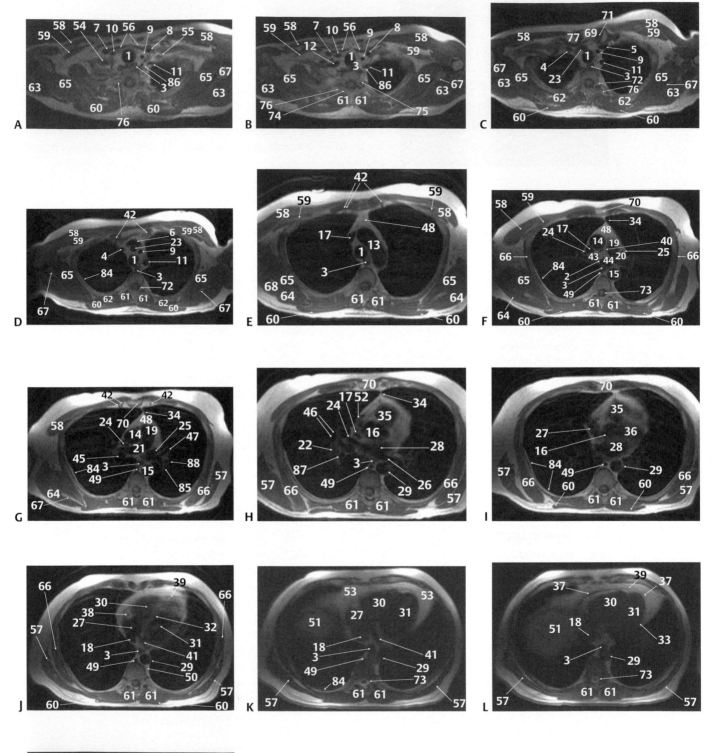

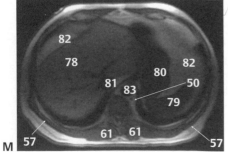

Figure I-7 (A–M) Sequential T1-weighted axial MRI spanning from the thoracic inlet to the upper abdomen illustrating normal hilar and mediastinal anatomy.

1. Trachea
2. Carina
3. Esophagus
4. Right brachiocephalic vein
5. Left brachiocephalic vein
6. Crossing brachiocephalic vein
7. Right jugular vein
8. Left jugular vein
9. Left common carotid artery
10. Right common carotid artery
11. Left subclavian artery
12. Right subclavian artery
13. Transverse aorta
14. Ascending aorta
15. Proximal descending thoracic aorta
16. Aortic root
17. Superior vena cava
18. Inferior vena cava
19. Main pulmonary artery
20. Left pulmonary artery
21. Right pulmonary artery
22. Right interlobar pulmonary artery
23. Brachiocephalic artery
24. Right superior pulmonary vein
25. Left superior pulmonary vein
26. Left inferior pulmonary vein
27. Right atrium
28. Left atrium
29. Descending thoracic aorta
30. Right ventricle
31. Left ventricle
32. Interventricular septum
33. Left ventricular free wall
34. Anterior junction line
35. Right ventricular outflow tract
36. Left ventricular outflow tract
37. Pericardium
38. Right coronary artery
39. Left anterior descending coronary artery
40. Transverse pericardial recess
41. Coronary sinus
42. Internal mammary vessels
43. Right main bronchus
44. Left main bronchus

45. Bronchus intermedius
46. Right middle lobe bronchi
47. Lingular bronchus
48. Mediastinal fat
49. Azygos vein
50. Hemiazygos vein
51. Dome of liver
52. Right atrial appendage
53. Fat pad
54. Right anterior scalene muscle
55. Left anterior scalene muscle
56. Sternothyroid-sternohyoid muscles
57. Latissimus dorsi muscles
58. Pectoralis major muscle
59. Pectoralis minor muscle
60. Trapezius muscle
61. Erector spinae muscle
62. Rhomboid major muscle
63. Supraspinatus muscle
64. Infraspinatus muscle
65. Subscapularis muscle
66. Serratus anterior muscle
67. Scapula
68. Teres minor muscle
69. Manubrium
70. Sternum
71. Sternoclavicular joint
72. Vertebral foramen
73. Spinal cord
74. Lamina
75. Pedicle
76. Transverse process
77. Clavicle
78. Liver
79. Spleen
80. Stomach
81. Intrahepatic inferior vena cava
82. Mesenteric fat
83. Abdominal aorta
84. Extrapleural (subcostal) fat
85. Left lower lobe bronchus
86. Left vertebral artery
87. Right lower lobe bronchus
88. Left interlobar pulmonary artery

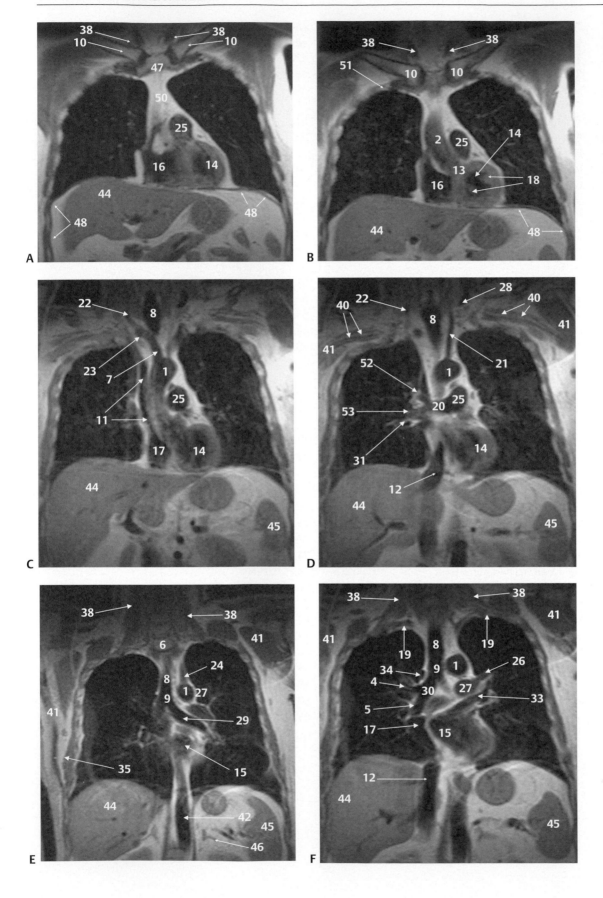

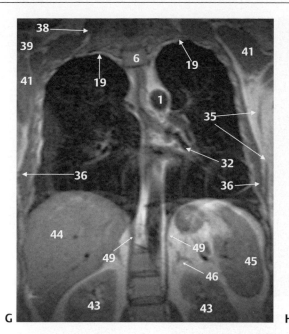
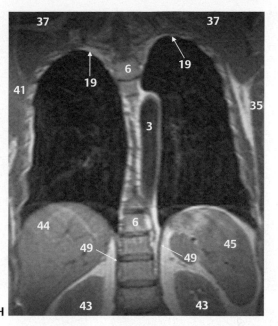

Figure I-8 (A–H) T1-weighted coronal MRI (anterior to posterior) of the chest illustrate normal hilar, mediastinal, and thoracic anatomy.

1.	Transverse aorta	28.	Left internal jugular vein
2.	Ascending aorta	29.	Left mainstem bronchus
3.	Descending aorta	30.	Right mainstem bronchus
4.	Right upper lobe bronchus	31.	Right middle lobe bronchus
5.	Bronchus intermedius	32.	Left lower lobe bronchus
6.	Thoracic spine	33.	Left superior pulmonary vein
7.	Brachiocephalic artery	34.	Right superior pulmonary vein
8.	Trachea	35.	Latissimus dorsi muscles
9.	Carina	36.	Serratus anterior muscles
10.	Clavicle	37.	Trapezius muscles
11.	Superior vena cava	38.	Sternocleidomastoid muscles
12.	Inferior vena cava	39.	Supraspinatus muscle
13.	Left ventricular outflow tract (aortic valve plane)	40.	Axillary vessels
14.	Left ventricle	41.	Subscapularis muscle
15.	Left atrium	42.	Abdominal aorta
16.	Right ventricle	43.	Kidney
17.	Right atrium	44.	Liver
18.	Papillary muscles	45.	Spleen
19.	Apical extrapleural fat	46.	Left adrenal gland
20.	Right pulmonary artery	47.	Manubrium
21.	Left common carotid artery	48.	Diaphragm
22.	Right common carotid artery	49.	Crus of diaphragm
23.	Right subclavian artery	50.	Anterior mediastinal fat
24.	Left subclavian artery	51.	Brachial plexus
25.	Main pulmonary artery	52.	Right upper lobe pulmonary artery
26.	Left upper lobe pulmonary artery	53.	Right interlobar pulmonary artery
27.	Left pulmonary artery		

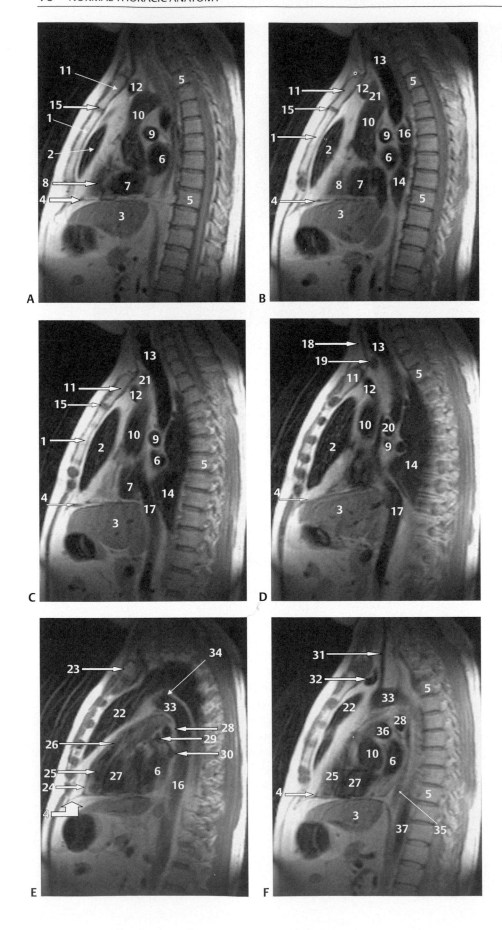

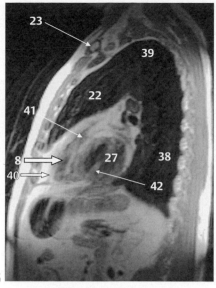

Figure I-9 (A–G) T1-weighted sagittal MRI (right to left) of the chest illustrates normal hilar, mediastinal, and thoracic anatomy.

1.	Sternum	22.	Left lung (anterior)
2.	Right lung (anterior)	23.	Clavicle
3.	Liver	24.	Pericardium
4.	Diaphragm	25.	Right ventricular cavity
5.	Thoracic spine	26.	Right ventricular outflow tract
6.	Left atrium	27.	Left ventricle
7.	Right atrium	28.	Left main bronchus
8.	Right ventricle	29.	Left superior pulmonary vein
9.	Right pulmonary artery	30.	Left inferior pulmonary vein
10.	Ascending aorta	31.	Left common carotid artery
11.	Manubrium	32.	Left brachiocephalic vein
12.	Brachiocephalic vein	33.	Aortic arch (transverse aorta)
13.	Trachea	34.	Left subclavian artery origin
14.	Right lung (posterior)	35.	Esophagus
15.	Sternomanubrial joint	36.	Main pulmonary artery
16.	Descending thoracic aorta	37.	Abdominal aorta
17.	Inferior vena cava	38.	Left lung (posterior)
18.	Internal jugular vein	39.	Left lung (apex)
19.	Right subclavian artery	40.	Fat pad
20.	Bronchus intermedius	41.	Interventricular septum
21.	Brachiocephalic artery (innominate artery)	42.	Papillary muscles

imaging (MRI) is comparable to CT and may be used in those patients in whom iodinated contrast media is contraindicated or ionizing radiation is a concern (e.g., children, pregnant women, serial exams).

Parenchyma

Acinus (Fig. I-10)

The acinus is the gas-exchanging unit of the lung. It is located distal to the terminal bronchiole (last conducting airway) and is composed of respiratory bronchioles, alveolar ducts, alveolar sacs, and alveoli.

Secondary Pulmonary Lobule (Fig. I-11)

This is the smallest discrete portion of the lung surrounded by connective tissue. It is polyhedral in shape, averages 1.0 to 2.5 cm in size, and is supplied by three to five terminal bronchioles. The

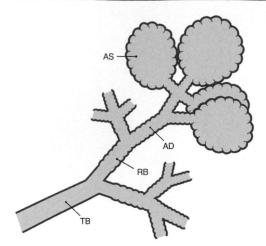

Figure I-10 The pulmonary acinus (illustration). TB, terminal bronchiole; RB, respiratory bronchiole; AD, alveolar duct; AS, alveolar sac.

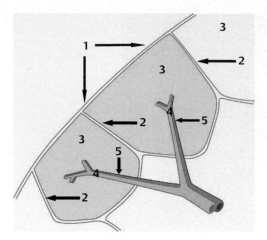

Figure I-11 The secondary pulmonary lobule (illustration).

1. Visceral pleura
2. Interlobular septum
3. Individual secondary pulmonary lobules
4. Centrilobular bronchus
5. Centrilobular artery

core structures include the centrilobular bronchus and its accompanying pulmonary artery, and lymphatics. The peripheral structures include the interlobular septa, which are continuous with the pleural surface, pulmonary veins, and lymphatics. The septa are not evenly distributed and are better developed in the lower lobes. Although inconspicuous on conventional imaging, the secondary pulmonary lobule is readily identified on high-resolution CT (HRCT).

Pleura

The pleura consists of two layers. The *parietal pleura* covers the nonpulmonary surfaces (e.g., ribs, mediastinum, diaphragm). It has a systemic blood supply (via branches of the subclavian artery, internal mammary artery, and intercostal arteries) and venous drainage (via branches of the azygos and hemiazygos systems, and the internal mammary veins). The parietal pleura contains pain fibers, the irritation and inflammation of which are responsible for pleuritic chest pain. The parietal pleura lymphatics also communicate with the pleural space. The *visceral pleura* covers the surface of the lung. It has a dual blood supply. It is believed that branches of the bronchial circulation supply the apical, hilar, mediastinal, and interlobar visceral pleura, whereas branches from the pulmonary arteries supply the costal and diaphragmatic pleura. The visceral pleura also has a dual venous drainage (e.g., pulmonary and bronchial veins). Branches of the vagus nerve and sympathetic trunk innervate the visceral pleura. However, it does not contain any pain fibers. Unlike the parietal pleura, the visceral pleura lymphatics do not communicate with the pleural space. Contiguous layers of visceral pleura form interlobar fissures that may be complete or incomplete.

Standard Fissures

The standard fissures divide the lung into lobes and include the minor (horizontal) fissure and the major (oblique) fissures.

MINOR FISSURE (FIG. I-12)

This fissure separates the anterior segment of the right upper lobe from the middle lobe. It is seen in 44 to 88% of normal chest radiographs (**Fig. I-12A,B**), and in two thirds of frontal radiographs

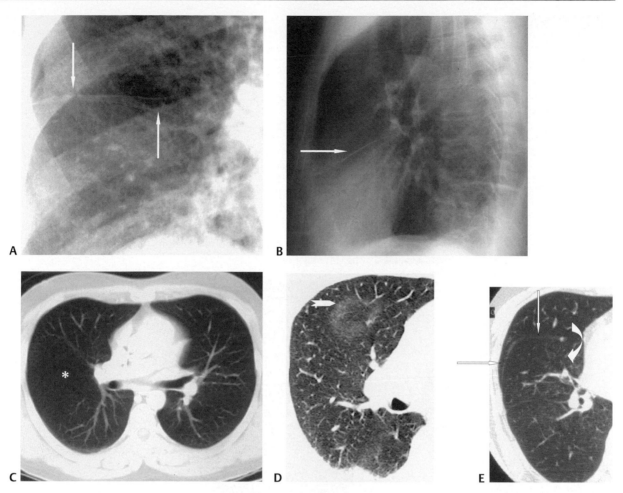

Figure I-12 Radiologic features of the minor fissure. Coned-down PA **(A)** and lateral **(B)** chest radiographs demonstrate the normal course and position of the minor fissure (arrows). **(C,D)** Minor fissure is a triangular area devoid of vasculature (*) or an oval area of ground-glass attenuation (arrowhead) on helical chest CT. **(E)** Incomplete minor fissure (arrows) with resulting fusion between the right upper and middle lobes (curved arrow).

lies at the level of the fourth anterior intercostal space. On helical CT, it is most often recognized as a triangular (**Fig. I-12C**) or oval lucent area devoid of vasculature. On 8% of studies, the fissure is seen as an oval area of ground-glass attenuation (**Fig. I-12D**). On HRCT, it appears as a curvilinear line or C-shaped band of increased attenuation. An incomplete minor fissure with resulting parenchymal fusion between the anterior segment of the upper lobe and the middle lobe (**Fig. I-12E**) is present in 60 to 90% of CT scans.

MAJOR FISSURES (FIGS. I-13 TO I-16)

The *right major fissure* separates the combined upper and middle lobes from the lower lobe. The *left major fissure* separates the combined upper and lingular lobes from the lower lobe. The major fissures are best seen on lateral chest radiography (**Fig. I-13**). The right oblique fissure originates at approximately the level of the fifth thoracic vertebra, and the left at approximately the level of the fourth thoracic vertebrae. The oblique fissures parallel the sixth rib as they course obliquely and inferiorly. The right fissure follows a more oblique, anterior, and inferior course than its counterpart. Major fissures may be seen on 80 to 90% of helical CT studies. Like the minor fissure, the major fissures most often appear as lucent bands devoid of vasculature. However, the major fissure may also appear as a well-defined line (**Fig. I-14A**) or as an ill-defined dense or somewhat fuzzy band (**Fig. I-14B**).

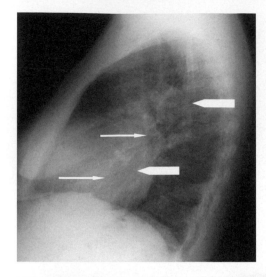

Figure I-13 Coned-down lateral chest radiograph demonstrate the normal course and position of the right (arrows) and left (arrowheads) major fissures.

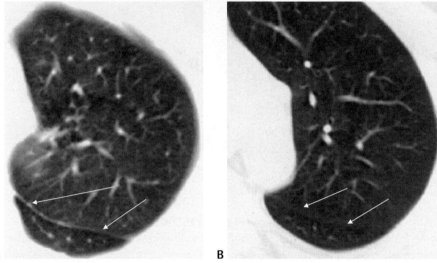

A   B

Figure I-14 Variable appearance of the major fissure on helical CT. **(A)** Well-defined line (arrows). **(B)** Ill-defined dense or fuzzy band (arrows).

On HRCT they are virtually always conspicuous, and may appear as single lines (**Fig. I-15A**), fuzzy ill-defined band (**Fig. I-15B**), or as two parallel lines (**Fig. I-15C**). The latter appearance is usually due to respiratory motion artifact. The fissures are incomplete on 12 to 75% of CT scans (**Fig. I-15D**). Incomplete fissures are more frequently seen on the right, especially between the upper and lower lobes, and are least common between the left upper and lower lobes. The major fissures undulate through the lungs and their morphology has been likened to that of a propeller blade or figure-8 pattern (**Fig. I-16A**), an appearance better appreciated on CT. In the upper thorax, the fissure is anteriorly concave (lateral facing orientation) (**Fig. I-16B**). In the inferior thorax, the fissure is anteriorly convex (medial facing orientation) (**Fig. I-16C**). Alterations in this orientation serve as clues to underlying volume loss or lung disease (**Fig. I-16D**).

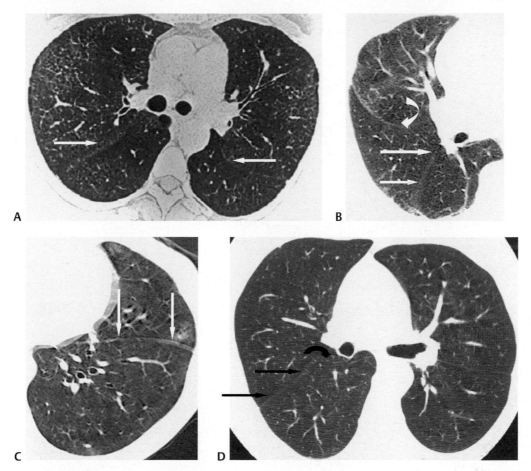

Figure I-15 Variable appearances of the major fissures on HRCT. **(A)** Single line (arrows). **(B)** Fuzzy ill-defined band (arrows). The minor fissure can also been seen (curved arrow). **(C)** Two parallel lines (arrows) artifactually created be respiratory and/or cardiac motion. **(D)** Incomplete right major fissure (arrows). Notice that the oblique fissure fails to reach the ipsilateral hilum, resulting in a parenchymal bridge of communication between the right middle and lower lobes (curved arrow).

Accessory Fissures (Fig. I-17)

Accessory fissures occur within a given lobe and may be seen on 10% of chest radiographs and 20% of CT examinations.

AZYGOS FISSURE (FIG. I-18)

Embryologically, this fissure results from abnormal migration of the right posterior cardinal vein (**Fig. I-18A**) into the lung apex, drawing in the layers of visceral and parietal pleura. The displaced azygos vein ultimately resides in a sling of four pleural layers (mesoazygos). This normal variant occurs in approximately 1% of the population and is twice as common in males as in females. It is seen on approximately 1% of imaging studies, and has the appearance of a curvilinear opacity that extends obliquely from the upper portion of the right lung, and terminates in a teardrop-shaped opacity about 2 to 4 cm above the hilum (**Fig. I-18B,C**), representing the displaced azygos vein. The lung residing medial to this fissure is referred to as the azygos lobe.

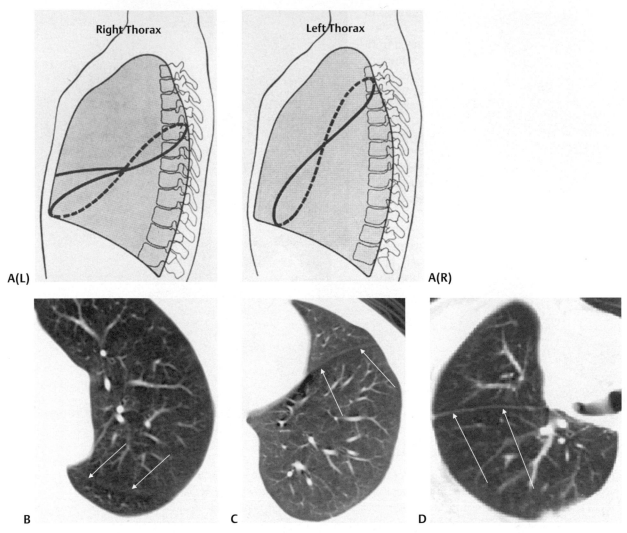

Figure I-16 Propeller-like morphology of the major fissure. **(A)** Artistic illustration depicts the undulating morphology of the major fissure. **(B)** Unenhanced chest CT through the upper thorax demonstrates the anterior concave (lateral facing orientation) (arrows) of the major fissure. **(C)** Unenhanced chest CT through the lower thorax demonstrates the anterior convex (medial facing orientation) (arrows) of the major fissure. **(D)** Unenhanced chest CT through the upper thorax illustrates an alteration in the normal lateral facing orientation of the right major fissure (arrows) secondary to right upper lobe volume loss from an obstructing endobronchial squamous cell carcinoma.

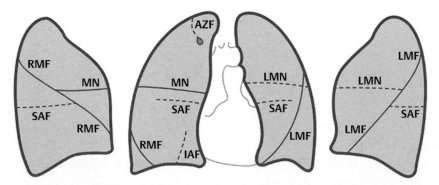

Figure I-17 Accessory fissures (illustration). The more commonly encountered accessory fissures are illustrated by the interrupted lines. Solid lines illustrate the standard fissures. AZF, azygos fissure; IAF, inferior accessory fissure; LMF, left major fissure; LMN, left minor fissure; MN, minor fissure; RMF, right major fissure; SAF, superior accessory fissure.

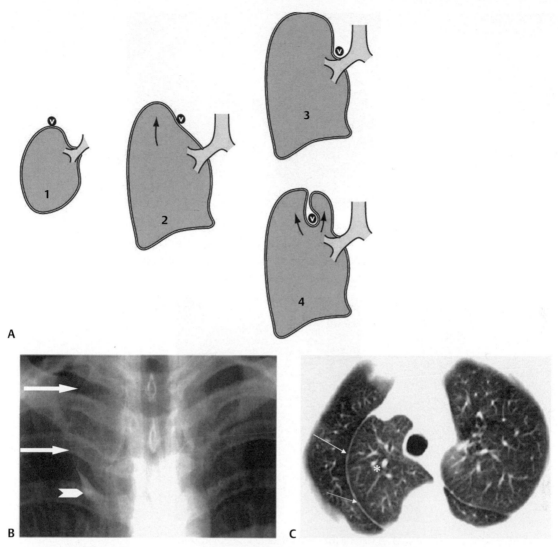

Figure I-18 Azygos fissure and lobe. **(A)** Abnormal migration of the right posterior cardinal vein results in formation of the azygos fissure and lobe (illustration). 1. The embryologic origin of the right posterior cardinal vein before its migration into the mediastinum. 2. The normal migration of the right posterior cardinal vein along the mediastinal pleural reflection. 3. The right posterior cardinal vein comes to reside at the tracheobronchial angle; the normal anatomic location of the azygos vein. 4. The abnormal migration of the right posterior cardinal vein into the lung apex drawing in the four layers of visceral and parietal pleura forming the mesoazygos or sling. **(B)** Coned-down PA chest radiograph demonstrates the azygos fissure (arrows). The teardrop opacity (arrowhead) represents the displaced azygos vein. **(C)** Unenhanced chest CT (lung window) demonstrates the appearance, course, and position of the azygos fissure (arrows) and the isolated azygos lobe (*).

INFERIOR ACCESSORY FISSURE (FIG. I-19)

This accessory fissure separates the medial basal segment of the lower lobe from the remaining basilar segments. It is the most common of the accessory fissures, seen in about 30 to 45% of anatomic specimens, 5 to 10% of frontal radiographs, and 15% of CT examinations. Although it occurs with equal frequency in the two hemithoraces, it is more conspicuous in the right hemithorax, extending superiorly and slightly medially from the hemidiaphragm toward the ipsilateral hilum (**Fig. I-19A**). The lung medial to this fissure is referred to as the cardiac lobe (**Fig. I-19B**).

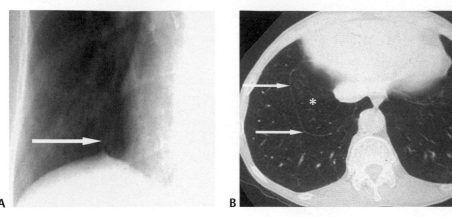

Figure I-19 Inferior accessory fissure and the cardiac lobe. **(A)** Coned-down PA chest radiograph demonstrates the typical location and course of this fissure (arrow). **(B)** Unenhanced chest CT (lung window) demonstrates the appearance, course, and orientation of the inferior accessory fissure (arrows) and the isolated cardiac lobe (*).

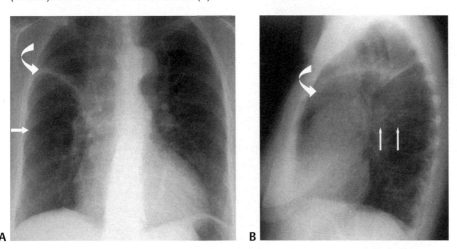

Figure I-20 Superior accessory fissure. PA **(A)** and lateral **(B)** chest radiographs demonstrate the typical location and course of this fissure (arrows). Note its relationship to the displaced minor fissure (curved arrow).

SUPERIOR ACCESSORY FISSURE (FIG. I-20)

This accessory fissure separates the superior segment of the lower lobe from the remainder of the lower lobe segments and is seen in approximately 6% of anatomic specimens. On imaging, it lies in a horizontal plane and may mimic the minor fissure, but it is typically lower, at the level of the lower lobe segmental bronchus (**Fig. I-20A**). On lateral chest radiography, it extends further posteriorly than the minor fissure, often overlying the spine (**Fig. I-20B**). The portion of lung isolated by this fissure is sometimes referred to as the dorsal lobe of Nelson.

LEFT MINOR FISSURE (FIG. I-21)

The left minor fissure is analogous to the right minor fissure. This accessory fissure separates the lingula from the left upper lobe. Although present in 8 to 18% of anatomic specimens, it is seen in only 1.5% of chest radiographs. It usually lies more cephalad than its counterpart and has a more medial sloping or more oblique course.

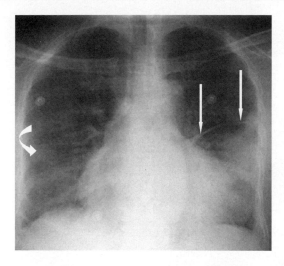

Figure I-21 Left minor fissure. AP chest radiograph demonstrates the typical location and course of this fissure (arrows). Note its relationship to the right minor fissure (curved arrow).

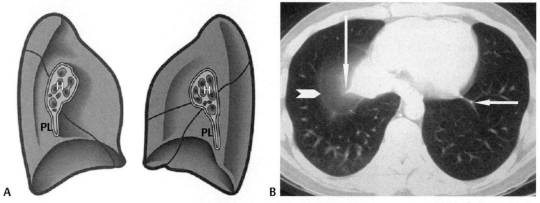

A B

Figure I-22 The pulmonary ligament. **(A)** Artistic depiction of the union of the visceral and parietal pleural layers at the hilum to form the pulmonary ligament. H, hilum; PL, pulmonary ligament. **(B)** Contrast-enhanced chest CT (lung window) demonstrates the right and left pulmonary ligaments (arrows). An inferior accessory fissure is also present (arrowhead). The dome of the diaphragm creates the ground-glass hazy opacity at the right lung base.

Pulmonary Ligament (Fig. I-22)

This septum represents the union at the hilum of the parietal and visceral pleural layers. It extends from the inferior margin of the hilum toward the ipsilateral hemidiaphragm. Although not conspicuous on chest radiography, the ligament is often seen on CT. The right pulmonary ligament lies adjacent to the azygos vein and the inferior vena cava and is seen on 40 to 60% of CT studies. The left pulmonary ligament lies adjacent to the esophagus and the descending thoracic aorta and is seen on 60 to 70% of CT examinations. The septum created by these pleural reflections contains bronchial veins, lymphatics, and lymph nodes [American Thoracic Society (ATS) station 9 nodes].

Mediastinum

Mediastinal Landmarks

Normal mediastinal landmarks may be divided into lines, stripes, and interfaces. Mediastinal lines include the anterior junction line, posterior junction line, and paraspinal lines. The *anterior junction line* may be observed on frontal chest radiography (**Fig. I-23A**) as an obliquely oriented line of variable thickness coursing from the right to the left thorax at the level of the transverse aorta. An alteration in the course of this junction line may indicate underlying anterior mediastinal pathology.

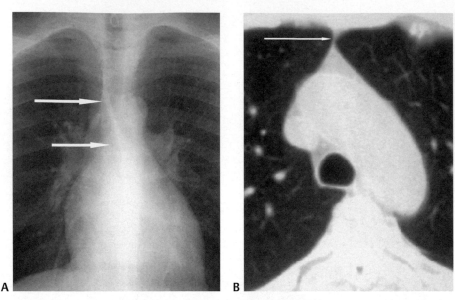

Figure I-23 Anterior junction line. Coned-down PA **(A)** chest radiograph demonstrates the obliquely oriented anterior junction line (arrows) coursing from the right to the left thorax. Compare its orientation and location with the posterior junction line in **Fig. I-24**. **(B)** Contrast-enhanced chest CT (lung window) demonstrates the junction line (arrow) as a thin septum interposed between the right and left anterior hemithoraces.

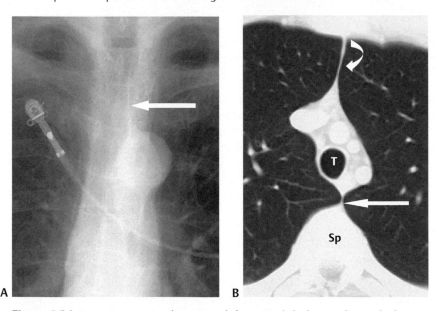

Figure I-24 Posterior junction line. Coned-down PA **(A)** chest radiograph demonstrates the vertically oriented posterior junction line (arrow) extending superiorly above the clavicles through the tracheal air column. **(B)** Contrast-enhanced chest CT (lung window) shows the posterior junction line (arrow) as a thin septum between the trachea (T) and the thoracic spine (Sp). An anterior junction line (curved arrow) is also demonstrated.

On CT (**Fig. I-23B**), the anterior junction line can be seen as a septum of variable thickness between the right and left lung at the transverse aorta level. The thickness of this septum varies depending on the amount of intervening fat between the apposed four layers of pleura. The *posterior junction line* may be observed on frontal chest radiography (**Fig. I-24A**) as a vertically oriented line projected through the tracheal air column and extending from the transverse aorta superiorly above the

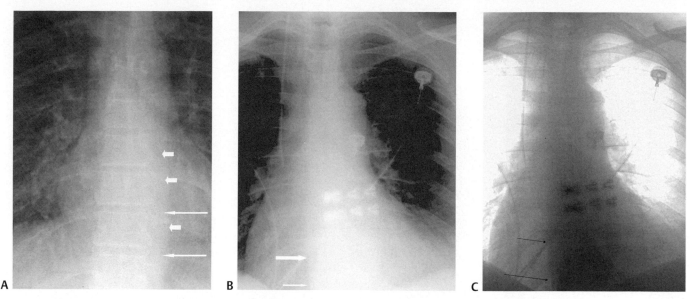

Figure I-25 Paraspinal lines. **(A)** Coned-down PA chest radiograph shows the left paraspinal stripe (long arrows) and its relationship to the descending thoracic aorta interface (short arrows). **(B)** Coned-down PA chest radiograph of another patient illustrates the normal, but less commonly seen, right paraspinal line (arrows). **(C)** This paraspinal line (arrows) is seen to better advantage on the accompanying inverted image.

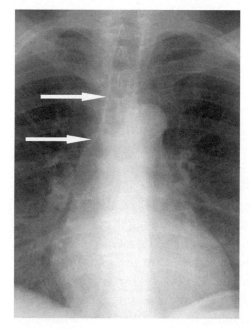

Figure I-26 Right paratracheal stripe. Coned-down PA chest radiograph shows the normal size and morphology of the right paratracheal stripe (arrows).

clavicles. An alteration in the position of this junction line may indicate underlying paravertebral or posterior mediastinal pathology. On CT (**Fig. I-24B**), the posterior junction line may be seen as a septum located between the trachea and esophagus anteriorly, and the thoracic spine posteriorly. The *paraspinal lines* (**Fig. I-25**) are best seen on well-penetrated frontal chest or anteroposterior (AP) thoracic spine radiography. Each line is approximately 1 cm wide, curvilinear, and maintains a constant relationship with the adjacent vertebral bodies. The *left paraspinal line* (**Fig. I-25A**) extends superiorly from the aorta and inferiorly to the diaphragm paralleling the lateral margin of the spine. This line normally lies medial to the descending aorta interface, but it may become displaced lateral to this interface in the setting of paraspinal abscesses. The *right paraspinal line* (**Fig. I-25B**) is less frequently visualized and usually is not seen in its entirety.

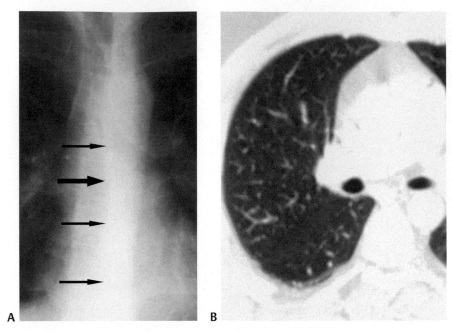

Figure I-27 Azygoesophageal interface. Coned-down PA **(A)** chest radiograph demonstrates the normal course and appearance of the azygoesophageal interface (arrows). **(B)** Contrast-enhanced chest CT (lung window) shows juxtaposition of aerated right lower lobe and the lateral walls of the azygos vein and esophagus form this interface.

The *right paratracheal stripe* (**Fig. I-26**) is formed by the apposition of the right upper lobe pleura and the adjacent lateral tracheal wall. It parallels the lateral tracheal border extending inferiorly to the azygos vein. The normal stripe is smooth and measures up to 3 mm in width. Widening of this paratracheal stripe may indicate underlying mediastinal disease (see Section XII).

Two juxtaposed tissues of differing opacity create interfaces. The two most important mediastinal interfaces are the *azygoesophageal interface* (**Fig. I-27**) and the *descending thoracic aorta interface* (**Fig. I-25**). On frontal chest radiography (**Fig. I-27A**) the azygoesophageal interface begins superiorly at the azygos vein and continues inferiorly to the diaphragm. It normally curves slightly toward the left. A focal convexity in this interface indicates underlying mediastinal disease. On CT (**Fig. I-27B**), the azygoesophageal interface is easily recognized by the juxtaposition of aerated lung within the superior segment of the right lower lobe and the lateral margin of the azygos vein and/or esophagus. The *descending thoracic aorta interface* is formed by the juxtaposition of the aerated left lower lobe and the lateral margin of the descending thoracic aorta. On frontal chest radiography (**Fig. I-25**) this interface can be seen extending from the top of the aortic arch to the diaphragm. Alterations in the contour of the interface suggest thoracic aorta vascular disease or paravertebral abnormalities. The normal mediastinum is illustrated on CT (**Fig. I-6**) and MRI (**Figs. I-7** to **I-9**). The mediastinal compartments are discussed further in Section XII.

Lymph Nodes

Most normal lymph nodes are ovoid, kidney bean–shaped, or flat in morphology with low attenuation centers or fatty hila. The short axis diameter is usually 7 mm or less. ATS station 10R nodes may be up to 15 mm. Most lymph nodes less than or equal to 10 mm are not considered pathologically

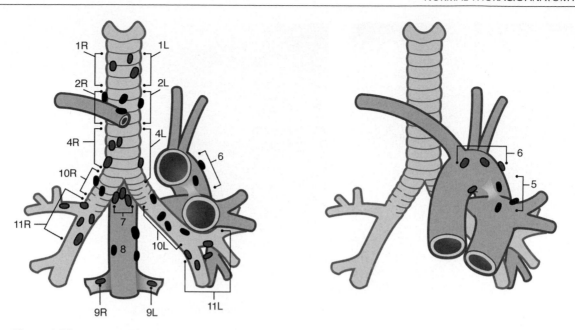

Figure I-28 American Thoracic Society map of the more commonly encountered mediastinal lymph nodes used in the staging of lung cancer (illustration).

Regional nodal stations for lung cancer staging
N2 nodes

Superior mediastinal nodes

1. Highest mediastinal
2. Upper paratracheal
3A. Prevascular (peribranch vessel) (not illustrated)
3P. Tracheal esophageal groove (related to posterior
    membranous trachea) (not illustrated)
4. Lower paratracheal

Aortic nodes

5. Aortic-pulmonary window
6. Paraaortic (parallel phrenic nerve, transverse aorta,
    ascending aorta)

Inferior mediastinal nodes

7. Subcarinal
8. Paraesophageal
9. Pulmonary ligament

N1 nodes

10. Hilar
11. Interlobar
12. Lobar bronchi (not illustrated)
13. Segmental bronchi (not illustrated)
14. Subsegmental bronchi (not illustrated)

enlarged. The ATS numbered map of mediastinal nodes used in the staging of lung cancer is illustrated in **Fig. I-28** and is further addressed in Section VI. N2 nodes include all lymph node stations within the mediastinal pleural reflection and are assigned single digits (i.e., 1–9). N1 nodes include all lymph nodes distal to the mediastinal pleural reflection and within the visceral pleura and are assigned double digits (i.e., 10–14).

Internal mammary lymph nodes include the parietal pleural lymph nodes located close to the anterior chest wall, paralleling the sternum, and internal mammary vessels. These nodes drain the chest wall and are of importance in breast cancer staging. They are usually 6 mm or less in short axis diameter and are rarely identified on chest radiography. Anterior diaphragmatic lymph nodes include those parietal lymph nodes located on the anterior surface of the diaphragm. The most medial lymph node is the pericardiophrenic lymph node. It is usually 8 mm or less in short-axis diameter and is not routinely identified on chest radiography.

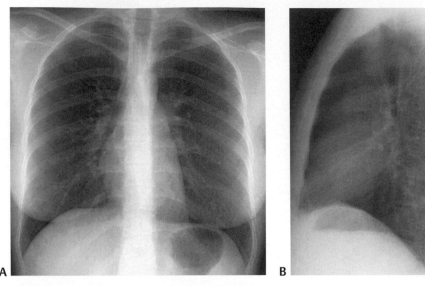

Figure I-29 PA **(A)** and lateral **(B)** chest radiographs demonstrate the normal relationships of the right and left hemidiaphragms.

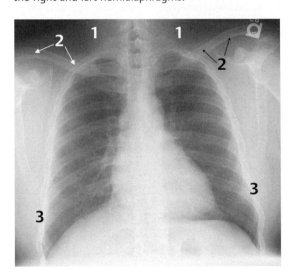

Figure I-30 PA chest radiograph demonstrates the normal soft tissues of the chest wall.

1. Sternocleidomastoid muscles
2. Companion shadows
3. Breast tissue

Diaphragm (Fig. I-29)

The diaphragm is a muscular tendinous sheath that separates the thorax from the abdomen. It is supplied by the phrenic and intercostal arteries and branches of the internal mammary artery, and innervated by the phrenic nerve. The right hemidiaphragm is usually one half an interspace higher than the left, and the heart usually obscures the anterior portion of the left hemidiaphragm. The diaphragm is usually smooth and uniform in contour, but arcuate elevations or scalloping are seen in 5% of normal individuals. Diaphragmatic abnormalities are further in Section XIII.

Chest Wall (Fig. I-30)

Various soft tissue structures of the chest wall may be seen on chest radiography. Those most frequently observed include the sternocleidomastoid muscles, the breast tissue, and the pectoralis muscles (anterior axillary fold). Companion shadows are smooth soft tissue opacities that parallel the ribs and clavicles and measure 1 to 2 mm in diameter. They are produced by visualization of the soft tissues and parietal pleura tangential to the x-ray beam and should not be confused with chest wall or pleural pathology. Costochondral calcification is a common finding that increases in frequency with age. The pattern of calcification varies with the patient's sex. In men, the superior and inferior borders of the cartilage tend to calcify, whereas in females the central cartilage calcifies.

Suggested Readings

Felson BF. In: Felson FB, ed. Chest Roentgenology. Philadelphia: WB Saunders, 1973:185–250

Fraser RS, Müller NL, Colman N, Paré PD. In: Fraser and Paré's Diagnosis of Diseases of the Chest, 4th ed. Philadelphia: WB Saunders, 1999:1–280

Jais P, Shah DC, Hocini M, Yamane T, Haissaguerre M, Clementy J. Radiofrequency catheter ablation for atrial fibrillation. J Cardiovasc Electrophysiol 2000;11:758–761.

Mountain CF, Dresler CM. Regional lymph node classification for lung cancer staging. Chest 1997;111:1718–1723

Proto AV, Speckman JM. The left lateral radiograph of the chest. I. Med Radiogr Photogr 1979; 55:30–42

Proto AV, Speckman JM. The left lateral radiograph of the chest. II. Med Radiogr Photogr 1980; 56:38–50

Webb WR, Jensen BG, Gamsu G, et al. Coronal magnetic resonance imaging of the chest: normal and abnormal. Radiology 1984;153:729–735

SECTION II
Developmental Anomalies

CASE 1 Tracheal Bronchus

Clinical Presentation

A 23-year-old woman with cough

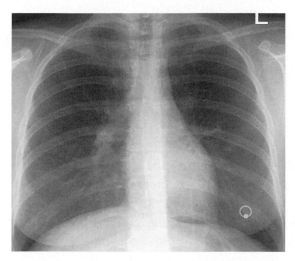

Figure 1A

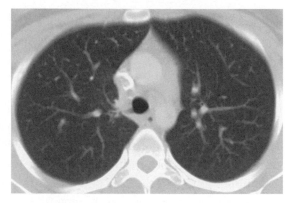

Figure 1B

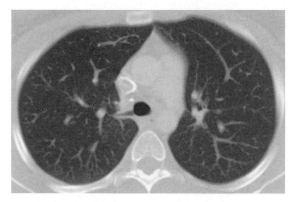

Figure 1C

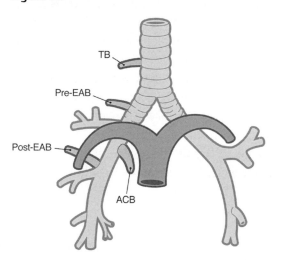

Figure 1D

Radiologic Findings

PA chest radiograph (**Fig. 1A**) demonstrates calcified right hilar lymph nodes from remote granulomatous infection. Contrast-enhanced chest CT (lung window) (**Figs. 1B** and **1C**) demonstrates a bronchus arising from the right lateral wall of the trachea. **Fig. 1D** depicts variations of right-sided anomalous bronchial branching. The tracheal bronchus (TB) arises from the lateral wall of the trachea. The pre-eparterial bronchus (pre-EAB) arises from the right mainstem bronchus proximal to the origin of the right upper lobe bronchus. The post-eparterial bronchus (post-EAB) arises distal to the origin of the right upper lobe bronchus. The accessory cardiac bronchus (ACB) arises from the medial wall of the right mainstem bronchus or the bronchus intermedius and is usually blind ending.

Diagnosis

Tracheal bronchus

Differential Diagnosis

- Tracheal diverticulum
- Tracheal fistula

Discussion

Background

Variations in bronchial branching are probably common, may affect all portions of the tracheo-bronchial tree, and are usually discovered incidentally. Tracheal bronchus is a rare anomaly that encompasses a spectrum of variant bronchial branching, manifests with anomalous bronchial origin from the trachea or bronchi, and typically affects the upper lobes. True tracheal bronchus is a rare anomaly in which the upper lobe bronchus (or one of its segmental bronchi) arises from the lateral wall of the trachea and is also known as "pig bronchus" or "bronchus suis" (the usual bronchial morphology in pigs and certain other mammals). A recently proposed modification in nomenclature classifies right-sided anomalous bronchi as pre-eparterial or post-eparterial if they arise proximal or distal to the origin of the right upper lobe bronchus, respectively (and distal to the carina) (**Fig. 1D**). The terms *prehyparterial* and *posthyparterial* are used for left-sided anomalous bronchi that arise proximal or distal to the left upper lobe bronchus, respectively. Upper lobe anomalous bronchi are seven times more common on the right side. Displaced (absent equivalent lobar, segmental, or sub-segmental bronchus) and supernumerary (coexistent normal upper lobe bronchial anatomy) anomalous bronchi occur; the former are more frequent. A displaced pre-eparterial bronchus arising from the right mainstem bronchus to supply the apical segment of the right upper lobe is the most common variant of anomalous bronchial branching.

Etiology

Tracheobronchial development occurs during the early embryonic period (26 days to 6 weeks) of fetal development. The normal five lobar bronchi appear by 32 days of gestation. Although the precise etiology of tracheal (and other anomalous) bronchi is not known, regression of anomalous bronchial buds, migration of primitive bronchi to anomalous positions, and induction of anomalous bronchial branches by surrounding primitive mesenchyme have all been suggested as possible mechanisms. Associated conditions include vascular abnormalities (such as anomalous pulmonary venous drainage) and accessory lobes and fissures. Other associations include rib anomalies, tracheoesophageal fistula, tracheobronchial stenosis, and trisomy 21.

Clinical Findings

Many patients with anomalous bronchi are asymptomatic and are diagnosed incidentally on cross-sectional imaging studies. The reported prevalence of tracheal bronchus in adult patients is 0.1%. Patients with tracheal bronchus may present in infancy or childhood with recurrent pulmonary infection, cough, stridor, hemoptysis, or respiratory distress. Recurrent upper lobe consolidation, bronchiectasis, atelectasis, and emphysema are reported in affected symptomatic children.

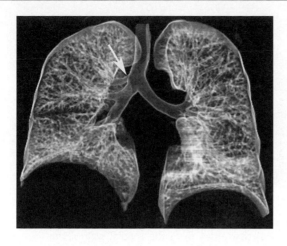

Figure 1E Unenhanced chest CT maximum intensity projection coronal image of an asymptomatic young man with a tracheal bronchus demonstrates the anomalous bronchus (arrow) as it originates from the lateral wall of the trachea and courses toward the right upper lobe.

Pathology

- Typically normal bronchial cartilage and distal lung
- Infection and/or inflammation, bronchiectasis

Imaging Findings

RADIOGRAPHY

- Normal chest radiograph (**Fig. 1A**)
- Visualization of anomalous bronchus
- Segmental or lobar right upper lobe atelectasis and/or consolidation

CT

- Visualization of anomalous bronchial origin from lateral trachea (**Figs. 1B** and **1C**)
- Spiral CT with multiplanar reconstruction, shaded surface display, minimum and maximum intensity projections (**Fig. 1E**), volume rendering and virtual bronchoscopy techniques useful in anatomic characterization and classification

Treatment

- None for asymptomatic individuals
- Excision of anomalous bronchus and associated lung tissue in patients with recurrent infection

Prognosis

- Good (particularly without associated anomalies)

PEARLS

- The typical bronchial branching depicted in anatomy texts is seldom encountered. A typical right upper lobe trifurcation was present in only 30% of all cases in one study.
- Recognition of asymptomatic tracheal bronchi is important in patients undergoing endotracheal intubation. An endotracheal tube may inadvertently occlude the lumen of a tracheal bronchus with resultant obstruction and potential infection.

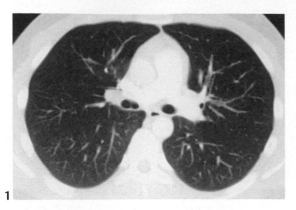 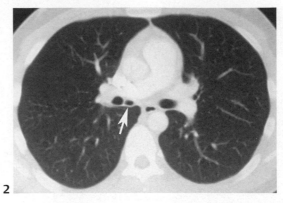

Figure 1F (1,2) Contrast-enhanced chest CT (lung window) of a 21-year-old man with hemoptysis and an accessory cardiac bronchus demonstrates an air-filled tubular structure (arrow) that arises from the medial wall of the bronchus intermedius and courses toward the mediastinum. (Courtesy of Maysiang Lesar, M.D., National Naval Medical Center, Bethesda, Maryland.)

- Tracheobronchial diverticula are distinct from anomalous bronchi. The latter have a normal mucosal lining and cartilage within their walls, and the former do not.
- Accessory cardiac bronchus is a rare type of supernumerary bronchus that arises from the medial aspect of the right mainstem or intermediate bronchus and courses caudally toward the mediastinum (hence the "cardiac" designation) (**Fig. 1F**). It is typically a blind-ending structure (**Fig. 1D**) but may be associated with normal or vestigial lung parenchyma. The lung parenchyma may be atelectatic and may manifest as a soft tissue mass surrounding the anomalous bronchus. Affected patients are usually asymptomatic but may present with hemoptysis or recurrent infection.

Suggested Readings

Evans ED, Kramer DS, Kravitz RM. Pediatric diseases of the lower airways. Semin Roentgenol 1998;33:136–150

Ghaye B, Szapiro D, Fanchamps J-M, Dondelinger RF. Congenital bronchial abnormalities revisited. Radiographics 2001;21:105–109

Middleton RM, Littleton JT, Brickey DA, Picone AL. Obstructed tracheal bronchus as a cause of post-obstructive pneumonia. J Thorac Imaging 1995;10:223–224

Wu JW, White CS, Meyer CA, Haramati LB, Mason AC. Variant bronchial anatomy: CT appearance and classification. AJR Am J Roentgenol 1999;172:741–744

CASE 2 Bronchial Atresia

Clinical Presentation

Asymptomatic 42-year-old woman

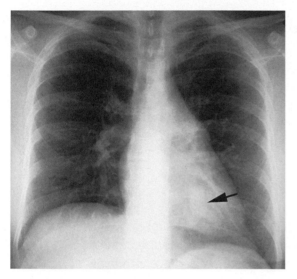

Figure 2A

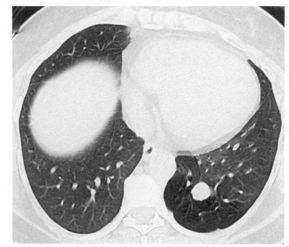

Figure 2B

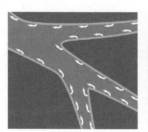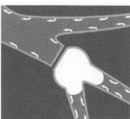

Figure 2C

Figure 2D

Radiologic Findings

PA chest radiograph (**Fig. 2A**) demonstrates a left lower lobe branching tubular opacity (arrow). Chest CT (lung window) (**Figs. 2B** and **2C**) shows the branching tubular lesion (**Fig. 2C**) surrounded by hyperlucent lung parenchyma. **Fig. 2D** depicts a normal bronchus (left) and the function of its mucociliary escalator (curved arrows); bronchial atresia (right) results in distal accumulation of secretions and mucocele formation.

Diagnosis

Bronchial atresia

Differential Diagnosis

- Mucous plug distal to bronchial obstruction (such as an endobronchial neoplasm)
- Focal bronchiectasis with mucous plugging
- Intralobar sequestration
- Allergic bronchopulmonary fungal disease
- Vascular malformation

Discussion

Background

Bronchial atresia is a rare congenital anomaly, which may affect lobar, segmental, or subsegmental bronchi. The left upper lobe bronchus (apical-posterior segment) is affected in approximately 64% of cases. Most cases of bronchial atresia are isolated, but associated anomalies have also been reported.

Etiology

Bronchial atresia is thought to result from an in-utero vascular insult that affects the blood supply to a small segment of the tracheobronchial tree with resultant complete interruption (atresia or stenosis) of the airway lumen and normal development of the distal airways. The surrounding alveoli may fail to develop normally and may overinflate because of collateral air drift through the pores of Kohn and canals of Lambert. Debris may accumulate distal to the atretic bronchus, forming a mucocele (**Fig. 2D**). Another theory postulates multiplying bronchial bud cells that lose connection with the proximal tracheobronchial tree.

Clinical Findings

Patients with bronchial atresia exhibit a wide age range but are often asymptomatic adults who are diagnosed incidentally on chest radiography. Up to 40% of patients present with cough, dyspnea, bronchospasm, or symptoms of pulmonary infection. Men are affected twice as often as women.

Pathology

GROSS

- Interrupted bronchial lumen and distended distal segmental bronchi
- Mucoid impaction
- Reduced size of affected pulmonary segment

MICROSCOPIC

- Reduced number of alveoli
- Alveolar overdistention

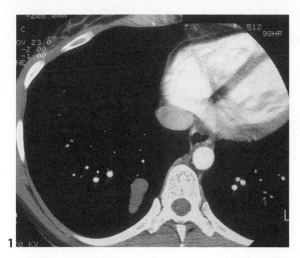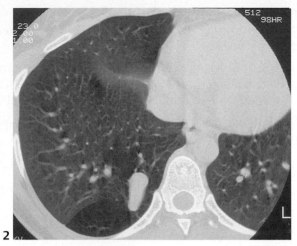

Figure 2E (1,2) Contrast-enhanced chest CT [mediastinal **(1)** and lung **(2)** window] of an asymptomatic 27-year-old woman with bronchial atresia demonstrates a nonenhancing, low-attenuation tubular opacity **(1)** and surrounding pulmonary overinflation **(2)**. (Courtesy of Jill D. Wruble, D.O., Mandel, M.D., and Blau, M.D., P.C, Hartford, Connecticut.)

Imaging Findings

RADIOGRAPHY

- Focal pulmonary overinflation
- Rounded, tubular or branching opacity (mucocele) (**Fig. 2A**)
- Focal overinflation surrounding mucocele
- Expiratory air trapping surrounding mucocele
- Air-fluid level within mucocele (with superimposed infection)

CT

- Rounded, tubular (**Fig. 2E**), or branching (**Figs. 2B** and **2C**) central opacity; low attenuation (–5 to 25 HU) (**Fig. 2E1**)
- Absence of contrast enhancement within bronchus or mucocele (**Fig. 2E1**)
- Overinflated lung surrounding mucocele (**Figs. 2B, 2C,** and **2E2**)

Treatment

- None for asymptomatic patients (clinical and/or radiographic follow-up)
- Consideration of surgical excision in patients with signs and symptoms of infection

Prognosis

- Excellent

PEARLS_____

- Bronchial atresia is a radiologic diagnosis based on the demonstration of a mucocele surrounded by hyperlucent lung (**Figs. 2B, 2C,** and **2E2**). The tubular morphology of the mucocele may suggest a vascular etiology, which is excluded by absence of contrast enhancement (**Fig. 2E1**) and absence of communication with pulmonary vessels.
- Mucoid impaction may result from a slow-growing obstructing endobronchial neoplasm. Thus, contrast-enhanced chest CT and/or endoscopic examination may be required to exclude an endo-luminal obstructing lesion.

Suggested Readings

Evans ED, Kramer DS, Kravitz RM. Pediatric diseases of the lower airways. Semin Roentgenol 1998;33:136–150

Fraser RS, Müller NL, Colman N, Paré PD. Developmental anomalies affecting the airways and lung parenchyma. In: Fraser RS, Müller NL, Colman N, Paré PD, eds. Fraser and Paré's Diagnosis of Diseases of the Chest, 4th ed. Philadelphia: WB Saunders, 1999:597–635

Ward S, Morcos SK. Congenital bronchial atresia—presentation of three cases and pictorial review. Clin Radiol 1999;54:144–148

CASE 3 Intralobar Sequestration

Clinical Presentation

A 37-year-old woman with recurrent pneumonia and productive cough

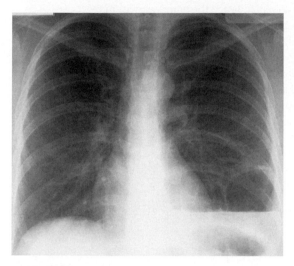

Figure 3A

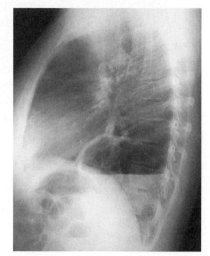

Figure 3B

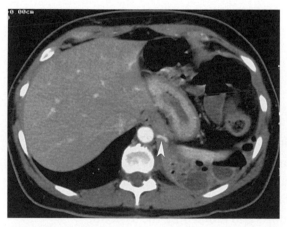

Figure 3C

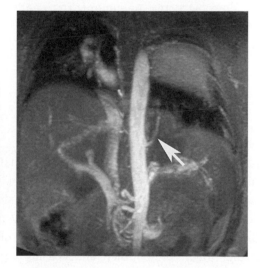

Figure 3D

Radiologic Findings

PA (**Fig. 3A**) and lateral (**Fig. 3B**) chest radiographs demonstrate a left lower lobe thin-walled multilocular cystic lesion with a large air-fluid level. Contrast-enhanced chest CT (mediastinal window) (**Fig. 3C**) demonstrates a heterogeneously enhancing left lower lobe lesion with soft tissue, air, and fluid components, supplied by a branch of the descending thoracic aorta (arrowhead). Gradient-echo magnetic resonance angiography (**Fig. 3D**) demonstrates the systemic artery (arrow) that supplies the lesion.

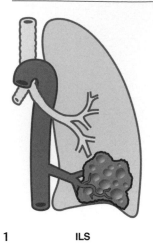
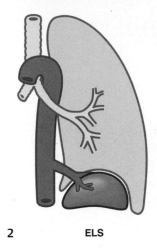

1   ILS   2   ELS

Figure 3E (1,2) The heterogeneous morphology and typical lower lobe location of intralobar sequestration (ILS, **1**) and the homogeneous morphology of extralobar sequestration (ELS, **2**), which is located outside the confines of the normal lung are illustrated. Systemic arteries supply both lesions **(1)** and **(2)**. Intralobar sequestration typically has a normal (pulmonary) venous drainage, and extralobar sequestration usually has a systemic (anomalous) venous drainage.

Diagnosis

Intralobar sequestration

Differential Diagnosis

- Pneumonia (including postobstructive pneumonia from endobronchial lesion)
- Lung abscess
- Bronchiectasis (with secondary infection)
- Infected bulla

Discussion

Background

The term *pulmonary sequestration* refers to lung parenchyma that does not communicate normally with the tracheobronchial tree and has a systemic blood supply. Intralobar sequestrations are four times more common than extralobar sequestrations and occur almost exclusively within the lower lobes (**Fig. 3E1**). Extralobar sequestrations represent accessory pulmonary lobes that result from abnormal foregut budding and are located outside the confines of the normal lung (**Fig. 3E2**). They may occur in the thorax, diaphragm, or abdomen, are typically supplied and drained by the systemic circulation, and represent true congenital anomalies.

Etiology

The majority of intralobar sequestrations are thought to represent acquired lesions, which result from lower lobe bronchial obstruction and subsequent distal infection. It is postulated that the inflammatory process obliterates the normal pulmonary arterial supply to these lesions, and that normal pulmonary ligament arteries (which arise from the thoracic aorta) are parasitized to provide a systemic blood supply. A small number of intralobar sequestrations probably do represent true congenital anomalies.

Clinical Findings

Patients with intralobar sequestration are often older children and adolescents, but approximately 50% are over the age of 20 years. Men and women are equally affected. Presenting symptoms include

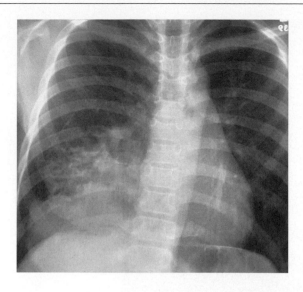

Figure 3F PA chest radiograph of a 13-year-old boy with cough, fever, and an intralobar sequestration demonstrates a heterogeneous right lower lobe consolidation with irregular borders.

chronic cough, sputum production, recurrent pneumonia, chest pain, bronchospasm, and hemoptysis. Some patients present with acute, chronic, or recurrent lower lobe infection. A small percentage of patients (15%) are asymptomatic and are diagnosed because of an incidentally discovered radiographic abnormality.

Pathology

GROSS

- Lower lobe location in 98% of cases, slightly more frequent on the left side
- Thickened overlying visceral pleura; may form adhesions with adjacent structures
- Dense, fibrous, consolidated lung with internal cysts filled with fluid, mucinous or purulent material; adjacent to normal nonsequestered lung
- Systemic arterial supply; typically coursing within the pulmonary ligament
- Normal (pulmonary) venous drainage in 95% of cases

MICROSCOPIC

- Acute and chronic inflammation, bronchopneumonia, bronchiectasis, fibrosis, and cystic change
- Lesion edges contiguous with nonsequestered adjacent lung; may sharply abut normal lung or may blend with it diffusely
- Elastic anomalous feeding arteries; may develop atherosclerotic changes

Imaging Findings

RADIOGRAPHY

- Lower lobe posterior basal segment location; more frequently the left lower lobe (**Figs. 3A, 3B,** and **3F**)
- Consolidation (**Fig. 3F**) or mass; may contain air, air-fluid levels (**Figs. 3A** and **3B**), and multilocular cysts (**Figs. 3A** and **3B**); irregular margins typical (**Fig. 3F**) but may also exhibit well-defined borders
- Predominantly cystic lesions may exhibit a single cyst or multiple cysts of variable size
- Rarely, branching tubular opacity representing impacted bronchi
- Surrounding lung may be hyperlucent
- May produce mass effect on adjacent structures (**Fig. 3F**)

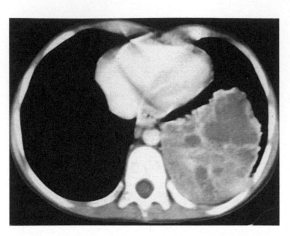

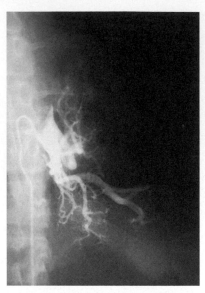

Figure 3G Contrast-enhanced chest CT (mediastinal window) of a 6-year-old boy with a left lower lobe intralobar sequestration demonstrates a heterogeneously enhancing multicystic mass with irregular borders.

Figure 3H Selective arteriogram of a 32-year-old woman with a left lower lobe intralobar sequestration demonstrates injection of contrast into the anomalous feeding artery, which originates from the descending thoracic aorta.

CT

- Posteromedial lower lobe location (**Figs. 3C** and **3G**)
- Heterogeneous or homogeneous mass (**Fig. 3G**)
- Heterogeneous or homogeneous consolidation
- Smooth, lobular, or irregular (**Fig. 3G**) borders against adjacent lung
- Typically heterogeneous attenuation with soft tissue, air, fluid, and/or air-fluid levels (**Figs. 3C** and **3G**)
- Heterogeneous enhancement (**Figs. 3C** and **3G**)
- Predominantly cystic lesion with single or multiple thin-walled cysts; may contain air and/or fluid
- Demonstration of anomalous systemic arterial supply (usually from descending thoracic aorta) in up to 80% of cases (**Fig. 3C**)

MR

- Heterogeneous intrapulmonary lower lobe lesion; may exhibit cystic areas
- Gradient-echo sequences may demonstrate systemic blood supply (**Fig. 3D**) and pulmonary venous drainage

ANGIOGRAPHY

- Aortography for demonstration of anomalous systemic arterial supply (single or multiple vessels) arising from the descending thoracic aorta (**Fig. 3H**) in up to 73% of cases, or other systemic abdominal arteries.
- Selective angiography of anomalous systemic artery may allow demonstration of pulmonary venous drainage.

Treatment

- Surgical excision of affected lobe and ligation of anomalous feeding vessels

Prognosis

- Excellent

PEARLS_____

- Intralobar sequestration must be considered in the differential diagnosis of any patient who presents with recurrent lower lobe infection or chronic radiologic abnormality. The diagnosis is supported by identification of systemic arterial supply to the lesion (**Figs. 3C, 3D,** and **3H**).
- Differentiation from extralobar sequestration is not always necessary but can usually be made based on clinical and morphologic features. Intralobar sequestration typically manifests in children and adults with signs and symptoms of infection, whereas extralobar sequestration usually affects neonates and infants who present with respiratory distress.
- As the term implies, intralobar sequestration is always located within lung, typically in a lower lobe (**Fig. 3E1**). As a result, it often exhibits irregular margins against the adjacent (nonsequestered) lung and may contain air. Extralobar sequestration occurs outside normal lung, typically exhibits a well-defined border (**Fig. 3E2**), and does not contain air.
- Both lesions are supplied by the systemic circulation (**Fig. 3E**), although the pulmonary arteries may partially supply both lesions.
- Preoperative imaging allows delineation of the number and location of systemic feeding arteries and may be helpful in surgical planning for ligation and control of these vessels.

Suggested Reading

Frazier AA, Rosado de Christenson ML, Stocker TJ, Templeton PA. Intralobar sequestration: radiologic-pathologic correlation. Radiographics 1997;17: 725–745

CASE 4 Right Aortic Arch

Clinical Presentation

A 43-year-old man evaluated prior to neck surgery

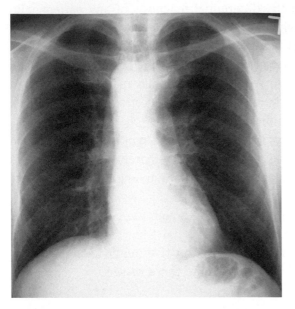

Figure 4A

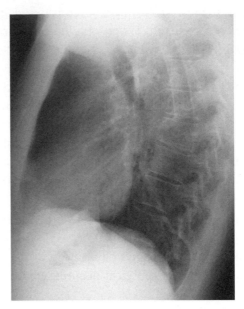

Figure 4B

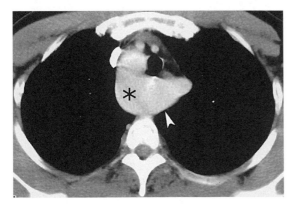

Figure 4C

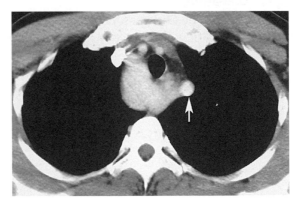

Figure 4D

Radiologic Findings

PA (**Fig. 4A**) and lateral (**Fig. 4B**) chest radiographs demonstrate a right aortic arch with a right descending aorta. There is mild mass effect on the posterior wall of the trachea on the lateral radiograph (**Fig. 4B**). Contrast-enhanced chest CT (mediastinal window) (**Figs. 4C** and **4D**) demonstrates the right aortic arch (*) and an aortic diverticulum (arrowhead) (**Fig. 4C**), which gives rise to an aberrant left subclavian artery (arrow) (**Fig. 4D**).

Diagnosis

Right aortic arch with aberrant left subclavian artery

48

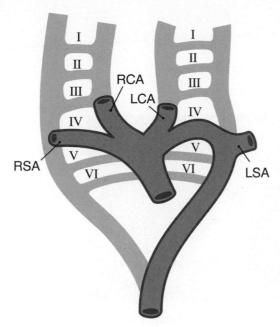

Figure 4E The normal embryologic development of the aortic arch requires the regression of several components of the primitive systems (depicted in a lighter tone of gray). There are paired dorsal aortae, which sequentially give rise to six paired arches (numbered with roman numerals). The normal left aortic arch results from persistence of the left fourth primitive arch and involution of part of the right fourth primitive arch. A portion of the right fourth primitive arch gives rise to the right subclavian artery. The precursors of the right subclavian artery (RSA), right carotid artery (RCA), left carotid artery (LCA), and left subclavian artery (LSA) are illustrated.

Differential Diagnosis

None

Discussion

Background

The aorta and great vessels develop embryologically from paired dorsal aortae, which sequentially give rise to six paired primitive arches (**Fig. 4E**), portions of which sequentially regress as new arches are formed. The normal left aortic arch results from persistence of the left fourth primitive arch (**Fig. 4E**), regression of the right fourth arch beyond the right subclavian artery, and persistence of the left dorsal aorta and the left ductus arteriosus (the latter forms from the left sixth primitive arch). The right brachiocephalic, left carotid, and left subclavian arteries arise in succession from the normal left aortic arch (**Fig. 4E**). Right aortic arch has an incidence of approximately 0.1 to 0.2%. A right aortic arch may exhibit mirror-image or non-mirror-image branching of the great vessels. In right aortic arch with mirror-image branching, the left brachiocephalic artery, right common carotid artery, and right subclavian artery arise in succession. The most common type of right aortic arch exhibits non-mirror-image branching. The left common carotid artery, right common carotid artery, right subclavian artery, and aberrant left subclavian artery arise from it in succession. There may be a left ductus arteriosus between the left subclavian and left pulmonary arteries and a resultant vascular ring.

Etiology

The most common type of right aortic arch (non-mirror-image branching) is thought to result from involution of the primitive left fourth arch between the left common carotid and left subclavian arteries (**Fig. 4E**). As a result, the left subclavian artery arises from the dorsal aorta as its fourth branch.

Clinical Findings

Right aortic arch with aberrant left subclavian artery (which produces a retroesophageal arterial segment) and left ductus arteriosus forms a true vascular ring but is not usually associated with

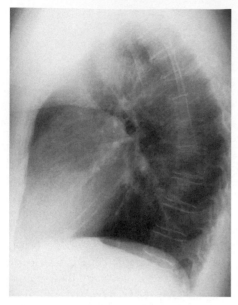

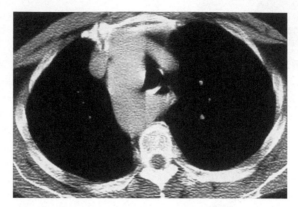

Figure 4F Lateral chest radiograph of a patient with a right aortic arch and an aberrant left subclavian artery who presented with cough and dysphagia demonstrates mass effect on the posterior trachea.

Figure 4G Unenhanced chest CT (mediastinal window) shows the relationship of the aorta and its diverticulum to the trachea and esophagus.

congenital heart disease. Affected patients may be asymptomatic or may present with cough, stridor, or dysphagia. Right aortic arch with mirror-image branching does not exhibit a retroesophageal arterial segment but is associated with congenital heart disease. Right aortic arch is present in 1.4% of patients with congenital cardiac anomalies, particularly tetralogy of Fallot, persistent truncus arteriosus, transposition of the great vessels with pulmonic stenosis, and ventricular septal defect with infundibular pulmonic stenosis.

Pathology

- Origin of aberrant left subclavian artery from aortic diverticulum
- Oblique course of aberrant left subclavian artery behind esophagus toward left upper extremity
- Development of atherosclerosis and aneurysms of the aortic arch and its branches as in left aortic arch

Imaging Findings

RADIOGRAPHY

- Right paratracheal soft tissue mass (**Fig. 4A**)
  - Vascular impression on the right side of the trachea
  - Rightward azygos vein displacement
- Retrotracheal soft tissue mass produced by the aortic diverticulum (which gives rise to aberrant left subclavian artery) (**Figs. 4B** and **4F**)
- Visualization of oblique tubular opacity projecting over the trachea on frontal radiography and coursing toward the left (aberrant left subclavian artery)

CT/MR

- Direct visualization of right aortic arch (**Figs. 4C, 4D,** and **4G**)
- Direct visualization of aortic diverticulum (**Figs. 4C** and **4G**)

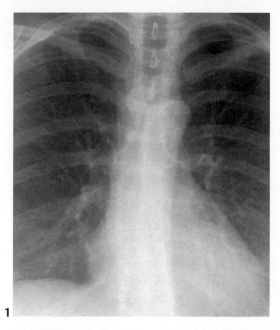
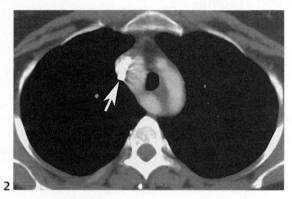

Figure 4H (1,2) Coned-down PA chest radiograph **(1)** and contrast-enhanced chest CT (mediastinal window) **(2)** of a 53-year-old woman with vague chest pain and a double aortic arch demonstrates bilateral indentations on the trachea produced by the two components of the double aortic arch **(1)**. Note that the right arch is located slightly more cephalad than the left **(1)**. The resultant vascular ring **(2)** produces mild mass effect on the trachea. Note the lateral displacement of the superior vena cava (arrow) by the right aortic arch **(2)**. (Courtesy of Diane C. Strollo, M.D., University of Pittsburgh, Pittsburgh, Pennsylvania.)

- Direct visualization of aberrant left subclavian artery origin (**Figs. 4D** and **4G**)
- Evaluation of mass effect on adjacent mediastinal structures (trachea, esophagus) (**Figs. 4C, 4D, and 4G**)
- Cardiac evaluation to exclude associated congenital heart disease

Treatment

- None for asymptomatic patients
- Division of the left ligamentum arteriosus, resection of aortic diverticulum, and reimplantation of the left subclavian artery onto the left carotid artery or reconstruction in symptomatic patients
- Consideration of arteriopexy, aortopexy, or tracheopexy in patients with recurrent symptoms

Prognosis

- Good for adults without associated congenital anomalies

PEARLS

- Patients with right aortic arch with non-mirror-image branching may have a large aortic diverticulum that may manifest as a left paratracheal soft tissue mass and may mimic a left aortic arch.
- Double aortic arch results from persistence of both embryonic fourth aortic arches (**Fig. 4E**), which encircle the trachea and join posteriorly as a left-sided descending aorta. The right arch is usually larger and situated more cephalad than the left (**Fig. 4H1**), and each arch gives rise to

ipsilateral common carotid and subclavian arteries. Double aortic arch is the most common cause of a symptomatic vascular ring in infants and young children. Radiographic findings may be similar to those of right aortic arch, but CT (**Fig. 4H2**) and MR demonstrate the patent left and right aortic arches and allow assessment of the origins of the great vessels.

Suggested Readings

Amplatz K, Moller JH. Anomalies of the aortic arch system. In: Amplatz K, Moller JH, eds. Radiology of Congenital Heart Disease. St Louis: Mosby, 1993:995–1049

Jaffe RB. Radiographic manifestations of congenital anomalies of the aortic arch. Radiol Clin North Am 1991;29:319–334

Raymond GS, Miller RM, Müller NL, Logan PM. Congenital thoracic lesions that mimic neoplastic disease on chest radiographs of adults. Am J Roentgenol 1997;168:763–769

Roberts CS, Othersen HB Jr, Sade RM, Smith CD III, Tagge EP, Crawford FA Jr. Tracheoesophageal compression from aortic arch anomalies: analysis of 30 operatively treated children. J Pediatr Surg 1994;29:334–338

CASE 5 Coarctation of the Aorta

Clinical Presentation

An 18-year-old woman with differential upper and lower extremity blood pressures and stronger radial than femoral pulses

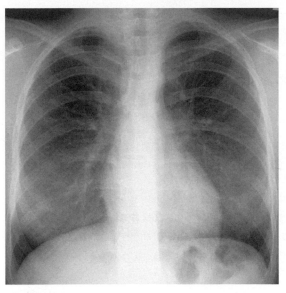

Figure 5A

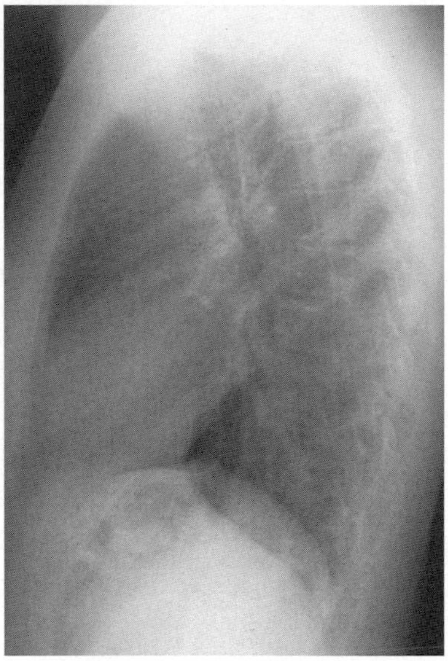

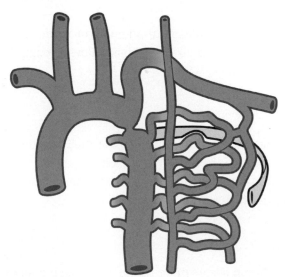

Figure 5B

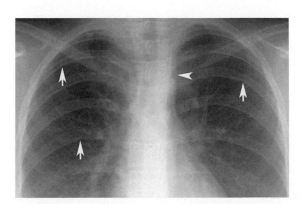

Figure 5C

Figure 5D

Radiologic Findings

PA (**Fig. 5A**) and lateral (**Fig. 5B**) chest radiographs and coned-down PA chest radiograph (**Fig. 5C**) demonstrate rib notching (arrows) and an inconspicuous aortic arch. The heart size and pulmonary vascularity are normal. The straight left superior mediastinal contour (arrowhead) is formed by an enlarged left subclavian artery. **Fig. 5D** depicts the collateral pathways that develop in coarctation of the aorta. Dilatation and tortuosity of the intercostal arteries produce the radiographic finding of rib notching, which results from benign pressure erosion by the pulsatile collateral vessels on adjacent ribs.

Diagnosis

Coarctation of the aorta

Differential Diagnosis

- Neurofibromatosis
- Pulmonary atresia with harvested systemic vessels communicating with pulmonary vessels

Discussion

Background

Coarctation of the aorta is a focal obstruction at the junction of the distal aortic arch and descending aorta near the ligamentum arteriosum. It accounts for approximately 6% of congenital cardiac anomalies. Although there is blood flow across the coarctation, it is supplemented by collateral flow that bypasses the obstruction through the spinal artery, intercostal arteries (**Fig. 5D**), epigastric arteries, lateral thoracic artery, and periscapular arteries. These collateral vessels are not usually present at birth and develop over time.

Etiology

Coarctation of the aorta is a congenital anomaly of unknown etiology. Diffuse aortic coarctation is thought to result from marked reduction of blood flow through the fetal aortic isthmus from associated congenital cardiac anomalies.

Pathology

- Localized coarctation—stenosis opposite the ductus arteriosus from a deformity of the media, which projects focally into the aortic lumen
- Diffuse coarctation—long segment hypoplastic stenosis extending from the left subclavian artery to the ductus arteriosus

Clinical Findings

Isolated aortic coarctation occurs more commonly in men than in women (2.5:1 ratio), but coarctation associated with congenital cardiac anomalies affects men and women equally. Approximately 20% of women with aortic coarctation also have Turner syndrome. Other associated conditions include bicuspid aortic valve (in approximately 50% of affected patients), mitral valve prolapse, patent ductus arteriosus, and ventricular septal defect. Patients with aortic coarctation and associated anomalies typically become symptomatic at birth and present with left heart failure. Patients with isolated coarctation may be entirely asymptomatic or may become symptomatic in childhood or young adulthood. Presenting symptoms include headache, claudication, and fatigue. Patients may also present with a murmur, systemic hypertension, or aortic dissection. Aortic coarctation in association with bicuspid aortic valve typically does not manifest with symptoms related to valvular stenosis but may manifest with bacterial endocarditis. On physical examination there are differential blood

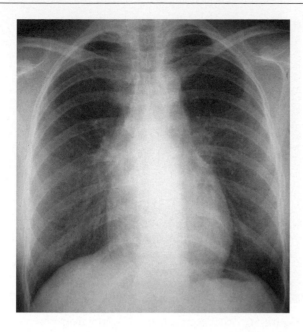

Figure 5E PA chest radiograph of a young woman with situs ambiguous (note bilateral hyparterial bronchi; see Case 13) and aortic coarctation shows a figure-of-3 contour of the left superior mediastinum. Note the dilatation of the ascending thoracic aorta secondary to associated stenotic bicuspid aortic valve with post-stenotic dilatation.

pressures between the upper and lower extremities (with differences of at least 20 mm Hg) and radial pulses that are stronger than femoral pulses.

Imaging Findings

RADIOGRAPHY

- Infants
  - Cardiomegaly related to heart failure
    - Left ventricular dilatation
    - Right ventricular dilatation
    - Left atrial enlargement
  - Accentuated pulmonary vasculature from pulmonary venous hypertension
  - Pulmonary edema
- Older children and adults
  - Normal heart size, normal pulmonary vascularity (**Figs. 5A** and **5B**)
  - Left ventricular cardiac configuration from left ventricular hypertrophy
  - Cardiomegaly from left ventricular failure
  - Narrow cardiac waist and inconspicuous pulmonary artery
  - Inconspicuous aortic arch (**Figs. 5A** and **5C**) obscured by enlarged left subclavian artery that forms a straight left superior mediastinal contour (**Figs. 5A** and **5C**)
  - Figure-of-3 configuration (**Fig. 5E**) of the left lateral border of the aortic arch from poststenotic dilatation distal to the coarctation
  - Aortic valve calcification and/or enlarged ascending aorta (**Fig. 5E**) from associated stenotic bicuspid aortic valve
  - Inferior rib notching (usually ribs 3 to 9) (**Figs. 5A** and **5C**)

CT

- Visualization of length and location of the coarctation and differential aortic size proximal and distal to the obstruction
- Visualization of aortic branches and their relationship to the coarctation
- Visualization of collateral internal mammary, intercostal, and paraspinal arteries

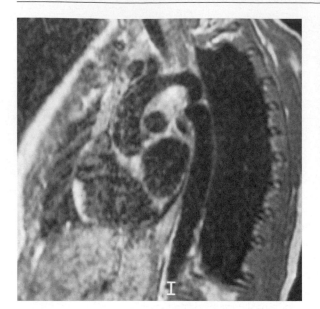

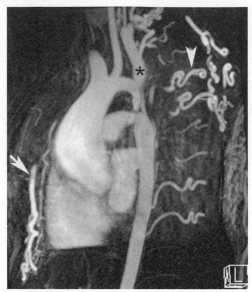

Figure 5F Sagittal T1-weighted MR of an 11-year-old boy with aortic coarctation demonstrates the location and degree of aortic stenosis and mild post-stenotic aortic dilatation.

Figure 5G Gadolinium-enhanced sagittal magnetic resonance angiography of the aorta of a young patient with aortic coarctation demonstrates the exact location of the lesion [distal to the origin of the left subclavian artery (*)], the major aortic branches, and numerous collateral vessels including internal mammary (arrow) and intercostal (arrowhead) arteries.

MR

- Oblique sagittal MR (**Fig. 5F**) and gadolinium-enhanced magnetic resonance angiography (**Fig. 5G**) for visualization and measurement of length and location of the coarctation and the degree of luminal narrowing
- Visualization of aortic branches and their relationship to the coarctation (**Fig. 5G**)
- Visualization of collateral internal mammary, intercostals, and paraspinal arteries (**Fig. 5G**)
- Velocity-encoded cine MR for estimation of flow gradient across the coarctation and estimation of collateral blood flow

ANGIOGRAPHY

- Demonstration of location and length of the coarctation
- Visualization of aortic branches and their relationship to the coarctation

Treatment

- Resection of the coarctation and graft placement
- Balloon dilatation of the coarctation for patients who are poor surgical candidates

Prognosis

- Good with surgical treatment
  - Early postsurgical complications: systemic hypertension and mesenteric arteritis
  - Late postsurgical complications: aneurysm, pseudoaneurysm, re-coarctation, and infective endocarditis
- Poor prognosis in patients who are not treated surgically; over 90% of these patients die by age 58 years

PEARLS

- Rib notching is produced by pulsation of dilated intercostal arteries (**Figs. 5A, 5C, 5D,** and **5G**), which provide collateral blood flow. It is rare before the age of 10 years and is most prominent along the posterior ribs and most visible in the upper ribs. The upper ribs (1 to 3) are usually free of notching because of communication between the intercostal arteries and the aorta above the coarctation (without a drop in systolic pressure). The lower ribs (10 to 12) are free of notching because of communication between intercostal arteries and superior epigastric arteries without additional collateral flow. Unilateral rib notching results when one of the subclavian arteries arises distal to the coarctation (as in aberrant right subclavian artery).

- The figure-of-3 sign (**Fig. 5E**) results from prominence of the left subclavian artery related to increased pressure (proximal to the coarctation) and the post-stenotic dilatation of the descending aorta. Esophageal displacement accounts for the reversed-3 sign on barium esophagography.

- Pseudocoarctation of the aorta represents a "kink" in the descending thoracic aorta at the ligamentum arteriosum without obstruction, pressure gradient, or collateral blood flow. It results from elongation of the ascending aorta and should be differentiated from true coarctation and cervical aortic arch. Chest radiographs may demonstrate mediastinal abnormalities similar to those seen in coarctation, but there is no obstruction and no symptoms or signs related to aortic obstruction or collateral blood flow.

Suggested Readings

Amplatz K, Moller JH. Coarctation of the aorta. In: Amplatz K, Moller JH, eds. Radiology of Congenital Heart Disease. St Louis: Mosby, 1993:469–497

Cole TJ, Henry DA, Jolles H, Proto AV. Normal and abnormal vascular structures that simulate neoplasms on chest radiographs: clues to the diagnosis. Radiographics 1995;15:867–891

Steiner RM, Reddy GP, Flicker S. Congenital cardiovascular disease in the adult patient: imaging update. J Thorac Imaging 2002;17:1–17

CASE 6 Marfan Syndrome

Clinical Presentation

An 18-year-old man with recurrent pneumothorax

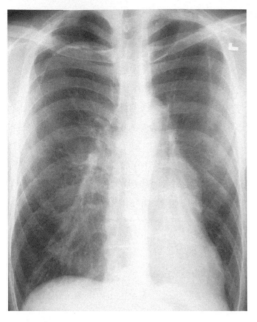

Figure 6A

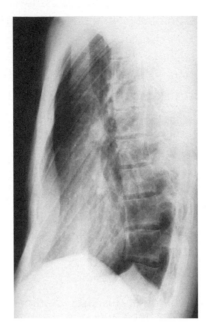

Figure 6B

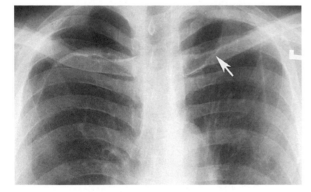

Figure 6C

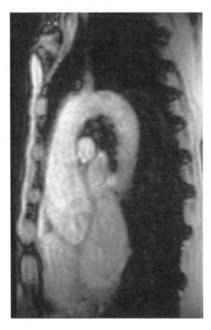

Figure 6D

Radiologic Findings

PA (**Fig. 6A**) and lateral (**Fig. 6B**) chest radiographs demonstrate a right pneumothorax and bilateral apical pleural thickening (**Fig. 6A**). Note the abnormal cardiac contour, enlargement of the main pulmonary artery, and pectus excavatum deformity. Coned-down PA chest radiograph (**Fig. 6C**) demonstrates bilateral apical pleural thickening and metallic sutures (arrow) from a previous lung resection for treatment of recurrent pneumothorax. Oblique sagittal gradient-echo magnetic resonance angiography (**Fig. 6D**) shows dilatation of the proximal ascending aorta and the sinuses of Valsalva. Note the narrow anteroposterior chest diameter produced by the pectus deformity.

Diagnosis

Marfan syndrome

Differential Diagnosis

- Primary spontaneous pneumothorax
- Annuloaortic ectasia of other etiology (Ehlers-Danlos syndrome, Turner syndrome, polycystic kidney disease, osteogenesis imperfecta)
- Ascending aortic aneurysm of other etiology (atherosclerosis, syphilis)
- Aortic stenosis with post-stenotic dilatation
- Aortic dissection

Discussion

Background

Marfan syndrome is a generalized connective tissue disorder involving primarily elastic tissues and affects the eye, skeleton, lung, and cardiovascular structures. Marfan syndrome is an autosomal-dominant disorder, but it may occur sporadically in up to 15% of cases.

Etiology

Marfan syndrome results from a genetic defect (linked to the *FBN1* gene on chromosome 15) in the production of glycoprotein fibrillin, which is important in the formation of elastic fibers found in normal connective tissue, and particularly affects the walls of major arteries. The resultant disruption of elastic fibers results in dilatation of the ascending aorta, sinuses of Valsalva (formed by the aortic valve leaflets), and the aortic annulus.

Pathology

GROSS

- Annuloaortic ectasia
  - Dilatation of the aortic annulus
  - Enlarged and redundant sinuses of Valsalva
  - Fusiform dilatation of the ascending aorta (spares the aortic arch and descending aorta)
- Redundant mitral valve
- Pulmonary artery dilatation

MICROSCOPIC

- Disruption of normal elastic fibers in the aortic media (and large pulmonary arteries) by abnormal mucoid material
  - "Cystic medial necrosis" descriptor no longer favored; no cystic changes or necrosis
- Myxomatous valvular degeneration, particularly the mitral and aortic valves

Clinical Findings

Patients with Marfan syndrome are typically tall and thin and may exhibit arachnodactyly. Chest wall anomalies occur frequently and include scoliosis and pectus deformities. Ocular involvement manifests with subluxation of the optic lens in up to 80% of patients. Approximately 50% of affected

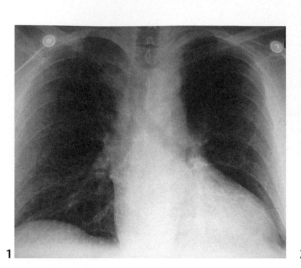
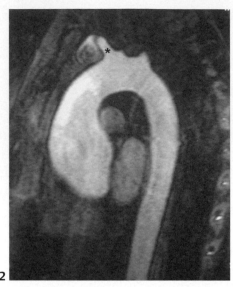

Figure 6E (1,2) Frontal chest radiograph **(1)** and oblique sagittal gradient-echo magnetic resonance angiography **(2)** of a young man with Marfan syndrome demonstrate cardiomegaly **(1)** secondary to left ventricular dilatation from aortic insufficiency and annuloaortic ectasia. Note that the distal ascending aorta rapidly tapers to a normal caliber before the origin of the right brachiocephalic artery **(2,***)** and that most of the aortic dilatation occurs proximally and at the sinuses of Valsalva **(2)**.

individuals have clinical evidence of cardiovascular disease by age 21 years. Children with Marfan syndrome typically exhibit auscultatory evidence of mitral insufficiency, whereas aortic insufficiency is more commonly diagnosed in affected adults. Approximately 10% of affected patients present because of spontaneous pneumothorax resulting from bullous disease.

Imaging Findings

RADIOGRAPHY

- Narrow anteroposterior chest diameter, pectus (excavatum or carinatum) deformity, scoliosis, and long, thin body habitus (**Figs. 6A** and **6B**)
- Dilatation of ascending thoracic aorta with normal caliber of the arch and descending aorta; may not be visible on radiography
- Cardiomegaly from aortic and less commonly mitral insufficiency and consequent left ventricular (**Fig. 6E1**) and left atrial enlargement
- Dilated main pulmonary artery (**Fig. 6A**)
- Spontaneous pneumothorax (may be recurrent) (**Figs. 6A** and **6C**)

CT

- Enlargement of ascending aorta from aortic valve to origin of brachiocephalic artery
- Normal aortic arch and descending aorta
- Left ventricular enlargement and hypertrophy
- Findings of aortic dissection: mediastinal hematoma, visualization of intimal flap

MR

- Enlargement of ascending aorta from aortic valve to origin of brachiocephalic artery (**Figs. 6D** and **6E2**)
- Left ventricular enlargement and hypertrophy

- Findings of aortic dissection: mediastinal hematoma, visualization of intimal flap
- Demonstration of aortic insufficiency

Treatment

- Propranolol for control of systemic hypertension to prevent further dilatation of ascending aorta and progression of aortic insufficiency
- Surgical graft placement within ascending aorta (wrapped with native aorta) and aortic valve replacement
- Anastomosis of coronary arteries to the graft

Prognosis

- Guarded; death from cardiovascular disease in over 90% of patients
- Good results with early surgical aortic repair prior to onset of dissection

PEARLS_____

- Marfan syndrome is one of the most common causes of ascending aortic aneurysm in young adults. Aortic aneurysm in patients with Marfan syndrome is differentiated from atherosclerotic aneurysm by absence of involvement of the descending thoracic aorta in the former and universal involvement of the descending aorta in the latter.
- Aortic aneurysm is defined as permanent dilatation with resultant diameter of at least 50% greater than normal. Normal aortic measurements in young adults on CT are as follows: 3.6 cm at the root, 3.5 cm at the ascending aorta, 2.6 cm at the proximal descending aorta, and 2.5 cm at the distal descending aorta. There is progressive diameter enlargement with increasing age (approximately 0.1 cm per decade).
- Syphilitic aortitis may mimic Marfan syndrome but is a rare cause of ascending aortic aneurysm in developed countries. It typically affects the elderly and infrequently results in severe aortic insufficiency.

Suggested Readings

Amplatz K, Moller JH. Marfan syndrome (cystic medial necrosis). In: Amplatz K, Moller JH, eds. Radiology of Congenital Heart Disease. St Louis: Mosby, 1993:1101–1117

Boxt LM, Katz J. Magnetic resonance of the thoracic aorta. In: Taveras JM, Ferrucci JT, eds. Taveras and Ferrucci on CD-ROM. Diagnosis. Imaging. Intervention, vol. 2. Philadelphia: Lippincott Williams & Wilkins, 2000

Fraser RS, Müller NL, Colman N, Paré PD. Hereditary anomalies of pulmonary connective tissue. In: Fraser RS, Müller NL, Colman N, Paré PD, eds. Fraser and Paré's Diagnosis of Diseases of the Chest, 4th ed. Philadelphia: WB Saunders, 1999;676–693

Nguyen BT. Computed tomography diagnosis of thoracic aortic aneurysms. Semin Roentgenol 2001;36:309–324

CASE 7 Aberrant Right Subclavian Artery

Clinical Presentation

Asymptomatic 42-year-old man

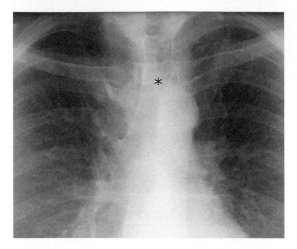

Figure 7A

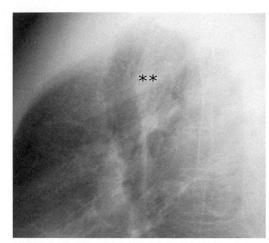

Figure 7B

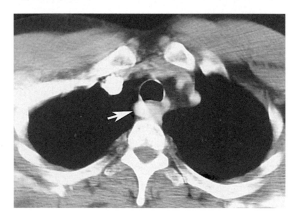

Figure 7C

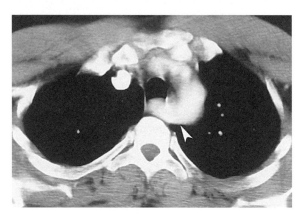

Figure 7D

(Figs. 7A, 7B, 7C, and 7D courtesy of Maysiang Lesar, M.D., National Naval Medical Center, Bethesda, Maryland.)

Radiologic Findings

Coned-down PA (**Fig. 7A**) and lateral (**Fig. 7B**) chest radiographs demonstrate a left aortic arch and a tubular opacity (*) that arises from its superior aspect, projects over the tracheal lumen, and courses obliquely toward the right upper extremity (**Fig. 7A**). Note the incidental presence of an azygos lobe. The lateral radiograph (**Fig. 7B**) demonstrates a soft tissue opacity (**) that produces mass effect on the dorsal aspect of the trachea. Contrast-enhanced chest CT (mediastinal window) (**Figs. 7C** and **7D**) demonstrates an aberrant right subclavian artery (arrow) (**Fig. 7C**) that arises from a diverticulum of Kommerell (arrowhead) (**Fig. 7D**).

Diagnosis

Aberrant right subclavian artery

Differential Diagnosis

None

Discussion

Background

An aberrant right subclavian artery arises as the last branch off a left-sided aortic arch and courses obliquely and superiorly behind the trachea and esophagus to resume its normal course. It is typically an isolated anomaly, represents the most common aortic arch malformation, and affects up to 2.3% of the population.

Etiology

An aberrant right subclavian artery results from interruption of the embryonic right fourth aortic arch between the right common carotid artery and the right subclavian artery (see Case 4, **Fig. 4E**) with regression of the right ductus arteriosus. The aortic arch branches arise in the following order: right common carotid artery, left common carotid artery, left subclavian artery, and right subclavian artery (**Fig. 7E**). The aberrant right subclavian artery may rarely arise from an aortic diverticulum that results from persistence of the dorsal portion of the embryonic right arch.

Clinical Findings

Affected patients are typically asymptomatic adults who are diagnosed incidentally. Patients with associated right ductus arteriosus have a complete vascular ring and may have symptoms. In addition, patients with associated common origin of the carotid arteries may present with symptoms of tracheal compression. Patients may present with symptoms of esophageal compression when there is aneurysmal dilatation of the aberrant vessel. In these cases, the aberrant vessel has been called "arteria lusoria" and the symptom "dysphagia lusoria" (from the Latin *lusus naturae*, meaning "game or freak of nature").

Pathology

- Atherosclerosis and aneurysms may develop as in the normal subclavian and/or brachiocephalic artery

Imaging Findings

RADIOGRAPHY

- Tubular opacity arising from the superior aspect of the aortic arch and coursing obliquely toward the right over the tracheal air column on frontal radiography (**Fig. 7A**)
- Soft tissue opacity above the aortic arch (**Fig. 7B**); may produce mass effect on the posterior trachea on lateral radiography (**Fig. 7B**)
- Lucent band coursing diagonally across the esophagus toward the right with focal mass effect on the dorsal esophagus on contrast esophagography

CT/MR

- Visualization of aberrant vessel arising from the distal posterior aortic arch and coursing toward the right behind the trachea and esophagus (**Figs. 7C** and **7D**)
- Visualization of aortic diverticulum when present (**Fig. 7D**)

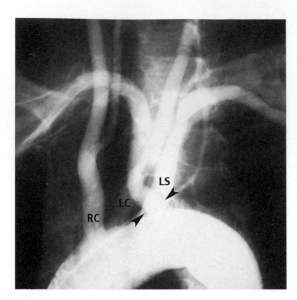

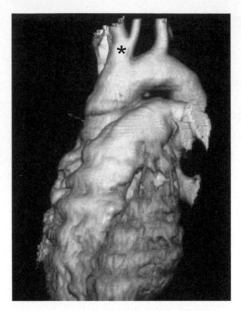

Figure 7E Thoracic aortogram of a patient with aberrant right subclavian artery demonstrates the right carotid (RC), left carotid (LC), left subclavian (LS), and aberrant right subclavian (arrowheads) arteries. Note that the aberrant right subclavian artery is the last branch off the aortic arch. (Courtesy of John J. Cronan, M.D., Brown Medical School, Rhode Island Hospital, Providence, Rhode Island.)

Figure 7F Contrast-enhanced chest CT (volume-rendered display) of a patient with a bovine arch demonstrates the common origin (*) of the right brachiocephalic and left carotid arteries. (Courtesy of Michael Atalay, M.D., Ph.D., Brown Medical School, Rhode Island Hospital, Providence, Rhode Island.)

ANGIOGRAPHY

- Demonstration of pattern of aortic branching: right carotid artery, left carotid artery, left subclavian artery, and right subclavian artery, the latter with an oblique course toward the right shoulder (**Fig. 7E**)

Treatment

- None for asymptomatic patients
- Division of right-sided ligamentum arteriosum and resection of aortic diverticulum in symptomatic patients with a vascular ring

Prognosis

- Excellent

PEARLS_____

- An aberrant right subclavian artery is a significant incidental finding in patients who will undergo cardiac catheterization through the right arm, as the catheter typically enters the descending aorta and cannot be maneuvered into the ascending aorta (**Fig. 7E**).
- The so-called diverticulum of Kommerell (**Fig. 7D**) was first described on an esophagram of an asymptomatic patient with a left aortic arch and an aberrant right subclavian artery arising from a vascular diverticulum, which produced mass effect on the esophagus. Interestingly, the aortic

diverticulum occurs more frequently in patients with right aortic arch and aberrant left subclavian artery (see Case 4, **Figs. 4C** and **4G**), and is also referred to as diverticulum of Kommerell in these instances.

- An aberrant right subclavian artery in a patient with aortic coarctation typically arises distal to the coarctation. In these cases, a right vertebral subclavian steal may result from retrograde flow from the right subclavian artery into the descending thoracic aorta. Affected patients may exhibit unilateral left rib notching.

- Other minor anomalies of aortic arch branching occur relatively frequently. The most frequent are common origin of the right brachiocephalic artery and the left common carotid artery (so-called bovine arch affecting up to 25% of patients with a left aortic arch) (**Fig. 7F**) and separate origin of the left vertebral artery proximal to the origin of the left subclavian artery (10% of patients).

Suggested Readings

Amplatz K, Moller JH. Anomalies of the aortic arch system. In: Amplatz K, Moller JH, eds. Radiology of Congenital Heart Disease. St Louis: Mosby, 1993:995–1049

Gross GW, Steiner RM. Radiographic manifestations of congenital heart disease in the adult patient. Radiol Clin North Am 1991;29:293–317

Jaffe RB. Radiographic manifestations of congenital anomalies of the aortic arch. Radiol Clin North Am 1991;29:319–334

van Son JA, Konstantinov IE, Burckhard F. Kommerell and Kommerell's diverticulum. Tex Heart Inst J 2002;29:109–112

CASE 8 Persistent Left Superior Vena Cava

Clinical Presentation

Asymptomatic 30-year-old man

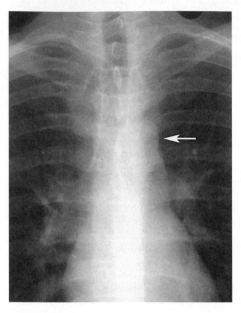

Figure 8A

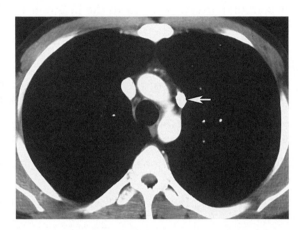

Figure 8B

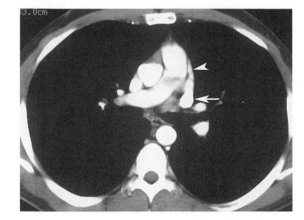

Figure 8C

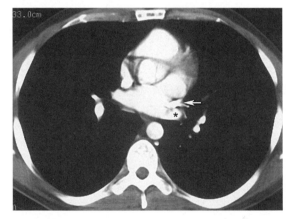

Figure 8D

(Figs. 8A, 8B, 8C, and 8D courtesy of Maysiang Lesar, M.D., National Naval Medical Center, Bethesda, M.D.)

Radiologic Findings

Coned-down PA chest radiograph (**Fig. 8A**) demonstrates a subtle vertically oriented soft tissue opacity lateral to the aortic arch (arrow). Contrast-enhanced chest CT (mediastinal window) (**Figs. 8B, 8C,** and **8D**) demonstrates a persistent left superior vena cava (arrow) coursing vertically along the left superior mediastinum (**Fig. 8B**). The vessel continues caudally coursing posterior to the left atrial appendage (arrowhead) (**Fig. 8C**) and anterior to the left superior pulmonary vein (*) (**Fig. 8D**). Note the normal right superior vena cava (**Figs. 8B** and **8C**).

Diagnosis

Persistent left superior vena cava

Differential Diagnosis

None

Discussion

Background

A persistent left superior vena cava (PLSVC) is a relatively common anomaly and represents the most frequent form of anomalous venous return to the heart. It occurs in approximately 0.3% of the general population, with an increased prevalence (4.4%) in patients with congenital heart disease.

Etiology

The embryonic sinus venosus has right and left horns that receive blood from three major venous structures—the vitelline, umbilical, and common cardinal veins—during the fourth week of embryonic development. The anterior cardinal veins are paired structures that drain the upper body, whereas the posterior cardinal veins drain the lower body. The left anterior cardinal vein normally joins the right anterior cardinal vein and forms the left brachiocephalic vein. The caudal portion of the right anterior cardinal vein forms the superior vena cava. The proximal left horn of the sinus venosus gives rise to the coronary sinus. The left anterior cardinal vein caudal to the brachiocephalic vein normally involutes, but its distal aspect persists as the so-called ligament or oblique vein of Marshall. Failure of involution of the left anterior cardinal vein results in PLSVC (**Fig. 8E**). In most cases (82%), a patent right superior vena cava coexists with PLSVC (**Fig. 8E**). Rarely, obliteration of the right anterior cardinal vein results in absence or atresia of the right superior vena cava.

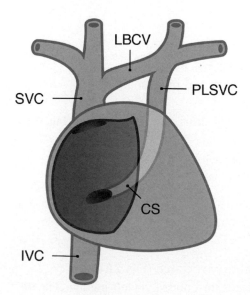

Figure 8E The course of the persistent left superior vena cava (PLSVC), which arises at the anastomosis of the left jugular and subclavian veins. Note that in the majority of cases the PLSVC drains into the right atrium via the coronary sinus (CS). A normal right superior vena cava (SVC) and a normal or atretic left brachiocephalic vein (LBCV) are typically found in association with a PLSVC.

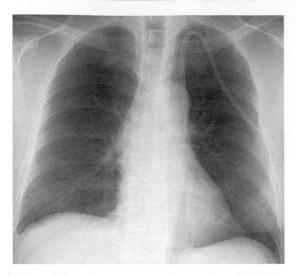

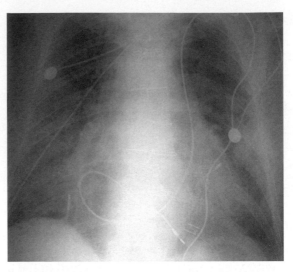

Figure 8F PA chest radiograph of a 67-year-old man with chronic renal failure demonstrates a dialysis catheter placed via left internal jugular vein approach with its tip in a PLSVC.

Figure 8G AP portable chest radiograph of an elderly man status–post median sternotomy and placement of a pacemaker lead via left subclavian vein approach shows the lead coursing from the left subclavian vein into a persistent left superior vena cava. The lead then enters the coronary sinus, the right atrium and finally reaches the right ventricle.

Clinical Findings

Affected patients are typically asymptomatic adults. The diagnosis is often made incidentally in patients who undergo central venous catheterization (**Fig. 8F**) or pacemaker placement/cardioverter defibrillator implantation when access to the heart is attempted via a left jugular/subclavian venous approach (**Fig. 8G**). PLSVC is associated with abnormal cardiac impulse formation and/or conduction related to abnormal development of the sinus node, the atrioventricular node and His bundle. Affected patients may be predisposed to arrhythmias and sudden death. Patients with PLSVC may have associated congenital heart disease, including abnormal atrioventricular connections, situs ambiguous, anomalous pulmonary venous return, Ebstein anomaly, common atrioventricular valves, tetralogy of Fallot, subaortic stenosis, and atrial and ventricular septal defects.

Pathology

- Left subclavian and jugular veins form left superior vena cava (**Fig. 8E**)
- Left superior vena cava descends vertically lateral to aortic arch and pulmonary artery
- Left superior vena cava receives hemiazygos vein
- Left superior vena cava typically (92%) drains into the coronary sinus and right atrium (**Fig. 8E**); may infrequently drain into the left atrium
- Normal (82%) (**Fig. 8E**), atretic or absent right superior vena cava
- Normal caliber (**Fig. 8E**), atretic or absent left brachiocephalic vein

Imaging Findings

RADIOGRAPHY

- Vertical left superior mediastinal soft tissue opacity lateral to aortic arch (**Fig. 8A**)
- Abnormal course of venous catheters and/or cardiac pacer leads introduced via left jugular (**Fig. 8F**) or subclavian (**Fig. 8G**) vein approach; vertical left paramediastinal catheter course (**Figs. 8F** and **8G**); continued course into the coronary sinus to enter the right heart (**Fig. 8G**)

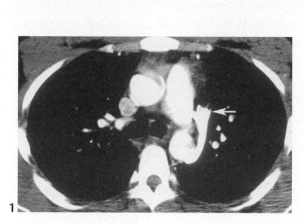 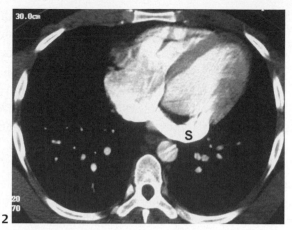

Figure 8H (1,2) Contrast-enhanced chest CT (mediastinal window) **(1,2)** of an asymptomatic 31-year-old man with persistent left superior vena cava (arrow) demonstrates communication between the PLSVC and the hemiazygos vein **(1)**. The PLSVC drains into an enlarged coronary sinus (S) **(2)**. (Courtesy of Maysiang Lesar, M.D., National Naval Medical Center, Bethesda, Maryland.)

CT/MR

- Left superior vena cava; course along left superior mediastinum lateral to aortic arch and pulmonary artery (**Fig. 8B**)
- Continued course posterior to left atrial appendage (**Fig. 8C**), anterior to left superior pulmonary vein (**Fig. 8D**)
- Drainage into the coronary sinus, which may be enlarged (**Fig. 8H2**)
- Identification and evaluation of coexistent right superior vena cava (**Figs. 8B, 8C,** and **8H1**)

ANGIOGRAPHY

- Venography for demonstration of existence and course of left superior vena cava
- Identification and evaluation of coexistent right superior vena cava

Treatment

- None

Prognosis

- Excellent (in the absence of associated anomalies)

PEARLS_____

- The recognition of PLSVC is important in patients undergoing placement of central venous lines (**Fig. 8F**), pacemaker electrodes, and cardioverter-defibrillator leads (**Fig. 8G**), as special techniques may have to be employed. In affected patients undergoing open-heart surgery, special techniques must be used to avoid flooding of the cardiac chambers by systemic blood entering through the coronary sinus. Surgical ligation of the LSVC may result in venous engorgement of the head and upper extremities in patients without a venous connection between the right and left superior vena cavae or absence of the right superior vena cava.

- PLSVC may be associated with atresia of the coronary sinus ostium without a left atrial connection, which results in retrograde flow of cardiac blood into the PLSVC. In these cases, surgical ligation of the PLSVC may result in myocardial ischemia and infarction.
- PLSVC may be associated with coronary sinus–left atrium fenestration (unroofing) with resultant right-to-left shunt or interatrial communication (coronary sinus atrial septal defect) at the mouth of the coronary sinus (see Case 14). In these cases the PLSVC drains into the left atrium and is associated with congenital cardiac malformations.

Suggested Readings

Amplatz K, Moller JH. Abnormalities of the venae cavae. In: Amplatz K, Moller JH, eds. Radiology of Congenital Heart Disease. St Louis: Mosby, 1993:1051–1060

Biffi M, Boriani G, Frabetti L, Bronzetti G, Branzi A. Left superior vena cava persistence in patients undergoing pacemaker or cardioverter-defibrillator implantation: a 10-year experience. Chest 2001;120:139–144

Jha NK, Gogna A, Tan TH, Wong KY, Shankar S. Atresia of coronary sinus ostium with retrograde drainage via persistent left superior vena cava. Ann Thorac Surg 2003;76:2091–2092

Miraldi F, di Gioia CRT, Proietti P, De Santis M, d'Amati G, Gallo P. Cardinal vein isomerism. An embryological hypothesis to explain a persistent left superior vena cava draining into the roof of the left atrium in the absence of coronary sinus and atrial septal defect. Cardiovasc Pathol 2002;11:149–152

Sarodia BD, Stoller JK. Persistent left superior vena cava: case report and literature review. Respir Care 2000;45:411–416

CASE 9 Arteriovenous Malformation

Clinical Presentation

A 22-year-old woman with postpartum dyspnea and hypoxemia

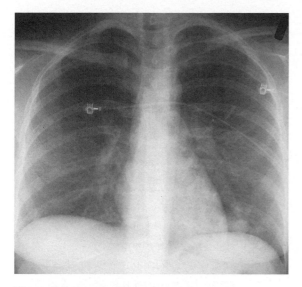

Figure 9A

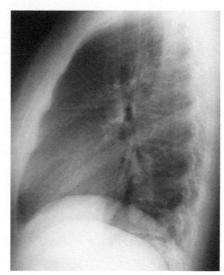

Figure 9B

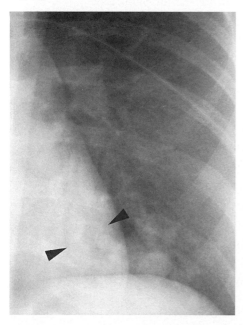

Figure 9C

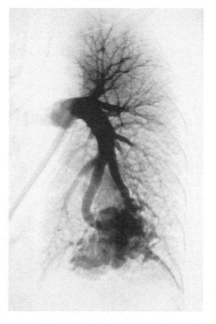

Figure 9D

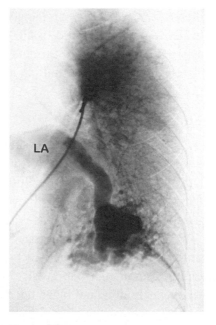

Figure 9E

(Figs. 9A, 9B, 9C, 9D, and 9E courtesy of Wanda M. Kirejczyk, M.D., New Britain General Hospital, New Britain, Connecticut.)

Radiologic Findings

PA (**Fig. 9A**) and lateral (**Fig. 9B**) chest radiographs demonstrate a left lower lobe mass of lobular contours. Coned-down PA chest radiograph (**Fig. 9C**) demonstrates tubular opacities (arrowheads) coursing between the mass and the left hilum. Left pulmonary arteriogram (**Figs. 9D** and **9E**) demonstrates a pulmonary arteriovenous malformation supplied by two branches of the left interlobar pulmonary artery (**Fig. 9D**) and drained into the left atrium (LA) via an enlarged pulmonary vein (**Fig. 9E**).

Diagnosis

Arteriovenous malformation

Differential Diagnosis

None

Discussion

Background

A pulmonary arteriovenous malformation (PAVM) is an abnormal communication between a pulmonary artery and a pulmonary vein without an intervening capillary bed and results in a right-to-left shunt.

Etiology

Arteriovenous malformations (AVMs) are thought to arise from congenital defects in the capillary bed, which result in a direct communication between the pulmonary arterial and venous circulations. Acquired arteriovenous communications also occur, usually result from trauma (noniatrogenic or iatrogenic) or inflammation, and are designated arteriovenous fistulae. Osler-Weber-Rendu syndrome or hereditary hemorrhagic telangiectasia (HHT) is an autosomal-dominant disorder with an estimated prevalence of one in 2000 to 40,000 persons. Approximately 60 to 90% of PAVM occur in patients with HHT, up to 35% of patients with HHT have one or more PAVM, and 60% of patients with HTT-related PAVM have multiple lesions.

Clinical Findings

Over 50% of patients with PAVM are asymptomatic. Symptomatic patients are usually adults between the fourth and sixth decades of life. Symptoms include fatigue and exertional dyspnea (which may relate to high-output heart failure) and neurologic complaints or fever from paradoxical emboli. Affected patients may develop myocardial infarction and mesenteric, renal, or limb ischemia. Stroke occurs in up to 40% of patients with PAVM, brain abscess in 20%, and hemoptysis and/or hemothorax in 10%. Affected patients may have a family history of PAVM or HHT and may exhibit digital clubbing, cyanosis, and mucosal telangiectasias. Approximately 40 to 60% of these patients have additional arteriovenous malformations in the skin and mucus membranes and may present with epistaxis, chronic gastrointestinal bleeding, and/or hematuria.

Pathology

GROSS

- Thin-walled dilated nonseptated vascular sac supplied by dilated and tortuous pulmonary artery or arteries and drained by pulmonary vein or veins
- Typical location in the lung periphery
- Majority (90%) are simple PAVM supplied by a single artery and drained by a single vein; complex (10%) lesions are supplied by two or more segmental arteries.
- Variable size ranging from less than 1 cm to several centimeters in diameter
- Approximately 33% are multiple; 20% are bilateral.

MICROSCOPIC

- Thin-walled, endothelial-lined blood-containing space within architecturally normal lung
- Alveolar hemorrhage in cases of PAVM rupture

Imaging Findings

RADIOGRAPHY

- Lobular, well-defined noncalcified nodule(s) and/or mass(es) (**Figs. 9A, 9B,** and **9C**)
- Typically located in peripheral lower lobe; often project below the dome of the diaphragm (**Figs. 9A** and **9C**)
- Associated tortuous tubular opacities coursing to and from hilum representing feeding and draining vessels (**Fig. 9C**)
- Rarely multiple pulmonary nodules/masses

CT

- Demonstration of PAVM and feeding and draining vessels (**Figs. 9F1, 9F2, 9G,** and **9I**)
- Evaluation of origin, number, length, and diameter of feeding vessels and internal structure of vascular sac (**Figs. 9F1, 9F2, 9G,** and **9I**)
- Rapid contrast enhancement and washout (**Figs. 9F1** and **9F2**)
- Unenhanced or enhanced 3D helical or multidetector CT for screening, characterization, and quantification of PAVM (**Figs. 9G** and **9I**)

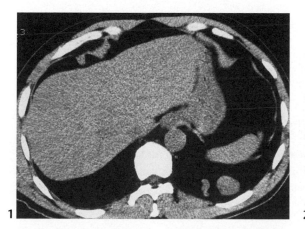
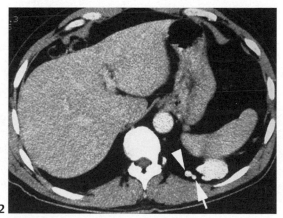

Figure 9F (1,2) Unenhanced **(1)** and contrast-enhanced **(2)** chest CT (mediastinal window) of a man with an asymptomatic left lower lobe simple PAVM demonstrates intense enhancement of the lesion and allows identification of the feeding artery (arrow) and draining vein (arrowhead).

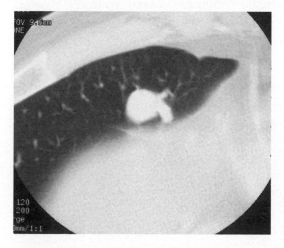

Figure 9G Unenhanced chest CT (lung window) of a 41-year-old woman with an incidentally discovered right middle lobe pulmonary nodule demonstrates a simple PAVM and allows visualization of its feeding and draining vessels. The smaller feeding artery enters the lesion anteriorly, and the larger draining vein is seen posteriorly. (Courtesy of William R. Corse, D.O., Parlee and Tatem Radiology Associates, Doylestown, Pennsylvania.)

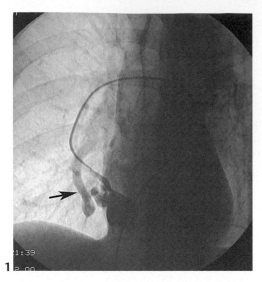 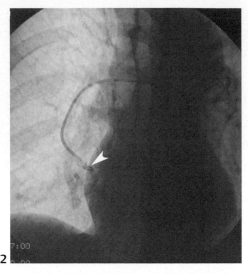

Figure 9H (1,2) Subtraction image from a pulmonary arteriogram **(1)** of a 47-year-old man who developed a left temporoparietal brain abscess secondary to a right middle lobe PAVM demonstrates selective injection of the feeding pulmonary artery and visualization of the tortuous draining vein (arrow). Frontal coned-down subtraction image from an embolotherapy procedure **(2)** demonstrates the pulmonary artery catheter within the feeding artery immediately after deployment of embolotherapy coils (arrowhead), which completely obliterated flow through the PAVM.

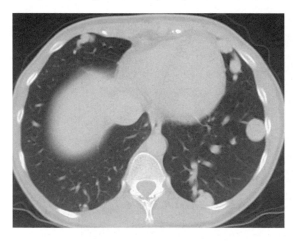

Figure 9I Chest CT (lung window) of a 32-year-old woman with HHT demonstrates at least five PAVM of various sizes affecting every visible lung lobe. The PAVMs manifest as peripheral juxtapleural pulmonary nodules with associated tubular opacities that represent the feeding pulmonary arteries and draining pulmonary veins.

MR

- Low signal flow-void in PAVM; low-to-intermediate signal in PAVM with internal thrombus
- Three-dimensional contrast-enhanced MR angiography for noninvasive diagnosis of PAVM larger than 5 mm; high-signal intensity nodule and associated vessels
- Evaluation of size and number of feeding vessels prior to embolotherapy

ANGIOGRAPHY

- Opacification of feeding vessels and draining veins (**Figs. 9D, 9E, and 9H1**)
- Confirmation of diagnosis, documentation of multiple lesions, and evaluation of origin, number, length, and diameter of the feeding vessels (**Figs. 9D and 9H1**), for coil embolization therapy planning (**Fig. 9H2**)

OTHER MODALITIES

- Contrast-enhanced two-dimensional echocardiography for screening (90% sensitivity for detection of intrapulmonary shunts)
- Lung perfusion scintigraphy for determination of shunt size

Treatment

- Embolotherapy with detachable coils (occasionally detachable balloons) for improvement of oxygenation and prevention of neurologic complications (**Fig. 9H2**)

Prognosis

- Guarded
- Significant morbidity and reported mortality rate of 10% for patients with HHT
- Complications of embolotherapy: paradoxical emboli, air emboli, transient ischemic attacks, angina, bradycardia, hypotension, and chest pain
- Complete obliteration of right-to-left shunt achieved in less than half of treated patients

PEARLS_____

- Patients with suspected HHT may undergo screening with arterial blood gas evaluation in room air and with 100% oxygen. Affected patients typically exhibit a 1 to 2% drop in O_2 saturation after standing and a further 8% drop in O_2 saturation after exercise. These findings are supplemented by imaging for definitive diagnosis.
- AVMs in patients with HHT typically affect the lungs, brain, nose, and gastrointestinal system (including the liver).
- PAVMs with feeding vessels larger than 3 mm in diameter are traditionally treated with embolotherapy (**Fig. 9H2**). However, a significant number of patients with smaller lesions suffer from clinically occult stroke. Thus, embolotherapy is often performed on all PAVMs that can be super-selectively cannulated. Embolotherapy catheters are ideally placed distal to branches supplying normal lung and as close as possible to the neck of the PAVM (**Fig. 9H2**). Recurrence from enlargement of a secondary feeding vessel missed during initial embolotherapy is reported.

Suggested Readings

Coley SC, Jackson JE. Pulmonary arteriovenous malformations. Clin Radiol 1998;53:396–404

Maki DD, Siegelman ES, Roberts DA, Baum RA, Gefter WB. Pulmonary arteriovenous malformations: three-dimensional gadolinium-enhanced MR angiography—initial experience. Radiology 2001;219: 243–246

Pugash RA. Pulmonary arteriovenous malformations: overview and transcatheter embolotherapy. Can Assoc Radiol J 2001;52:92–102

CASE 10 Partial Anomalous Pulmonary Venous Return

Clinical Presentation

A 36-year-old woman with cough and fever

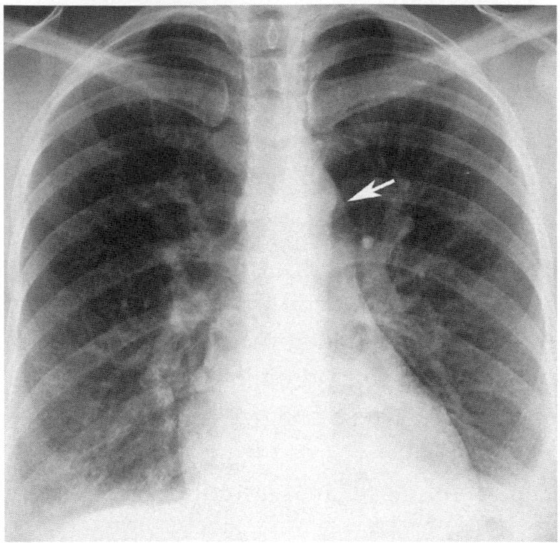

Figure 10A

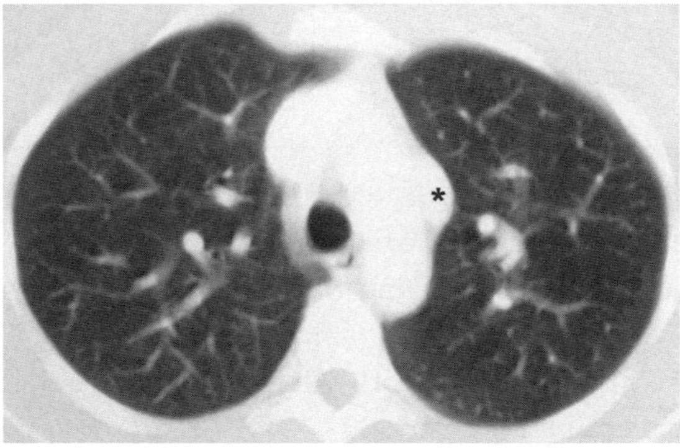

Figure 10B

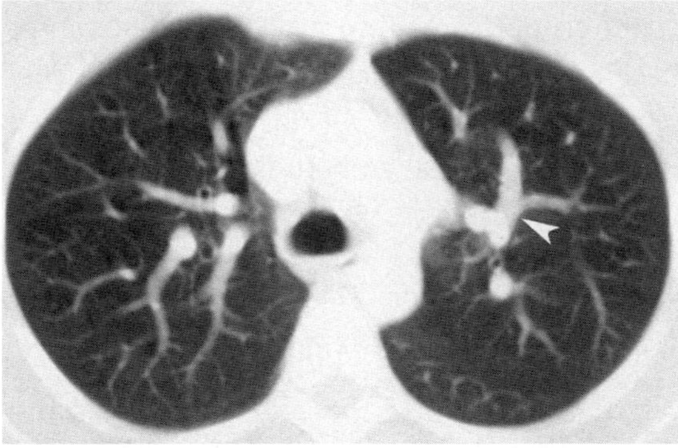

Figure 10C

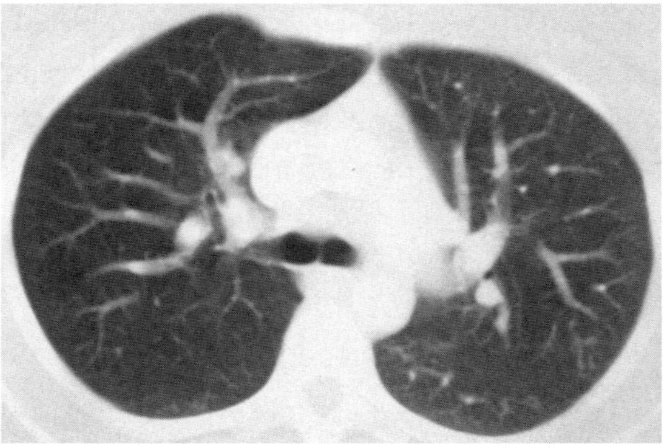

Figure 10D

(Figs. 10A, 10B, 10C, and 10D courtesy of Maysiang Lesar, M.D., National Naval Medical Center, Bethesda, M.D.)

Radiologic Findings

PA chest radiograph (**Fig. 10A**) demonstrates bibasilar parenchymal consolidations, a left pleural effusion, and an abnormal contour of the left superior mediastinum (arrow). Contrast-enhanced chest CT (lung window) (**Figs. 10B, 10C,** and **10D**) demonstrates an anomalous pulmonary vein (arrowhead) (**Fig. 10C**) coursing medially toward the mediastinum to anastomose with a vertical vein (*) (**Fig. 10B**), which drains into the left brachiocephalic vein. The vertical vein (*) (**Fig. 10B**) is responsible for the abnormal mediastinal contour.

Diagnosis

Partial anomalous pulmonary venous return, left upper lobe

Differential Diagnosis

Persistent left superior vena cava

Discussion

Background

Anomalous pulmonary venous connections are congenital anomalies in which one or more pulmonary veins drain into the right-sided circulation with a resultant left-to-right shunt. These anomalous connections may be total (the entire pulmonary venous return) or partial. Partial anomalous pulmonary venous connections may affect left or right pulmonary veins and are reported in up to 0.7% of autopsies and in approximately 0.2% of adults studied with CT.

Etiology

The primitive pulmonary veins begin to drain into the heart early in embryogenesis by joining the pulmonary portion of the splanchnic plexus. Partial anomalous pulmonary venous return is thought to result from premature atresia of the right or left primitive pulmonary veins while there are still primitive pulmonary-systemic connections.

Pathology

- Right-sided partial anomalous pulmonary venous return to the vena cava, right atrium, azygos vein, coronary sinus, or portal vein
- Left-sided partial anomalous pulmonary venous return to an anomalous vertical vein that drains into the left brachiocephalic vein

Clinical Findings

Patients with partial anomalous pulmonary venous return and a significant left-to-right shunt present with symptoms. Symptomatic patients are typically male children and young adults in whom the anomalous venous return is right-sided. Up to 90% of these patients have an associated sinus venosus or ostium secundum atrial septal defect (see Case 14). These patients may present with fatigue, exertional dyspnea, and heart failure. Asymptomatic patients are usually women without known atrial septal defect who exhibit a left-sided anomalous vein. These patients are often diagnosed incidentally with CT.

Imaging Findings

RADIOGRAPHY

- Abnormal left superior mediastinal contour (**Fig. 10A**)
- Abnormal or anomalous course of pulmonary veins

CT/MR

- Demonstration of anomalous pulmonary veins (**Figs. 10C** and **10D**)
- Demonstration of anomalous vascular connections
  - Dilated left brachiocephalic vein (**Fig. 10E1**)
  - Left upper lobe anomalous pulmonary vein drainage into a vertical vein (**Figs. 10B, 10D,** and **10E2**), which drains into a dilated left brachiocephalic vein (**Fig. 10E1**)

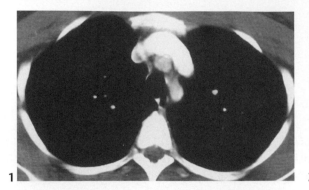

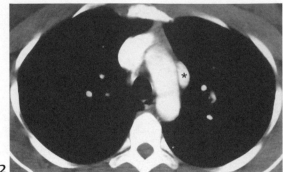

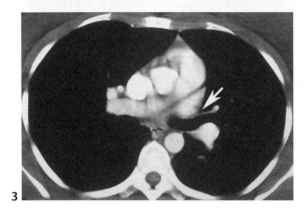

Figure 10E (1,2,3) Contrast-enhanced chest CT (mediastinal window) **(1,2,3)** of the same patient illustrated in **Figures 10A, 10B, 10C,** and **10D** demonstrates the anastomosis of the anomalous vertical vein (*) **(2)** with a mildly enlarged left brachiocephalic vein **(1)**. Note the absence of the left superior pulmonary vein in its expected normal location (arrow) **(3)**. (Courtesy of Maysiang Lesar, M.D., National Naval Medical Center, Bethesda, Maryland.)

- Absence of left upper lobe pulmonary vein from its normal location anterior to the left mainstem bronchus (**Fig. 10E3**)
- Right upper lobe anomalous pulmonary venous drainage into the vena cava, azygos vein, or right atrium; may exhibit absence of right upper lobe pulmonary vein in its normal location

Treatment

- Surgical repair of partial anomalous venous connection when ratio of pulmonary-to-systemic shunt exceeds 1.5:1
- Surgical repair of associated anomalies such as atrial septal defect

Prognosis

- Excellent in patients without associated anomalies
- Dependent on severity and number of associated conditions in patients with congenital heart disease

Suggested Reading

Haramati LB, Moche IE, Rivera VT, et al. Computed tomography of partial anomalous pulmonary venous connection in adults. J Comput Assist Tomogr 2003;27:743–749

CASE 11 Scimitar Syndrome

Clinical Presentation

Asymptomatic 29-year-old woman

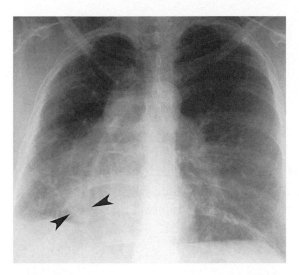

Figure 11A

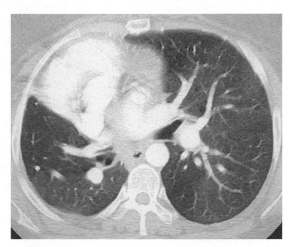

Figure 11B

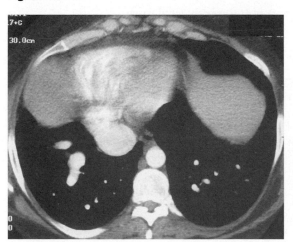

Figure 11C

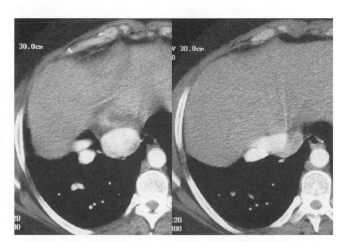

Figure 11D

Radiologic Findings

PA (**Fig. 11A**) chest radiograph demonstrates a small right lung with a hyparterial bronchus, ipsilateral mediastinal shift, and arcuate tubular opacities that course toward the right cardiophrenic angle (arrowheads). Contrast-enhanced chest CT (lung window) (**Fig. 11B**) demonstrates the small volume of the bilobed right lung. Contrast-enhanced chest CT (mediastinal window) (**Figs. 11C** and **11D**) demonstrates paired anomalous pulmonary veins (**Fig. 11C**) that drain into the inferior vena cava (**Fig. 11D**).

79

Diagnosis

Scimitar syndrome; congenital pulmonary venolobar syndrome

Differential Diagnosis

- Arteriovenous malformation
- Pulmonary varix
- Intralobar sequestration
- Mucoid impaction; bronchial atresia

Discussion

Background

Scimitar syndrome is a complex disorder also known as congenital pulmonary venolobar syndrome and hypogenetic lung syndrome. It characteristically affects the right lung and manifests with a variety of cardiopulmonary anomalies. The term *scimitar* refers to the arcuate course followed by the anomalous pulmonary vein, which resembles the shape of a scimitar (a Turkish sword).

Etiology

Scimitar syndrome is a rare congenital anomaly of the right lung and pulmonary vasculature.

Pathology

- Hypogenetic right lung with errors in segmentation/bronchial branching/lobation (lobar agenesis, aplasia or hypoplasia)
- Anomalous pulmonary venous return affecting all or part of the right lung; single or multiple anomalous veins drain into inferior vena cava, hepatic or portal circulation, azygos vein, coronary sinus, or right atrium
- Additional findings:
  - Right pulmonary artery aplasia or hypoplasia
  - Systemic blood supply to the right lung
  - Absence or interruption of the inferior vena cava
  - Anomalous superior vena cava
  - Duplication, eventration, or partial absence of right hemidiaphragm
  - Tracheal trifurcation
  - Esophageal and/or gastric communication with the lung; horseshoe lung

Clinical Findings

Patients with scimitar syndrome may be diagnosed as infants or neonates because of associated symptomatic congenital cardiovascular disease (seen in approximately 25 to 50% of affected patients). Associated congenital cardiac anomalies may include ostium secundum atrial septal defect, ventricular septal defect, patent ductus arteriosus, tetralogy of Fallot, coarctation of the aorta, hypoplastic left heart, double-outlet right ventricle, double-chambered right ventricle, and endocardial cushion defect. Affected patients may also exhibit pulmonary arterial hypertension. Patients with significant left-to-right shunts (typically 2:1 or greater) may present with fatigue and dyspnea. Patients with scimitar syndrome may also present with hemoptysis and/or recurrent pulmonary infection.

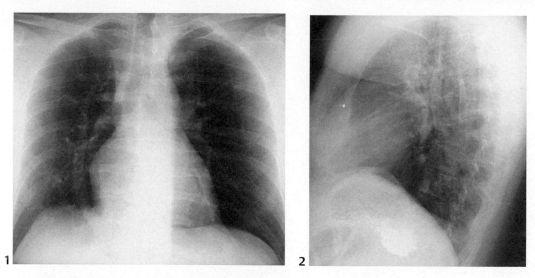

Figure 11E (1,2) PA **(1)** and lateral **(2)** chest radiographs of an asymptomatic 22-year-old man demonstrate the scimitar sign in association with mild right pulmonary hypoplasia. Note the retrosternal soft tissue opacity produced by the interface between the hypoplastic right lung and the dextroposed portion of heart **(2)**.

Approximately 50% of affected patients are entirely asymptomatic and are diagnosed incidentally because of an abnormal chest radiograph. Pulmonary artery pressures are normal or slightly elevated in the majority of patients who present as adults. Women are slightly more commonly affected with a female-to-male ratio of 1.4:1.

Imaging Findings

RADIOGRAPHY

- Small right lung and hemithorax (**Figs. 11A** and **11E**), mediastinal shift to the right (dextroposition of the heart) (**Fig. 11A**), indistinct right cardiac border (**Fig. 11A**); increased right lung opacity (**Fig. 11A**); apical pleural cap (**Fig. 11A**)
- Blunt costophrenic angle (**Fig. 11A**)
- Vertically oriented curved tubular opacity (anomalous draining vein) in right inferior hemithorax coursing toward right cardiophrenic angle (**Figs. 11A** and **11E1**); may be obscured by the heart in cases with pronounced cardiac dextroposition (**Fig. 11A**)
- Diminished right pulmonary vascularity (**Figs. 11A** and **11E**)
- Broad retrosternal band-like opacity (**Fig. 11E2**)

CT/MR

- Small right lung; mediastinal shift to the right (**Fig. 11B**)
- Optimal visualization of anomalous vessel (variable size and number), its course and drainage into inferior vena cava (**Figs. 11C, 11D,** and **11F**), right atrium, coronary sinus, or hepatic circulation
- Evaluation/identification of other components of the syndrome (**Fig. 11F2**)
- Noninvasive assessment of left-to-right shunt with velocity-encoded cine MR

Treatment

- None for asymptomatic patients without associated anomalies
- Surgical correction for symptomatic patients with significant shunts (ligation, coil embolization)

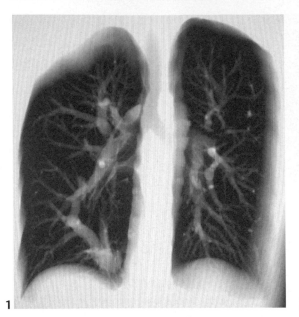
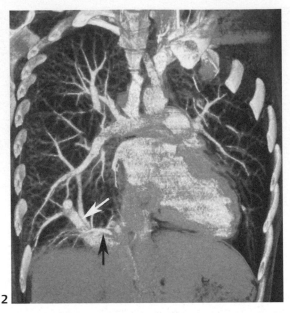

Figure 11F (1,2) Contrast-enhanced chest CT maximum intensity projection coronal image **(1)** and volume-rendered coronal image **(2)** of an asymptomatic 19-year-old man with chest pain and scimitar syndrome demonstrate the course of the anomalous vein (white arrow) **(1,2)**. Note the systemic arterial supply to the right lower lobe (black arrow) that arose from the celiac axis **(2)**. Note that in this case the right bronchi exhibit eparterial morphology **(1)**.

- Lung resection for patients with recurrent hemoptysis and/or pulmonary infection
- Correction of significant associated congenital cardiovascular disease

Prognosis

- Excellent in the absence of associated anomalies
- Relates to presence or absence of associated congenital heart disease and its severity

PEARLS_____

- The most frequent anomalies in patients with congenital pulmonary venolobar (scimitar) syndrome are hypogenetic lung and partial anomalous pulmonary venous return.
- The radiographic visualization of the anomalous pulmonary vein with its typical curved configuration is known as the scimitar sign (**Figs. 11A** and **11E1**).
- Partial anomalous pulmonary venous return occurs in up to 0.7% of patients with congenital heart disease. It is most commonly associated with atrial septal defect (see Cases 10 and 14). Atrial septal defect occurs in approximately 90% of patients with partial anomalous pulmonary venous return to the superior vena cava or right atrium (see Case 10), and in only 15% of patients with anomalous drainage to the inferior vena cava.
- Some investigators classify cases of scimitar syndrome with abnormal bronchial communications and systemic blood supply to the affected lung as variants of intralobar sequestration. There are also reports of congenital venolobar syndrome in association with extralobar sequestration. In some cases of scimitar syndrome there is systemic blood supply to the hypogenetic lung without other typical features of pulmonary sequestration (**Fig. 11F2**).

Suggested Readings

Cirillo RL Jr. The scimitar sign. Radiology 1998;206:623–624

Gilkeson RC, Basile V, Sands MJ, Hsu JT. Chest case of the day. Scimitar syndrome. AJR Am J Roentgenol 1997;169:267, 270–273

Henk CB, Prokesch R, Grampp S, Strasser G, Mostbeck GH. Scimitar syndrome: MR assessment of hemodynamic significance. J Comput Assist Tomogr 1997;21:628–630

Mulligan ME. History of scimitar syndrome. Radiology 1999;210:288–290

Woodring JH, Howard TA, Kanga JF. Congenital pulmonary venolobar syndrome revisited. Radiographics 1994;14:349–369

CASE 12 Pulmonary Varix

Clinical Presentation

A 65-year-old woman with chest pain

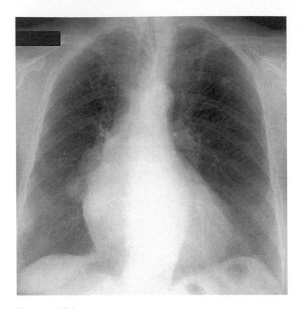

Figure 12A

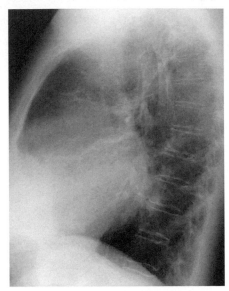

Figure 12B

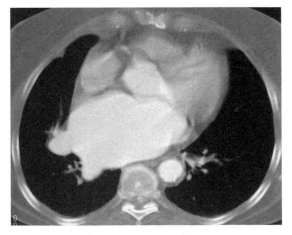

Figure 12C

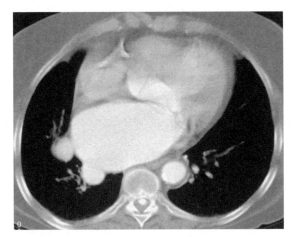

Figure 12D

Radiologic Findings

PA (**Fig. 12A**) and lateral (**Fig. 12B**) chest radiographs demonstrate cardiomegaly, a multilobular soft tissue mass that projects over the right hilum (**Fig. 12A**), and focal enlargement of the superior aspect of the left atrium (**Fig. 12B**). Nodular upper lobe parenchymal opacities relate to remote granulomatous infection. Contrast-enhanced chest CT (mediastinal window) (**Figs. 12C** and **12D**) shows that the lobular opacities seen on radiography correspond to focal dilatation of the pulmonary veins as they enter an enlarged left atrium.

Diagnosis

Pulmonary varix

Differential Diagnosis

None

Discussion

Background

Pulmonary varix is a rare lesion characterized by focal nonobstructive aneurysmal enlargement of one or more pulmonary veins prior to entering the left atrium.

Etiology

Both acquired and congenital etiologies of pulmonary varix have been proposed. Pulmonary varix is typically associated with mitral valve dysfunction, usually insufficiency. In these cases, the right pulmonary veins are typically affected.

Pathology

- Dilatation and tortuosity of one or more pulmonary veins
- Normal anatomic structure

Clinical Findings

Affected patients are often asymptomatic and are diagnosed incidentally because of a radiographic abnormality. Some patients present with symptoms related to mitral valve disease. Hemoptysis and chronic lobar collapse are also reported. Rarely, patients present with systemic embolization of endoluminal thrombus.

Imaging Findings

RADIOGRAPHY

- Single or multiple rounded or ovoid lobular mass(es) or nodule(s) (**Fig. 12A**) projecting over the medial lower lobe; may only be visible on one radiographic projection (PA or lateral) (**Fig. 12A**)
- Round mass or nodule related to the left atrium on lateral radiography (**Fig. 12B**)
- May enlarge with onset of pulmonary venous hypertension
- Cardiomegaly; left atrial enlargement (**Figs. 12A** and **12B**)

CT/MR

- Demonstration of vascular nature of the nodules or masses seen on radiography (**Figs. 12C** and **12D**)
- Demonstration of communication with the left atrium (**Figs. 12C** and **12D**)
- Both prompt (**Figs. 12C** and **12D**) and delayed vascular enhancement reported
- Left atrial enlargement related to mitral insufficiency (**Figs. 12C** and **12D**)

Treatment

- None in asymptomatic patients
- Management of mitral valve dysfunction in symptomatic patients

Prognosis

- Good
- One death reported from associated hemoptysis

PEARLS

- Pulmonary varix typically affects the right inferior pulmonary and/or the lingular vein.
- Pulmonary varix is also known as hilar pseudotumor. Imaging abnormalities typically relate to enlargement of the right venous confluence.

Suggested Readings

Cole TJ, Henry DA, Jolles H, Proto AV. Normal and abnormal vascular structures that simulate neoplasms on chest radiographs: clues to the diagnosis. Radiographics 1995;15:867–891

Fraser RS, Müller NL, Colman N, Paré PD. Developmental anomalies affecting the pulmonary vessels. In: Fraser RS, Müller NL, Colman N, Paré PD, eds. Fraser and Paré's Diagnosis of Diseases of the Chest, 4th ed. Philadelphia: WB Saunders, 1999:637–675

Gaeta M, Volta S, Vallone A. Hilar pseudonodule due to varix of the inferior pulmonary vein. AJR Am J Roentgenol 1995;165:1305

CASE 13 Heterotaxy Syndrome

Clinical Presentation

A 68-year-old woman admitted for pacemaker placement

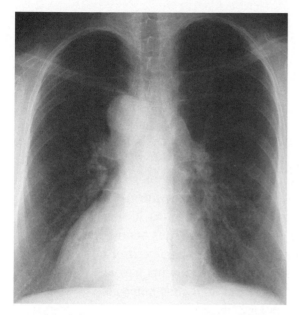

Figure 13A

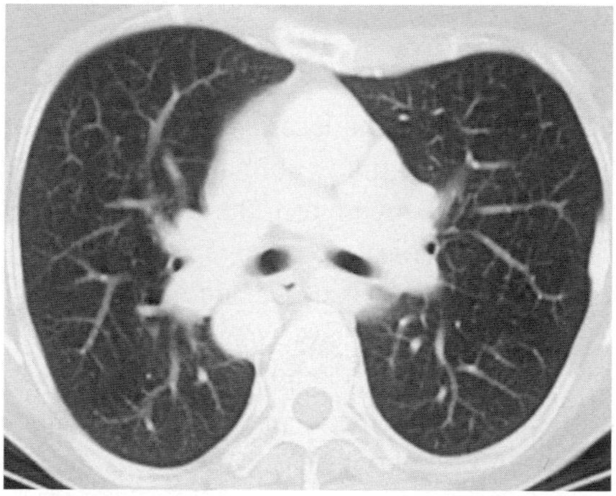

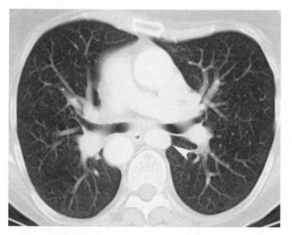

Figure 13B

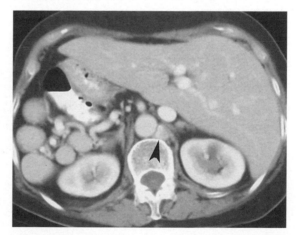

Figure 13C

Figure 13D

Radiologic Findings

PA chest radiograph (**Fig. 13A**) demonstrates dextrocardia, a right aortic arch, and bilateral hyparterial bronchi. Contrast-enhanced chest CT (lung window) (**Figs. 13B** and **13C**) demonstrates bilateral hyparterial bronchi and an enlarged hemiazygos vein (arrowhead) (**Fig. 13C**) consistent with hemiazygos continuation of the inferior vena cava. Contrast-enhanced abdominal CT (soft tissue window) (**Fig. 13D**) demonstrates a left-sided liver, a right-sided stomach, and multiple right-sided spleens (polysplenia). Note the enlarged hemiazygos vein (arrowhead) (**Fig. 13C**).

Diagnosis

Heterotaxy syndrome: dextrocardia, polysplenia, hemiazygos continuation of the inferior vena cava

Differential Diagnosis

None

Discussion

Background

Situs (location, position) refers to the location of the viscera and atria with respect to the midline. The majority of the population exhibits normal visceroatrial situs (situs solitus) characterized by a morphologic right (systemic) atrium on the right side and a contralateral morphologic left (pulmonary) atrium. The pulmonary anatomy is characterized by a trilobed right lung with ipsilateral liver, gallbladder, and inferior vena cava and a bilobed left lung with ipsilateral stomach, single spleen, and aortic arch. The incidence of congenital heart disease in patients with situs solitus is approximately 0.8%. Approximately 0.1% of the population exhibits situs inversus characterized by mirror-image location of the atria, major vessels, and abdominal structures. These patients have a 3 to 5% incidence of congenital heart disease. The terms *heterotaxy, isomerism,* and *situs ambiguous* refer to absence of an orderly arrangement of viscera and atrial morphology (in one or the other side of the body). Patients with heterotaxy or situs ambiguous have a high incidence (50 to 100%) of congenital heart disease.

Etiology

The primitive heart and its vascular connections form early in embryogenesis (between 20 and 30 days of gestation). Alterations in development during this stage when there is incomplete septation of the cardiac chambers may result in the complex anatomic relationships observed in heterotaxy syndrome. Genetic studies suggest a multifactorial inheritance pattern for these anomalies.

Pathology

- Asplenia
  - Bilateral right-sidedness; bilateral trilobed lungs and eparterial (upper lobe bronchus superior to ipsilateral pulmonary artery) bronchi
  - Bilateral systemic atria
  - Absent spleen
  - Left inferior vena cava
- Polysplenia
  - Bilateral left-sidedness; bilateral bilobed lungs and hyparterial (upper lobe bronchus inferior to ipsilateral pulmonary artery) bronchi
  - Bilateral pulmonary atria
  - Multiple spleens
  - High incidence of azygos and/or hemiazygos continuation of the inferior vena cava, intrahepatic segment typically present

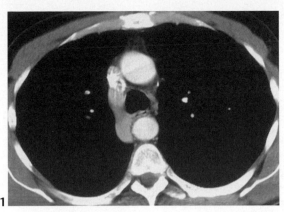 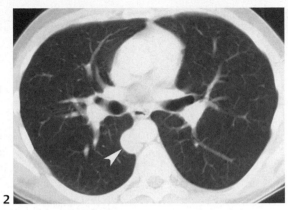

Figure 13E (1,2) Contrast-enhanced chest CT (mediastinal and lung window) **(1,2)** of an asymptomatic 35-year-old man with polysplenia evaluated for an incidentally discovered right paratracheal soft tissue mass demonstrates an enlarged azygos arch **(1)** and an enlarged azygos vein (arrowhead) **(2)** coursing along the right side of the descending aorta. Note bilateral symmetric hyparterial bronchi **(2)**.

- Asplenia and polysplenia
  - Variable laterality of the heart, aorta, major hepatic lobe, and stomach (and multiple spleens in polysplenia)
  - Intestinal malrotation
  - Bridging liver

Clinical Findings

Polysplenia more commonly affects females than males. Patients with polysplenia may be diagnosed as infants or neonates because of associated symptomatic (typically noncyanotic) congenital cardiovascular disease. However, congenital heart disease may manifest with milder cardiac defects such as partial anomalous pulmonary venous return, atrial septal defect, and atrioventricular canal. Symptomatic patients may present with heart failure. Approximately 10% of patients with polysplenia have mild or no congenital heart disease. These patients are asymptomatic and are diagnosed incidentally (**Figs. 13E** and **13F**). Patients with asplenia typically present with symptoms of cyanosis and severe respiratory distress from severe complex congenital heart disease, usually total anomalous pulmonary venous return, but also common atrioventricular canal and univentricular heart. They may also present with symptoms of immune deficiency related to absence of the spleen. Patients with heterotaxy may present in infancy because of volvulus with malrotation.

Imaging Findings

RADIOGRAPHY

- Bilateral hyparterial bronchi (**Fig. 13A**)
- Variable position of the heart (cardiac apex) (**Fig. 13A**), aortic arch (**Fig. 13A**), and stomach
- Soft tissue mass in azygos region from enlarged azygos arch (with associated azygos continuation of the inferior vena cava)

CT/MR

- Demonstration of bilateral hyparterial bronchial morphology (**Figs. 13B, 13C,** and **13E2**); bilateral bilobed lungs on CT
- Variable position of the heart

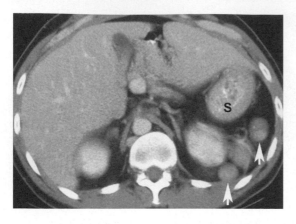

Figures 13F Contrast-enhanced abdominal CT (soft tissue window) of a 35-year-old man with polysplenia demonstrates a right-sided liver, a left-sided stomach (S), a midline gallbladder, and multiple spleens (arrows). Note the prominent (retrocrural) azygos vein.

- Multiple spleens or single multilobate spleen (**Figs. 13D** and **13F**)
- Variable positions of spleen(s), stomach, liver, and gallbladder (**Figs. 13D** and **13F**)
- Demonstration of azygos (**Figs. 13E2** and **13F**) or hemiazygos (**Figs. 13B, 13C,** and **13D**) continuation of the inferior vena cava; hepatic vein drainage into atrium
- Demonstration of atrial morphology through evaluation of atrial appendage morphology on MR; morphologic left atrial appendage with tubular shape and curved downward apex
- Evaluation of associated cardiac anomalies

Treatment

- None for asymptomatic patients
- Surgical correction of symptomatic or significant congenital heart disease and associated conditions

Prognosis

- Polysplenia: relates to severity and number of associated anomalies; excellent without associated anomalies; high mortality with associated biliary atresia
- Asplenia: poor; death in the first year of life in up to 80% of affected patients

PEARLS

- The morphology of the tracheobronchial tree is a reliable indicator of underlying atrial morphology. An eparterial bronchus exists when the main bronchus is superior to the ipsilateral pulmonary artery (see Case 11), and a hyparterial bronchus exists when the main bronchus is inferior to the ipsilateral pulmonary artery (see Case 5, **Fig. 5E,** Case 11, **Fig. 11A,** and Case 13, **Fig. 13A**). The morphologic right (systemic) atrium is usually ipsilateral to an eparterial bronchus, while the morphologic left (pulmonary) atrium is usually ipsilateral to a hyparterial bronchus.
- Determination of situs is the first step in the assessment of patients with complex congenital heart disease.

Suggested Readings

Applegate KE, Goske MJ, Pierce G, Murphy D. Situs revisited: imaging of the heterotaxy syndrome. Radiographics 1999;19:837–852

Hong YK, Park YW, Ryu SJ, et al. Efficacy of MRI in complicated congenital heart disease with visceral heterotaxy syndrome. J Comput Assist Tomogr 2000;24:671–682

CASE 14 Atrial Septal Defect

Clinical Presentation

A 35-year-old man evaluated for a murmur found on a routine physical examination

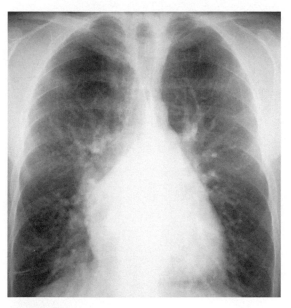

Figure 14A

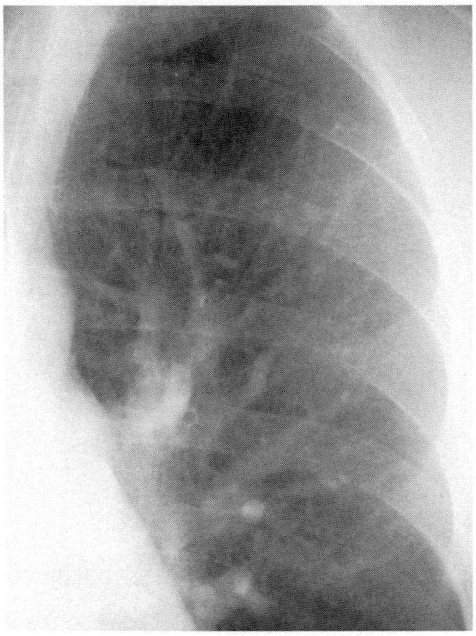

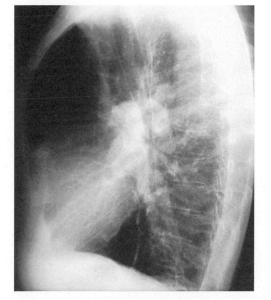

Figure 14B

Figure 14C

Radiologic Findings

PA (**Fig. 14A**), coned-down PA (**Fig. 14B**), and lateral (**Fig. 14C**) chest radiographs demonstrate cardiomegaly and overcirculation. Note the enlarged central and peripheral pulmonary arteries.

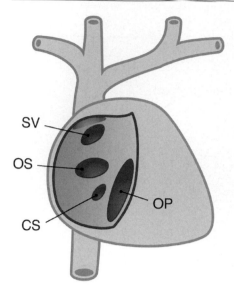

Figure 14D Illustration of the different types of ASD and their location within the atrial septum. The most common type is the ostium secundum (OS) ASD. Sinus venosus (SV) ASD occurs near the orifice of the superior vena cava, and ostium primum (OP) ASD occurs inferiorly. Coronary sinus (CS) ASD occurs near the ostium of the coronary sinus.

Diagnosis

Atrial septal defect

Differential Diagnosis

- Other left-to-right shunt; ventricular septal defect, patent ductus arteriosus
- Pulmonary arterial hypertension

Discussion

Background

Atrial septal defect (ASD) accounts for approximately 10% of congenital heart disease and is a common congenital cardiac lesion among those that initially manifest in adulthood. It represents approximately 30% of all congenital heart disease in patients over the age of 40 years. ASD may be an isolated condition or may be associated with other cardiovascular anomalies.

Etiology

Atrial septal defect represents a congenital defect in the interatrial septum that results in communication between the two atrial chambers.

Pathology

- Typically large defect; may measure up to 4 cm in diameter
- ASD classification based on anatomic location (**Fig. 14D**)
  - Ostium secundum (**Fig. 14D**)
    - Most common
    - Located at the fossa ovalis
    - Only true septal defect (completely surrounded by septal tissue)
  - Sinus venosus (**Fig. 14D**)
    - Located at superior atrial septum beneath superior vena cava orifice
    - Strong association with anomalous venous connection of the right superior pulmonary vein to the superior vena cava

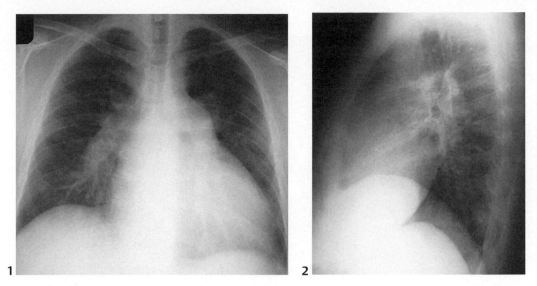

Figure 14E (1,2) PA **(1)** and lateral **(2)** chest radiographs of a 33-year-old man with ASD and Eisenmenger physiology who presented with a brain abscess following an episode of bacteremia demonstrate cardiomegaly and marked enlargement of the central pulmonary arteries. Note the poor visualization of peripheral pulmonary arteries and right ventricular enlargement with filling of the retrosternal clear space.

- Ostium primum (**Fig. 14D**)
  - Located at inferior atrial septum
  - Associated with endocardial cushion defect
- Coronary sinus (**Fig. 14D**)
  - Unroofing of coronary sinus resulting in interatrial communication

Clinical Findings

Patients with ostium secundum ASD may remain asymptomatic until the second or third decades of life. Females are more commonly affected than males with a female-to-male ratio of 3:2. Many of these patients are diagnosed incidentally because of a murmur, typically a systolic murmur along the left sternal border with a split fixed second heart sound. Approximately half of affected patients over the age of 40 years are symptomatic and present with exertional dyspnea, fatigue, chest pain from atrial flutter or fibrillation, fever from infective endocarditis, paradoxical emboli, clinical right heart failure, or pulmonary hypertension. Palpitations and recurrent pulmonary infections are also reported. Approximately 15% of affected patients also have mitral valve insufficiency. Associated anomalies include persistent left superior vena cava, partial anomalous pulmonary venous connections, and mitral valve prolapse. ASD is described as part of the autosomal-dominant Holt-Oram syndrome.

Imaging Findings

RADIOGRAPHY

- Cardiomegaly (**Figs. 14A, 14E,** and **14F**)
- Right ventricular enlargement with filling of retrosternal space (**Fig. 14E2**)
- Enlarged central and peripheral pulmonary arteries from shunt circulation (**Figs. 14A** and **14B**)
- Pulmonary arterial hypertension (untreated patients) and Eisenmenger physiology
  - Enlarged central pulmonary arteries and pulmonary trunk (**Figs. 14E** and **14F**)
  - Decreased visualization ("pruning") of peripheral pulmonary arteries (**Figs. 14E1** and **14F**)
  - Calcification of central pulmonary arteries (with sustained pulmonary hypertension) (**Fig. 14F**)

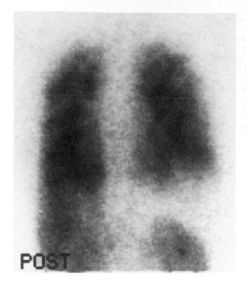

Figure 14F Technetium 99m–labeled MAA perfusion lung scan (posterior projection) of a young man with ASD demonstrates renal activity secondary to the intracardiac right-to-left shunt.

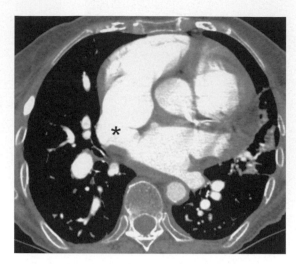

Figure 14G Contrast-enhanced chest CT (mediastinal window) of a patient with an ASD demonstrates discontinuity of the atrial septum (*) at the site of the ASD. (Courtesy of Diane C. Strollo, M.D., University of Pittsburgh Medical Center, Pittsburgh, Pennsylvania.)

- Normal or small left atrium, normal pulmonary valve
- Left atrial enlargement and pulmonary venous hypertension in older adults

ECHOCARDIOGRAPHY

- Demonstration of ASD
- Evaluation of associated valvular dysfunction
- Accurate measurement of chamber size

MR/CT

- Demonstration of ASD (**Fig. 14G**)
- Demonstration of anomalous right superior pulmonary vein
- Measurement of size of shunt with velocity-encoded cine MR
- Turbulent pulmonary artery flow in patients with pulmonary arterial hypertension

Treatment

- Elective surgical repair (closure) for children with ASD and a left-to-right shunt greater than 50% at approximately 5 years of age
- Surgical repair for adults without severe pulmonary arterial hypertension

Prognosis

- Good for surgically treated patients; 10-year survival, of 95%
- Relates to degree of mitral valve dysfunction and associated arrhythmias in patients with ostium secundum ASD

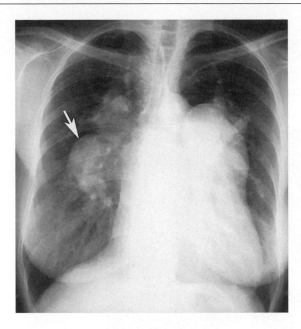

Figure 14H PA chest radiograph of a 45-year-old woman with an ASD and Eisenmenger physiology demonstrates findings consistent with long-standing pulmonary arterial hypertension: cardiomegaly with massive enlargement and mural calcification (arrow) of the central pulmonary arteries and vascular pruning.

PEARLS

- Echocardiography with color flow Doppler is the modality of choice for the evaluation of ASD.
- Lung perfusion scintigraphy may demonstrate the presence of a shunt (**Fig. 14H**).
- Pulmonary hypertension in patients with ASD is thought ultimately to result from thrombosis in dilated pulmonary arteries.
- Surgery for correction of ASD is not indicated before the age of 1 year as many ASD close spontaneously.
- ASD with endocardial cushion defect is the most frequent cardiac anomaly diagnosed in patients with Down syndrome.

Suggested Readings

Amplatz K, Moller JH. Atrial septal defect. In: Amplatz K, Moller JH, eds. Radiology of Congenital Heart Disease. St Louis: Mosby, 1993:321–338

Gross GW, Steiner RM. Radiographic manifestations of congenital heart disease in the adult patient. Radiol Clin North Am 1991;29:293–317

Nath H, Soto B. Acyanotic congenital cardiac malformations. In: Taveras JM, Ferrucci JT, eds. Radiology on CD-ROM: Diagnosis, Imaging, Intervention, vol 2. Philadelphia: Lippincott Williams & Wilkins, 2000

Steiner RM, Reddy GP, Flicker S. Congenital cardiovascular disease in the adult patient. Imaging update. J Thorac Imaging 2002;17:1–17

CASE 15 Pulmonic Stenosis

Clinical Presentation

A 22-year-old man evaluated for newly diagnosed leukemia

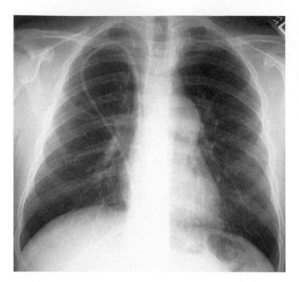

Figure 15A

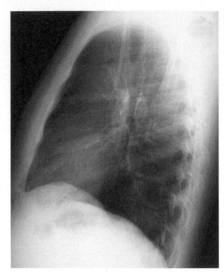

Figure 15B

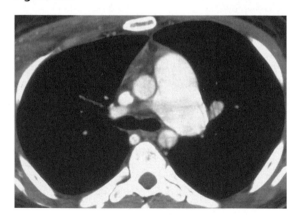

Figure 15C

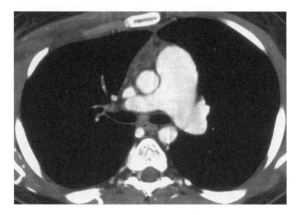

Figure 15D

(Figs. 15A, 15B,15C, and 15D courtesy of Diane C. Strollo, M.D., University of Pittsburgh, Pittsburgh, Pennsylvania.)

Radiologic Findings

PA (**Fig. 15A**) and lateral (**Fig. 15B**) chest radiographs demonstrate enlargement of the main pulmonary artery. The heart and peripheral pulmonary vasculature are normal. Note the central venous catheter with its tip in the superior vena cava. Contrast-enhanced chest CT (mediastinal window) (**Figs. 15C** and **15D**) demonstrates marked enlargement of the main and left pulmonary arteries and a normal right pulmonary artery (**Fig. 15D**).

Diagnosis

Pulmonic stenosis

Differential Diagnosis

- Patent ductus arteriosus
- Hypoplasia of the right pulmonary artery

Discussion

Background

Pulmonic stenosis is the most common congenital anomaly that produces obstruction of the right ventricular outflow tract. It occurs as an isolated anomaly in up to 7% of patients with congenital heart disease. It is a common congenital cardiac lesion among those that initially manifest in adulthood.

Etiology

Pulmonic stenosis results from a congenital malformation of the pulmonary valve.

Pathology

- Typically a valve with three leaflets, fused commissures, a small central orifice, and dome-shaped morphology; also bicuspid or dysplastic valve morphology
- Mild to moderate main pulmonary artery enlargement; left pulmonary artery enlargement
- Global right ventricular hypertrophy from chronic pressure overload

Clinical Findings

Patients with pulmonic stenosis are acyanotic. Many are entirely asymptomatic, and most present in the third to fourth decades of life. Physical examination typically reveals a harsh long (diamond-shaped) systolic ejection murmur. Patients with severe obstruction from pulmonic stenosis may present in childhood with easy fatigability and right ventricular failure.

Imaging Findings

RADIOGRAPHY

- Mild to moderate main pulmonary artery enlargement (**Figs. 15A** and **15E**)
- Left pulmonary artery enlargement (**Figs. 15A** and **15E**)
- Normal right pulmonary artery, peripheral pulmonary arteries and pulmonary veins (**Figs. 15A, 15B**, and **15E**)
- Normal heart size (**Figs. 15A, 15B**, and **15E**)
- Rarely, pulmonic valve calcification
- Right ventricular enlargement in cases with right ventricular failure

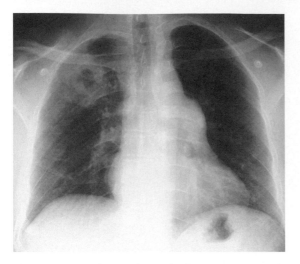

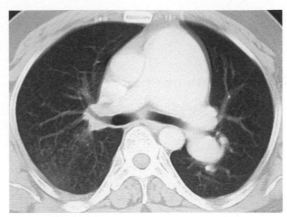

Figure 15E PA chest radiograph of a young man with post–primary tuberculosis and asymptomatic pulmonic stenosis demonstrates a cavitary lesion in the right upper lobe and enlargement of the main and left pulmonary arteries (initially thought to represent lymphadenopathy).

Figure 15F Contrast-enhanced chest CT (lung window) demonstrates marked enlargement of the main and left pulmonary arteries. Note the normal right pulmonary artery and the tree-in-bud opacities in the right lung secondary to transbronchial dissemination of tuberculosis.

CT/MR

- Main and left pulmonary artery enlargement (**Figs. 15C, 15D,** and **15F**)
- Demonstration of normal right pulmonary artery (**Figs. 15D** and **15F**)
- Velocity-encoded cine MR imaging; demonstration of differential blood flow in the pulmonary arteries and estimation of gradient across the stenotic valve
- Turbulent flow on gradient-echo cine sequences

Treatment

- Balloon dilatation for reduction of transvalvular gradient
- Repeat dilatation or open surgical correction (valve replacement) in approximately 20% of treated patients

Prognosis

- Good with appropriate treatment
- Survival beyond 50 years unusual in untreated patients
- Mortality and morbidity from infective endocarditis

PEARLS_____

- Pulmonary artery enlargement in pulmonic stenosis results from post-stenotic dilatation secondary to the high velocity jet of blood forced through the stenotic valve. However, the degree of dilatation is not related to the severity of the obstruction.
- Trilogy of Fallot refers to pulmonic stenosis complicated by right ventricular hypertrophy and a right-to-left shunt through an incompetent foramen ovale.
- Pulmonic stenosis and pulmonary arterial hypertension may both manifest with pulmonary artery enlargement. The two conditions are differentiated based on the fact that the right pulmonary artery is normal in pulmonic stenosis and enlarged in pulmonary arterial hypertension.

Suggested Readings

Amplatz K, Moller JH. Pulmonary stenosis. In: Amplatz K, Moller JH, eds. Radiology of Congenital Heart Disease. St Louis: Mosby, 1993:499–536

Gross GW, Steiner RM. Radiographic manifestations of congenital heart disease in the adult patient. Radiol Clin North Am 1991;29:293–317

Schiebler GI, Elliott LP. Pathophysiology and roentgenologic findings in pulmonary valve stenosis. In: Taveras JM, Ferrucci JT, eds. Radiology on CD-ROM: Diagnosis, Imaging, Intervention, vol. 2. Philadelphia: Lippincott Williams & Wilkins, 2000

Steiner RM, Reddy GP, Flicker S. Congenital cardiovascular disease in the adult patient. Imaging update. J Thorac Imaging 2002;17:1–17

SECTION III
Airways Disease

CASE 16 Tracheal Stricture

Clinical Presentation

A 57-year-old man with stridor

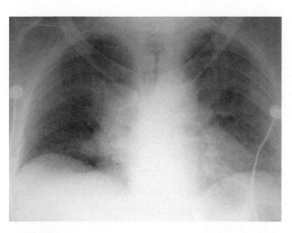

Figure 16A

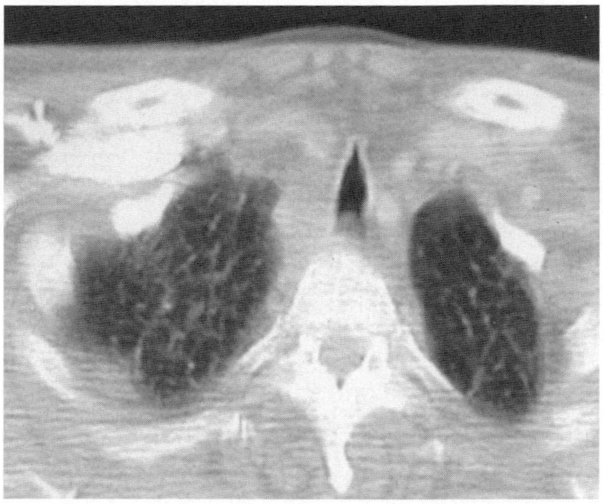

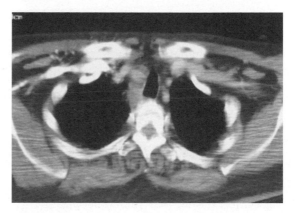

Figure 16B

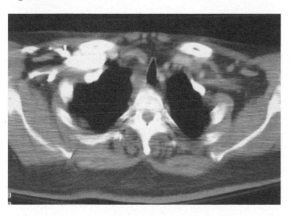

Figure 16C

Figure 16D

Radiologic Findings

PA chest radiograph (**Fig. 16A**) demonstrates symmetric narrowing of the tracheal lumen. Contrast-enhanced chest CT [lung (**Fig. 16B**) and mediastinal (**Figs. 16C** and **16D**) window] demonstrates tracheal narrowing with a reduced coronal diameter and anterior luminal tapering.

Diagnosis

Tracheal stenosis, postintubation

Differential Diagnosis

- Benign and malignant tracheal neoplasm
- Wegener granulomatosis
- Amyloidosis

Discussion

Background

Tracheal stenosis is defined as narrowing of the tracheal lumen by more than 10% of its normal diameter. It is a relatively uncommon condition with a frequently insidious onset. Early signs and symptoms may be disregarded or confused with other disorders.

Etiology

Congenital tracheal stenosis manifests during infancy. The most common cause of benign tracheal stenosis in adults is trauma, usually related to endotracheal intubation or tracheostomy. Stricture typically occurs at the site of an inflatable endotracheal tube cuff but may also develop at the site of a tracheotomy stoma. The portions of the trachea most susceptible to stenosis are those where mucosa overlies the cartilaginous rings. Inflation of the endotracheal tube cuff to pressures exceeding 20 mm Hg (the mean capillary pressure in the tracheal mucosa) may obstruct blood flow and cause ischemic necrosis and subsequent fibrosis. Strictures may occur as early as 36 hours postintubation. Utilization of endotracheal tubes with low-pressure cuffs has reduced the prevalence of tracheal stenosis to less than 1% as compared with a prevalence of 20% when high-pressure cuffs were in use.

Clinical Findings

Affected patients with tracheal stenosis may present with dyspnea on exertion, stridor, and wheezing. Stridor typically develops 5 weeks or more after extubation.

Pathology

GROSS

- Luminal narrowing
- Variable thickening of the tracheal wall
- Endoluminal granulation tissue; may mimic neoplasm
- Distortion of cartilaginous plates

MICROSCOPIC

- Granulation tissue (early)
- Dense mucosal and submucosal fibrosis (late)

Imaging Findings

RADIOGRAPHY

- Circumferential, symmetric or eccentric tracheal narrowing, often with an hourglass configuration (**Fig. 16A**)
- Narrowed segment is typically less than 2 cm in length (**Fig. 16A**)
- Typical location above thoracic inlet (**Fig. 16A**)

CT

- Circumferential or eccentric tracheal narrowing (**Figs. 16B, 16C, and 16D**)
- Variable tracheal wall thickness (**Figs. 16B, 16C, and 16D**)

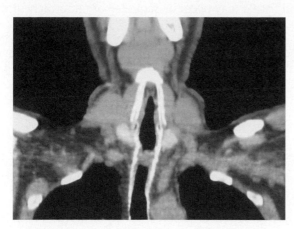

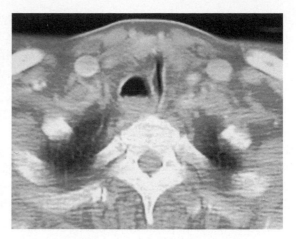

Figure 16E Unenhanced chest CT (mediastinal window) with coronal reformation of a 42-year-old man 1 year status post–temporary tracheostomy demonstrates a soft tissue nodule within the tracheal lumen at the thoracic inlet. Surgical resection revealed granuloma surrounding a retained surgical suture fragment.

Figure 16F Unenhanced expiratory chest CT (lung window) of a 52-year-old woman with chronic obstructive pulmonary disease and tracheomalacia demonstrates severe narrowing of the tracheal lumen. An air-fluid level is demonstrated in the adjacent esophagus.

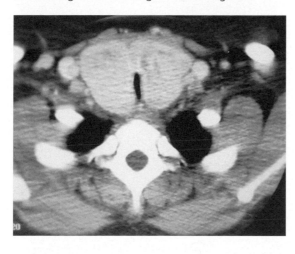

Figure 16G Contrast-enhanced chest CT (mediastinal window) of a 39-year-old woman with goiter demonstrates diffuse enlargement of the thyroid gland, which produces extrinsic mass effect on the trachea with resultant luminal narrowing.

Treatment

- Surgical excision of stenotic segment and reconstruction
- Endoscopic mechanical dilatation
- Tracheal stenting
- Laser photoablation for focal mucosal lesions

Prognosis

- Excellent; sleeve resection curative in 91% of patients

PEARLS

- Tracheal stenosis may occur as a result of granuloma formation caused by surgical sutures related to tracheostomy (**Fig. 16E**) and may mimic an endoluminal tracheal neoplasm.
- Tracheomalacia results from an abnormal degree of compliance of the tracheal wall and its supporting cartilage. The resultant flaccidity is usually apparent during forced expiration (**Fig. 16F**).

- Tracheomalacia and/or ulcerative tracheoesophageal fistula may occur as sequelae of endotracheal intubation.
- Tracheal stenosis may result from extrinsic compression by vascular anomalies (aberrant right subclavian artery, double aortic arch, pulmonary artery sling) or thyroid enlargement related to goiter or neoplasia (**Fig. 16G**).

Suggested Readings

Grenier PA, Beigelman-Aubry C, Fetita C, Martin-Bouyer Y. Multidetector-row CT of the airways. Semin Roentgenol 2003;38:146–157

Grillo HC, Donahue DM. Postintubation tracheal stenosis. Chest Surg Clin N Am 1996;6:725–731

Lee KS, Yoon JH, Kim TK, Kim JS, Chung MP, Kwon OJ. Evaluation of tracheobronchial disease with helical CT with multiplanar and three dimensional reconstruction: correlation with bronchoscopy. Radiographics 1997;17:555–567

Stark P. Imaging of tracheobronchial injuries. J Thorac Imaging 1995;10:206–219

Stauffer JL, Olson DE, Petty TL. Complications and consequences of endotracheal intubation and tracheostomy: a prospective study of 150 critically ill patients. Am J Med 1981;70:65–76

CASE 17 Saber Sheath Trachea

Clinical Presentation

A 57-year-old man with chronic obstructive pulmonary disease

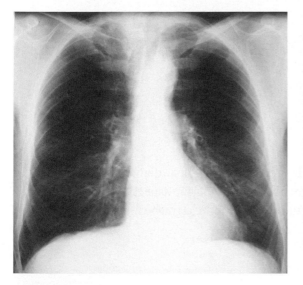

Figure 17A

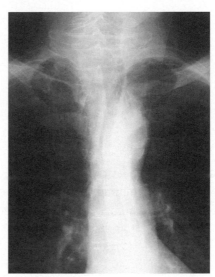

Figure 17B

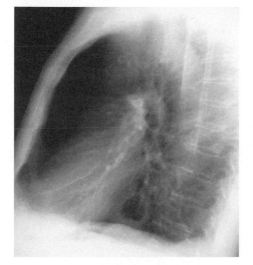

Figure 17C

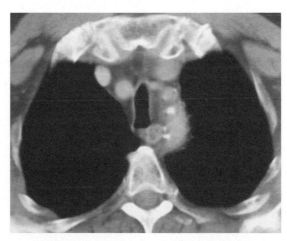

Figure 17D

Radiologic Findings

PA (**Fig. 17A**), coned-down PA (**Fig. 17B**), and lateral (**Fig. 17C**) chest radiographs demonstrate narrowing of the tracheal coronal diameter (**Figs. 17A** and **17B**) to less than half of its sagittal diameter (**Fig. 17C**). Contrast-enhanced chest CT (mediastinal window) (**Fig. 17D**) demonstrates the deformity of the tracheal lumen. The tracheal wall is of normal thickness. The cross-sectional morphology of the tracheal lumen resembles that of a saber sheath.

Diagnosis

Saber sheath trachea

Differential Diagnosis

- Tracheal stricture
- Relapsing polychondritis
- Amyloidosis
- Tracheobronchopathia osteochondroplastica

Discussion

Background

Saber sheath trachea is defined as a tracheal deformity in which the coronal tracheal diameter is equal to or less than one half the sagittal diameter, measured 1 cm above the superior aspect of the aortic arch. The deformity begins at the thoracic inlet, only affects the intrathoracic trachea, and is considered a sign of chronic obstructive pulmonary disease.

Etiology

Saber sheath trachea is thought to result from repeated coughing and abnormal increased intrathoracic pressures, which may cause tracheal collapse and fixed coronal narrowing.

Clinical Findings

Most individuals with saber sheath trachea have chronic obstructive pulmonary disease and may have chronic cough. Affected patients are typically older men with emphysema. There are no specific symptoms associated with saber sheath trachea.

Pathology

- Normal wall thickness
- Smooth, irregular, or nodular inner tracheal margins
- Frequent cartilage ring calcification

Imaging Findings

RADIOGRAPHY

- Abrupt coronal narrowing of the intrathoracic tracheal diameter on frontal radiography (**Figs. 17A** and **17B**)
- Normal to increased sagittal tracheal diameter on lateral radiography (**Fig. 17C**)

CT

- Characteristic "saber sheath" intrathoracic tracheal deformity; narrow coronal diameter (**Fig. 17D**), widened sagittal diameter (**Fig. 17D**)
- Normal tracheal wall thickness (**Fig. 17D**)
- Smooth (**Fig. 17D**), irregular, or nodular inner tracheal margins
- Calcification of cartilaginous tracheal rings

Treatment

- None

Prognosis

- Good

PEARL_____

- Chest CT of patients with saber sheath trachea, when performed during forced expiration, may show further tracheal narrowing or tracheomalacia.

Suggested Readings

Fraser RS, Müller NL, Colman N, Paré PD. Large airway disease. In: Fraser RS, Müller NL, Colman N, Paré PD, eds. Fraser and Paré's Diagnosis of Diseases of the Chest, 4th ed. Philadelphia: Saunders, 1999:264–286

Trigaux JP, Hermes G, Dubois P, Van Beers B, Delaunois L, Jamart J. CT of saber-sheath trachea: correlation with clinical, chest radiographic and functional findings. Acta Radiol 1994;35:247–250

Webb EM, Elicker BM, Webb WR. Using CT to diagnose nonneoplastic tracheal abnormalities: appearance of the tracheal wall. AJR Am J Roentgenol 2000;174:1315–1321

CASE 18 Tracheobronchomegaly; Mounier-Kuhn Syndrome

Clinical Presentation

A 38-year-old woman with recurrent respiratory infections

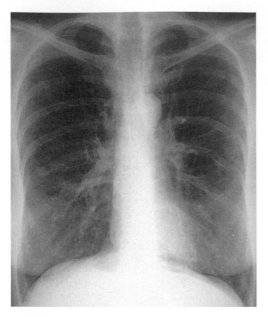

Figure 18A

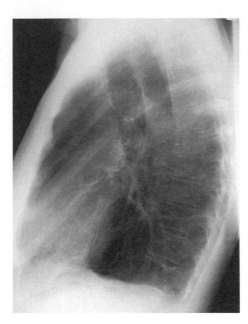

Figure 18B

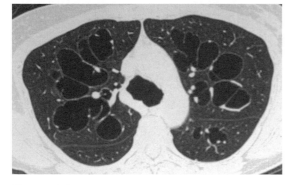

Figure 18C

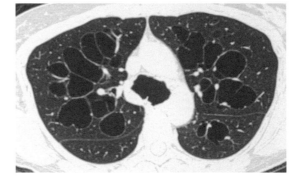

Figure 18D

Radiologic Findings

PA (**Fig. 18A**) and lateral (**Fig. 18B**) chest radiographs demonstrate enlargement of the tracheal lumen and bilateral central thin-walled pulmonary cystic lesions. HRCT (lung window) (**Figs. 18C** and **18D**) demonstrates marked tracheal enlargement involving the origins of the mainstem bronchi. Note the corrugated contour of the tracheal wall and bilateral branching thin-walled cystic lesions located centrally in the lung consistent with bronchiectasis.

Diagnosis

Tracheobronchomegaly; Mounier-Kuhn syndrome

Differential Diagnosis

- Bronchiectasis
- Williams-Campbell syndrome
- Chronic airway inflammation and/or infection with tracheobronchomalacia
- Allergic bronchopulmonary fungal disease

Discussion

Background

Tracheobronchomegaly or Mounier-Kuhn syndrome is a rare condition also known as tracheal diverticulosis and tracheobronchiectasis.

Etiology

The etiology of tracheobronchomegaly is unknown. Some authors have postulated a congenital etiology related to connective tissue disease because of associated conditions such as Ehlers-Danlos syndrome in affected adults and cutis laxa in affected children with reported associations of double carina, tracheal trifurcation, and a congenitally foreshortened right upper lobe bronchus. A familial form of the disease with autosomal-recessive inheritance has also been reported. Other authors postulate an acquired etiology, as the disease has been reported in infants after intensive ventilatory support. Cigarette smoking may also be implicated in the development of the disease. Tracheobronchomegaly is thought to result from weakness of cartilaginous and membranous components of the trachea and main bronchi.

Clinical Findings

Affected patients are often men who are diagnosed in the third to fifth decades of life. Most affected adults present with recurrent pulmonary infection and marked sputum production, but symptoms usually date back to childhood. These patients may develop dyspnea on exertion and respiratory failure. Hemoptysis may occur. Spontaneous pneumothorax and digital clubbing have also been described. Some patients are entirely asymptomatic and are diagnosed incidentally.

Pathology

GROSS

- Dilatation of the trachea and main bronchi
- Mucosal herniation between adjacent cartilage rings results in airway diverticulosis; diverticula may contain retained secretions
- Normal caliber of fourth- and fifth-order airways

MICROSCOPIC

- Atrophy and/or absence of longitudinal elastic fibers in the airway wall
- Thinning of muscularis mucosa
- Absent myenteric plexus
- Absence of cartilaginous elements

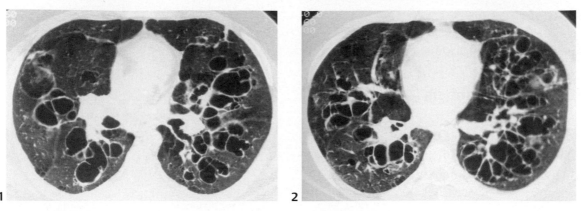

Figure 18E (1,2) Unenhanced chest CT (lung window) of a 27-year-old man with recurrent pulmonary infection and Williams-Campbell syndrome demonstrates extensive bronchiectasis. The central bronchi were of normal caliber. (Courtesy of H. Page McAdams, M.D., Duke University Medical Center, Durham, North Carolina.)

Imaging Findings

RADIOGRAPHY

- Dilatation of trachea and main bronchi (**Figs. 18A** and **18B**); may be limited to the trachea

CT

- Dilatation of trachea and main bronchi (**Figs. 18C** and **18D**)
- Diameter of trachea, right main bronchus or left main bronchus exceeding 30 mm, 24 mm, and 23 mm, respectively (**Figs. 18C** and **18D**)
- Corrugated appearance of airway walls due to mucosal prolapse through adjacent cartilaginous rings (**Figs. 18C** and **18D**)
- Perihilar cystic spaces representing bronchial diverticulosis (**Figs. 18C** and **18D**)
- Proximal airway collapse on expiration due to tracheobronchomalacia

Treatment

- Antibiotics
- Postural drainage
- Bronchoscopy for clearance of secretions
- Tracheostomy and possible tracheal stenting
- Lung transplantation

Prognosis

- Recurrent lower respiratory tract infections
- Development of dyspnea and respiratory failure as the lungs become progressively damaged.

PEARL_____

- Williams-Campbell syndrome results from absence of cartilage rings beyond the first and second bronchial divisions with resultant bronchiectasis that typically affects the fourth- to sixth-order bronchi (**Fig. 18E**). Affected patients have normal caliber trachea and central bronchi.

Suggested Readings

Blake MA, Clarke PD, Fenlon HM. Thoracic case of the day. Mounier-Kuhn syndrome (tracheobronchomegaly). AJR Am J Roentgenol 1999;173:822,824–825

Lazzarini-de-Oliveira LC, Costa de Barros Franco CA, Gomes de Salles CL, de Oliveira AC Jr. A 38-year-old man with tracheomegaly, tracheal diverticulosis, and bronchiectasis. Chest 2001; 120:1018–1020

Maron EM, Goodman PC, McAdams HP. Diffuse abnormalities of the trachea and main bronchi. AJR Am J Roentgenol 2001;176:713–717

Sorenson SM, Moradzadeh E, Bakhda R. Repeated infections in a 68-year-old man. Chest 2002; 121:644–646

CASE 19 Tracheoesophageal Fistula

Clinical Presentation

A 27-year-old man who sustained a stab wound to the chest

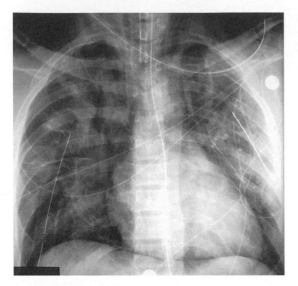

Figure 19A

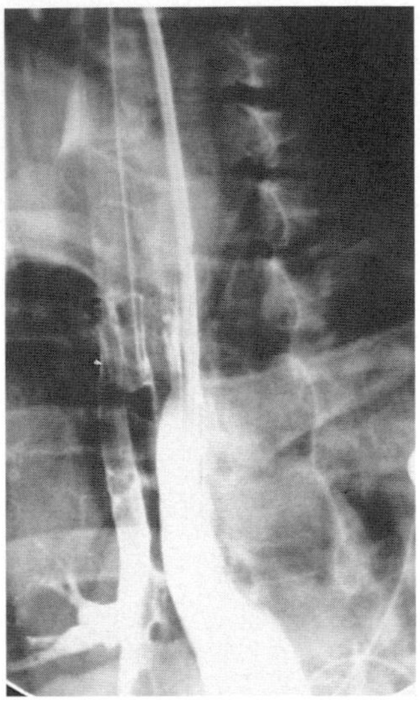

Figure 19B

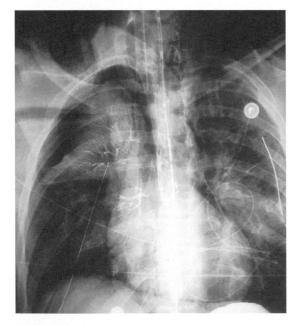

Figure 19C

Radiologic Findings

Supine AP chest radiograph (**Fig. 19A**) demonstrates a pneumomediastinum and bilateral pneumothoraces. Note appropriately positioned endotracheal tube, bilateral pleural tubes, and nasogastric tube. Coned-down AP chest radiograph (**Fig. 19B**) during Gastrografin instillation into the nasogastric tube (tip at the midesophagus) shows simultaneous opacification of the distal esophagus, the trachea, and the right mainstem bronchus through a tracheoesophageal fistula. Delayed AP chest radiograph (**Fig. 19C**) demonstrates opacification of the right tracheobronchial tree.

Diagnosis

Tracheoesophageal fistula, traumatic

Differential diagnosis

None

Discussion

Background

Most tracheoesophageal fistulas in adults are acquired lesions. In the pediatric population, they are most commonly associated with congenital lesions (e.g., esophageal atresia). Tracheoesophageal fistula (TEF) should be excluded in all patients with a history of penetrating trauma to the mediastinum or neck.

Etiology

TEF may occur as a complication of intrathoracic malignancy (60%), prolonged tracheal intubation, esophageal instrumentation, infection, or trauma. TEF occurs in 5 to 10% of patients with advanced esophageal cancer and is more prevalent in those who have had prior irradiation. The diagnosis is usually made with a fluoroscopic contrast esophagram. CT may be useful in demonstrating an occult TEF in patients at risk who have a normal esophagram.

Clinical Findings

Symptoms related to TEF vary depending on the size of the fistula. Affected patients may cough after swallowing or may present with indirect signs related to the fistula such as pneumonia, gaseous distention of the esophagus, pneumomediastinum, and subcutaneous air.

Pathology

- Abnormal communication between the trachea and esophagus

Imaging Findings

RADIOGRAPHY

- Normal chest radiographs
- Pneumomediastinum (common) (**Fig. 19A**)
- Pneumothorax (**Fig. 19A**)
- Consolidation related to aspiration
- Air-distended esophagus
- Airway opacification on contrast esophagography (**Figs. 19B** and **19C**)

CT

- Direct visualization of fistula
- Assessment of fistula size and location

- Pneumomediastinum
- Pneumothorax
- Consolidation
- Air-distended esophagus

Treatment

- Esophageal stenting
- Surgical repair

Prognosis

- Favorable with prompt stenting or repair
- Morbidity and mortality from secondary infection

PEARLS_____

- When the esophagus and trachea are injured simultaneously, failure to recognize TEF may jeopardize surgical airway repair, as contamination with saliva may persist from an unrecognized esophageal communication.
- Endotracheal cuff-related tracheal injury is the most common cause of nonmalignant TEF.
- TEF secondary to malignancy carries a bleak prognosis, but improved survival and quality of life may be gained by prompt esophageal bypass or stenting.

Suggested Readings

Gimenez A, Franquet T, Erasmus JJ, Martinez S, Estrada P. Thoracic complications of esophageal disorders. Radiographics 2002;22:S247–S258

Kanne JP, Stern EJ, Pohlman TH. Trauma cases from Harborview Medical Center. Tracheoesophageal fistula from a gunshot wound to the neck. AJR Am J Roentgenol 2003;180:212

Reed MF, Mathisen DJ. Tracheoesophageal fistula. Chest Surg Clin N Am 2003;13:271–289

CASE 20 Amyloidosis

Clinical Presentation

A 56-year old woman with cough

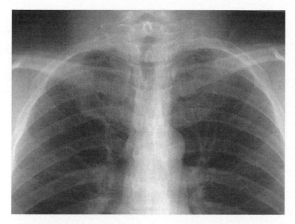

Figure 20A

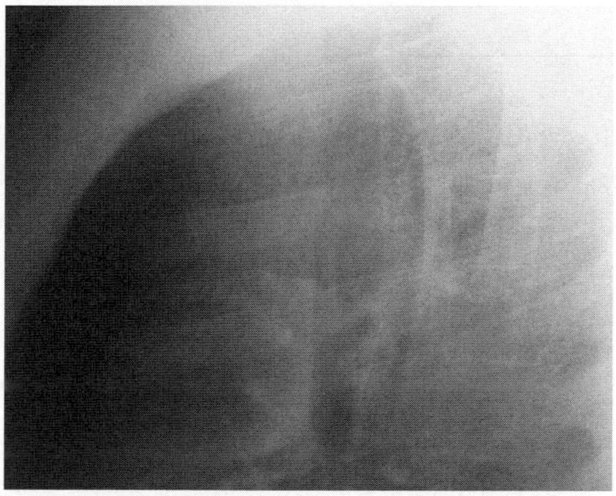

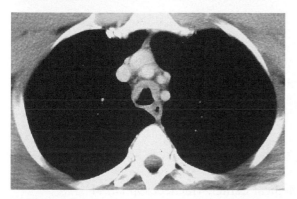

Figure 20C

Figure 20B

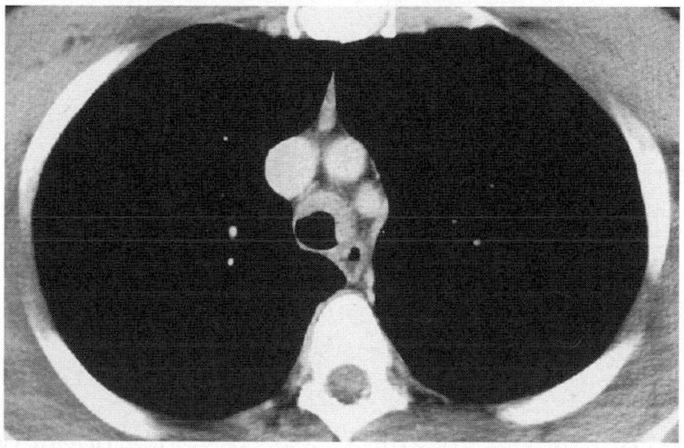

Figure 20D

Radiologic Findings

Coned-down PA (**Fig. 20A**) and coned-down lateral (**Fig. 20B**) chest radiographs demonstrate symmetric tracheal narrowing. Contrast-enhanced chest CT (mediastinal window) (**Figs. 20C** and **20D**) demonstrates a soft tissue mass of the anterolateral tracheal wall, which narrows the tracheal lumen. Note absence of soft tissue infiltration and obliteration of peritracheal tissue planes.

Diagnosis

Tracheobronchial amyloidosis

Differential Diagnosis

- Primary and secondary neoplasia (adenoid cystic carcinoma, tracheal metastasis)
- Wegener granulomatosis
- Tracheobronchopathia osteochondroplastica

Discussion

Background

Amyloidosis is a rare disease that may affect the lung or tracheobronchial tree. It may occur as a primary lesion or as secondary amyloid deposition in association with chronic disease. Tracheobronchial involvement is the most common and severe form of thoracic amyloidosis. Primary tracheal amyloidosis is rare and usually involves the trachea in a slow and indolent manner.

Etiology

The etiology of tracheobronchial amyloidosis is unknown. Chronic diseases associated with secondary amyloidosis include rheumatoid arthritis, Crohn's disease, ankylosing spondylitis, tuberculosis, bronchiectasis, and familial Mediterranean fever.

Clinical Findings

Affected patients may be asymptomatic or may present with dyspnea, cough, hemoptysis, and/or hoarseness. Patients with severe proximal disease may have significantly decreased airflow, air trapping, and fixed upper airway obstruction on pulmonary function tests. Symptoms may develop over a period of months or years.

Pathology

GROSS

- Focal or diffuse tracheal wall thickening with resultant airway narrowing and deformity
- Irregular nodules or masses
- Irregular airway thickening

MICROSCOPIC

- Submucosal amyloid forms irregular masses or sheets in airway walls with sparing of airway cartilage
- Positive Congo red stain and apple-green birefringence on polarized microscopy
- Small submucosal vessels often demonstrate amyloid in their walls
- Osseous metaplasia, giant cells, macrophages, and plasma cells may be present

Imaging Findings

RADIOGRAPHY

- Nodular, irregular or smooth narrowing of tracheal lumen (**Figs. 20A** and **20B**)
- Lobar or segmental atelectasis and consolidation from endobronchial obstruction

CT

- Nodular or plaque-like (**Figs. 20C** and **20D**) thickening of the airway wall; focal or circumferential
- Irregular narrowing or occlusion of airway lumen (**Figs. 20C** and **20D**)

- Calcification within areas of mural thickening or masses
- Associated paratracheal and/or peribronchial lymphadenopathy; may calcify

Treatment

- Bronchoscopic recanalization (laser resection, stent placement)
- External radiation
- Systemic therapy (melphalan, corticosteroids, colchicines)

Prognosis

- Unpredictable; severe morbidity and mortality with increasing airway obstruction; 30% mortality within 7 to 12 years postdiagnosis in one study
- Common recurrences; may require repeated bronchoscopic recanalization; airway compromise may persist posttreatment

PEARLS

- Serial pulmonary function tests and CT may offer the best assessment of airway involvement and disease progression in patients with tracheobronchial amyloidosis.
- Tracheobronchial amyloidosis does not spare the posterior tracheal membrane (unlike tracheobronchopathia osteochondroplastica) and is not associated with tracheomalacia on expiratory imaging.

Suggested Readings

Capizzi SA, Betancourt E, Prakash UB. Tracheobronchial amyloidosis. Mayo Clin Proc 2000;75: 1148–1152

Kim HY, Im JG, Song KS, et al. Localized amyloidosis of the respiratory system: CT features. J Comput Assist Tomogr 1999;23:627–631

Lechner GL, Jantsch HS, Greene RE. Radiology of the trachea. In: Taveras JM, Ferrucci JT, eds. Radiology: Diagnosis-Imaging-Intervention, vol. 1. Philadelphia: Lippincott Williams & Wilkins, 1998:1–31

McCarthy MJ, Rosado-de-Christenson ML. Tumors of the trachea. J Thorac Imaging 1995;10:180–198

Travis WD, Colby TV, Koss MN, Rosado-de-Christenson ML, Müller NL, King TE Jr. Miscellaneous diseases of uncertain etiology. In: King DW, ed. Atlas of Nontumor Pathology: Non-Neoplastic Disorders of the Lower Respiratory Tract, first series, fascicle 2. Washington, DC: American Registry of Pathology; 2002:857–900

CASE 21 Tracheobronchial Papillomatosis

Clinical Presentation

A 27-year-old man with fever and malaise and known tracheobronchial papillomatosis

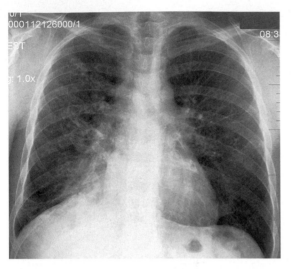

Figure 21A

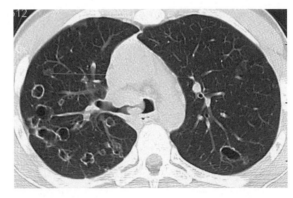

Figure 21B

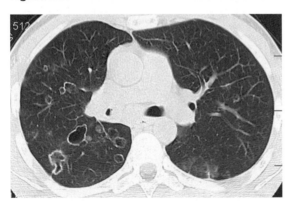

Figure 21C

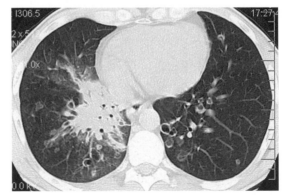

Figure 21D

Radiologic Findings

PA chest radiograph (**Fig. 21A**) demonstrates a right lower lobe consolidation and bilateral irregular cystic lung lesions more numerous in the right lung. Unenhanced chest CT (lung window) (**Figs. 21B, 21C,** and **21D**) demonstrates multifocal thin-walled cystic lung lesions with variable shapes and endobronchial soft tissue masses affecting the carina, the right mainstem bronchus, and the bronchus intermedius (**Figs. 21B** and **21C**). Note the near-complete obstruction and circumferential thickening of the bronchus intermedius by an endobronchial papilloma (**Fig. 21C**) and right lower lobe consolidation (**Fig. 21D**). At endoscopy, squamous cell carcinoma was diagnosed.

Diagnosis

Tracheobronchial papillomatosis; squamous cell carcinoma

Differential Diagnosis

- Pulmonary metastases
- Multifocal cavitary primary lung cancer
- *Pneumocystis jiroveci* pneumonia
- Vasculitis

Discussion

Background

Papillomas are the most common laryngeal tumor of young children. Tracheobronchial papillomatosis is a premalignant condition that results from tracheobronchial dissemination of laryngeal papillomas. It is also known as recurrent respiratory papillomatosis. The lesions typically involve the larynx, but they extend into the trachea and proximal bronchi in 5% of cases and into the small airways and pulmonary parenchyma in less than 1%.

Etiology

Tracheobronchial papillomatosis is caused by infection with the human papilloma virus, typically types 6 and 11. The infection may be transmitted to the newborn during passage through a birth canal previously colonized by the papilloma virus. Papillomas typically affect the larynx, but they may extend distally to the tracheobronchial tree and lung parenchyma, particularly after treatment with laser or endoscopic fulguration or after local resection or tracheostomy. The mechanism of distal dissemination is thought to relate to aspiration of infected fragments or multicentric infection. Distal dissemination of papillomas typically occurs approximately 10 years following laryngeal involvement. Malignant transformation is thought to be associated with human papilloma virus types 16 and 18.

Clinical Findings

Tracheobronchial papillomatosis usually affects young children, and men are more frequently affected than women. Hoarseness is a common initial symptom of laryngeal involvement. Patients with pulmonary disease may present with recurrent infection, hemoptysis, or obstructive effects of endoluminal papillomas such as wheezing and atelectasis. These patients are at risk of malignant degeneration of the papillomas into squamous cell carcinoma.

Pathology

GROSS

- Polypoid or sessile papillary nodules or masses projecting into airway lumen; variable size and number; may completely obstruct airway lumen
- Distal airway and lung parenchyma dissemination; pulmonary nodules or masses; may exhibit cavitation due to necrosis or expectoration of keratinized material

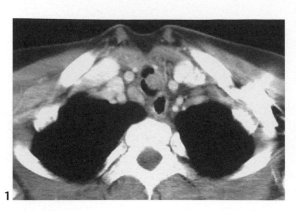 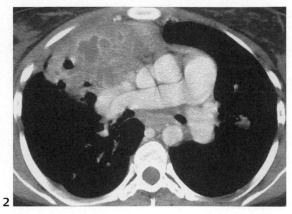

Figure 21E (1,2) Contrast-enhanced chest CT (mediastinal window) of a 29-year-old man with cough, hemoptysis, and tracheobronchial papillomatosis demonstrates an endoluminal soft tissue nodule within the trachea and a heterogeneously enhancing right upper lobe mass with direct mediastinal invasion, which represented a squamous cell carcinoma.

MICROSCOPIC

- Squamous papillomas; well-differentiated squamous epithelium over a central fibrovascular core
- Parenchymal lesions; sheets of squamous cells
- Potential for malignant degeneration into squamous cell carcinoma

Imaging Findings

RADIOGRAPHY

- Multiple endoluminal airway nodules or irregular airway walls; may be limited to the trachea or main bronchi
- Multiple bilateral pulmonary nodules or masses; thin-walled cavitary nodules or masses
- Atelectasis, consolidation (**Fig. 21A**), bronchiectasis from obstructing endobronchial papillomas
- Consolidation or mass related to malignant degeneration (**Fig. 21A**)

CT

- Multifocal pulmonary nodules (**Figs. 21B, 21C,** and **21D**)
- Multifocal thin-walled cavitary pulmonary nodules or masses (**Figs. 21B, 21C,** and **21D**)
- Endoluminal soft tissue nodules or masses of variable size (**Figs. 21B, 21C,** and **21E1**); may significantly occlude airway lumen
- Postobstructive atelectasis or consolidation (**Fig. 21D**)
- Enlarging consolidation (**Fig. 21D**) or mass (**Fig. 21E2**) in cases of malignant transformation to squamous cell carcinoma (**Figs. 21D** and **21E2**)

Treatment

- Antibiotics
- Clearance of secretions with postural drainage and/or bronchoscopy
- Laser or endoscopic fulguration of papillomas
- Tracheostomy or tracheal stenting
- Lung transplantation

PEARL

- An increase in the size or change in the morphology of a pulmonary lesion in a patient with known papillomatosis requires further imaging or tissue sampling to exclude malignant degeneration.

Suggested Readings

Gruden JF, Webb WR, Sides DM. Adult-onset disseminated tracheobronchial papillomatosis: CT features. J Comput Assist Tomogr 1994;18:640–642

Kotylak TB, Barrie JR, Raymond GS. Answer to case of the month # 81. Tracheobronchial papillomatosis with spread to pulmonary parenchyma and the development of squamous cell carcinoma. Can Assoc Radiol J 2001;52:126–128

Prince JS, Duhamel DR, Levin DL, Harrell JH, Friedman PJ. Non-neoplastic lesions of the tracheobronchial wall: radiologic findings with bronchoscopic correlation. Radiographics 2002;22:S215–S230

Rady PL, Schnadig VJ, Weiss RL, Hughes TK, Tyring SK. Malignant transformation of recurrent respiratory papillomatosis associated with integrated human papillomavirus type 11 DNA and mutation of p53. Laryngoscope 1998;108:735–740

Wilde E, Duggan MA, Field SK. Bronchogenic squamous cell carcinoma complicating localized recurrent respiratory papillomatosis. Chest 1994;105:1887

CASE 22 Adenoid Cystic Carcinoma

Clinical Presentation

A 30-year-old woman with cough and stridor

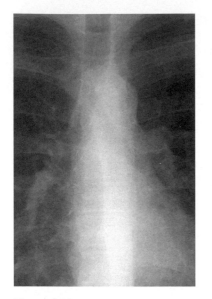

Figure 22A

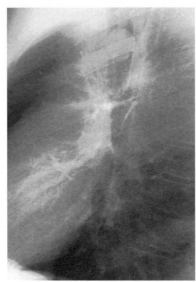

Figure 22B

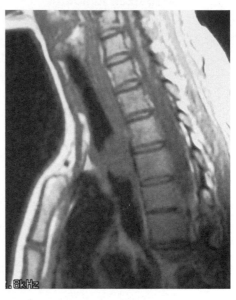

Figure 22E

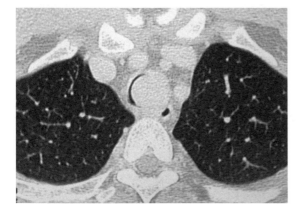

Figure 22C

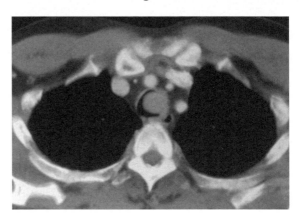

Figure 22D

Radiologic Findings

Coned-down PA (**Fig. 22A**) and coned-down lateral (**Fig. 22B**) chest radiographs demonstrate a well-defined ovoid mass within the distal tracheal lumen. Contrast-enhanced chest CT [lung (**Fig. 22C**) and mediastinal (**Fig. 22D**) window] demonstrates an endoluminal spherical soft tissue mass arising from the posterolateral tracheal wall that almost completely obstructs the airway lumen. There is circumferential tracheal wall thickening, which suggests local invasion. Sagittal T1-weighted MR image (**Fig. 22E**) demonstrates the endoluminal tracheal mass and the longitudinal extent of airway involvement.

124

Diagnosis

Adenoid cystic carcinoma

Differential Diagnosis

- Mucoepidermoid carcinoma
- Carcinoid
- Squamous cell carcinoma
- Other mesenchymal (benign or malignant) neoplasm

Discussion

Background

Adenoid cystic carcinoma represents the second most common primary malignant neoplasm of the trachea, although some argue that it may be the most common. Adenoid cystic carcinoma and mucoepidermoid carcinoma (another malignant neoplasm that typically affects the proximal bronchi) are primary malignancies of the airway that exhibit histologic features identical to those of primary salivary gland neoplasms of the same name.

Etiology

Adenoid cystic carcinoma and mucoepidermoid carcinoma are malignant neoplasms of unknown etiology thought to originate from the submucosal bronchial glands. A relationship between cigarette smoking and these neoplasms has not been identified.

Clinical Findings

Patients with adenoid cystic carcinoma are usually young adults who are typically symptomatic and present with clinical features of airway obstruction including cough, hemoptysis, and respiratory infection. Rarely, affected patients may present because of symptoms related to distant metastases.

Pathology

GROSS

- Well-defined polypoid endoluminal nodule or mass or annular constriction of the airway lumen
- Typically located in the distal trachea; may also occur within the large central bronchi
- Airway wall invasion and growth along the airway

MICROSCOPIC

- Small cells arranged in cylindrical or glandular patterns surrounding mucin-filled spaces and solid areas
- Often covered by normal airway epithelium
- Local invasion

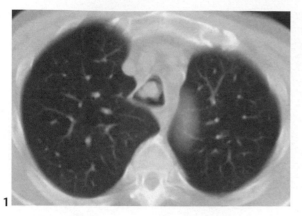
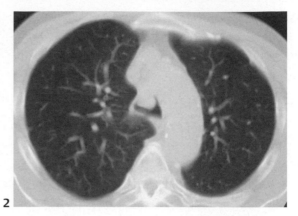

Figure 22F (1,2) Unenhanced chest CT [lung **(1,2)** window] of a 56-year-old man with stridor and squamous cell tracheal carcinoma demonstrates an endoluminal soft tissue nodule with lobular irregular borders arising from the anterior tracheal wall.

Imaging Findings

CHEST RADIOGRAPHY

- Focal endoluminal nodule or mass (**Figs. 22A** and **22B**)
- Focal circumferential airway narrowing
- Secondary obstruction; atelectasis, consolidation

CT/MR

- Well-defined endoluminal nodule or mass (**Figs. 22C, 22D,** and **22E**)
- May extend longitudinally or circumferentially along airway wall (**Figs. 22C, 22D,** and **22E**)
- May invade peritracheal soft tissues

Treatment

- Complete excision, which may be difficult in cases of locally invasive tumors
- Lung-sparing excision (sleeve resection) if tumor-free margins can be attained

Prognosis

- Guarded because of local recurrence and distant metastases
- Best for completely excised localized tumors

PEARLS

- Tracheal masses may become quite large before the onset of symptoms. Silent growth of an endotracheal lesion may produce compromise of up to 75% of the airway lumen (**Fig. 22C**).
- CT imaging tends to underestimate the longitudinal extent of the tumor. Maximum intensity projection coronal and sagital images are more informative.
- Squamous cell carcinoma of the trachea (**Fig. 22F**) is considered in some reports the most frequent primary tracheal malignancy and may account for approximately 45% of tracheal neoplasms. Affected patients are typically men (male-to-female ratio of 4:1) and are usually cigarette smokers. These lesions are exophytic ulcerative endoluminal nodules or masses. Imaging studies demonstrate endoluminal nodules (**Fig. 22F**), masses, or annular constriction of the trachea with or without local mediastinal invasion.

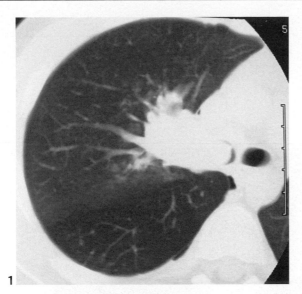 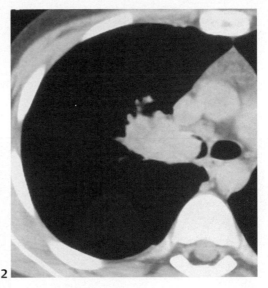

Figure 22G (1,2) Contrast-enhanced chest CT [lung **(1)** and mediastinal **(2)** window] of a 9-year-old boy with wheezing and a mucoepidermoid carcinoma demonstrates an endoluminal ovoid mass within the right main stem bronchus. Note the well-defined margin of the lesion, the linear orientation of the mass along the bronchial lumen and early postobstructive effects **(1)**.

- Mucoepidermoid carcinoma (**Fig. 22G**) consists of mucin-secreting, squamous, and intermediate cells with little mitotic activity or necrosis. It is a polypoid, well-defined endoluminal nodule typically found in the central bronchi. Patients with mucoepidermoid carcinoma are usually young adults and children who present with cough, hemoptysis, and/or wheezing. Imaging studies demonstrate a well-defined ovoid or lobular endoluminal mass that parallels the orientation of the airway in which it originates (**Fig. 22G**). Intrinsic foci of high attenuation or calcification are described. Associated mucoid impaction, bronchial dilatation, air trapping, consolidation (**Fig. 22G1**), and/or atelectasis may be seen.

Suggested Readings

Colby T, Koss M, Travis WD. Tumors of salivary gland type. In: Colby T, Koss M, Travis WD, eds. Atlas of Tumor Pathology: Tumors of the Lower Respiratory Tract, fascicle 13, series 3. Washington, DC: Armed Forces Institute of Pathology, 1995:65–89

Kim TS, Lee KS, Han J, et al. Mucoepidermoid carcinoma of the tracheobronchial tree: radiographic and CT findings in 12 patients. Radiology 1999;212:643–648

McCarthy MJ, Rosado de Christenson ML. Tumors of the trachea. J Thorac Imaging 1995;10:180–198

CASE 23 Bronchiectasis

Clinical Presentation

A 36-year-old man with chronic productive cough and recurrent pneumonia

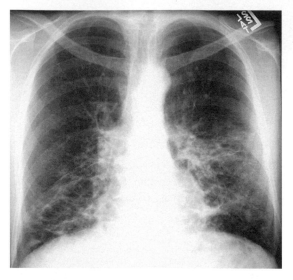

Figure 23A

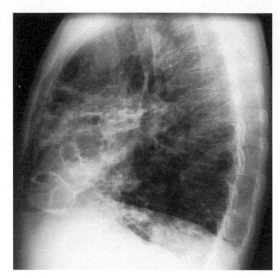

Figure 23B

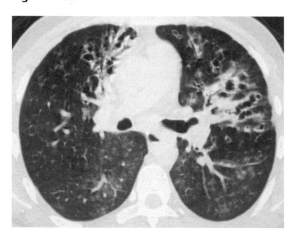

Figure 23C

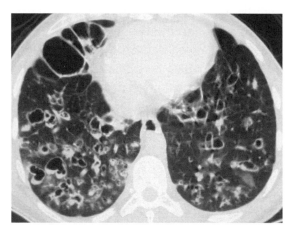

Figure 23D

Radiologic Findings

PA (**Fig. 23A**) and lateral (**Fig. 23B**) chest radiographs demonstrate bilateral central coarse linear and interstitial opacities with ring-like and cystic morphology and a bronchial distribution affecting primarily the right middle lobe, lingula, and both lower lobes. Unenhanced chest CT (lung window) (**Figs. 23C** and **23D**) demonstrates bilateral areas of moderate and severe bronchiectasis with bronchial wall thickening. Note multiple areas of mucoid impaction and endoluminal air-fluid levels in the lower lobes (**Fig. 23D**).

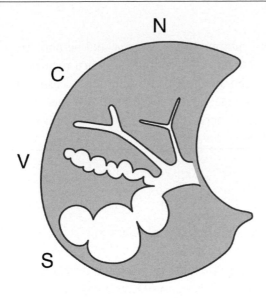

Figure 23E A normal bronchus (N) compared with the three grades of severity of bronchiectasis: cylindrical (C), varicose (V), and saccular (cystic) (S).

Diagnosis

Bronchiectasis with mucous plugging secondary to infection

Differential Diagnosis

Bronchiectasis secondary to other etiologies

Discussion

Background

Bronchiectasis is defined as chronic irreversible bronchial dilatation and may be secondary to a variety of inflammatory and destructive bronchial wall disorders. It is typically graded according to its severity as mild, moderate, and severe forms, which are respectively termed cylindrical, varicose, and saccular (cystic) (**Fig. 23E**). Cylindrical bronchiectasis is characterized by mild bronchial dilatation with preservation of bronchial morphology (**Fig. 23E**). Varicose bronchiectasis is characterized by areas of bronchial dilatation alternating with foci of luminal constriction that result in a beaded bronchial morphology (**Fig. 23E**). The most severe form of bronchiectasis is characterized by cystic or saccular bronchial dilatation measuring over 1 cm in diameter (**Fig. 23E**). All forms of bronchiectasis are associated with bronchial wall thickening.

Etiology

The underlying mechanism behind most forms of bronchiectasis is bronchial wall injury. Etiologies include childhood viral and bacterial infections, cystic fibrosis, immunodeficiency disorders, dyskinetic cilia syndrome, allergic bronchopulmonary fungal disease, and lung and bone marrow transplantation. Pulmonary fibrosis may cause bronchiectasis by retraction of peribronchial fibrous tissue (traction bronchiectasis) and is usually a localized process (e.g., tuberculosis, sarcoidosis, pulmonary fibrosis, radiation fibrosis).

Clinical Findings

Affected patients are often symptomatic with cough, purulent sputum, fever, dyspnea, and hemoptysis (which may be severe), and many have coexisting sinusitis. Patients commonly experience recurrent acute pneumonia and exacerbations of bronchitis. Until the mid-20th century, most cases of bronchiectasis were related to postinfectious bronchial damage. Since the advent of antibiotic therapy, there has been a marked decline in the incidence of bronchiectasis in developed countries. However, bronchiectasis remains a significant health problem in developing countries.

Pathology

GROSS

- Thickened and dilated bronchi; mild to marked (3 mm to 3 cm) bronchial dilatation
- Cylindrical bronchiectasis: cylinder-like ectasia
- Varicose bronchiectasis: alternating dilatation and constriction with bulbous bronchial terminations
- Cystic (saccular) bronchiectasis: involvement of first three to four segmental bronchial divisions with progressive spherical distal dilatation toward the lung periphery

MICROSCOPIC

- Minimal to severe acute and chronic inflammation
- Bronchial wall thickening and infiltration by mononuclear inflammatory cells and fibrous tissue
- Loss of mucosal elastic tissue and muscle; cartilage destruction in advanced disease
- Bronchiolitis
- Hypertrophy of bronchial arteries and veins

Imaging Findings

RADIOGRAPHY

- Visible bronchial walls (**Figs. 23A** and **23B**)
  - Single or parallel "tram track" lines (thickened airway walls seen longitudinally)
  - Poorly defined ring-like or curvilinear opacities (thickened airway walls seen on-end or obliquely)
- Variable lung volume (atelectasis or hyperinflation)
- Round, oval, or tubular Y- or V-shaped opacities (dilated airways filled with secretions, mucoid impaction)
- Multiple thin-walled ring-like opacities in cystic bronchiectasis, often with air-fluid levels (**Figs. 23A** and **23B**)
- Normal chest radiographs in 7% of affected patients

CT/HRCT

- Absence of normal distal tapering of bronchial lumen (**Figs. 23C, 23D, 23F, 23G,** and **23H**)
- Internal diameter of bronchial lumen greater than that of adjacent pulmonary artery (**Figs. 23C, 23D, 23F, 23H,** and **23I**)
- Visible bronchi within 1 cm of costal pleura or abutting mediastinal pleura (**Figs. 23C, 23D, 23F, 23H,** and **23K1**)
- Mucus-filled dilated bronchi (**Figs. 23C, 23D, 23H, 23I,** and **23K1**)
- Associated bronchiolitis in 75% of patients (decreased lung attenuation and vascularity, bronchiolectasis and centrilobular tree-in-bud opacities) (**Figs. 23G** and **23H**)

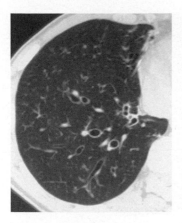

Figure 23F Unenhanced chest CT (lung window) of a 54-year-old man with recurrent pneumonia demonstrates cylindrical bronchiectasis in the right middle and lower lobes. The dilated airways are larger than their respective adjacent pulmonary arteries and exhibit the "signet ring" sign of bronchiectasis. Some of the dilated airways have mildly thickened walls.

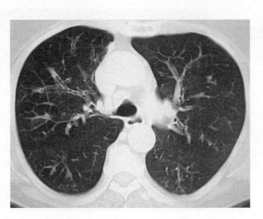

Figure 23G Unenhanced chest CT (lung window) of an 84-year-old woman with chronic productive cough demonstrates moderate right upper lobe bronchiectasis manifesting with "tram track" lines. There is also mild right lower lobe bronchiectasis and left lower lobe bronchiolitis manifesting with centrilobular "tree-in-bud" opacities.

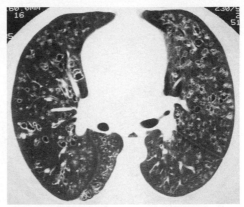

Figure 23H Unenhanced chest CT (lung window) of a 30-year-old man with primary ciliary dyskinesia (PCD) referred for lung transplantation demonstrates diffuse cylindrical and varicose bronchiectasis, nodular opacities representing mucus-filled dilated bronchi, and centrilobular opacities consistent with bronchiolitis.

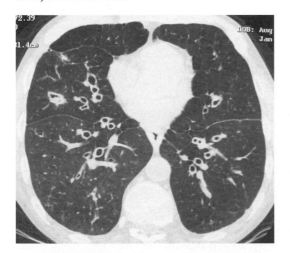

Figure 23I Unenhanced chest CT (lung window) of a 49-year-old HIV-positive man demonstrates bilateral bronchiectasis and bronchial wall thickening.

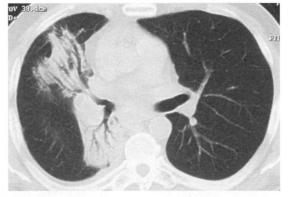

Figure 23J Unenhanced chest CT (lung window) of a 45-year-old man who received radiation therapy for lung cancer demonstrates parenchymal fibrosis and atelectasis with internal cylindrical and varicose (traction) bronchiectasis.

Treatment

- Antibiotics
- Treatment of underlying condition
- Surgical excision for patients with localized disease and recurrent or severe persistent symptoms
- Lung transplantation for selected patients with severe, diffuse, advanced disease
- Bronchial artery embolization or surgery in patients with severe hemoptysis

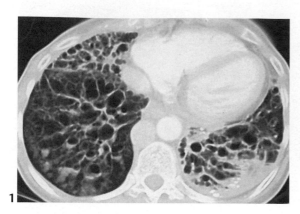 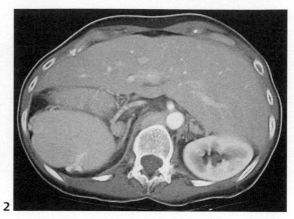

Figure 23K (1,2) Contrast-enhanced chest CT (lung window) **(1)** of a 51-year-old woman with Kartagener syndrome demonstrates extensive cystic (saccular) bronchiectasis that predominantly involves the lower lung zones. Note air-fluid levels within dilated airways consistent with acute infection. Contrast-enhanced abdominal CT (soft tissue window) **(2)** reveals transposition of the abdominal viscera.

Prognosis

- Good; response to conservative treatment in mild cases
- Reported mortality rate of 19% during a 14-year follow-up period; mean age at death of 54 years
- Progression of disease in some patients who undergo surgical excision of localized postinfectious bronchiectasis

PEARLS_____

- Reversible bronchial dilatation may occur in patients with pneumonia and typically resolves within 4 to 6 months. This is not considered bronchiectasis.
- High-resolution CT is the "gold standard" for the diagnosis and characterization of bronchiectasis, with a sensitivity of 98%.
- Bronchiectasis may occur in the setting of radiation pneumonitis and is secondary to surrounding pulmonary fibrosis. Radiation fibrosis typically manifests with dense consolidation and volume loss with internal traction bronchiectasis (**Fig. 23J**). These abnormalities typically conform to the radiation port.
- Kartagener syndrome is a variant of primary ciliary dyskinesia (PCD) characterized by bronchiectasis (**Fig. 23K1**), chronic sinusitis, and situs inversus (**Fig. 23K2**). Only 50% of patients with PCD have situs inversus (**Fig. 23K2**). PCD is associated with male infertility, a distinguishing clinical feature that may be useful in the differential diagnosis of patients with bronchiectasis. The disorder results from an ultrastructural abnormality in the cilia, although these disorders have been described in patients with structurally normal cilia.

PITFALLS_____

- Pulsation ("star") artifact commonly occurs at the left lung base on CT/HRCT and produces thin streaks that radiate from the edges of vessels and may simulate bronchiectasis.
- Doubling artifact on CT/HRCT causes fissures, vessels, and airways to be seen as double structures due to cardiac pulsation or respiration. The resultant imaging findings may mimic bronchiectasis. Doubling artifact may be reduced by utilizing ECG gating, very rapid scan times, and/or spirometrically controlled respiration.

Suggested Readings

Fraser RS, Müller NL, Colman N, Paré PD. Large airway disease. In: Fraser RS, Müller NL, Colman N, Paré PD, eds. Fraser and Paré's Diagnosis of Diseases of the Chest, 4th ed. Philadelphia: Saunders, 1999:264–286

Grenier PA, Beigelman-Aubry C, Fetita C, Martin-Bouyer Y. Multidetector-row CT of the airways. Semin Roentgenol 2003;38:146–157

Hansell DM. Bronchiectasis. Radiol Clin North Am 1998;36:107–128

Kim JS, Müller NL, Park CS, Grenier P, Herold CJ. Cylindrical bronchiectasis: diagnostic findings on thin-section CT. AJR Am J Roentgenol 1997;168:751–754

CASE 24 Cystic Fibrosis

Clinical Presentation

A 33-year-old man with wheezing, dyspnea, and productive cough

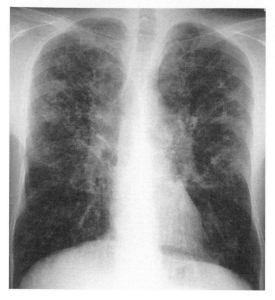

Figure 24A

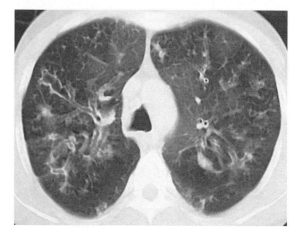

Figure 24B

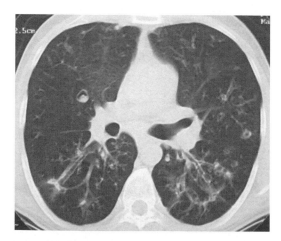

Figure 24C

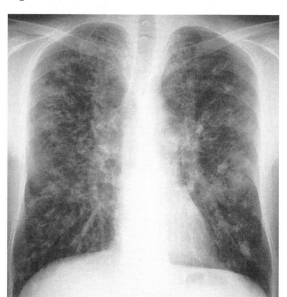

Figure 24D

Radiologic Findings

PA chest radiograph (**Fig. 24A**) demonstrates increased lung volumes and extensive bilateral bronchiectasis manifesting as ring, tram track, nodular, and reticular opacities most severe in the upper lungs. Unenhanced chest CT (lung window) (**Figs. 24B** and **24C**) demonstrates extensive bronchiectasis in the right upper lobe (**Fig. 24B**). Note cystic bronchiectasis with internal mucous plug in right upper lobe (**Fig. 24C**). PA chest radiograph (**Fig. 24D**) obtained 1 month later demonstrates additional multiple bilateral ill-defined nodular opacities that represent mucous plugs in the dilated airways.

Diagnosis

Cystic fibrosis

Differential Diagnosis

- Williams-Campbell syndrome
- Allergic bronchopulmonary fungal disease
- Other causes of bronchiectasis (e.g., chronic aspiration, healed tuberculosis)

Discussion

Background

Cystic fibrosis is a hereditary multisystem genetically transmitted disease that affects exocrine tissues in the lung, pancreas, gastrointestinal tract, liver, salivary glands, and the male reproductive system.

Etiology

Cystic fibrosis is transmitted as an autosomal-recessive trait. The responsible gene is located on the long arm of chromosome 7. The protein product of the cystic fibrosis transmembrane conductance regulator gene (*CFTR*) may undergo many different mutations that can lead to cystic fibrosis. Phenotypic variations occur in the magnitude of sweat chloride elevation, the presence and degree of pancreatic insufficiency, the age of onset, and the severity of pulmonary disease.

In the lung, dysfunction of an amino acid protein impairs the ability of airway epithelial cells to secrete salt (and thus water), with resultant excessive reabsorption of salt and water. This leads to desiccation of luminal secretions with mucous plugging. Mucociliary clearance decreases, predisposing to colonization by bacteria and recurrent infection.

Clinical Findings

Patients with cystic fibrosis may present during infancy (meconium ileus) or as young adults, reflecting variations in underlying genetic factors. Patients with thoracic involvement present with recurrent infections with associated wheezing, dyspnea, productive cough, and/or hemoptysis. Recurrent infection is associated with malnutrition and protein depletion. Common complications include hemoptysis, pneumothorax, and asthma, with an increased prevalence of allergic bronchopulmonary fungal disease such as aspergillosis. Many patients with cystic fibrosis now survive into adulthood.

Pathology

GROSS

- Bronchiectasis
- Airway plugging by mucus or purulent material
- Acute and organizing pneumonia, often with abscess formation
- Multifocal areas of atelectasis and overinflation
- Patchy distribution with more severe involvement of the upper lungs

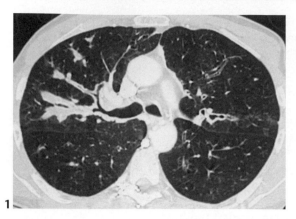 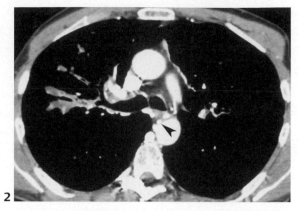

Figure 24E (1,2) Contrast-enhanced chest CT [lung **(1)** and mediastinal **(2)** window] of a 29-year-old man with cystic fibrosis demonstrates bronchiectasis and mucous plugging that predominantly involves the upper lobes **(1)**. The mucous plugs manifest as low-attenuation material within dilated bronchi **(2)**. Note the numerous dilated bronchial arteries **(2**, arrowhead), a common finding in patients with advanced cystic fibrosis.

MICROSCOPIC

- Chronic bronchial wall inflammation
- Focal epithelial ulceration
- Cartilage destruction

Imaging Findings

RADIOGRAPHY

- Large lung volumes (**Figs. 24A** and **24D**)
- Atelectasis with or without mucous plugging
- Widespread bronchiectasis most severe in the upper lobes (**Figs. 24A** and **24D**)
- Nodular or tubular opacities (mucoid impaction) (**Fig. 24D**)
- Recurrent consolidation
- Lymphadenopathy
- Advanced disease
  - Pulmonary arterial hypertension
  - Cardiomegaly (cor pulmonale)

CT/HRCT

- Bronchiectasis; cylindrical, diffuse, bilateral with preferential upper lobe involvement (**Figs. 24B** and **24C**)
- Centrilobular nodules and associated linear opacities with "tree-in-bud" morphology
- Geographic lung attenuation (**Figs. 24B** and **24C**)
- Air trapping
- Mucous plugs within dilated airways (**Figs. 24B, 24C,** and **24E**)

Treatment

- Maintenance of airway clearance (chest physiotherapy)
- Antibiotics for the treatment of secondary infection
- Nutritional support
- Lung transplantation in selected cases

Prognosis

- Variable; depends on clinical severity
- Significantly increased life expectancy in recent decades; predicted mean life expectancy of 40 years

PEARLS_____

- Hilar enlargement in patients with cystic fibrosis may be due to lymphadenopathy (in 30 to 50% of adults) or central pulmonary artery enlargement due to pulmonary arterial hypertension.
- HRCT is the imaging modality of choice for diagnosing bronchiectasis and is more sensitive than radiography in detecting early disease in patients with cystic fibrosis.
- The upper lobe predominance of bronchiectasis in cystic fibrosis is a distinguishing imaging feature from bronchiectasis secondary to impaired mucociliary clearance, which has lower lobe predominance.

Suggested Readings

Fraser RS, Müller NL, Colman N, Paré PD. Cystic fibrosis. In: Fraser RS, Müller NL, Colman N, Paré PD, eds. Fraser and Paré's Diagnosis of Diseases of the Chest, 4th ed. Philadelphia: Saunders, 1999:2298–2320

Mason AC, Nakielna BE. Newly diagnosed cystic fibrosis in adults: patterns and distribution of bronchiectasis in 12 cases. Clin Radiol 1999;54:507–512

Stevens DA, Moss RB, Kurup VP, et al. Allergic bronchopulmonary aspergillosis in cystic fibrosis—state of the art: Cystic Fibrosis Foundation Consensus Conference. Clin Infect Dis 2003;37(suppl 3): S225–S264

Travis WD, Colby TV, Koss MN, Rosado-de-Christenson ML, Müller NL, King TE Jr. Bronchial disorders. In: King DW, ed. Atlas of Nontumor Pathology: Non-Neoplastic Disorders of the Lower Respiratory Tract, first series, fascicle 2. Washington, DC: American Registry of Pathology; 2002:81–433

CASE 25 Allergic Bronchopulmonary Aspergillosis

Clinical Presentation

A 57-year-old woman with a long history of asthma

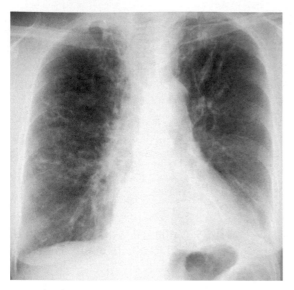

Figure 25A

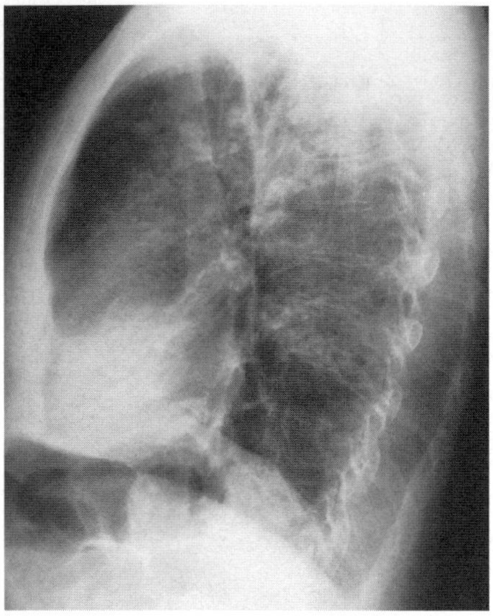

Figure 25B

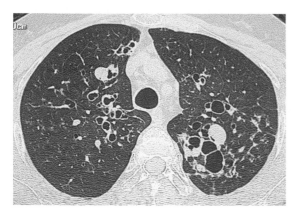

Figure 25C

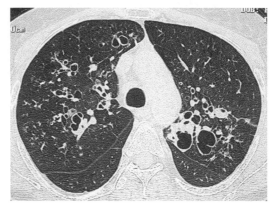

Figure 25D

Radiologic Findings

PA (**Fig. 25A**) and lateral (**Fig. 25B**) chest radiographs demonstrate ring-like opacities in the perihilar regions and upper lobes and a left upper lobe tubular opacity that appears to emanate from the hilum. Unenhanced chest CT (lung window) (**Figs. 25C** and **25D**) demonstrates cystic bronchiectasis that predominantly involves the central aspects of the lungs with relative sparing of the lung periphery. Well-defined soft tissue upper lobe nodules (**Fig. 25C**) represent mucoid impaction within dilated bronchi.

Diagnosis

Allergic bronchopulmonary aspergillosis

Differential Diagnosis

Bronchiectasis of other etiology.

Discussion

Background

Allergic bronchopulmonary aspergillosis (ABPA) is also known as allergic bronchopulmonary fungal disease, because species other than *Aspergillus fumigatus* are sometimes implicated. Typically, *Aspergillus fumigatus* colonizes the airway lumen in patients with asthma. The retained bronchial secretions initiate immune complex and complement formation with resultant tissue injury. Acutely, the injury may manifest as transient subsegmental or lobar consolidation. Chronic changes damage the larger bronchi and produce central bronchiectasis, which is the imaging hallmark of ABPA.

Etiology

ABPA is caused by type I and type III [immunoglobulin E (IgE) and IgG] immunologic responses to the fungal (usually *Aspergillus*) species in the airway lumen. Excessive mucus production and abnormal ciliary function result in mucoid impaction.

Clinical Findings

Affected patients may present with recurrent wheezing, malaise, low-grade fever, cough, sputum production, and chest pain. ABPA typically affects patients with asthma but also occurs in 2 to 5% of patients with cystic fibrosis. Patients with ABPA characteristically have blood and sputum eosinophilia and elevated total serum IgE. Serum levels of IgE may be used to confirm the diagnosis and to confirm acute exacerbations of the disease.

Pathology

GROSS

- Bronchiectasis, predominantly in segmental and subsegmental upper lobe airways
- Bronchial wall thickening
- Mucous plugs
- Atelectasis and peripheral consolidation

MICROSCOPIC

- Inspissated mucus containing macrophages, eosinophils, and hyphal fragments
- Inflammatory infiltrates in bronchial walls (eosinophils, lymphocytes, and plasma cells)
- Occasional chondritis and cartilage destruction
- Bronchocentric necrotizing granulomatosis in some cases
- Normal lung parenchyma or obstructive pneumonitis

Imaging Findings

RADIOGRAPHY

- Central (proximal) bronchiectasis predominantly involving the upper lobes (**Figs. 25A** and **25B**)
- Parallel linear opacities and ring shadows (central and upper zone predominance) (**Figs. 25A** and **25B**)

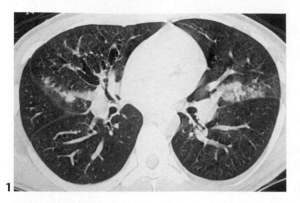 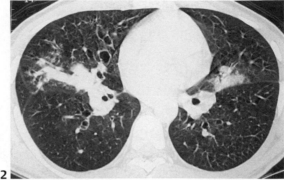

Figure 25E (1,2) Unenhanced chest CT (lung window) of a 44-year-old man with asthma demonstrates central bronchiectasis and atelectasis and consolidation involving the right middle lobe and lingula. A tubular opacity in the lateral segment of the right middle lobe **(2)** represents mucoid impaction.

- Tubular opacities from mucoid impaction (**Figs. 25A** and **25B**)
- Atelectasis in 50% of patients (lobe or entire lung)

CT/HRCT

- Central bronchiectasis, often severe and widespread (**Figs. 25C, 25D,** and **25E**)
- Mucoid impaction (**Figs. 25C** and **25E**); may exhibit high-density mucus (30%) and occasional calcification
- Bronchial wall thickening
- Linear or branching centrilobular opacities (tree-in-bud)
- Air-fluid levels within dilated bronchi; may indicate infection
- Peripheral consolidation or diffuse ground-glass opacity (subacute) (**Fig. 25E**)
- Atelectasis (**Fig. 25E**)
- Air trapping on expiration

Treatment

- Corticosteroids

Prognosis

- Resolution of acute disease
- Prevention of disease progression with corticosteroid therapy
- Recurrence
- Progression to diffuse pulmonary fibrosis
- Steroid dependence

PEARLS

- Chest CT in patients with asthma may be normal or may demonstrate bronchial wall thickening, which may extend to the centrilobular structures. Expiratory chest CT may demonstrate a mosaic pattern of attenuation related to air trapping with focal or diffuse hyperlucency interposed with areas of normally aerated and perfused lung. Central pulmonary arteries may undergo irreversible enlargement.
- Patients with ABPA typically have cystic bronchiectasis, in comparison to patients with cystic fibrosis who often have diffuse cylindrical bronchiectasis.

Suggested Readings

Franquet T, Müller NL, Oikonomou A, Flint JD. Aspergillus infection of the airways: computed tomography and pathologic findings. J Comput Assist Tomogr 2004;28:10–16

Fraser RS, Müller NL, Colman N, Paré PD. Fungi and actinomyces. In: Fraser RS, Müller NL, Colman N, Paré PD, eds. Fraser and Paré's Diagnosis of Diseases of the Chest, 4th ed. Philadelphia: Saunders, 1999:875–978.

McGuinness G, Naidich DP. CT of airways disease and bronchiectasis. Radiol Clin North Am 2002; 40:1–19

Webb WR, Müller NL, Naidich DP. Airways disease. In: Webb WR, Müller NL, Naidich DP, eds. High-Resolution CT of the Lung, 3rd ed. Philadelphia: Lippincott Williams & Wilkins, 2001:467–546

CASE 26 Proximal Acinar Emphysema

Clinical Presentation

A 58-year-old man with dyspnea and a 30-pack-year history of cigarette smoking

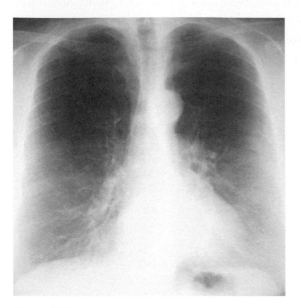

Figure 26A

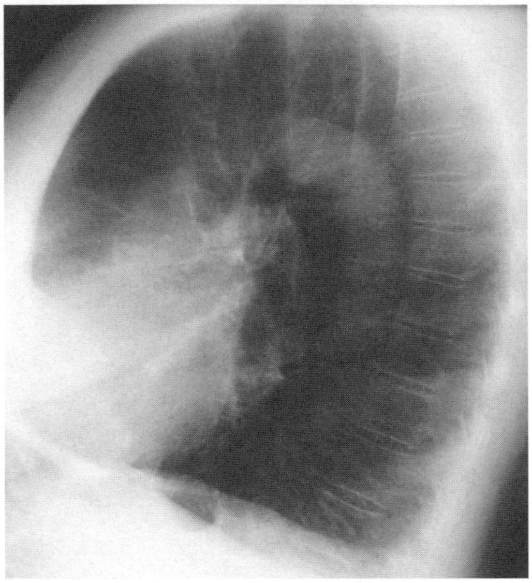

Figure 26B

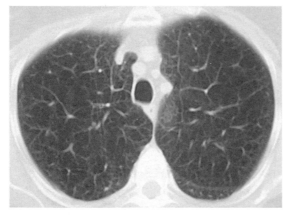

Figure 26C

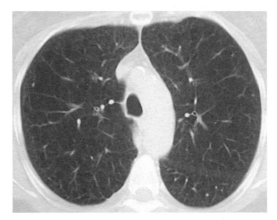

Figure 26D

Radiologic Findings

PA (**Fig. 26A**) and lateral (**Fig. 26B**) chest radiographs demonstrate increased lung volumes, hyperlucency, and paucity of vascular markings in the upper lung zones (**Fig. 26A**). Note increased anteroposterior diameter of the chest and flattening of the hemidiaphragms (**Fig. 26B**). Unenhanced chest CT (lung window) (**Figs. 26C** and **26D**) demonstrates abnormal centrilobular lucencies with imperceptible walls that diffusely affect the upper lung zones. Some pulmonary arteries appear straightened and small in caliber (**Fig. 26D**).

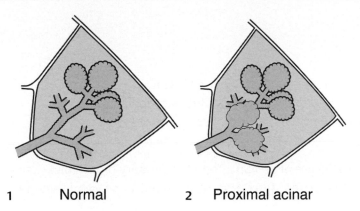

1   Normal   2   Proximal acinar

Figure 26E (1) A normal pulmonary acinus contained within a secondary pulmonary lobule. Each acinus is composed of respiratory bronchioles, alveolar ducts, and alveolar sacs. Proximal acinar emphysema **(2)** predominantly affects the proximal elements of the pulmonary acinus.

Diagnosis

Proximal acinar emphysema (syn. centrilobular, centriacinar)

Differential Diagnosis

None

Discussion

Background

Emphysema is defined as abnormal permanent enlargement of the airspaces distal to the terminal bronchiole accompanied by destruction of their walls with minimal or absent fibrosis. Emphysema is categorized according to the affected part of the pulmonary acinus. Proximal acinar (syn. centrilobular, centriacinar) emphysema involves the proximal aspect of the acinus with distention and destruction that primarily affects the respiratory bronchioles (**Fig. 26E**).

Etiology

Proximal acinar (centrilobular) emphysema occurs primarily in cigarette smokers and is related to an imbalance between elastolytic and antielastolytic processes in the lung. Cigarette smoke impairs α_1-antitrypsin's protease inhibitory function and results in increased elastolytic activity with subsequent loss of the connective tissue attachments of the terminal bronchiole and damage to the lung's elastic framework. These changes are responsible for terminal bronchiolar collapse and resultant airflow obstruction.

Clinical Findings

Patients with proximal acinar (centrilobular) emphysema are typically adults between the ages of 55 and 75 years. They present with dyspnea and less commonly with cough. These patients may be thin and appear to be in respiratory distress. They exhibit prolonged expiration, breathe with pursed lips, and may sit leaning forward. Pulmonary function test results are characterized by increased total lung capacity (TLC) and residual volume (RV). The diffusing capacity is characteristically decreased.

Pathology

GROSS

- Enlarged overinflated lungs
- Emphysematous airspaces between the center and the periphery of acini
- Variable severity within the same lobule and among affected pulmonary lobules
- Most severe in upper lobes and superior segments of lower lobes

MICROSCOPIC

- Dilated respiratory bronchioles (early); confluence of several affected respiratory bronchioles (late)
- Progression to respiratory bronchiole destruction, formation of enlarged airspaces in central aspects of the acinus
- Relatively normal distal acinus
- More prominent involvement of second- and third-order respiratory bronchioles

Imaging Findings

RADIOGRAPHY

- Increased lung volumes (**Figs. 26A** and **26B**)
- Flattening of the diaphragms (**Fig. 26B**)
- Enlarged retrosternal space (**Fig. 26B**)
- Abnormal lucency in the upper lung zones (**Fig. 26A**)
- Reduction in number and caliber of pulmonary vessels (**Figs. 26A** and **26B**); vessels may be displaced by bullae or emphysematous spaces; may exhibit widened branching angles with loss of side branches
- Crowding of vessels in the middle and lower lungs in moderate and severe emphysema
- Focal lucencies, decreased vascularity and bullae (**Fig. 26A**)
- Normal in mild cases

CT/HRCT

- Focal areas (3–10 mm) of centrilobular low attenuation with imperceptible walls (**Figs. 26C, 26D, 26F,** and **26G**)
- Central nodular opacity (centrilobular arteriole) within area of low attenuation (**Figs. 26F** and **26G**)
- Most severe involvement of upper lobes and superior segments of lower lobes (**Fig. 26G, 26I**)
- Large confluent areas of emphysema may progress to panlobular involvement (**Fig. 26G**)
- Associated paraseptal emphysema and/or bullae (**Fig. 26G**)

Treatment

- Cessation of smoking
- Supplemental oxygen
- Lung volume reduction surgery in selected patients
- Lung transplantation in end-stage disease

Prognosis

- Poor; progressive, disabling dyspnea
- Reports of improvement in lung function, exercise tolerance, and quality of life following lung volume reduction surgery

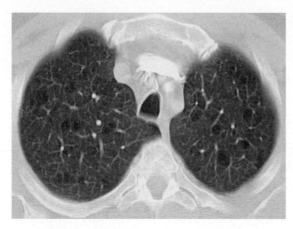

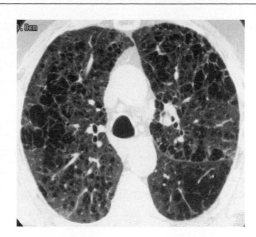

Figure 26F Contrast-enhanced chest CT (lung window) of a 48-year-old woman with proximal acinar emphysema demonstrates multifocal areas of low attenuation with imperceptible walls scattered throughout otherwise normal lung. The abnormalities predominantly affected the upper lung zones.

Figure 26G Unenhanced chest CT (lung window) of a 61-year-old man with advanced emphysema demonstrates scattered areas of proximal acinar emphysema in both upper lobes, distal acinar (paraseptal) emphysema in the juxtapleural left upper lobe, and confluent panacinar (panlobular) areas of parenchymal destruction.

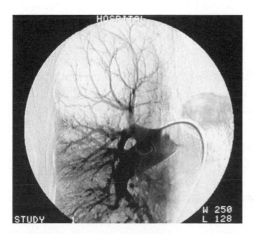

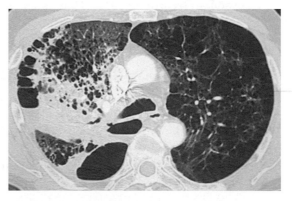

Figure 26H Selective right pulmonary arteriogram of a 61-year-old woman with marked upper lobe emphysema demonstrates straightening and separation of pulmonary arteries in the upper lung with associated crowding of vessels (passive atelectasis) in the middle and lower lung zones.

Figure 26I Contrast-enhanced chest CT (lung window) of a 62-year-old man with emphysema and pneumonia demonstrates marked emphysematous and bullous changes in the left upper lobe and pneumonia in the right lung. Areas of lucency within the consolidation represent numerous foci of emphysema that result in a "Swiss cheese" appearance. Note an arcade of paraseptal emphysema along the juxtapleural right upper lobe.

PEARLS_____

- Thin-section CT and HRCT are useful in detection of early proximal acinar emphysema and in the assessment of severity and extent of disease in patients undergoing evaluation for lung volume reduction surgery.
- Bullae are emphysematous spaces in the lung that measure over 1 cm in diameter. They may occur in association with any type of emphysema but are most common in patients with distal acinar (paraseptal) and proximal acinar (centrilobular) emphysema.

- The upper zone predominance of proximal acinar emphysema may relate to several factors, including a slower transit time of neutrophils in the upper as compared with the lower lungs, decreased perfusion of the upper (**Fig. 26H**) as compared with lower zones (gravity related), and increased mechanical stress in the upper lungs caused by more negative pleural pressures and relative hyperinflation.
- Emphysema may affect the imaging manifestations of other lung diseases. Vascular findings of pulmonary edema are more prominent in the middle and lower lung than in the upper lung in patients with moderate or severe emphysema. Pneumonia may exhibit atypical appearances with foci of low attenuation (emphysematous lung) within areas of confluent opacity (pneumonia) in a pattern sometimes referred to as "Swiss cheese lung" (**Fig. 26I**).

Suggested Readings

Collins J. CT signs and patterns of lung disease. Radiol Clin North Am 2001;39:1115–1135

Copley SJ, Wells AU, Müller NL, et al. Thin-section CT in obstructive pulmonary disease: discriminatory value. Radiology 2002;223:812–819

Fraser RS, Müller NL, Colman N, Paré PD. Emphysema. In: Fraser RS, Müller NL, Colman N, Paré PD, eds. Fraser and Paré's Diagnosis of Diseases of the Chest, 4th ed. Philadelphia: Saunders, 1999: 239–254

Meyers BF, Yusen RD, Guthrie TJ, et al. Results of lung volume reduction surgery in patients meeting a National Emphysema Treatment and Trial high-risk criterion. J Thorac Cardiovasc Surg 2004;127:829–835

Travis WD, Colby TV, Koss MN, Rosado-de-Christenson ML, Müller NL, King TE Jr. Obstructive pulmonary diseases. In: King DW, ed. Atlas of Nontumor Pathology: Non-Neoplastic Disorders of the Lower Respiratory Tract, first series, fascicle 2. Washington, DC: American Registry of Pathology; 2002:435–471

Webb WR, Müller NL, Naidich DP. Diseases characterized primarily by cysts and emphysema. In: Webb WR, Müller NL, Naidich DP, eds. High-Resolution CT of the Lung, 3rd ed. Philadelphia: Lippincott Williams & Wilkins, 2001:421–466

CASE 27 Panacinar Emphysema

Clinical Presentation

A 72-year-old woman with exertional dyspnea

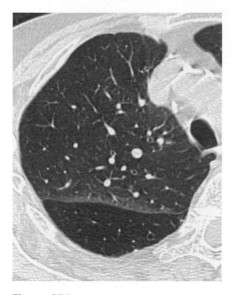

Figure 27A

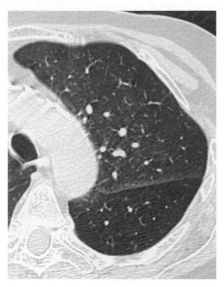

Figure 27B

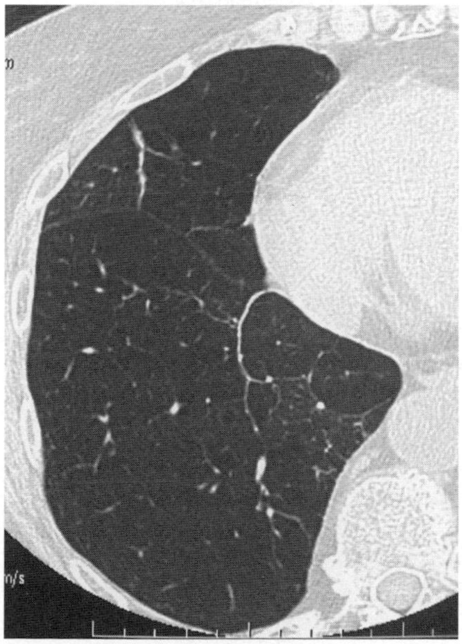

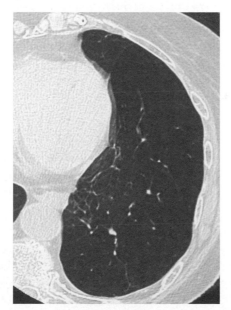

Figure 27C

Figure 27D

(Figs. 27A, 27B, 27C, and 27D courtesy of Rakesh Shah, M.D., North Shore University Hospital, Manhasset, New York.)

Radiologic Findings

Unenhanced chest CT (lung window) (**Figs. 27A, 27B, 27C,** and **27D**) demonstrates bilateral decreased attenuation affecting the lower lobes with simplification of lung architecture and hypovascularity.

147

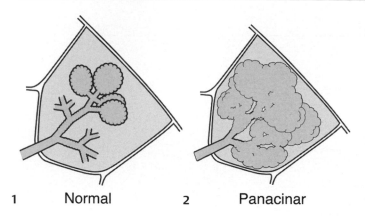

Figure 27E 1,2 A normal pulmonary acinus contained within a secondary pulmonary lobule **(1)**. Each acinus is composed of respiratory bronchioles, alveolar ducts, and alveolar sacs. Panacinar emphysema **(2)** destroys the entire acinus and all acini within the secondary pulmonary lobule.

Diagnosis

Panacinar (panlobular) emphysema

Differential Diagnosis

α_1-antitrypsin deficiency

Discussion

Background

Panacinar (syn. panlobular) emphysema affects each acinus in its entirety and all acini within the secondary pulmonary lobule (**Figs. 27A, 27B, 27C,** and **27E**). It is the characteristic finding in patients with α_1-antitrypsin deficiency. Although panacinar emphysema may involve the lung diffusely, predominant lower lung involvement is characteristic. This is in contradistinction to proximal acinar emphysema, which predominantly involves the upper lungs. Panacinar emphysema is less common than proximal acinar (centrilobular) emphysema.

Etiology

The familial form of panacinar emphysema is seen in association with α_1-antitrypsin deficiency. Panacinar emphysema also occurs as a result of intravenous drug abuse (e.g., talc, Ritalin) and in segments of lung affected by congenital bronchial atresia.

Clinical Findings

The clinical manifestations of panacinar emphysema are similar to those of proximal acinar emphysema. Affected patients may present with a nonproductive cough and progressive exertional dyspnea. The degree of disability relates to the severity of the emphysema.

Pathology

GROSS

- Large airspaces with intervening strands of tissue and blood vessels ("cotton candy" lung)
- Greatest severity of involvement in the lower lung zones

MICROSCOPIC

- Enlargement and destruction of entire acinus
- Absence of alveolar septa

- No normal intervening lung
- Talc granulomas and fibrosis in cases of intravenous drug abuse

Imaging Findings

RADIOGRAPHY

- Large lung volumes
- Decreased pulmonary vascularity
- Predominant lower lobe involvement

CT/HRCT

- Extensive areas of abnormal low attenuation (**Figs. 27A, 27B, 27C,** and **27D**)
- Paucity of vascular markings (**Figs. 27A, 27B, 27C,** and **27D**)
- Involvement of entire secondary pulmonary lobule (**Figs. 27A, 27B, 27C,** and **27D**)
- Diffuse or lower lobe predominance (**Figs. 27A, 27B, 27C,** and **27D**)
- Absence of focal lucencies or bullae (**Figs. 27A, 27B, 27C,** and **27D**)

Treatment

- Supportive
- Replacement therapy with α_1-protease inhibitor purified from human blood

Prognosis

- Dependent on pulmonary function
- Variable disease progression; worst prognosis in patients with α_1-antitrypsin deficiency who are also smokers

PEARLS_____

- α_1-antitrypsin deficiency, the most common cause of panacinar emphysema, is an autosomal-codominant genetic disorder in which reduced levels of α_1-antitrypsin allow neutrophil elastase to damage pulmonary elastic fibers and other connective tissues with resultant emphysema. Symptoms occur at an earlier age (third or fourth decades of life) and are exacerbated in patients with α_1-antitrypsin deficiency who are cigarette smokers.

Suggested Readings

Copley SJ, Wells AU, Müller NL, et al. Thin-section CT in obstructive pulmonary disease: discriminatory value. Radiology 2002;223:812–819

Fraser RS, Müller NL, Colman N, Paré PD. Emphysema. In: Fraser RS, Müller NL, Colman N, Paré PD, eds. Fraser and Paré's Diagnosis of Diseases of the Chest, 4th ed. Philadelphia: Saunders, 1999:239–254.

Spouge D, Mayo JR, Cardoso W, Müller N. Panacinar emphysema: CT and pathologic findings. J Comput Assist Tomogr 1993;17:710–713

Travis WD, Colby TV, Koss MN, Rosado-de-Christenson ML, Müller NL, King TE Jr. Obstructive pulmonary diseases. In: King DW, ed. Atlas of Nontumor Pathology: Non-Neoplastic Disorders of the Lower Respiratory Tract, first series, fascicle 2. Washington, DC: American Registry of Pathology; 2002:435–471

Webb WR, Müller NL, Naidich DP. Diseases characterized primarily by cysts and emphysema. In: Webb WR, Müller NL, Naidich DP, eds. High-Resolution CT of the Lung, 3rd ed. Philadelphia: Lippincott Williams & Wilkins, 2001:421–466

CASE 28 Bullous Lung Disease and Distal Acinar Emphysema

Clinical Presentation

A 46-year-old man with dyspnea

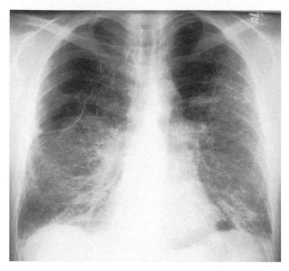

Figure 28A

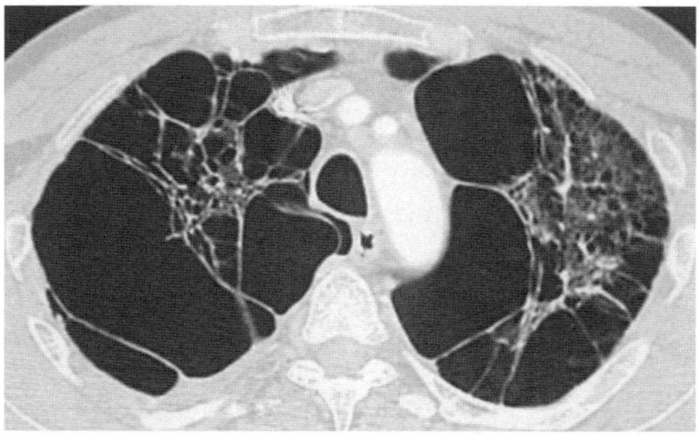

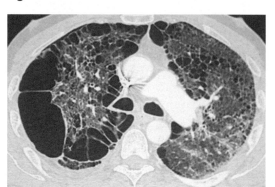

Figure 28B

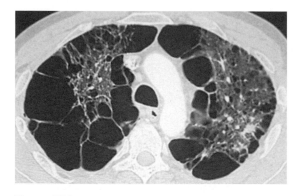

Figure 28C

Figure 28D

Radiologic Findings

PA chest radiograph (**Fig. 28A**) demonstrates hyperinflation with bilateral upper lobe hyperlucency secondary to bilateral large apical bullae that compress adjacent lung. Bands of atelectasis are demonstrated at both lung bases. High-resolution CT (lung window) (**Figs. 28B, 28C,** and **28D**) demonstrates bilateral large bullae that preferentially affect the right lung and produce mediastinal shift to the left. Note the miniscule anterior right-sided secondary spontaneous pneumothorax (**Fig. 28D**). Scattered areas of proximal acinar emphysema and a single juxtapleural arcade of distal acinar emphysema are demonstrated in the left upper lobe (**Fig. 28C**).

Diagnosis

Bullous lung disease and distal acinar emphysema

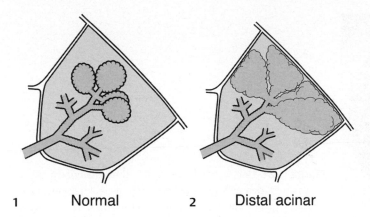

1   Normal   **2**   Distal acinar

Figure 28E (1,2) A normal pulmonary acinus contained within a secondary pulmonary lobule **(1)**. Each acinus is composed of respiratory bronchioles, alveolar ducts, and alveolar sacs. Distal acinar emphysema destroys the distal portion of the acinus in the periphery of the secondary pulmonary lobule **(2)**.

Differential Diagnosis

None

Discussion

Background

Distal acinar (paraseptal) emphysema is the least common type of emphysema and, together with proximal acinar emphysema, is frequently associated with the formation of bullae. It affects the periphery of the acinus (**Fig. 28E**) adjacent to the juxtapleural upper lobe interlobular septa and is usually an incidental imaging finding. Adjacent foci of paraseptal emphysema may coalesce to form bullae. A bulla is defined as a sharply demarcated air-containing space measuring 1 cm in diameter or more in the distended state. They are characteristically thin-walled (1 mm) and may be unilocular or compartmentalized by thin septa. Bullae may be solitary or multiple and most commonly occur in the lung apex. Multiple adjacent juxtapleural bullae may mimic distal acinar emphysema. The term *giant bullous emphysema* (syn. vanishing lung syndrome) refers to bullae that occupy at least one third of a hemithorax. These giant bullous lesions tend to be asymmetric and occur in cigarette-smoking, young, dyspneic men.

Etiology

The pathogenesis of distal acinar emphysema is uncertain but is probably related to a relative paucity of vascular and elastic fibers in juxtapleural pulmonary lobules.

Clinical Findings

Bullous lung disease is most commonly detected in patients who have concomitant emphysema but also occurs in patients with connective-tissue diseases such as Marfan syndrome and Ehlers-Danlos syndrome. Affected patients may be asymptomatic but commonly complain of dyspnea on exertion. Distal acinar emphysema rarely causes functional abnormalities. Rupture of juxtapleural bullae may result in spontaneous pneumothorax in tall, asthenic individuals (**Fig. 28F**).

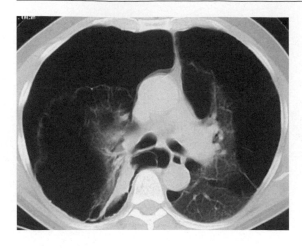

Figure 28F Unenhanced chest CT (lung window) of a 51-year-old man with giant bullous lung disease demonstrates bilateral giant bullae and a secondary spontaneous right pneumothorax.

Pathology

GROSS

- Characteristic single juxtapleural arcade of cystic areas, often with visible walls, most commonly in the periphery of the upper lobes
- Emphysematous spaces measure from less than 1 mm to over 2 cm in diameter
- Mass effect on adjacent lung

MICROSCOPIC

- Enlarged destroyed alveolar ducts

Imaging Findings

RADIOGRAPHY

- Thin-walled, well-defined avascular areas in lung parenchyma (bullae) (**Fig. 28A**)
- Mass effect on adjacent lung (**Fig. 28A**)
- Air-fluid levels within secondarily infected bullae
- Associated pneumothorax

CT/HRCT

- Focal juxtapleural cystic areas near interlobular septa, large vessels, and bronchi (**Figs. 28B, 28C, 28D,** and **28F**)
- Frequent associated proximal acinar emphysema (**Fig. 28D**)
- Large bullae, usually between 2 and 8 cm in diameter (giant bullous emphysema) (**Figs. 28B, 28C, 28D,** and **28F**)

Treatment

- Smoking cessation and preoperative pulmonary rehabilitation
- Surgical resection of the affected lobe for patients with incapacitating dyspnea and large bullae that fill more than 30% of the affected hemithorax, and for patients with recurrent infection and/or pneumothorax

Prognosis

- Good

- Bullae typically increase progressively in size, but may also become infected and subsequently disappear. Patient selection remains one of the most important aspects of successful surgery for bullous lung disease. Compressed, atelectatic lung may reexpand following resection of bullae.
- Distal acinar emphysema may be an isolated finding or may be associated with chronic bronchitis and chronic airflow obstruction.

Suggested Readings

Copley SJ, Wells AU, Müller NL, et al. Thin-section CT in obstructive pulmonary disease: discriminatory value. Radiology 2002;223:812–819

Fraser RS, Müller NL, Colman N, Paré PD. Emphysema: diseases of the airways. In: Fraser RS, Müller NL, Colman N, Paré PD, eds. Fraser and Paré's Diagnosis of Diseases of the Chest, 4th ed. Philadelphia: Saunders, 1999:2168–2263

Greenberg JA, Singhal S, Kaiser LR. Giant bullous lung disease: evaluation, selection, techniques, and outcomes. Chest Surg Clin N Am 2003;13:631–649

Travis WD, Colby TV, Koss MN, Rosado-de-Christenson ML, Müller NL, King TE Jr. Obstructive pulmonary diseases. In: King DW, ed. Atlas of Nontumor Pathology: Non-Neoplastic Disorders of the Lower Respiratory Tract, first series, fascicle 2. Washington, DC: American Registry of Pathology; 2002:435–471

Webb WR, Müller NL, Naidich DP. Diseases characterized primarily by cysts and emphysema. In: Webb WR, Müller NL, Naidich DP, eds. High-Resolution CT of the Lung, 3rd ed. Philadelphia: Lippincott Williams & Wilkins, 2001:421–466

CASE 29 Bronchiolitis Obliterans

Clinical Presentation

A 33-year-old man with cough and dyspnea

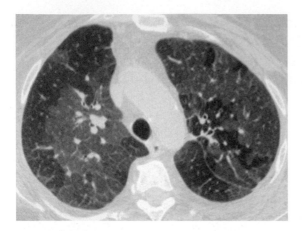

Figure 29A

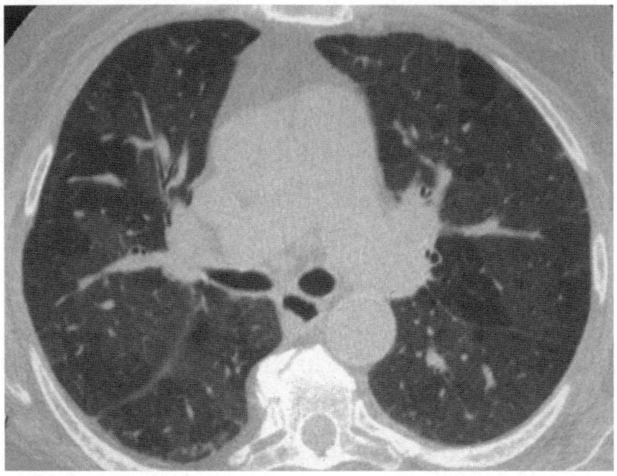

Figure 29B

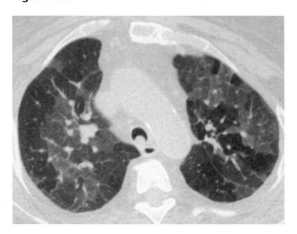

Figure 29C

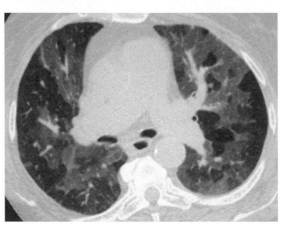

Figure 29D

Radiologic Findings

Inspiratory high-resolution chest CT (lung window) (**Figs. 29A** and **29B**) demonstrates heterogeneous lung attenuation with geographic areas of low attenuation and intervening normal lung. Vessels within the areas of low attenuation appear reduced in caliber. Corresponding expiratory HRCT (lung window) (**Figs. 29C** and **29D**) shows accentuation of lung heterogeneity and increased contrast between the geographic areas of increased and decreased attenuation.

Diagnosis

Bronchiolitis obliterans

Differential Diagnosis

- Extrinsic allergic alveolitis
- Infection
- Hemorrhage
- Chronic pulmonary arterial hypertension (including chronic thromboembolic disease)

Discussion

Background

Bronchiolitis obliterans (BO) (syn. constrictive bronchiolitis) is a clinical syndrome caused by airflow obstruction and air trapping as a result of concentric peribronchiolar inflammation and fibrosis involving the small airways (i.e., terminal bronchioles, respiratory bronchioles, and alveolar ducts). It is a nonspecific reaction to a variety of insults.

Etiology

Bronchiolitis obliterans may be idiopathic or related to a variety of disorders including collagen vascular diseases (e.g., rheumatoid arthritis), toxic gas inhalation, viral or bacterial pneumonia, graft-versus-host disease (e.g., from heart-lung or bone marrow transplantation), and drug-induced disease. Damage to bronchiolar epithelium results in peribronchiolar inflammation and fibrosis in the airway wall, airway lumen, or both.

Clinical Findings

Affected patients with bronchiolitis obliterans typically present with subacute or chronic symptoms of dyspnea, malaise, fatigue, cough, and occasional wheezing.

Pathology

- Concentric mucosal fibrosis of terminal and respiratory bronchioles
- Luminal narrowing or obliteration of respiratory and terminal bronchioles
- Chronic peribronchiolar inflammation
- Bronchiolar ectasia with mucus stasis

Imaging Findings

RADIOGRAPHY

- Often normal
- Mild hyperinflation
- Subtle peripheral attenuation of vascular markings

CT/HRCT

- Mosaic attenuation (air trapping and oligemia); typical patchy distribution (**Figs. 29A, 29B, 29C, and 29D**)
- Air trapping on expiration (**Figs. 29C** and **29D**); may occur in conjunction with normal inspiratory scans
- Bronchiectasis and/or bronchiolectasis

Treatment

- Corticosteroids

Prognosis

- Poor prognosis in bronchiolitis obliterans related to connective tissue disease
- Potentially fatal in heart-lung, lung, or bone marrow transplantation

PEARLS_____

- The histologic changes in bronchiolitis obliterans are subtle in contrast to the more striking clinical and radiologic features.
- High-resolution CT findings in bronchiolitis obliterans are similar regardless of the underlying cause of the disease.
- Bronchiolitis obliterans should be distinguished from cryptogenic organizing pneumonia (previously known as bronchiolitis obliterans organizing pneumonia). The former typically manifests with mosaic attenuation and air trapping, while the latter is characterized by multifocal consolidation, nodules, or masses.

Suggested Readings

Boehler A, Kesten S, Weder W, Speich R. Bronchiolitis obliterans after lung transplantation—a review. Chest 1998;114:1411–1426

Heng D, Sharples LD, McNeil K, Stewart S, Wreghitt T, Wallwork J. Bronchiolitis obliterans syndrome: incidence, natural history, prognosis, and risk factors. J Heart Lung Transplant 1998;17:1255–1263

Travis WD, Colby TV, Koss MN, Rosado-de-Christenson ML, Müller NL, King TE Jr. Diffuse parenchymal lung diseases. In: King DW, ed. Atlas of Nontumor Pathology: Non-Neoplastic Disorders of the Lower Respiratory Tract, first series, fascicle 2. Washington, DC: American Registry of Pathology; 2002:47–160

Webb WR, Müller NL, Naidich DP. Airways disease. In: Webb WR, Müller NL, Naidich DP, eds. High-Resolution CT of the Lung, 3rd ed. Philadelphia: Lippincott Williams & Wilkins, 2001:467–546

SECTION IV
Atelectasis

CASE 30 Resorption Atelectasis

Clinical Presentation

A 2-year-old child status post–patent ductus arteriosus repair with decreased oxygen saturations and decreased right breath sounds following extubation

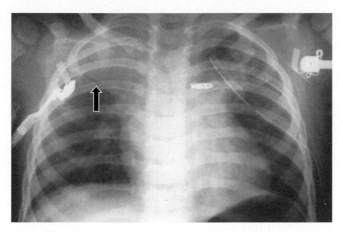

Figure 30A

Radiologic Findings

AP chest radiograph (**Fig. 30A**) demonstrates opacity in the upper right thorax without air bronchograms. The minor fissure (arrow) is displaced cephalad.

Diagnosis

Right upper lobe atelectasis (resorption) from endobronchial mucous plug

Discussion

Background

This is the most common and complex mechanism of atelectasis and results from obstruction in airflow somewhere between the trachea and the alveoli. In acute endobronchial obstruction, the total partial pressure of gases in mixed venous blood becomes less than that in alveolar air. As blood passes through the alveolar capillaries, the partial pressures equilibrate, and the alveoli diminish in volume in proportion to the quantity of oxygen absorbed. The partial pressures of alveolar carbon dioxide and nitrogen then increase relative to those in the capillary bed. These gases diffuse into the capillary bed to maintain gaseous equilibrium with a proportional decrease in alveolar volume. The partial pressure of alveolar oxygen increases relative to that in the capillary bed. Oxygen subsequently diffuses into the capillary bed to maintain equilibrium with a resultant proportional decrease in the alveolar volume. The cycle is repeated until all alveolar gas is absorbed and the alveoli collapse.

159

Clinical Findings

Complete collapse may occur in 18 to 24 hours while breathing room air. Because oxygen is absorbed 60 times more rapidly than nitrogen, total collapse may occur in less than 1 hour while breathing 100% oxygen at the time of airflow occlusion (e.g., general anesthesia, malpositioned endotracheal tube, etc.).

Imaging Findings

- Acute development of segmental, lobar, or total lung collapse (**Fig. 30A**)
- Absent air bronchograms (**Fig. 30A**)
- Rapid reexpansion following relief of the obstruction

Treatment

- Respiratory physiotherapy, bronchiolytics, and bronchodilators
- Bronchoscopy in selected cases

PEARLS_____

- In children, obstruction is often due to a mucous plug or aspirated foreign body.
- In young adults (< 35 years), obstruction is often due to a mucous plug, foreign body, or benign tumor.
- In older adults, primary and secondary lung carcinomas must be excluded.

Suggested Readings

Fraser RS, Müller NL, Colman N, Paré PD. Atelectasis. In: Fraser RS, Müller NL, Colman N, Paré PD, eds. Fraser and Paré's Diagnosis of Diseases of the Chest, 4th ed. Philadelphia: Saunders, 1999: 513–517

Woodring JH, Reed JC. Types and mechanisms of pulmonary atelectasis. J Thorac Imaging 1996; 11:92–108

CASE 31 Relaxation Atelectasis

Clinical Presentation

A 42-year-old woman who is 1 year status post–total abdominal hysterectomy and bilateral salpingo-oophorectomy for ovarian carcinoma, now with several weeks of progressive dyspnea

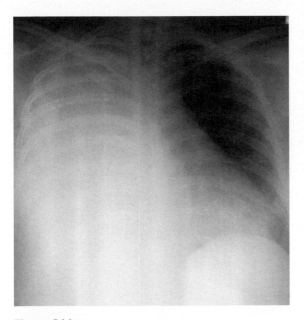

Figure 31A

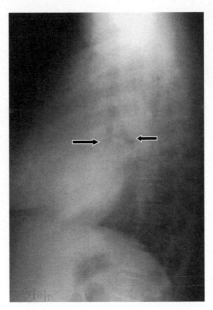

Figure 31B

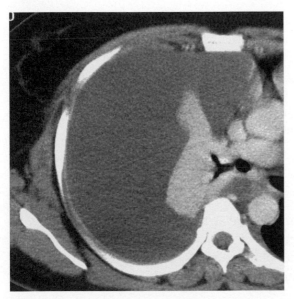

Figure 31C

Radiologic Findings

PA (**Fig. 31A**) and lateral (**Fig. 31B**) chest radiographs show an opaque right hemithorax and contralateral cardiomediastinal shift. Notice the posterior displacement of the bronchi (arrows). Chest CT with contrast-enhanced chest CT (**Fig. 31C**; mediastinal window) reveals a massive right hydrothorax, right lung atelectasis, and contralateral mediastinal shift.

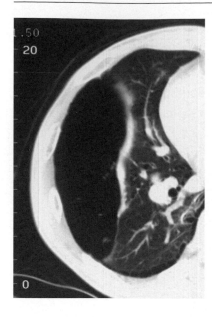

Figure 31D Contrast-enhanced chest CT image (lung window) of a 62-year-old man with dyspnea reveals a large bullous lesion in the peripheral right lung with adjacent relaxation atelectasis.

Diagnosis

Massive malignant pleural effusion with relaxation atelectasis of the right lung

Differential Diagnosis

- Right lung atelectasis
- Parenchymal consolidation

Discussion

Background

Relaxation atelectasis (passive atelectasis) occurs in response to a pneumothorax, pleural effusion, or other space-occupying lesion (**Fig. 31D**). In the absence of pleural adhesions, the degree of atelectasis is proportional to the volume of air or fluid in the pleural space.

Clinical Findings

If the atelectasis is secondary to a massive pleural effusion, the affected hemithorax is dull to percussion with diminished breath sounds on auscultation. The severity of dyspnea depends on the patient's underlying respiratory reserve and the rate at which the fluid accumulated. The gradual accumulation of fluid over time allows the patient to accommodate for the volume loss.

Imaging Findings

- The upper lobes demonstrate a greater degree of relaxation atelectasis in cases of pneumothorax.
- The lower lobes exhibit a greater degree of relaxation atelectasis in cases of pleural effusion (**Fig. 31A, 31B,** and **31C**).
- The cartilaginous support of lobar and larger segmental bronchi allows them to resist collapse, remain air-filled, and manifest as air bronchograms.

Treatment

- Directed toward the underlying disease process and evacuation of the pleural air or fluid when necessary

Prognosis

- In the absence of pleural adhesions, once the abnormal pleural air or fluid collection is evacuated, the elastic recoil properties of the chest wall and affected lung will allow the lung to reexpand and function normally

PEARL_____

- An endobronchial tumor must be excluded if air bronchograms are absent.

Suggested Readings

Fraser RS, Müller NL, Colman N, Paré PD. Atelectasis. In: Fraser RS, Müller NL, Colman N, Paré PD, eds. Diagnosis of Diseases of the Chest, 4th ed. Philadelphia: Saunders, 1999:517–52.

Woodring JH, Reed JC. Types and mechanisms of pulmonary atelectasis. J Thorac Imaging 1996; 11:92–108

CASE 32 Cicatrization Atelectasis

Clinical Presentation

A 51-year-old man who is 5 months status post–radiation therapy for unresectable adenocarcinoma of the lung

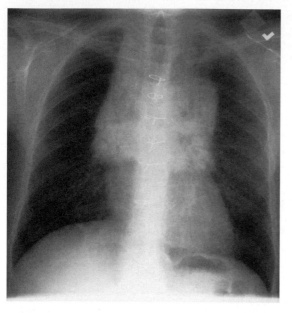

Figure 32A

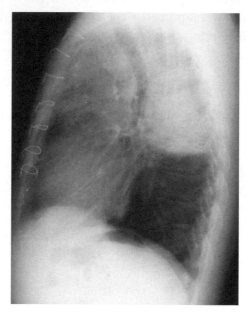

Figure 32B

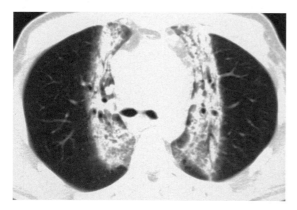

Figure 32C

Radiologic Findings

PA (**Fig. 32A**) and lateral (**Fig. 32B**) chest radiographs demonstrate well-defined opacities with sharp borders involving the superior mediastinum and the paramediastinal lung zones. The bronchi within the affected lung are distorted and dilated. Notice the hilar retraction, diaphragmatic elevation, and compensatory overinflation of the uninvolved lower lungs. Contrast-enhanced chest CT (**Fig. 32C**; lung window) reveals a sharply demarcated band of increased attenuation in the medial anterior and posterior lung zones. Notice the traction bronchiectasis and bronchovascular reorientation in the affected lung.

Diagnosis

Iatrogenic pulmonary fibrosis with localized cicatrization atelectasis corresponding to the radiation therapy portal

Discussion

Background

Localized fibrosis is associated with volume loss. The prototypical example is fibrosis secondary to chronic infection (e.g., long-standing tuberculosis). Idiopathic pulmonary fibrosis is the prototype for a generalized form of cicatrization atelectasis.

Clinical Findings

Chronic radiation damage begins 3 to 4 months following initiation of therapy. The fibrosis and volume loss develop gradually and stabilize 9 to 12 months after completion of therapy. Many patients are asymptomatic. Symptoms, when present, may be insidious and include cough and dyspnea. Forced vital and diffusion capacity may be reduced.

Imaging Findings

- Parenchymal opacity with loss of volume (**Figs. 32A** and **32C**)
- Parenchymal opacity conforming to the radiation portal (**Figs. 32A** and **32C**)
- Affected lung appears dense and heterogeneous because of architectural distortion, dilated bronchi, and bronchioles (**Figs. 32A, 32B,** and **32C**)
- Compensatory signs of chronic volume loss are usually evident (e.g., localized mediastinal shift, compensatory overinflation of unaffected lung) (**Figs. 32A** and **32C**)

Treatment

- Corticosteroids

Prognosis

- Dependent on the underlying disease process

PEARL_____

- Late complications of radiation therapy also include pericardial effusion, pericardial calcification, accelerated atherosclerosis, airway strictures, and bone demineralization.

Suggested Readings

Fraser RS, Müller NL, Colman N, Paré PD. Atelectasis In: Fraser and Paré's Diagnosis of Diseases of the Chest, 4th ed. Philadelphia: Saunders, 1999:522–525

Fraser RS, Müller NL, Colman N, Paré PD. Irradiation. In: Fraser and Paré's Diagnosis of Diseases of the Chest, 4th ed. Philadelphia: Saunders, 1999:2595–2606

Westcott JL, Cole SR. Traction bronchiectasis in end-stage pulmonary fibrosis. Radiology 1986;161:665–669

Woodring JH, Reed JC. Types and mechanisms of pulmonary atelectasis. J Thorac Imaging 1996;11:92–108

CASE 33 Adhesive Atelectasis

Clinical Presentation

Premature infant with cyanosis and acute respiratory distress

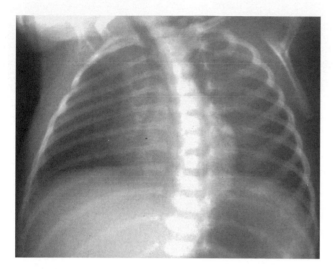

Figure 33A

Radiologic Findings

AP chest radiograph (**Fig. 33A**) demonstrates bilateral, symmetrical, perihilar opacities with a fine granular pattern. There are bilateral low lung volumes.

Diagnosis

Respiratory distress syndrome of the newborn; adhesive atelectasis

Differential Diagnosis

- Pneumonia
- Volume overload or heart failure
- Massive aspiration
- Pulmonary hemorrhage

Discussion

Background

This is the least understood type of atelectasis. It is related to the production of abnormal or insufficient surfactant, which results in increased surface tension within the alveoli and alveolar collapse (e.g., microatelectasis). It may produce significant arteriovenous shunting in spite of a relatively normal chest radiograph.

Clinical Findings

Adhesive atelectasis may also be seen in the setting of acute respiratory distress syndrome, post-operative states, bronchopneumonia, acute radiation pneumonitis, smoke inhalation, pulmonary thromboembolic disease, pulmonary contusion, and hemorrhage.

Imaging Findings

- Chest radiograph may be relatively normal.
- Patent bronchi and bronchioles may manifest as air bronchograms (i.e., nonobstructive atelectasis).

Treatment

- Directed toward the underlying disease process
- Supplemental oxygen therapy and mechanical ventilation as needed
- Surfactant (Curosurf) administration

Prognosis

- Variable

PEARL

- Prototypical examples of adhesive atelectasis include respiratory distress syndrome of the newborn and acute radiation pneumonitis.

Suggested Readings

Fraser RS, Müller NL, Colman N, Paré PD. Atelectasis. In: Fraser RS, Müller NL, Colman N, Paré PD, eds. Fraser and Paré's Diagnosis of Diseases of the Chest, 4th ed. Philadelphia: Saunders, 1999:522

Plavka R, Kopecky P, Sebron V, et al. Early versus delayed surfactant administration in extremely premature neonates with respiratory distress syndrome ventilated by high-frequency oscillatory ventilation. Intensive Care Med 2002;28:1483–1490

Wilcox P, Baile EM, Hards J, et al. Phrenic nerve function and its relationship to atelectasis after coronary artery bypass surgery. Chest 1988;93:693–698

Woodring JH, Reed JC. Types and mechanisms of pulmonary atelectasis. J Thorac Imaging 1996;11: 92–108

CASE 34 Right Lower Lobe Atelectasis: Obstructing Small Cell Lung Cancer

Clinical Presentation

A 52-year-old woman with a long history of tobacco abuse now with progressive cough and fatigue

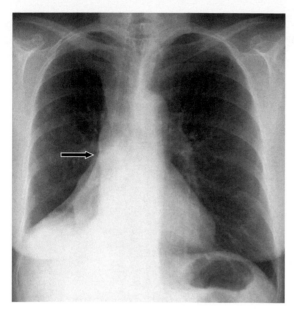

Figure 34A

Radiologic Findings

PA chest radiograph (**Fig. 34A**) demonstrates inferior displacement of the oblique fissure and right hilum. Notice the convex bulge in the medial aspect of the displaced oblique fissure (i.e., reverse-S sign of Golden; arrow). A right basilar opacity obscures part of the hemidiaphragm.

Diagnosis

Right lower lobe atelectasis secondary to an obstructing non–small cell lung cancer

Differential Diagnosis

Right lower lobe atelectasis secondary to other endobronchial lesions

Discussion

Background

Fissural displacement is the most easily recognized and most reliable *direct* sign of lobar atelectasis. The position and morphology of the displaced fissures vary with the degree of volume loss. Crowding of the bronchovascular markings is another important *direct* sign of atelectasis. If the affected lobe or segment is atelectatic but contains some air, bronchovascular markings will be visible but are crowded into a smaller space (one of the earliest signs of volume loss). This sign is most easily recognized when comparison radiographs are available. Crowding of bronchovascular markings occurs in all varieties of collapse except for resorption atelectasis. However, opacification of the affected lung may obscure their visualization. This case also illustrates the reverse-S sign of Golden, which suggests a central neoplasm (also see Case 42), as the etiology for the volume loss.

Clinical Findings

Patients may have a change in a preexistent cough or have weight loss and intermittent hemoptysis. The affected hemithorax may be dull to percussion with diminished breath sounds on auscultation.

Treatment

- Directed toward the underlying disease (Section VI)

Prognosis

- Variable depending on the cell type of obstructing neoplasm and stage at presentation (Section VI)

Suggested Reading

Woodring JH, Reed JC. Types and mechanisms of pulmonary atelectasis. J Thorac Imaging 1996; 11:92–108

CASE 35 Right Upper Lobe Atelectasis: Obstructing Mucous Plug

Clinical Presentation

A 38-year-old man status post–abdominal surgery who required ventilator support, had an abrupt drop in oxygen saturations, and decreased breath sounds

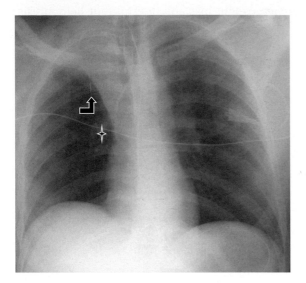

Figure 35A

Radiologic Findings

AP chest radiograph (**Fig. 35A**) shows cephalad displacement of the minor fissure (arrow) and elevation of the right hilum (*) and right hemidiaphragm. Notice the decrease in volume of the right hemithorax.

Diagnosis

Right upper lobe atelectasis from an obstructing mucous plug

Discussion

Background

Hilar displacement is an *indirect* sign of volume loss. In 97% of individuals, the left hilum is higher than the right. In 3% of individuals, the hila lie at approximately the same level. The normal left hilum never lies lower than the normal right hilum. An alteration in normal hilar relationships is the most reliable *indirect* sign of atelectasis. Hilar displacement is more common in upper lobe than lower lobe atelectasis, and is usually more marked in cases of chronic volume loss.

Clinical Findings

Affected patients may exhibit an abrupt drop in oxygen saturations, altered A-a gradient, and diminished breath sounds over the affected region.

Imaging Findings

- Alteration in normal hilar relationships (**Fig. 35A**)
- Alteration in the normal course and position of interlobar fissures (**Fig. 35A**)
- Increased opacity in the affected lung parenchyma (**Fig. 35A**)
- Signs of compensatory overinflation

Treatment

- Respiratory physiotherapy, bronchiolytics, and bronchodilators
- Bronchoscopy in selected cases

Prognosis

- Good if recognized and treated early
- Delayed recognition and treatment may result in secondary bacterial infection

PEARL_____

- Because the normal right hilum lies lower than the left, downward displacement of the right hilum in lower lobe collapse is often more difficult to recognize radiographically than downward displacement of the left hilum.

Suggested Readings

Felson B. The lobes. In: Felson B, ed. Chest Roentgenology. Philadelphia: Saunders, 1973:92–133

Fraser RS, Müller NL, Colman N, Paré PD. Atelectasis. In: Fraser and Paré's Diagnosis of Diseases of the Chest, 4th ed. Philadelphia: Saunders, 1999:532–533

CASE 36 Left Lower Lobe Atelectasis: Obstructing Neoplasm

Clinical Presentation

A 65-year-old woman with a long history of tobacco abuse developed intermittent hemoptysis and progressive cough.

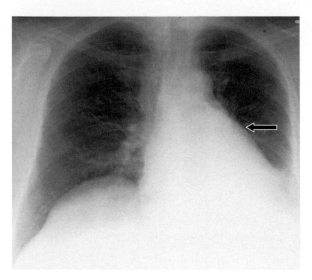

Figure 36A

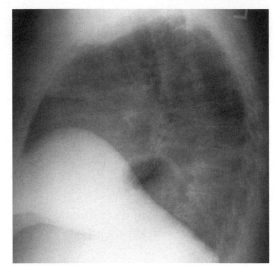

Figure 36B

Radiologic Findings

PA (**Fig. 36A**) and lateral (**Fig. 36B**) chest radiographs demonstrate a localized basilar opacity overlying the lower thoracic spine and obscuring the posterolateral hemidiaphragm. The trachea and major bronchi are displaced posteriorly. There is loss of definition of the left hilum and the interlobar pulmonary artery with leftward mediastinal shift and a decrease in the volume of the left hemithorax. Notice the focal convexity in the medial aspect of the displaced oblique fissure (i.e., reverse-S sign of Golden) (arrow).

Diagnosis

Left lower lobe atelectasis from an obstructing small cell lung carcinoma

Differential Diagnosis

Atelectasis secondary to other obstructing lesions

Discussion

Background

As lung loses volume and becomes airless, its relative density increases because of gas resorption and fluid accumulation. However, a given lobe or segment must be almost "totally" collapsed before an increase in opacity is perceptible. The overall volume of an airless lobe or segment depends on the order bronchus affected and the volume of sequestered fluid within the obstructed lung.

Clinical Findings

Affected patients may exhibit hypoxemia, altered A-a gradient, digital clubbing, diminished breath sounds over the affected region, and various paraneoplastic syndromes (see Section VI).

Imaging Findings

- Increased opacity in the affected lung parenchyma (**Fig. 36B**)
- Alteration in normal hilar relationships (**Fig. 36A**)
- Alteration in the normal course and position of interlobar fissures
- Signs of compensatory overinflation

Treatment (See Section VI)

- Platinum-based chemotherapy
- Possible concurrent radiotherapy for patients with limited-stage small cell lung cancer
- Surgical excision with combination chemotherapy for patients with very limited-stage disease (T1/T2 and No)

Prognosis (See Section VI)

- Poor prognosis; 5-year survival of 1 to 5%
- Median survival without treatment of 2 to 4 months

PEARL

- The reverse-S sign of Golden suggests that a central neoplasm is responsible for the volume loss.

Suggested Readings

Fraser RS, Müller NL, Colman N, Paré PD. Atelectasis. In: Fraser RS, Müller NL, Colman N, Paré PD, eds. Fraser and Paré's Diagnosis of Diseases of the Chest, 4th ed. Philadelphia: Saunders, 1999:528

Woodring JH, Reed JC. Types and mechanisms of pulmonary atelectasis. J Thorac Imaging 1996; 11:92–108

CASE 37 Chronic Left Lower Lobe Atelectasis with Recurrent Pneumonia

Clinical Presentation

A 43-year-old woman with recurrent pneumonia

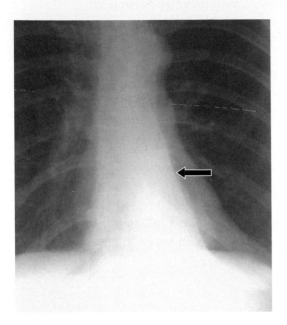

Figure 37A

Radiologic Findings

Coned-down PA (**Fig. 37A**) chest radiograph demonstrates a triangular retrocardiac opacity with its apex directed toward the ipsilateral hilum and its base toward the hemidiaphragm. There is caudal displacement of the oblique fissure (arrow). The left hilum appears small, is inferiorly displaced, and the left interlobar artery is not perceptible.

Diagnosis

Chronic left lower lobe atelectasis with recurrent pneumonia

Discussion

Background

The reorientation of normal vascular structures is a subtle, but very helpful, *indirect* sign of volume loss. The normal right hilum has a concave lateral border, formed by the convergence of the superior pulmonary vein from above and the descending pulmonary artery from below. As the upper lobe collapses, the superior pulmonary vein rotates medially and flattens this hilar concavity. Loss of visualization of the interlobar artery is a reliable sign of lower lobe atelectasis. This sign is especially valuable in the left hemithorax when a pleural effusion creates a triangular paravertebral opacity

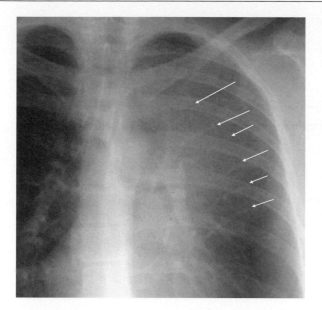

Figure 37B Coned-down PA chest radiograph shows an ill-defined left-sided parahilar opacity and a "parallel" pattern of vascular reorientation (arrows) in the left superior hemithorax. Diagnosis: left upper lobe atelectasis from an endobronchial carcinoid tumor.

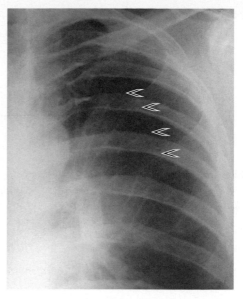

Figure 37C Coned-down PA chest radiograph of the upper thorax demonstrates an ill-defined left perihilar opacity and a "divergent" pattern of vascular reorientation (arrowheads) in the left superior hemithorax. Diagnosis: left upper lobe collapse from an obstructing endobronchial squamous cell carcinoma.

simulating lower lobe atelectasis. The interlobar artery is not visible in lower lobe collapse, but is visible with pleural effusion. "Parallel" (**Fig. 37B**) and "divergent" (**Fig. 37C**) patterns of vascular reorientation may be seen with upper lobe volume loss, are related to compensatory overinflation of nonatelectatic lower lung, and are more often appreciated with left upper lobe than right upper lobe volume loss.

Clinical Findings

Patients may present because of recurrent unexplained pneumonia, productive cough, weight loss, and hemoptysis.

Imaging Findings

- Reorientation of normal vascular structures and relationships (**Figs. 37A, 37B,** and **37C**)
- "Parallel" or "divergent" patterns of vascular reorientation (**Figs. 37B** and **37C**)
- Small or inapparent ipsilateral hilum (**Fig. 37A**)
- Loss of definition of the ipsilateral interlobar pulmonary artery (**Fig. 37A**)

Treatment

- Respiratory physiotherapy, bronchiolytics, and bronchodilators
- Prophylactic antibiotics
- Lobectomy when necessary

Prognosis

- Variable

- Vascular reorientation is a subtle but helpful indirect sign of volume loss.

Suggested Readings

Fraser RS, Müller NL, Colman N, Paré PD. Atelectasis. In: Fraser RS, Müller NL, Colman N, Paré PD, eds. Fraser and Paré's Diagnosis of Diseases of the Chest, 4th ed. Philadelphia: Saunders, 1999:533

Proto AV, Moser ES. Upper lobe volume loss: divergent and parallel patterns of vascular reorientation. Radiographics 1987;7:875–887

Woodring JH, Reed JC. Types and mechanisms of pulmonary atelectasis. J Thorac Imaging 1996; 11:92–108

CASE 38 Left Lower Lobe Collapse Caused by Bronchorrhea

Clinical Presentation

A 28-year-old man was in a recent motor vehicle accident had no audible breath sounds at the left lung base

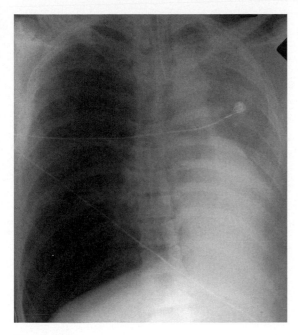

Figure 38A

Radiologic Findings

AP chest radiograph (**Fig. 38A**) demonstrates an opaque left lower hemithorax, abrupt cutoff of the left lower lobe bronchus, and marked leftward shift of the trachea and mediastinum. Notice the approximation of the left posterior ribs.

Diagnosis

Left lower lobe atelectasis caused by bronchorrhea relieved by bronchoscopy

Differential Diagnosis

Atelectasis secondary to other posttraumatic etiologies

Discussion

Background

Mediastinal shift is an *indirect* sign of volume loss and is usually a feature of acute atelectasis. The normal mediastinum is fairly mobile and reacts promptly to differences in pressure between the right and left hemithoraces. The anterior and middle mediastinal compartments are more mobile than the posterior mediastinum. Thus, the former two compartments shift to a greater extent than the latter. Tracheal and upper mediastinal displacement are more prominent features of upper lobe collapse, whereas inferior mediastinal displacement is more typical of lower lobe collapse.

Clinical Findings

Affected patients may exhibit decreased oxygen saturations, altered A-a gradient, and diminished or absent breath sounds over the affected area.

Imaging Findings

- Shift in normal mediastinal relationships (**Fig. 38A**)
- Signs of compensatory overinflation in the nonaffected lung
- Increased opacity in the affected lung parenchyma (**Fig. 38A**)

Treatment

- Respiratory physiotherapy
- Bronchiolytics
- Occasionally bronchoscopy

Prognosis

- Good

PEARL_____

- Mediastinal shift is typically a feature of acute atelectasis and a helpful indirect sign of volume loss.

Suggested Reading

Fraser RS, Müller NL, Colman N, Paré PD. Atelectasis. In: Fraser RS, Müller NL, Colman N, Paré PD, eds. Fraser and Paré's Diagnosis of Diseases of the Chest, 4th ed. Philadelphia: Saunders, 1999:529

CASE 39 Left Upper Lobe Atelectasis: Central Hilar Neoplasm

Clinical Presentation

A 50-year-old woman with progressive dyspnea and new onset of chest pain

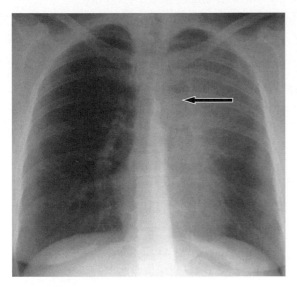

Figure 39A

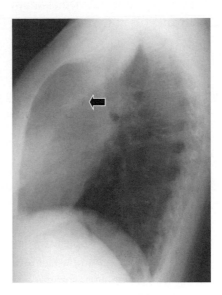

Figure 39B

Radiologic Findings

PA (**Fig. 39A**) and lateral (**Fig. 39B**) chest radiographs show an ill-defined left perihilar opacity and anterior displacement of the major fissure (short arrow). There is a discrepancy in volume between the right and left hemithoraces with compensatory overinflation of the right lung and attenuation of the pulmonary vasculature. Notice the hyperlucent air crescent (long arrow) between the left perihilar opacity and the aorta.

Diagnosis

Left upper lobe atelectasis from a central small cell carcinoma

Differential Diagnosis

Atelectasis from an endobronchial lesion

Discussion

Background

As lung collapses, the surrounding parenchyma overexpands to compensate for the volume loss. Compensatory overinflation is a reliable and important *indirect* sign of atelectasis. It is often inapparent in early lobar atelectasis but increases in conspicuity with progressive volume loss. Alterations in the normal vascular markings (e.g., wide separation in vessels and decrease in number of blood vessels per unit of lung volume) are helpful radiographic findings and often result in a

179

relative increased lucency in the affected lung. When the degree of volume loss is relatively small, compensatory overinflation is usually limited to the ipsilateral lung. Greater degrees of volume loss may be associated with overinflation of the contralateral lung and mediastinal displacement toward the atelectatic lung. The contralateral lung shifts across the mediastinum in one of three locations: (1) anterior mediastinum at the level of first three or four costal cartilages manifesting as displacement of the anterior junction line; (2) posterior-superior mediastinum (supra-aortic triangle) at the level of the third to fifth thoracic vertebrae; and (3) posterior-inferior mediastinum (retrocardiac space).

Clinical Findings

Patients may present with hypoxemia, progressive dyspnea, digital clubbing, diminished or absent breath sounds over the affected area, and various paraneoplastic syndromes (see Section VI).

Imaging Findings

- Increased left perihilar opacity that obscures left cardio-mediastinal border (**Fig. 39A**)
- Increased retrosternal opacity and anterior displacement of left major fissure on lateral radiography (**Fig. 39B**)
- Lüftsichel sign created by the overinflated superior segment of the lower lobe insinuating between the upper mediastinum and the opaque atelectatic upper lobe (**Fig. 39A**).
- Well-delineated crisp-appearing transverse aorta produced by the adjacent overinflated superior segment of the left lower lobe (**Fig. 39A**).

Treatment

- Directed toward the underlying disease process and relief of the obstruction (see Section VI)

Prognosis

- Good in cases of simple obstruction and atelectasis
- Complicated in cases of atelectasis from obstructing neoplasms (see Section VI)

PEARLS_____

- The radiologist must be careful not to misinterpret the Lüftsichel sign as right upper lobe herniation across the midline or as a left apical pneumothorax.
- The Lüftsichel sign is rarely seen in right upper lobe collapse.

Suggested Readings

Blankenbaker DG. The Lüftsichel sign. Radiology 1998;208:319–320

Fraser RS, Müller NL, Colman N, Paré PD. Atelectasis. In: Fraser RS, Müller NL, Colman N, Paré PD, eds. Fraser and Paré's Diagnosis of Diseases of the Chest, 4th ed. Philadelphia: Saunders, 1999: 529–532

Isbell D, Grinnan D, Patel MR. Lüftsichel sign in upper lobe collapse. Am J Med 2002;112:676–677

Woodring JH, Reed JC. Radiographic manifestations of lobar atelectasis. J Thorac Imaging 1996; 11:109–144

CASE 40 Right Middle Lobe Atelectasis: Central Neoplasm

Clinical Presentation

A 68-year-old man with a long history of tobacco abuse and a recent change in the nature of his chronic cough

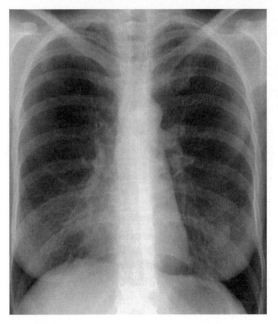

Figure 40A

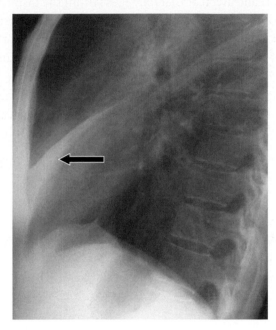

Figure 40B

Radiologic Findings

PA (**Fig. 40A**) chest radiograph reveals an ill-defined right perihilar opacity that partially obscures the right heart border and contains no air bronchograms. On the coned-down lateral radiograph (**Fig. 40B**), there is a corresponding triangular opacity with its base abutting the sternum and its apex directed toward the hilum. Notice the anterior displacement of the major fissure (arrow) and elevation of the right hemidiaphragm.

Diagnosis

Right middle lobe atelectasis from an endobronchial squamous cell carcinoma

Differential Diagnosis

- Simple right middle lobe atelectasis
- Right middle lobe pneumonia

181

Discussion

Background

Air bronchograms are a reliable sign that a process is in the lung parenchyma. The most common causes are pneumonia and pulmonary edema. Air bronchograms may also be seen in atelectatic lobes if the airway is patent. Compensatory signs of volume loss may be absent, as collapse is prevented by accumulation of fluid and alveolar macrophages within the distal airspaces, and by chronic inflammatory cells and fibrous tissue within the interstitium (e.g., obstructive pneumonitis). Resorption atelectasis is excluded if air is visible within the bronchial tree. If the obstruction is severe enough to cause absorption of air from the affected lobe, it must also result in absorption of gas from the airways. The normal right diaphragm is 1 to 2 cm higher than the left. In 2% of individuals it may be 3 cm higher or more. In 9% of individuals, the two hemidiaphragms lie at the same level, or the left diaphragm is slightly higher than the right. Diaphragmatic elevation is more often seen in acute as opposed to chronic atelectasis and is a more prominent feature of lower lobe than upper lobe atelectasis.

Clinical Findings

Patients may have a change in a preexistent cough or experience weight loss and intermittent hemoptysis. The affected hemithorax may be dull to percussion with diminished breath sounds on auscultation.

Treatment

- Directed toward the underlying disease process and relief of the obstruction (see Section VI)

Prognosis

- Dependent on the stage at presentation (Section VI)

PEARLS_____

- In the absence of air bronchograms, an underlying obstructing endobronchial mass must be excluded.
- Acute confluent bronchopneumonia (e.g., *Staphylococcus aureus*) with homogeneous opacification of a lobe or segment and bronchi filled with inflammatory exudate may also result in absent air bronchograms.

Suggested Readings

Fraser RS, Müller NL, Colman N, Paré PD. Atelectasis. In: Fraser RS, Müller NL, Colman N, Paré PD, eds. Fraser and Paré's Diagnosis of Diseases of the Chest, 4th ed. Philadelphia: Saunders, 1999: 533–534

Proto AV, Tocino I. Radiographic manifestations of lobar collapse. Semin Roentgenol 1980;15:117–173

CASE 41 Right Upper Lobe Atelectasis: Aspirated Tooth Fragment

Clinical Presentation

A 16-year-old in a motorcycle accident sustained significant maxillofacial trauma, and has diminished breath sounds over the right upper thorax.

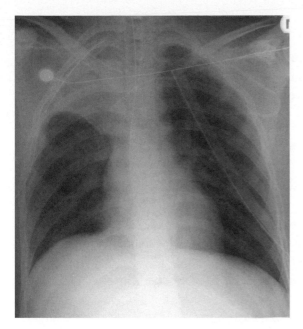

Figure 41A

Radiologic Findings

AP chest radiograph (**Fig. 41A**) shows a homogeneous opacity occupying the superior one third of the right lung with a curvilinear inferior border and an inconspicuous superior border. There is slight elevation of the right hemidiaphragm.

Diagnosis

Right upper lobe atelectasis from an aspirated tooth fragment

Differential Diagnosis

- Right upper lobe atelectasis secondary to posttraumatic bronchorrhea
- Right upper lobe atelectasis secondary to blood clot

Discussion

Background

The right upper lobe is bound inferiorly by the minor fissure and posteriorly by the major fissure. In upper lobe atelectasis, the middle and lower lobes overexpand and displace the collapsing upper lobe in a superior, anterior, and medial direction.

Clinical Findings

Affected patients may exhibit an altered A-a gradient, diminished oxygen saturations, and decreased breath sounds over the affected region. The physical examination may also reveal absent or fractured teeth, orthodontic hardware, or a foreign body, which may have been aspirated, leading to the endobronchial obstruction and subsequent volume loss.

Imaging Findings

- Minor fissure moves superiorly and medially and bows upward with its lateral border often higher than its medial border (**Fig. 41A**).
- Early stages: the displaced fissure may appear as a thin arcuate line.
- Progressive atelectasis: the displaced fissure appears as an arcuate interface between the opaque atelectatic lobe and the lucent overexpanded middle and lower lobes.
- Right hilum is often elevated, and the bronchus intermedius and descending pulmonary artery rotate laterally (**Fig. 41A**).
- Right upper lobe atelectasis may obscure the ipsilateral superior mediastinum (**Fig. 41A**).

Treatment

- Relief of the obstruction via bronchoscopy

Prognosis

- Good if recognized and treated promptly
- Delayed recognition may be complicated by recurrent infection, sepsis, bronchiectasis, and/or hemoptysis

PEARL_____

- Complete or near-complete upper lobe atelectasis may mimic an apical or superior mediastinal mass. Recognition of other indirect signs of volume loss is critical in making the appropriate diagnosis.

Suggested Readings

Felson B. The lobes. In: Felson B, ed. Chest Roentgenology. Philadelphia: Saunders, 1973:92–133

Fraser RS, Müller NL, Colman N, Paré PD. Atelectasis. In: Fraser and Paré's Diagnosis of Diseases of the Chest, 4th ed. Philadelphia: Saunders, 1999:539–543

Mintzer RA, Sakowicz BA, Blonder JA. Lobar collapse: usual and unusual forms. Chest 1988;94:615–620

Proto AV, Tocino I. Radiographic manifestations of lobar collapse. Semin Roentgenol 1980;15:117–173

Woodring JH, Reed JC. Radiographic manifestations of lobar atelectasis. J Thorac Imaging 1996;11:109–144

CASE 42 Right Upper Lobe Atelectasis with Reverse-S Sign of Golden

Clinical Presentation

A 58-year-old man with a long history of tobacco abuse, a worsening cough, and a recent episode of hemoptysis

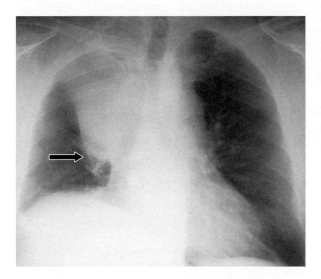

Figure 42A

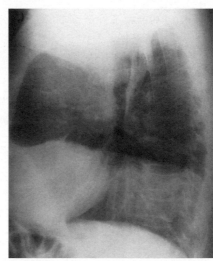

Figure 42B

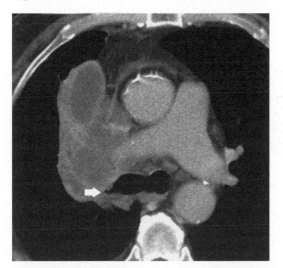

Figure 42C

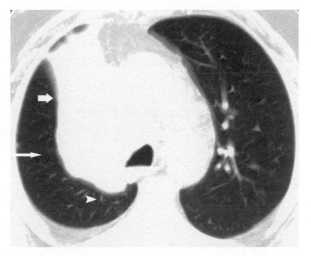

Figure 42D

Radiologic Findings

PA (**Fig. 42A**) and lateral (**Fig. 42B**) chest radiographs show a mass-like opacity involving the anterior-superior right hemithorax with well-defined borders. There is a focal convex bulge in the medial portion of the minor fissure at the bronchus intermedius (arrow) and elevation of the right hemidiaphragm. Contrast-enhanced chest CT (**Fig. 42C,** mediastinal window, and **Fig. 42D,** lung window) reveal an encased right upper lobe bronchus (arrow) with associated postobstructive changes, volume loss in the right hemithorax, and ipsilateral mediastinal shift. Notice the upward (short arrow) and medial (arrowhead) displacement of the minor fissure and the upward and forward displacement of the major fissure (long arrow).

Diagnosis

Right upper lobe atelectasis with reverse-S sign of Golden from small cell lung carcinoma

Differential Diagnosis

- Postobstructive upper lobe atelectasis from an endobronchial lesion
- Postobstructive upper lobe atelectasis from extrinsic bronchial compression by reactive or neoplastic lymphadenopathy

Discussion

Background

In noncomplicated right upper lobe atelectasis, the inferior border of the minor fissure should be concave on frontal and lateral radiographs. Right upper lobe atelectasis caused by a hilar mass (e.g., small cell carcinoma) is often associated with a convex bulge in the medial aspect of the fissure. The lateral aspect of the fissure is appropriately concave. The result is a reverse-S–shaped configuration of the minor fissure (i.e., reverse-S sign of Golden), a sign highly suggestive of a central neoplasm as the etiology of the atelectasis.

Clinical Findings

Affected patients may present with hypoxemia, progressive dyspnea, and hemoptysis, diminished or absent breath sounds over the affected area, and various paraneoplastic syndromes (see Section VI)

Imaging Findings

- Opaque right upper thorax
- Convex bulge medial aspect of displaced minor fissure (**Figs. 42A, 42B,** and **42C**)

Treatment

- Surgical resection
- Palliative chemotherapy and/or radiation therapy (see Section VI)

Prognosis

- Dependent on stage at presentation (i.e., limited vs extensive) (see Section VI)

PEARL_____

- The reverse-S sign of Golden may be exhibited by atelectasis of any lobe.

Suggested Readings

Golden R. The effect of bronchostenosis upon the roentgen-ray shadows in carcinoma of the bronchus. Am J Roentgenol Radiat Ther 1925;13:21–30

Proto AV, Tocino I. Radiographic manifestations of lobar collapse. Semin Roentgenol 1980;15:117–173

Reinig JW, Ross P. Computed tomography appearance of Golden's "S" sign. J Comput Tomogr 1984;8: 219–223

Woodring JH, Reed JC. Types and mechanisms of pulmonary atelectasis. J Thorac Imaging 1996;11: 92–108

CASE 43 Right Middle Lobe Atelectasis: Central Neoplasm

Clinical Presentation

A 68-year-old woman with cough and progressive dyspnea

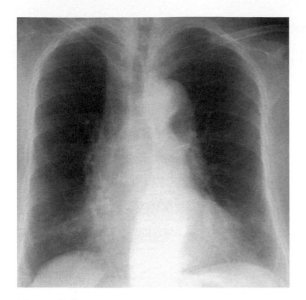

Figure 43A

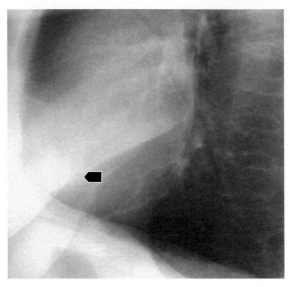

Figure 43B

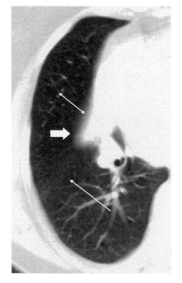

Figure 43C

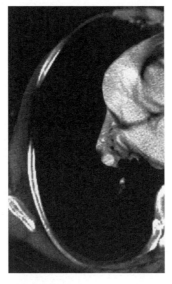

Figure 43D

Radiologic Findings

PA (**Fig. 43A**) chest radiograph reveals an ill-defined opacity in the right lower hemithorax that obscures the heart border. A corresponding triangular-shaped opacity (arrow), the base of which abuts the sternum, is seen on the coned-down lateral radiograph (**Fig. 43B**). Notice the concave configuration of the inferior margin of the anteriorly displaced major fissure (arrowhead). Contrast-enhanced chest CT (**Fig. 43C,** lung window, and **Fig. 43D,** mediastinal window) shows a triangular opacity with its apex pointing toward the lateral chest wall (short arrow). Note the anterior displacement of the major fissure (long arrow) and posterior displacement of the minor fissure (double arrow). No patent middle lobe bronchi are visualized.

Diagnosis

Right middle lobe atelectasis from an endobronchial carcinoid tumor

Differential Diagnosis

- Simple right middle lobe atelectasis
- Right middle lobe syndrome (e.g., remote granulomatous disease, bronchiectasis)

Discussion

Background

Middle lobe atelectasis is one of the most difficult diagnoses on frontal chest radiography and the easiest on lateral chest radiography. With progressive volume loss, the minor fissure and lower half of the major fissure approximate one another and nearly abut in complete middle lobe atelectasis.

Clinical Findings

The majority of central carcinoid tumors are associated with signs and symptoms of bronchial obstruction (e.g., cough, fever, chest pain, hemoptysis) (see Section VI).

Imaging Findings

RADIOGRAPHY

- Frontal radiography may demonstrate only obscuration of the right heart border (**Fig. 43A**)
- Lateral chest radiography demonstrates a well-defined, curved opacity bordered by the major and minor fissures, and extending anteriorly and inferiorly from the hilum (**Fig. 43B**)
- The collapsed middle lobe may be very thin and misinterpreted as a thickened fissure

CT

- Triangular opacity bounded posteriorly by the major fissure, medially by the mediastinum (i.e., right atrium) and anteriorly by the minor fissure (**Figs. 43C** and **43D**)
- Anterior margin is usually less defined than the posterior border
- Middle lobe bronchus enters the posteromedial corner of the triangular opacity (**Figs. 43C** and **43D**)

Treatment

- Conservative local therapies [e.g., segmentectomy, sleeve resection, neodymium:yttrium-aluminum-garnet (Nd-YAG) laser]
- Surgical lobectomy (see Section VI)

Prognosis

- 10-year survival rates: 90–95%
- Regional lymph node metastases < 5% cases (see Section VI)

PEARLS

- Lingular atelectasis resembles middle lobe atelectasis. Frontal chest radiography may reveal obscuration of the left heart border. Lateral chest radiography may show a thin triangular opaque band similar to that observed with middle lobe collapse. Mediastinal shift and signs of compensatory overinflation are usually absent.
- Because the collapsed middle lobe is oriented obliquely, it may only be appreciated on one or two axial CT images.

Suggested Readings

Naidich DP, Ettinger N, Leitman BS, et al. CT of lobar collapse. Semin Roentgenol 1984;19:222–235

Proto AV, Tocino I. Radiographic manifestations of lobar collapse. Semin Roentgenol 1980;15:117–173

CASE 44 Multilobar Collapse: Allergic Bronchopulmonary Aspergillosis

Clinical Presentation

A 68-year-old woman with a history of asthma and chronic cough empirically treated for pneumonia without clinical improvement

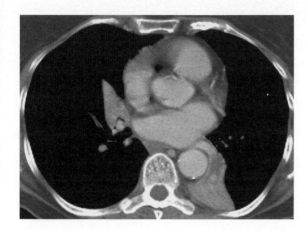

Figure 44A (Courtesy of Malcolm K. Sydnor, M.D., Medical College of Virginia Hospitals–Virginia Commonwealth University Health System, Richmond, Virginia.)

Radiologic Findings

Chest CT (**Fig. 44A**; mediastinal window) reveals total collapse of the right middle and left lower lobes. Notice the mucus-filled bronchi in the collapsed left lower lobe.

Diagnosis

Multilobar collapse from allergic bronchopulmonary aspergillosis (ABPA)

Differential Diagnosis

- Nonneoplastic causes of multilobar collapse (e.g., mucous plugs, aspirated foreign bodies, postinfectious or postinflammatory airway stenosis)
- Neoplastic disease

Discussion

Background

The double-lesion sign was originally described by Felson. The basic premise is that if a single endobronchial lesion cannot explain the collapse of multiple lobes or segments, then one has a reasonable level of confidence that a neoplasm is not responsible. For example, one might expect that because of the independent anatomic relationship of the right upper and middle lobe bronchi, it would be unusual for a single endobronchial lesion to cause simultaneous collapse of both lobes. However, most cases do indeed prove to be the result of a malignancy. A single endobronchial lesion in the bronchus intermedius could explain combined middle and lower lobe collapse, but lung cancer is unlikely to be responsible for combined collapse of the left lower lobe and any other segment of the upper lobe. Similarly, the simultaneous collapse of lobes or segments in different lungs is invariably the result of nonneoplastic disease.

Clinical Findings

Patients with ABPA may suffer from asthma and often present with bronchospasm, initially episodic but later becoming more chronic. Affected patients may expectorate brown mucous plugs and experience intermittent fever, hemoptysis, and recurrent pneumonia.

Imaging Findings

- Each individual collapsed lobe or segment demonstrates its own typical radiographic pattern of volume loss (**Fig. 44A**) (also see Cases 41–47).

Treatment

- Bronchoscopy
- Corticosteroids
- Itraconazole

Prognosis

- Most patients with ABPA respond well to treatment.
- Multilobar obstruction and collapse secondary to malignancy: prognosis is poor due to its advanced stage and invasion.

PEARLS_____

- The double-lesion sign does not always invalidate primary lung cancer as the cause of multilobar collapse. Combined right upper and middle lobe collapse may occur with tumor infiltration of both lobar bronchi. The tumor may obstruct one bronchus, and metastatic adenopathy may obstruct the second bronchus. It is also possible to have simultaneous multicentric neoplasms or a benign lesion affecting one bronchus (e.g., tuberculosis) and malignancy affecting the second bronchus.
- Think about ABPA in asthmatic patients with no other explanation for lobar collapse.

Suggested Readings

Felson B. The lobes. In: Felson B, ed. *Chest Roentgenology*. Philadelphia: Saunders, 1973:128–133

Franguet T, Muller NL, Gimenez A, Guembe P, de La Torre J, Bague S. Spectrum of pulmonary aspergillosis: histologic, clinical, and radiologic findings. Radiographics 2001;21:825–837

Gotway MB, Dawn SK, Caoili EM, Reddy GP, Araoz PA, Webb WR. The radiologic spectrum of pulmonary aspergillus infection. J Comput Assist Tomogr 2002;26:159–173

CASE 45 Left Upper Lobe Atelectasis: An Obstructing Central Small Cell Lung Carcinoma

Clinical Presentation

A 50-year-old woman with chest pain

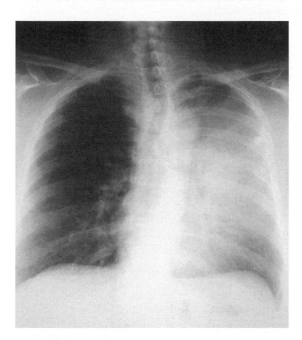

Figure 45A

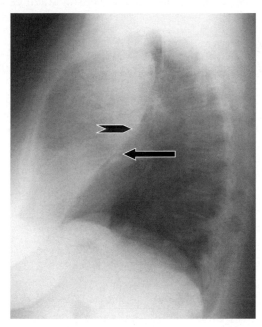

Figure 45B

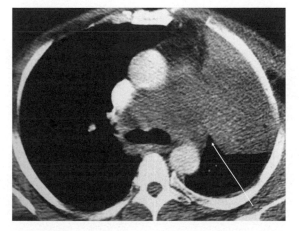

Figure 45C

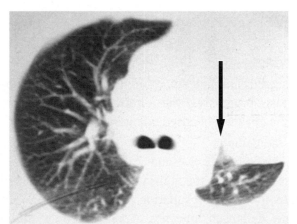

Figure 45D

Radiologic Findings

PA (**Fig. 45A**) and lateral (**Fig. 45B**) chest radiographs show an ill-defined left perihilar and upper lobe opacity without perceptible air bronchograms. There is marked anterior displacement of the oblique fissure (arrow). A hyperlucent crescent insinuates between the opacity and the transverse aorta on the PA radiograph and outlines the aortic arch on the lateral radiograph. A focal convexity (arrowhead) is in the left hilar region at the expected location of the inconspicuous upper lobe bronchus. Contrast-enhanced chest CT (**Fig. 45C**, mediastinal window, and **Fig. 45D**, lung window) reveals a precarinal and aorticopulmonary window mass producing the focal convexity in the left hilum (Golden S sign). The overinflated superior segment of the lower lobe (long arrow) accounts for the radiographic Lüftsichel sign.

Diagnosis

Left upper lobe atelectasis from an obstructing central small cell lung carcinoma

Differential Diagnosis

Left upper lobe atelectasis secondary to other endobronchial lesions

Discussion

Background

Atelectasis of the entire left upper lobe is more common than isolated lingular atelectasis. The left upper lobe collapses in a superior and anterior direction, while pushed by the overexpanding lower lobe, and is easier to recognize on lateral chest radiography. Anterior displacement of the major fissure is the most helpful and reliable sign.

Clinical Findings

Affected patients may present with hypoxemia, progressive dyspnea, digital clubbing, diminished or absent breath sounds over the affected area, and various paraneoplastic syndromes (Section VI).

Imaging Findings

RADIOGRAPHY

- Lateral chest radiography
  - The displaced fissure and collapsing upper lobe first appear as a thin arcuate line.
  - As atelectasis progresses, the anteriorly displaced fissure is seen as an arcuate interface between the opaque, collapsed upper lobe and the lucent, overexpanded lower lobe (**Fig. 45B**).
- Frontal chest radiography
  - Crowding of the bronchovascular markings may be the only early radiographic sign.
  - As collapse progresses, the atelectatic lobe appears as a homogeneous opacity, radiating from the ipsilateral hilum in a superior, lateral, and inferior direction.
  - The opaque collapsed lobe has a poorly defined lateral edge and obscures the superior mediastinum (**Fig. 45A**).
- Additional signs on frontal chest radiography include
  - Elevation of the left hilum
  - A more horizontal lie of the left mainstem bronchus
  - Superior displacement of the lower lobe bronchus and descending pulmonary artery
  - Lüftsichel sign is more often present than absent (**Fig. 45A**).
- Severe atelectasis
  - Upper lobe may become flattened against the anterior chest wall and inapparent on frontal radiography.
  - Collapsed lobe may be visualized only as a narrow band-like opacity paralleling the sternum on lateral radiography.

CT

- Wedge-shaped opacity with apex directed posteriorly, and its base against the anterior chest wall, representing the atelectatic left upper lobe (**Figs. 45C** and **4D**).
- Offending or causative lesion may be visualized.

Treatment

- Surgical resection
- Palliative chemotherapy and/or radiation therapy (see Section VI)

Prognosis

- Dependent on stage at presentation (i.e., limited vs extensive) (see Section VI)

PEARL_____

- Atelectasis from simple obstruction should not be considered when a focal convexity (Golden S sign) and a drowned lobe are present.

Suggested Readings

Fraser RS, Müller NL, Colman N, Paré PD. Atelectasis. In: Fraser RS, Müller NL, Colman N, Paré PD, eds. Fraser and Paré's Diagnosis of Diseases of the Chest, 4th ed. Philadelphia: Saunders, 1999:539–543

Mintzer RA, Sakowicz BA, Blonder JA. Lobar collapse: usual and unusual forms. Chest 1988;94:615–620

Woodring JH, Reed JC. Radiographic manifestations of lobar atelectasis. J Thorac Imaging 1996;11: 109–144

CASE 46 Right Lower Lobe Atelectasis: Small Cell Lung Cancer

Clinical Presentation

A 37-year-old woman with new onset of seizures and brain metastases

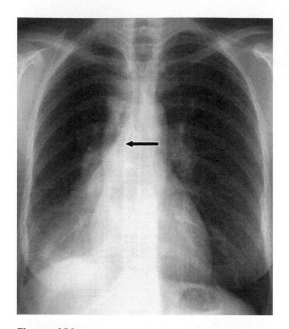

Figure 46A

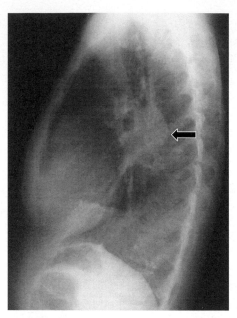

Figure 46B

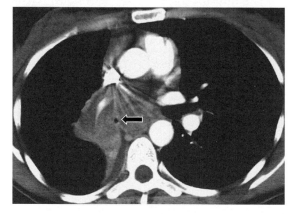

Figure 46C

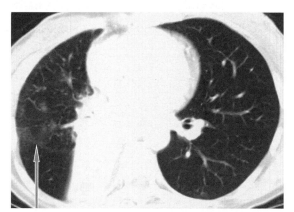

Figure 46D

Radiologic Findings

PA (**Fig. 46A**) and lateral (**Fig. 46B**) chest radiographs show a mass in the azygoesophageal recess (arrow), medial to the bronchus intermedius on the frontal radiograph, and a convex retrohilar mass (arrow), related to the bronchus intermedius and proximal lower lobe bronchi on the lateral exam. There is inferior displacement of the right hilum. The right interlobar artery and the proximal lower lobe bronchus are inconspicuous. The major fissure is displaced inferiorly and caudad. Contrast-enhanced chest CT (**Fig. 46C,** mediastinal window, and **Fig. 46D,** lung window) reveals a heterogeneous subcarinal and right infrahilar mass that encases the bronchus intermedius (arrow) and the interlobar artery. The middle lobe bronchi are narrowed but patent. There is obliteration of the lower lobe bronchi with distal atelectasis and consolidation as well as inferior, medial, and posterior displacement of the major fissure (long arrow).

Diagnosis

Right lower lobe atelectasis from small cell lung cancer

Differential Diagnosis

Right lower lobe atelectasis from other lesions

Discussion

Background

Both lower lobes collapse in a posterior, inferior, and medial direction. The lower lobes are bound anteriorly by the major fissure and attached to the mediastinum and medial diaphragm by the pulmonary ligament. Thus, collapse occurs posteromedially and inferiorly against the lower mediastinum.

Clinical Findings

Affected patients may present with hypoxemia, progressive dyspnea, and hemoptysis, diminished or absent breath sounds over the affected area, and various paraneoplastic syndromes (see Section VI).

Imaging Findings

- Upper half of the major fissure shifts inferiorly and the lower half posteriorly (**Figs. 46A** and **46D**).
- Minor fissure may or may not shift inferiorly.
- Atelectatic right lower lobe obscures the hemidiaphragm, paraspinal interface, and inferior vena cava; right heart border remains visible (**Figs. 46A** and **46B**).
- Atelectatic left lower lobe obscures the hemidiaphragm, paraspinal interface, and descending thoracic aorta; left heart border remains visible.
- Other radiographic features include
  - Inferior and medial displacement of the ipsilateral hilum and mainstem bronchus
  - Reorientation of the mainstem and lower lobe bronchi into a more vertical plane.
  - Narrowing of the carinal angle (**Fig. 46A**)
  - Interlobar pulmonary artery is incorporated into the atelectatic lower lobe, becomes inconspicuous, and the hilum appears small (**Fig. 46A**).
- As the degree of lower lobe atelectasis progresses
  - Opaque atelectatic lobe assumes a triangular morphology (**Fig. 46A**).
  - Apex is directed toward the hilum (**Fig. 46A**).
  - Base toward the hemidiaphragm (**Fig. 46A**)

Treatment

- Surgical resection
- Palliative chemotherapy and/or radiation therapy (see Section VI)

Prognosis

- Dependent on stage at presentation (i.e., limited vs extensive) (see Section VI)

PEARLS

- Loss of definition of the ipsilateral interlobar artery and a small or inapparent ipsilateral hilum are cardinal signs of lower lobe atelectasis.
- Because both lower lobes are large in volume, compensatory signs of volume loss are present, and their recognition may prevent the misdiagnosis of pleural effusion.

Suggested Readings

Fraser RS, Müller NL, Colman N, Paré PD. Atelectasis. In: Fraser RS, Müller NL, Colman N, Paré PD, eds. Fraser and Paré's Diagnosis of Diseases of the Chest, 4th ed. Philadelphia: Saunders, 1999:552

Mintzer RA, Sakowicz BA, Blonder JA. Lobar collapse: usual and unusual forms. Chest 1988;94: 615–620

Woodring JH, Reed JC. Radiographic manifestations of lobar atelectasis. J Thorac Imaging 1996;11: 109–144

CASE 47 Combined Right Middle and Lower Lobe Atelectasis

Clinical Presentation

A 47-year-old woman had a recent hysterectomy and now has tachypnea and diminished breath sounds on the right.

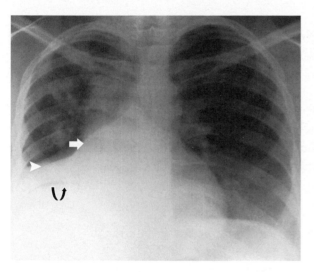

Figure 47A

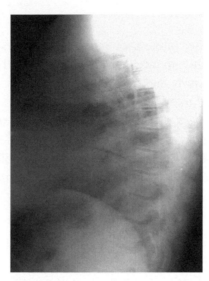

Figure 47B

Radiologic Findings

PA (**Fig. 47A**) and lateral (**Fig. 47B**) chest radiographs show inferior and caudal displacement of the major fissure (straight arrow), and inferior displacement of the minor fissure (arrowhead). A radiopacity obscures the right heart border, the hemidiaphragm, and the posteroinferior thorax. There is significant right-sided volume loss and ipsilateral mediastinal shift. Postoperative pneumoperitoneum (curved arrow) demonstrates the degree of diaphragmatic elevation.

Diagnosis

Combined right middle and lower lobe atelectasis from a mucous plug in the bronchus intermedius

Differential Diagnosis

- Isolated right lower lobe atelectasis
- Right subpulmonic pleural effusion

Discussion

Background

Simultaneous collapse of the right middle and lower lobes localizes the obstructing lesion to the bronchus intermedius.

199

Clinical Findings

Affected patients may present with hypoxia, altered A-a gradient, diminished or absent breath sounds over the affected area.

Imaging Findings

RADIOGRAPHY

FRONTAL CHEST

- Obscured right atrial border (atelectatic middle lobe) (**Fig. 47A**)
- Obscured right hemidiaphragm (atelectatic lower lobe) (**Fig. 47A**)
- Major fissure moves inferiorly and medially and maintains a convex lateral border. (**Fig. 47A**).
- Minor fissure is displaced inferiorly (**Fig. 47A**).
- Both fissures are more inferiorly displaced laterally than medially (**Fig. 47A**).
- Combination may be misinterpreted as isolated lower lobe collapse.
  - If the opacity extends to the costophrenic angle, combined lobar collapse is likely (**Fig. 47A**).
  - If the minor fissure is visualized in its normal anatomic position, isolated lower lobe atelectasis is favored.

LATERAL CHEST

- Atelectatic lobes create an opacity over the inferior hemithorax extending from the anterior to posterior chest wall (**Fig. 47B**).
- Opacity may demonstrate either a convex or concave superior border that can be misinterpreted as a subpulmonic effusion.
  - Identification of both the major and minor fissures in their normal locations favors a subpulmonic effusion.
  - Superior border of a subpulmonic effusion is usually flat where the fluid interfaces with the lung base.

Treatment

- Respiratory physiotherapy, bronchiolytics, and bronchodilators
- Bronchoscopy when indicated

Prognosis

- Good

PEARLS_____

- Compensatory signs of volume loss and ipsilateral mediastinal shift are invariably present because of the large volume lost when the two lobes collapse.
- Combined lobar atelectasis produces opacity higher medially at the hilum and lower laterally at the costophrenic angle. Pleural effusion creates opacity higher laterally against the chest wall.

Suggested Readings

Fraser RS, Müller NL, Colman N, Paré PD. Atelectasis. In: Fraser and Paré's Diagnosis of Diseases of the Chest, 4th ed. Philadelphia: Saunders, 1999:554

Mintzer RA, Sakowicz BA, Blonder JA. Lobar collapse: usual and unusual forms. Chest 1988;94:615–620

Woodring JH, Reed JC. Radiographic manifestations of lobar atelectasis. J Thorac Imaging 1996;11:109–144

CASE 48 Total Atelectasis of the Left Lung from Malpositioned Endotracheal Tube

Clinical Presentation

A pediatric burn victim with an acute onset of respiratory distress and oxygen desaturation

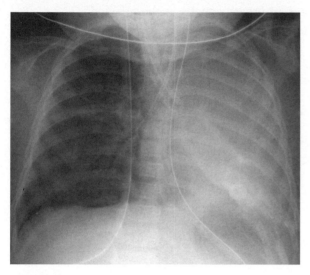

Figure 48A

Radiologic Findings

AP chest radiograph (**Fig. 48A**) demonstrates an opaque left hemithorax with marked overinflation of the right lung and ipsilateral mediastinal shift. The endotracheal tube is malpositioned with the tip in the right mainstem bronchus.

Diagnosis

Total atelectasis of the left lung from inadvertent right mainstem bronchus intubation

Differential Diagnosis

None

Discussion

Background

Atelectasis of an entire lung is common and more often affects the left lung. Mainstem bronchus obstruction from any etiology may produce ipsilateral atelectasis. Complete atelectasis of either lung is usually associated with complete opacification of the ipsilateral hemithorax, ipsilateral mediastinal shift, diaphragmatic elevation, and compensatory overinflation of the contralateral lung, and may be misinterpreted as a massive unilateral pleural effusion or pneumonia. Massive unilateral pleural effusion behaves as a space-occupying lesion and enlarges the affected hemithorax. Thus, the ipsilateral hemidiaphragm is depressed or inverted, and the mediastinum shifts to the contralateral side. Diffuse unilateral pneumonia may completely opacify a hemithorax and obscures the ipsilateral hemidiaphragm and mediastinal borders, but the lung volume remains the same, and signs of atelectasis are absent.

Clinical Findings

Complete atelectasis of a lung is associated with diminished or absent breath sounds in the affected hemithorax. Patients may experience tachypnea, tachycardia, and an abrupt drop in oxygen saturations.

Imaging Findings

- Opacification of the affected hemithorax (**Fig. 48A**)
- Ipsilateral mediastinal shift (**Fig. 48A**)
- Ipsilateral diaphragmatic elevation (**Fig. 48A**)
- Compensatory overinflation of the contralateral lung (**Fig. 48A**)

Treatment

- Correction of the malpositioned tube

Prognosis

- Good if recognized early and treated promptly
- Delayed recognition and treatment may be complicated by barotrauma

PEARLS_____

- Malpositioned endotracheal tube should be excluded in critical care patients with isolated upper lobe or complete lung atelectasis. In these settings, atelectasis occurs rapidly.
- Understanding direct and indirect signs of volume loss allows the radiologist to exclude massive unilateral effusion or diffuse unilateral pneumonia in cases of complete lung atelectasis.

Suggested Readings

Fraser RS, Müller NL, Colman N, Paré PD. Atelectasis. In: Fraser RS, Müller NL, Colman N, Paré PD, eds. Fraser and Paré's Diagnosis of Diseases of the Chest, 4th ed. Philadelphia: Saunders, 1999:517–539

Proto AV, Tocino I. Radiographic manifestations of lobar collapse. Semin Roentgenol 1980;15:117–173

Woodring JH, Reed JC. Radiographic manifestations of lobar atelectasis. J Thorac Imaging 1996; 11:109–144

CASE 49 Rounded Atelectasis

Clinical Presentation

A 63-year-old man employed as a construction worker with a 50-pack-year history of tobacco abuse complains of chronic cough.

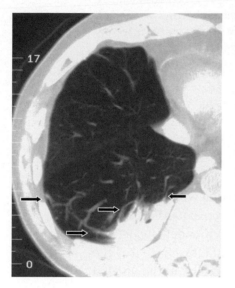

Figure 49A

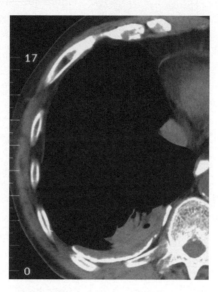

Figure 49B

Radiologic Findings

Unenhanced chest CT (**Fig. 49A,** lung window, and **Fig. 49B,** mediastinal window) reveals an ovoid soft tissue mass in the medial posterior basal segment right lower lobe abutting the costovertebral pleura. The mass contains air bronchograms, and several vessels (arrows) are drawn in toward its superior and lateral borders. There is focal pleural thickening and calcification adjacent to the mass.

Diagnosis

Rounded atelectasis, a manifestation of asbestos-related pleural disease

Synonyms

- Round atelectasis
- Folded lung
- Asbestos pseudotumor

Differential Diagnosis

- Primary lung cancer
- Pneumonia

203

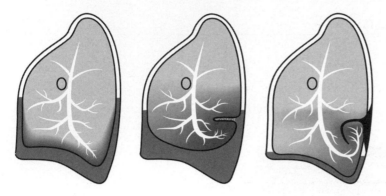

Figure 49C Artistic rendition illustrating the formation of rounded atelectasis as a sequela to an antecedent pleural effusion. See discussion in text.

Discussion

Background

Rounded atelectasis is a distinct form of relaxation atelectasis seen in association with focal pleural thickening. Decortication of the adjacent pleura is often associated with reexpansion of the atelectatic lung. Two hypotheses have been proposed for the development of rounded atelectasis. The first is predicated on a preexistent pleural effusion (**Fig. 49C**). The pleural effusion causes the adjacent lower lobe to float upward and compresses the lung. A cleft or fold occurs in the visceral pleura if the rate of pleural fluid accumulation exceeds the rate of alveolar air resorption. The lung then begins to tilt and curl on itself in a concentric fashion along this cleft. Fibrinous adhesions along this cleft suspend the atelectatic segment of lung. As the effusion resorbs, aerated lung fills in the space around the rounded atelectasis. Organization of the fibrinous exudate and fibrous contraction causes the affected lung to remain "balled up" as a mass-like lesion. The second, and currently more accepted, theory suggests an irritant, such as asbestos, induces local pleuritis that causes the pleura to thicken and contract. The adjacent lung "shrinks," and the atelectasis develops in a rounded configuration.

Clinical Findings

Most cases of rounded atelectasis occur in patients with a history of asbestos exposure. Other manifestations of asbestos exposure may be observed in such patients (e.g., pleural plaques). However, rounded atelectasis has also been described in association with pleural effusions of tuberculous and nontuberculous etiologies, pulmonary infarction, iatrogenic pneumothorax, heart failure, following surgical coronary artery revascularization, malignant pleural disease, etc. Rounded atelectasis itself is not associated with any symptoms.

Imaging Findings

RADIOGRAPHY

- 2 to 8 cm focal juxtapleural mass with adjacent pleural thickening in the posterolateral or posteromedial aspect of the lower lobes
- Adjacent bronchovascular bundles drawn together in a curvilinear fashion toward the medial margin of the mass
- Adjacent lung overexpands and is oligemic
- Remains relatively stable in size and shape over time

CT

- Ovoid or rounded parenchymal lesion that ranges from 2 to 8 cm in diameter (**Figs. 49A** and **49B**)
- Adjacent pleural thickening and hypertrophy of the subcostal fat
- Adjacent bronchi and vessels are tethered together and converge on the medial margin of the mass, creating the "parachute cord" or "comet tail" sign (**Fig. 49A**).
- Central or hilar aspect of the mass is often ill defined where the vessels are drawn together, lateral margin of the mass is better defined (**Fig. 49A**).
- Air bronchograms visualized in approximately 18% lesions
- Additional signs of asbestos exposure (e.g., plaques) observed in 20 to 60% of cases (**Fig. 49B**)

Treatment

- None
- Pleural decortication for patients with restrictive physiology

Prognosis

- Good; benign process with no malignant potential
- Majority of lesions remain stable for years.
- Occasionally, the region of "folded" lung may slightly decrease or even increase in size.
- Total regression sometimes occurs but is unusual in patients with asbestos-related pleural disease.

PEARLS

- Although most cases occur in patients with a history of asbestos exposure, rounded atelectasis is not pathognomonic of such exposure, and may result from a variety of pleural and parenchymal insults.
- It may be necessary to differentiate rounded atelectasis from carcinoma in problematic cases.
- Rounded atelectasis is metabolically inactive on PET imaging which can be used to differentiate atypical/or problematic cases from potential peripheral lung cancer.

Suggested Readings

Batra P, Brown K, Hayashi K, Mori M. Rounded atelectasis. J Thorac Imaging 1996;11:187–197

Hillerdal G. Rounded atelectasis: clinical experience with 74 patients. Chest 1989;95:836–841

McHugh K, Blaquiere RM. CT features of rounded atelectasis. AJR Am J Roentgenol 1989;153:257–260

CASE 50 Right Middle Lobe Syndrome

Clinical Presentation

A 48-year old man with a long history of tobacco abuse and chronic cough

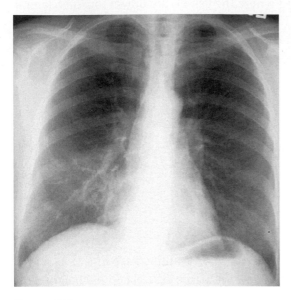

Figure 50A

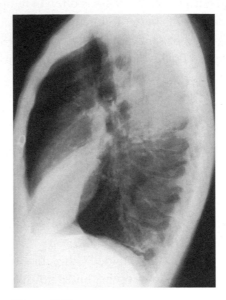

Figure 50B

Radiologic Findings

PA (**Fig. 50A**) chest radiograph demonstrates a vague opacity in the lower right hemithorax that obscures the right heart border. A retrosternal triangular opacity with its base against the sternum and apex directed toward the hilum is seen on the lateral chest radiograph (**Fig. 50B**). The lungs are hyperexpanded, consistent with underlying chronic obstructive lung disease. PA and lateral chest radiographs from 3 years earlier (not illustrated) demonstrated the same findings.

Diagnosis

Right middle lobe syndrome (RMLS)

Synonyms

- Brock syndrome
- Middle lobe syndrome

Differential Diagnosis

- Middle lobe pneumonia
- Middle lobe obstruction secondary to an endobronchial lesion

206

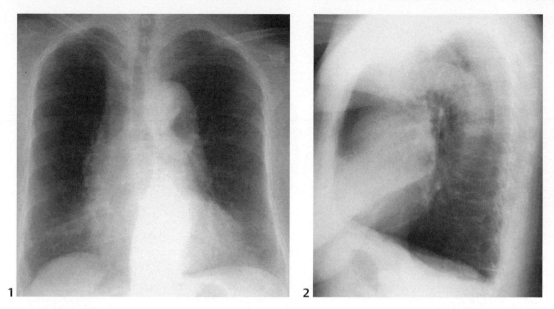

Figure 50C (1) PA chest radiograph of a 68-year-old woman with chronic cough shows an ill-defined opacity in the lower right thorax that obliterates the right heart border. **(2)** The lateral radiograph reveals the characteristic retrosternal triangular opacity of middle lobe collapse. Note the concave configuration of the undersurface of the inferior major fissure. This exam was unchanged when compared with chest radiographs from 3 years earlier.

Discussion

Background

Middle lobe syndrome is an uncommon lung disorder associated with recurrent atelectasis, pneumonias, or bronchiectasis of the right middle lobe, lingula, or both. The relative narrow diameter of the middle lobe bronchus and its acute angle off the tracheobronchial tree hinder drainage and clearance of secretions. The middle lobe syndrome is characterized as either obstructive or nonobstructive. Bronchial obstruction can result from aspiration of foreign bodies, endobronchial tumors, mucous plugs, postinflammatory granulation tissue and broncholithiasis, or extrinsic compression from hilar lymphadenopathy. Asthma-associated edema, inflammation, and bronchospasm are the most common nonobstructive causes, especially in children.

Clinical Findings

The most common symptoms include a persistent or recurrent cough, recurrent or chronic pneumonia, intermittent wheezing, and dyspnea. Less common symptoms include hemoptysis, low-grade fever, chest pain, and weight loss. Some patients are asymptomatic. Rales, fine wheezes, and diffuse rhonchi may be heard on auscultation.

Imaging Findings
RADIOGRAPHY

- Frontal radiography
  - Obscuration of the right heart border (**Figs. 50A** and **50C**) with right middle lobe collapse
  - Obscuration of the left heart border with lingular collapse

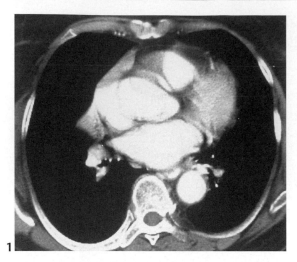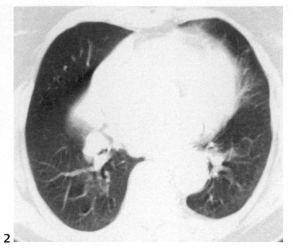

Figure 50D 1,2 Contrast enhanced chest CT [mediastinal (1) and lung window (2)] demonstrates a triangular opacity, the apex of which points peripherally. Notice the anterior displacement of the major fissure and the posterior displacement of the minor fissure.

- Lateral chest radiography
  - Well-defined curved opacity bordered by the major and minor fissures, and extending anteriorly and inferiorly from the hilum (**Figs. 50B** and **50C**)
- Collapsed middle lobe may be very thin and misinterpreted as a thickened fissure
- Consolidation or volume loss in middle lobe or lingula
- Patchy airspace opacity in middle lobe or lingula
- Middle lobe or lingular bronchiectasis

CT

- Patchy airspace opacity in middle lobe or lingula
- Consolidation or volume loss in middle lobe or lingula (**Fig. 50D1**)
- Triangular opacity bounded posteriorly by the major fissure, medially by the mediastinum (i.e., right atrium), and anteriorly by the minor fissure (**Fig. 50D2**)
  - Anterior margin is usually less defined than the posterior border.
  - Middle lobe bronchus enters the posteromedial corner of the triangular opacity (**Figs. 50D1** and **D2**).
- Middle lobe and lingular bronchiectasis seen to better advantage than with radiography

Treatment

- Directed toward underlying cause
- Respiratory therapy, bronchodilators, mucolytics, and postural drainage
- Bronchoscopy
- Low-dose roxithromycin
- Lobectomy is indicated in cases of malignancy, bronchial stenosis, and recurrent infection or hemoptysis refractory to medical management.
- 22% of patients require lobectomy.

Prognosis

- Resolution in one third of pediatric patients after bronchoscopy
- Resolution in one third of patients with medical management alone

PEARL_____

- Serial radiographs demonstrating chronic right middle lobe or lingular volume loss are critical to making the correct diagnosis.

Suggested Readings

Ayed Adel K. Resection of the right middle lobe and lingula in children with middle lobe/lingula syndrome. Chest 2004;125:38–42

De Boeck K, Williams T, Van Gysel D, Corbeel L, Eeckels R. Outcome after right middle lobe syndrome. Chest 1995;108:150–152

Gudmundsson G, Gross TJ. Middle lobe syndrome. Am Fam Physician 1996;53:2547–2550

Kawamura M, Arai Y, Tani M. Improvement in right lung atelectasis (middle lobe syndrome) following administration of low-dose roxithromycin. Respiration 2001;68:210–214

Kwon KY, Myers JL, Swenson SJ, Colby TV. Middle lobe syndrome: a clinicopathological study of 21 patients. Hum Pathol 1995;26:302–307

SECTION V
Pulmonary Infections and Aspiration Pneumonia

CASE 51 Streptococcus Pneumoniae Pneumonia

Clinical Presentation

A 38-year-old man with fever and cough productive of rusty blood-streaked sputum

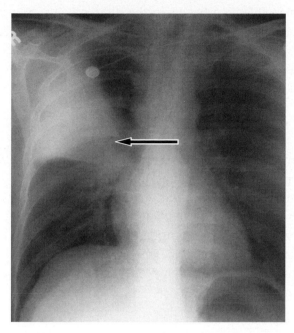

Figure 51A

Radiologic Findings

AP chest radiograph (**Fig. 51A**) shows dense, nonsegmental homogeneous right upper lobe consolidation abutting the minor fissure. Note the subtle air bronchograms medially (arrow).

Diagnosis

Pneumococcal pneumonia

Differential Diagnosis

Other community-acquired pneumonias

Discussion

Background

Most pneumococcal pulmonary infections occur in the winter and early spring. The organism is acquired through person-to-person transmission by aerosolized droplets, physical contact, or both. Risk factors for infection include very young or advanced age, chronic heart and/or lung disease, alcoholism and/or cirrhosis, sickle cell anemia, lymphoma, leukemia, multiple myeloma, HIV infection, intravenous drug abuse, and prior splenectomy.

Etiology

Pneumococcal pneumonia is caused by the gram-positive, diplococcal bacterium *Streptococcus pneumoniae*. It is the most common pathogen identified in patients admitted to the hospital and is likely responsible for > 50% of all community-acquired pneumonias. Infection begins in the distal airspaces, edema fluid rapidly accumulates, and the inflammatory exudate spreads contiguously and centrifugally from acinus to acinus, across segmental boundaries, resulting in confluent airspace consolidation confined only by pleural surfaces. Because alveolar air is replaced by exudate, there is little volume loss. Pneumococcal pneumonia is the prototype of lobar or airspace pneumonia.

Clinical Findings

Seventy percent of patients that develop pneumococcal pneumonia have had a recent upper respiratory tract infection. Additionally, pneumococcal pneumonia often complicates influenza. In fact, it is the most common bacterial pneumonia that occurs following infection with influenza. Patients with pneumococcal pneumonia often present with an abrupt onset of rigors, followed by fever, cough productive of rusty sputum, dyspnea, and pleuritic chest pain. Leukocytosis is usually present, but severe infection may be associated with white blood counts of less than 3000 cells/mm^3. Metastatic infection (e.g., endocarditis, meningitis, arthritis), pericarditis, and rarely empyema may occur as complications of pneumococcal pneumonia.

Pathology

GROSS

- Lobar consolidation

MICROSCOPIC

- Pulmonary infiltration by neutrophils
- Inflammatory exudate surrounded by edema

Imaging Findings

RADIOGRAPHY

- Homogeneous, nonsegmental, parenchymal consolidation typically involving one lobe, with a predilection for the lower lobes or posterior segments of the upper lobes (**Fig. 51A**)
- Mass-like rounded consolidation (i.e., round pneumonia) (**Fig. 51B**)
- Airspace disease abutting surrounding visceral pleura (**Fig. 51A**)
- Frequent air bronchograms (**Figs. 51A** and **51B**)
- Rare cavitation
- Minimal volume loss (**Figs. 51A** and **51B**)
- Pleural effusion common (60%); empyema is unusual

Treatment

- Antibiotic of choice: penicillin
- Antibiotic of choice for penicillin-resistant strains (30% of isolates): vancomycin

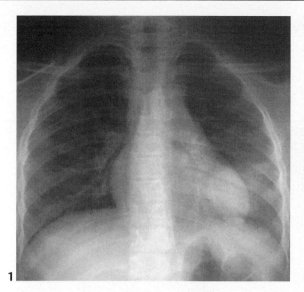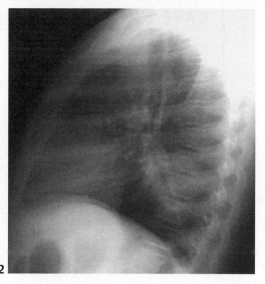

Figure 51B (1,2) PA **(1)** and lateral **(2)** chest radiographs of a 5-year-old child with round (pneumococcal) pneumonia reveal a homogeneous, ovoid opacity that partially obscures the left heart border and the T8–T10 vertebrae. Subtle air bronchograms are present, but there is no volume loss. (Courtesy of Stephanie E. Spottswood, M.D., Children's Hospital of the King's Daughters; Medical Center Radiologists, Norfolk, Virginia.)

Prognosis

- Onset of recovery within 24 to 48 hours of initiation of antibiotic therapy; resolution after 2 weeks
- Slow clearance in elderly patients, those requiring hospitalization, smokers, and patients with significant underlying lung disease and bacteremia; 4 to 8 week disease course in these cases
- Increased mortality in patients over 50 years, those with cirrhosis, cardiac or chronic pulmonary disease, asplenia, malignancy, bacteremia, and penicillin-resistant disease

PEARLS

- Absence of air bronchograms argues against the diagnosis of pneumococcal pneumonia.
- Round pneumonias are more frequently seen in children less than 8 years of age, but may be seen in adults. Adult infection rapidly progresses to more typical lobar pneumonia. Failure to do so should suggest underlying malignant neoplasia.

Suggested Readings

Fraser RS, Müller NL, Colman N, Paré PD. Pulmonary infection. In: Fraser and Paré's Diagnosis of Diseases of the Chest, 4th ed. Philadelphia: Saunders, 1999:736–743

Marrie TJ. Pneumococcal pneumonia: epidemiology and clinical features. Semin Respir Infect 1999;14:227–236

Reimer LG. Community-acquired bacterial pneumonias. Semin Respir Infect 2000;15:95–100

Travis WD, Colby TV, Koss MN, Rosado-de-Christenson ML, Müller NL, King TE Jr. Lung infections. In: King DW, ed. Atlas of Nontumor Pathology: Non-Neoplastic Disorders of the Lower Respiratory Tract, first series, fascicle 2. Washington, DC: American Registry of Pathology; 2002:541–544

Wagner AL, Szabunio M, Hazlett KS, Wagner SG. Radiologic manifestations of round pneumonia in adults. AJR Am J Roentgenol 1999;172:549–550

CASE 52 Staphylococcal Pneumonia

Clinical Presentation

An 11-year-old girl with fever, cough, and purulent sputum production

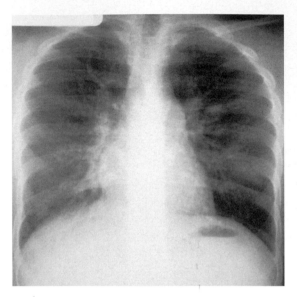

Figure 52A

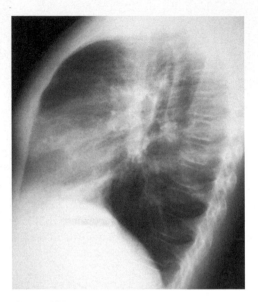

Figure 52B

Radiologic Findings

PA (**Fig. 52A**) and lateral (**Fig. 52B**) chest radiographs show multifocal, patchy consolidations in the anterior basal segment of the right lower lobe and the lateral segment of the right middle lobe.

Diagnosis

Staphylococcal pneumonia

Differential Diagnosis

Other community-acquired bronchopneumonias

Discussion

Background

Pulmonary infection occurs through hematogenous spread or aspiration of contaminated oral secretions; 20 to 40% of older children and adults and more than 50% of health care workers are nasal carriers of staphylococci. Staphylococcal pneumonia often complicates viral pneumonias (e.g., influenza) in adults and measles in children. Aspiration can lead to staphylococcal pneumonia in intubated patients and in those with underlying chronic obstructive lung disease and/or or lung cancer. Patients with contaminated vascular catheters and those with endocarditis (**Fig. 52C**) or intravenous drug abuse histories (**Fig. 52D**) may have hematogenous spread to the lungs. *Staphylococcus*

216

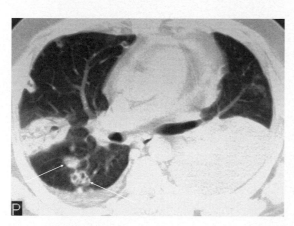

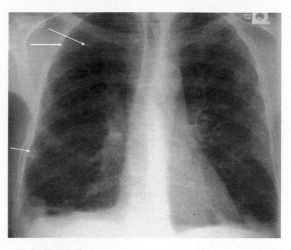

Figure 52C Contrast-enhanced chest CT (lung window) of a 41-year-old patient with a tricuspid valve murmur, fever, and endocarditis shows multiple parenchymal and juxtapleural nodules and consolidations of variable size. Many lesions are cavitated, and some exhibit associated feeding vessels (arrows).

Figure 52D PA chest radiograph of a 37-year-old intravenous drug abuser with hematogenous spread of staphylococcal infection reveals multiple, diffuse, bilateral, ill-defined nodules, some of which have cavitated (arrows). Note the right pleural effusion.

causes approximately 5% of community-acquired pneumonias, but it is responsible for more than 10% of hospital-acquired pneumonias.

Etiology

The gram-positive bacteria *Staphylococcus* sp., and most often *S. aureus*, cause the majority of cases of staphylococcal bronchopneumonia. Staphylococci produce toxins causing significant tissue destruction and the potential development of abscesses. The inflammatory exudate is multifocal and fills the large airways, following the course of the tracheobronchial tree. The consolidation is usually segmental and characterized by segmental volume loss and the lack of air bronchograms.

Clinical Findings

Patients with staphylococcal pneumonia may present with fever, cough, and purulent sputum production. Those with complicating pulmonary infarcts may complain of chest pain and may experience hemoptysis. Leukocytosis is common. Abscesses develop in 15 to 20% of patients with staphylococcal pneumonia (**Fig. 52E**). Pneumatoceles are uncommon in adults but occur in up to 40% of children with staphylococcal pneumonia (**Fig. 52F**). These thin-walled cystic spaces usually resolve over weeks to months but may rupture into the pleural space, causing spontaneous pneumothoraces. Empyema complicates staphylococcal pulmonary infection in 20% of affected adults (**Fig. 52G**) and 75% of affected children.

Pathology

GROSS

- Yellow-tan, pus-containing nodules related to the airways (e.g., aspiration) or the vasculature (e.g., hematogenous spread)
- Abscesses common
- Pleural invasion and/or empyema may or may not be present.

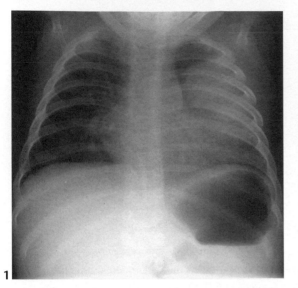
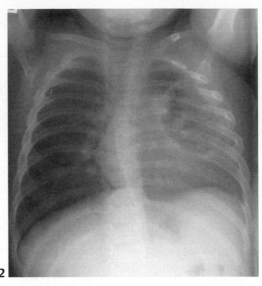

Figure 52E (1,2) AP chest radiograph **(1)** of a 9-month-old child with staphylococcal pneumonia who is toxic with a high fever following a 2-week course of antibiotics for otitis media shows a focal, ill-defined consolidation in the left upper lobe with volume loss. AP chest radiograph 6 days later **(2)** shows irregular cavitation in the consolidated upper lobe consistent with a lung abscess. (Courtesy of Das Narla, M.D., Medical College of Virginia Hospitals–Virginia Commonwealth University Health System, Richmond, Virginia.)

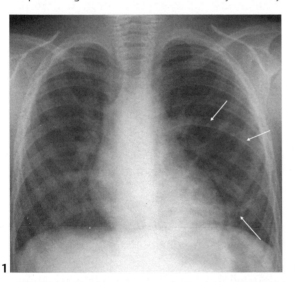
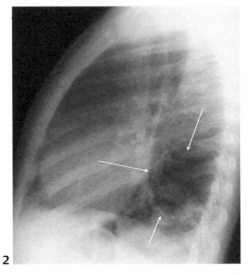

Figure 52F (1,2) AP **(1)** and lateral **(2)** chest radiographs of a 5-year-old child, 6 months after treatment for staphylococcal pneumonia, show a well-defined, thin-walled 6.0 cm pneumatocele (arrows) at the site of previous consolidation (not shown).

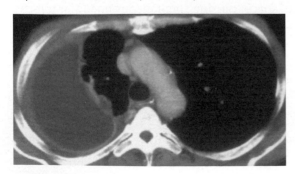

Figure 52G Contrast-enhanced chest CT (mediastinal window) of a 53-year-old man with empyema complicating staphylococcal pneumonia shows a right-sided lentiform fluid collection that exhibits the "split pleura" sign.

MICROSCOPIC

- Neutrophils in the airways and alveoli

Imaging Findings

RADIOGRAPHY

- Patchy, heterogeneous, multifocal, segmental airspace consolidation that usually affects the lower lobes (**Figs. 52A** and **52B**)
- Absence of air bronchograms (**Figs. 52A, 52B,** and **52E**)
- May develop abscess(es) with cavitation, irregular, shaggy, internal walls, and air-fluid levels (**Fig. 52E2**)
- Subpleural nodule(s) or mass(es), with associated feeding vessels, in cases with hematogenous spread of infection (e.g., septic emboli) (**Figs. 52D**)
- Volume loss (**Fig. 52E1**)
- Pleural effusion common (30–50%); progression to empyema in 50% of cases

CT/HRCT

- Any of the above radiographic findings
- Centrilobular nodules and "tree-in-bud" opacities may be visualized.
- Pleural effusion may be present.
- Empyema in untreated or complicated cases (**Fig. 52G**)

Treatment

- Intravenous β-lactam agents (e.g., nafcillin, oxacillin) or a first-generation cephalosporin (e.g., cefazolin)
- Vancomycin in cases of methicillin-resistant strains

Prognosis

- Mortality rate of 25 to 30%; increases to 80% with bacteremia

PEARLS_____

- Bronchopneumonia is the most common of the three patterns of pneumonia, the others being lobar pneumonia and interstitial pneumonia.
- If air bronchograms are present, bronchopneumonia is less likely.
- Septic emboli manifest as poorly defined juxtapleural opacities. Two thirds of such lesions have associated feeding vessels appreciated on CT (**Fig. 52C**). Juxtapleural wedge-shaped consolidations represent septic emboli complicated by pulmonary infarction.

Suggested Readings

Fraser RS, Müller NL, Colman N, Paré PD. Pulmonary infection. In: Fraser and Paré's Diagnosis of Diseases of the Chest, 4th ed. Philadelphia: Saunders, 1999:702–703,743–748

MacFarlane J, Rose D. Radiographic features of staphylococcal pneumonia in adults and children. Thorax 1996;51:539–540

Reimer LG. Community-acquired bacterial pneumonias. Semin Respir Infect 2000;15:95–100

Travis WD, Colby TV, Koss MN, Rosado-de-Christenson ML, Müller NL, King TE Jr. Lung infections. In: King DW, ed. Atlas of Nontumor Pathology: Non-Neoplastic Disorders of the Lower Respiratory Tract, first series, fascicle 2. Washington, DC: American Registry of Pathology; 2002:541–544.

CASE 53 *Haemophilus* Pneumonia

Clinical Presentation

A 22-year-old woman with a history of diabetes mellitus, cough, and fever

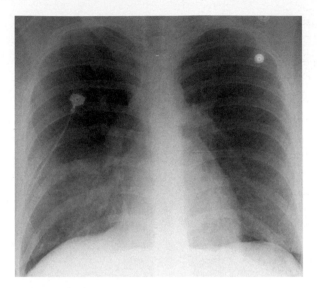

Figure 53A

Radiologic Findings

AP chest radiograph (**Fig. 53A**) shows patchy segmental right lower lobe consolidation.

Diagnosis

Haemophilus influenzae pneumonia

Differential Diagnosis

Other community-acquired bronchopneumonias

Discussion

Background

Haemophilus influenzae pulmonary infection is acquired through person-to-person transmission by aerosolized droplets deposited in the nasopharynx. The nasopharynx is colonized in up to 90% of children by 5 years of age. Many patients with chronic obstructive lung disease are also colonized. Those persons at most risk for pulmonary infection by *Haemophilus influenzae* include children 2 months to 3 years of age, adults over 50 years of age, and patients with chronic obstructive lung disease, alcoholism, diabetes mellitus, sickle cell anemia, HIV infection, various immunoglobulin deficiencies, multiple myeloma, and asplenia.

Etiology

The pleomorphic, gram-negative bacterium *Haemophilus influenzae* causes *Haemophilus* pneumonia. Most organisms that colonize the nasopharynx are unencapsulated and nontypeable. Most strains that infect the lung are encapsulated and typeable. Type b is the most common strain responsible for *Haemophilus* pneumonia, and is responsible for 5 to 20% of community-acquired pneumonias. Type b is also a major cause of nosocomial *Haemophilus influenzae* pneumonia in hospitals and nursing homes.

Clinical Findings

Haemophilus bronchopneumonia is often preceded by an upper respiratory tract infection. Presenting symptoms include fever, productive cough, and dyspnea. Leukocytosis is mild or absent. *Haemophilus* pneumonia may be complicated by lung abscess and empyema. Bacteremia and meningitis may also occur.

Pathology

GROSS

- Acute bronchiolitis and bronchopneumonia

MICROSCOPIC

- Purulent exudate with neutrophils, necrotic cellular debris, and fibrin in the bronchi and bronchioles

Imaging Findings

- Patchy airspace opacities (i.e., bronchopneumonia) (**Fig. 53A**)
- Combination of reticular-nodular opacities and lobar consolidation (15–30%)
- Cavitation in less than 15% of infections; may complicate lobar consolidation
- Pleural effusion (40–50%)
- Empyema rare in adults; 10% of children
- Slow radiologic resolution

Treatment

- Third-generation cephalosporins and combinations of penicillin with an β-lactamase inhibitor
- Vaccination of all children and high-risk patients against *Haemophilus influenzae* type b

Prognosis

- Overall mortality 28% in adults; 5% in children
- Fetal death rate over 50% in infections occurring during pregnancy

PEARL_____

- *Haemophilus* pneumonia may demonstrate a radiographic pattern of lobar consolidation in patients with altered immunity.

Suggested Readings

Fraser RS, Müller NL, Colman N, Paré PD. Pulmonary infection. In: Fraser RS, Müller NL, Colman N, Paré PD, eds. Fraser and Paré's Diagnosis of Diseases of the Chest, 4th ed. Philadelphia: Saunders, 1999:767–770

Travis WD, Colby TV, Koss MN, Rosado-de-Christenson ML, Müller NL, King TE Jr. Lung infections. In: King DW, ed. Atlas of Nontumor Pathology: Non-Neoplastic Disorders of the Lower Respiratory Tract, first series, fascicle 2. Washington, DC: American Registry of Pathology; 2002:541–544

CASE 54 *Klebsiella* Pneumonia

Clinical Presentation

A 42-year-old alcoholic man with fever, chills, and pleuritic chest pain

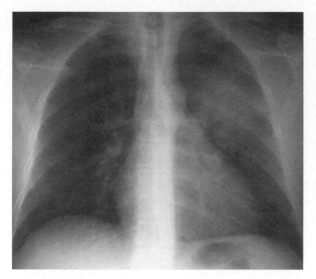

Figure 54A

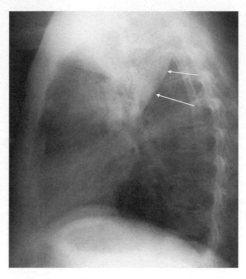

Figure 54B

Radiologic Findings

PA (**Fig. 54A**) and lateral (**Fig. 54B**) chest radiographs reveal a homogeneous, nonsegmental left upper lobe consolidation with air bronchograms. The upper lobe is overexpanded, and the oblique fissure bulges posteriorly (arrows).

Diagnosis

Klebsiella pneumoniae pneumonia (Friedländer's pneumonia after the German pathologist Karl Friedländer)

Differential Diagnosis

- Mixed anaerobic infection
- *Haemophilus influenzae* pneumonia
- Staphylococcal pneumonia

Discussion

Background

Klebsiella pneumonia usually results from aspiration of infected secretions. Risk factors for *Klebsiella* pneumonia include alcoholism, diabetes mellitus, and chronic obstructive lung disease.

223

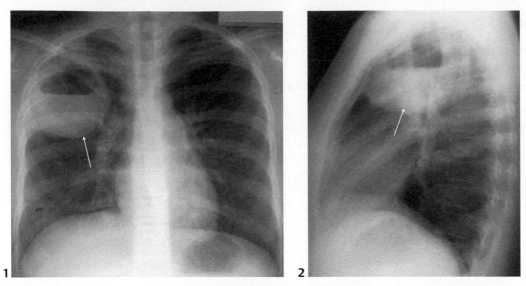

Figure 54C (1,2) PA **(1)** and lateral **(2)** chest radiographs of a teenage intravenous drug abuser with *Klebsiella* pneumonia reveals a right upper lobe pneumonia with complicating cavitation and lung abscess formation. A large air-fluid level can also be identified. Note the "bulging" minor fissure (arrows).

Etiology

Klebsiella pneumonia is caused by the gram-negative bacterium *Klebsiella pneumoniae*. Although found in the normal intestinal flora, *K. pneumoniae* causes approximately 5% of community-acquired and up to 30% of nosocomial pneumonias. *K. pneumoniae* produces a large volume of inflammatory exudate. The exudate infiltrates the entire affected lobe, which enlarges, overexpands, and causes the abutting fissure to bulge toward the adjacent unaffected lobe.

Clinical Findings

Klebsiella pneumonia more often affects men (90%) and patients over 40 years of age. Affected patients present with sudden onset of fever, rigors, dyspnea, pleuritic chest pain, and cough productive of thick, mucoid, bloody sputum (i.e., currant jelly). Prostration and hypotension may occur. The white blood cell count may be elevated, diminished, or normal. *Klebsiella* pneumonia may be complicated by multicentric abscesses, cavitation, pulmonary gangrene, bronchiectasis, and empyema. Chronic pneumonia may be associated with interstitial fibrosis, organizing pneumonia, bronchiolitis, and necrotizing bronchitis.

Pathology

GROSS

- Extensive inflammatory infiltrate throughout an enlarged, overexpanded lung lobe
- Necrosis and abscess formation

MICROSCOPIC

- Alveoli and bronchioles filled with neutrophils and macrophages
- Areas of acute vasculitis and thrombosis

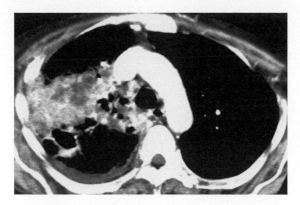

Figure 54D Contrast-enhanced chest CT (mediastinal window) of an elderly alcoholic patient with right upper lobe *Klebsiella* pneumonia shows intermingled enhancing consolidation and poorly marginated low-attenuation areas with numerous small air-containing cavities consistent with necrotizing pneumonia. Note the ipsilateral pleural effusion.

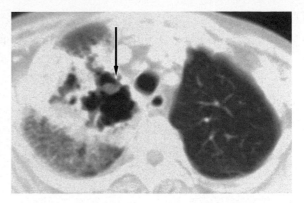

Figure 54E Contrast-enhanced chest CT (lung window) of a 48-year-old woman with complicated right upper lobe *Klebsiella* pneumonia reveals a large irregular cavity with intracavitary sloughed lung (arrow) consistent with pulmonary gangrene.

Imaging Findings

RADIOGRAPHY

- Homogeneous, nonsegmental lobar consolidation with air bronchograms (**Figs. 54A** and **54B**)
- Lobar expansion, "bulging fissure sign" (**Figs. 54A** and **54B**)
- Lung abscess(es) (occur in up to 50% of cases) (**Fig. 54C**)
- Pulmonary gangrene
  - Begins as a lobar consolidation, usually in the upper lobes
  - Coalescence of intrinsic lucencies to form a large cavity
  - "Mass within a mass" or "air crescent" sign secondary to sloughed lung parenchyma or lung necrosis
- Pleural effusion (70%) and/or empyema

CT

- Necrotizing pneumonia
  - Enhancing consolidations and poorly marginated low-attenuation areas with multiple small air-containing cavities (**Fig. 54D**)
  - Scattered enhancing linear branching structures representing pulmonary vessels in atelectatic or consolidated lung (e.g., "CT angiogram sign") (**Fig. 54D**)
  - Centripetal resolution from the periphery to the center with residual fibrosis
- Pulmonary gangrene
  - Coalescence of multiple small abscesses into a large cavity containing sloughed or necrotic lung (**Fig. 54E**)
  - Narrowed or obliterated feeding bronchus impeding drainage of necrotic and infected lung material
  - Large-vessel thrombosis
- Pleural effusion and empyema (**Fig. 54D**)

Treatment

- Aminoglycosides with either a cephalosporin or broad-spectrum penicillin
- Surgical resection of infected lung in patients with pulmonary gangrene

Prognosis

- Mortality rate: 25 to 50%

PEARLS_____

- Because of the high prevalence of pneumococcal pneumonia in most communities, the majority of patients with pneumonia that manifests with lobar expansion and a "bulging fissure sign" are infected with *Streptococcus pneumoniae* rather than with *Klebsiella pneumoniae*.
- The radiologic hallmark of pulmonary gangrene is a soft tissue mass within a cavity that develops in a preexistent consolidation.

Suggested Readings

Curry CA, Fishman EK, Buckley JA. Pulmonary gangrene: radiological and pathological correlation. South Med J 1998;91:957–960

Fraser RS, Müller NL, Colman N, Paré PD. Pulmonary infection. In: Fraser RS, Müller NL, Colman N, Paré PD, eds. Fraser and Paré's Diagnosis of Diseases of the Chest, 4th ed. Philadelphia: Saunders, 1999:752–753

Moon WK, Im JG, Yeon KM, Han MC. Complication of Klebsiella pneumonia: CT evaluation. J Comput Assist Tomogr 1995;19:176–181

Schmidt AJ, Stark P. Radiographic findings in Klebsiella (Friedländer's) pneumonia: the bulging fissure sign. Semin Respir Infect 1998;13:80–82

Travis WD, Colby TV, Koss MN, Rosado-de-Christenson ML, Müller NL, King TE Jr. Lung infections. In: King DW, ed. Atlas of Nontumor Pathology: Non-Neoplastic Disorders of the Lower Respiratory Tract, first series, fascicle 2. Washington, DC: American Registry of Pathology; 2002:549–550

CASE 55 *Pseudomonas* Pneumonia

Clinical Presentation

A 63-year-old woman with fever, chills, and cough productive of purulent sputum

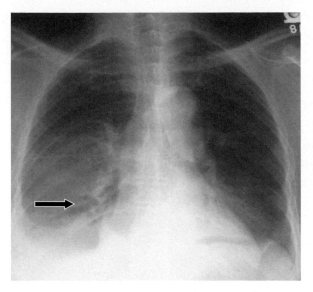

Figure 55A

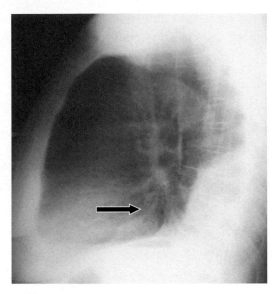

Figure 55B

Radiologic Findings

PA (**Fig. 55A**) and lateral (**Fig. 55B**) chest radiographs reveal a nonsegmental right lower lobe consolidation without associated volume loss. Note the air bronchograms (arrows) and the ipsilateral pleural effusion.

Diagnosis

Pseudomonas pneumonia

Differential Diagnosis

- Community-acquired pneumonia
  - *Staphylococcus aureus*
  - *Streptococcus pyogenes* (group A streptococcus)
  - *Klebsiella pneumoniae*
- Opportunistic pneumonia
  - *Escherichia coli*
  - *Proteus* sp.
  - *Enterobacter*
  - *Serratia marcescens*

227

Discussion

Background

Nonbacteremic *Pseudomonas* infection is usually acquired through aspiration of infected oropharyngeal secretions. Risk factors for *nonbacteremic* infection include advanced age, debilitation, chronic cardiopulmonary disease, cystic fibrosis, and contaminated respiratory therapy equipment. Bacteremic infection may be acquired through breaks in the skin, the gastrointestinal mucosa, or the respiratory tract. Risk factors for *bacteremic* infection include debilitation, underlying hematologic or lymphoreticular malignancy, immunosuppression, HIV infection, neutropenia, and severe burns.

Etiology

The gram-negative aerobic bacteria *Pseudomonas* sp. cause *Pseudomonas* pneumonia, and *Pseudomonas aeruginosa* is responsible for most pulmonary infections. *Pseudomonas* sp. survives in water, vegetation, and soil. Infection may result from exposure to contaminated hot tubs, whirlpools, vegetables, and flowers. Because of its resistance to many disinfectants, it is a common cause of nosocomial infection. *Pseudomonas* sp. also colonizes the gastrointestinal tracts of 5% of adults and of 50% of hospitalized patients with underlying malignancy.

Clinical Findings

Nonbacteremic infections are characterized by systemic toxicity, fever, chills, and cough productive of purulent sputum. The white blood count is initially normal, but leukocytosis eventually develops in most patients. Bacteremic infections are associated with high fever, systemic toxicity, confusion, and cough productive of scant, nonpurulent sputum. *Pseudomonas* pneumonia may be complicated by lung abscess and empyema.

Pathology

- Nonbacteremic
  - Bronchocentric pneumonitis
  - Neutrophilic infiltrate with abscess formation and necrosis
- Bacteremic
  - Vasocentric pneumonitis
  - Necrosis, hemorrhage, vasculitis, and organisms in vessel walls
  - Hemorrhagic infarcts and thromboemboli

Imaging Findings

RADIOGRAPHY

- Nonbacteremic infection
  - Bronchopneumonia pattern of consolidation (**Figs. 55A** and **55B**)
  - Multifocal, bilateral, segmental consolidation with a lower lobe predilection
  - Nodular and reticular opacities may be identified
  - Abscess formation within regions of consolidation (**Figs. 55C** and **55D**)
  - Small pleural effusions common (**Figs. 55A** and **55B**); empyema unusual

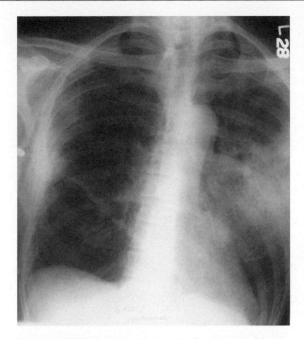 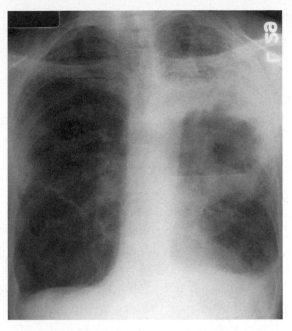

Figure 55C PA chest radiograph of a 61-year-old man with *Pseudomonas* pneumonia who presented with fever, cough, and purulent sputum shows a patchy left upper lobe segmental consolidation with concomitant volume loss. No air bronchograms are seen.

Figure 55D PA chest radiograph obtained 12 days latter shows progression of the consolidation and the formation of a thick-walled abscess cavity and a new left pleural effusion. Small nodular and reticular opacities are seen in the left apex and lower lobe.

- Bacteremic infection
  - Multifocal pulmonary nodules or nodular opacities (> 2 cm diameter)
  - Coalescence of nodules into consolidations
  - Frequent cavitation

CT/HRCT

- Bacteremic infection
  - Multilobar airspace consolidation with upper lung zone predilection (82%)
  - Nodular opacities (50%)
    - Centrilobular and tree-in-bud opacities (64%)
    - Larger, randomly distributed nodules (36%)
  - Ground-glass opacities (31%)
  - Peribronchial thickening (57%)
  - Necrosis (29%)
  - Pleural effusions
    - Unilateral (18%)
    - Bilateral (46%)

Treatment

- Aminoglycoside and antipseudomonal penicillin, cephalosporin, carbapenem, or monobactam antibiotic

Prognosis

- Mortality: 36 to 81%

PEARL

- Patients with bacteremic *Pseudomonas* infections are usually more ill clinically than the chest radiograph would suggest.

Suggested Readings

Arancibia F, Bauer TT, Ewig S, et al. Community-acquired pneumonia due to gram-negative bacteria and *Pseudomonas aeruginosa*: incidence, risk, and prognosis. Arch Intern Med 2002;162:1849–1858

Bodey GP. *Pseudomonas aeruginosa* infections in cancer patients: have they gone away? Curr Opin Infect Dis 2001;14:403–407

Shah RM, Wechsler R, Salazar AM, Spirn PW. Spectrum of CT findings in nosocomial *Pseudomonas aeruginosa* pneumonia. J Thorac Imaging 2002;17:53–57

Travis WD, Colby TV, Koss MN, Rosado-de-Christenson ML, Müller NL, King TE Jr. Lung infections. In: King DW, ed. Atlas of Nontumor Pathology: Non-Neoplastic Disorders of the Lower Respiratory Tract, first series, fascicle 2. Washington, DC: American Registry of Pathology; 2002:550–553

CASE 56 *Legionella* Pneumonia

Clinical Presentation

A 69-year-old woman on chronic corticosteroid therapy for remote kidney transplant, with new fever, rigors, nonproductive cough, headache, and diarrhea

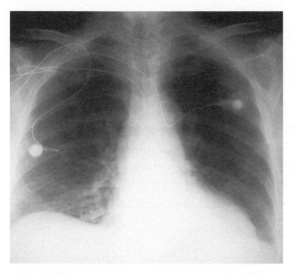

Figure 56A

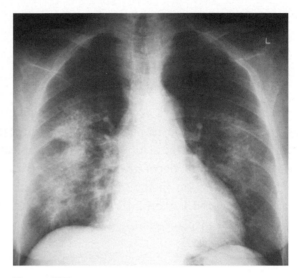

Figure 56B

Figure 56C

Radiologic Findings

AP chest radiograph (**Fig. 56A**) shows subtle, patchy, nonsegmental heterogeneous right lower lobe opacities. AP chest radiograph obtained 3 days later (**Fig. 56B**) reveals rapid disease progression. Patchy consolidations occupy most of the right perihilar region, right lower lobe, and the contralateral perihilar region. AP chest radiograph obtained 9 days later (**Fig. 56C**) shows extensive airspace consolidation with contiguous spread to the right upper and middle lobes, near complete opacification of the right hemithorax, and progression of the left perihilar involvement.

Diagnosis

Legionella pneumonia

Differential Diagnosis

Other community-acquired bronchopneumonias

Discussion

Background

Pulmonary infection with *Legionella* is acquired through contaminated aerosolized water droplets. There have been no cases of person-to-person transmission. Most cases of *Legionella* pneumonia are traced to water, the natural habitat of *Legionella* sp. Typical sources include lakes, rivers, air-conditioning towers, contaminated decorative fountains, hot water storage tanks, showerheads, and hot tubs. Risk factors for infection include male gender (male to female ratio: 2-3:1), advanced age, malignancy (e.g., hairy cell leukemia), chronic obstructive pulmonary disease, renal failure, corticosteroid therapy, and transplantation.

Etiology

Legionella pneumonia is caused by the gram-negative bacteria *Legionella* sp., most commonly *Legionella pneumophila*. It is responsible for 2 to 25% of community-acquired pneumonias requiring hospitalization and 1 to 40% of nosocomial pneumonias.

Clinical Findings

Affected patients usually present after a 2- to 10-day incubation period with constitutional symptoms (e.g., lethargy, fever, headache). Fevers may be high and unremitting. Respiratory symptoms include nonproductive cough or cough productive of watery or purulent sputum, dyspnea (50%), pleuritic chest pain (33%), and hemoptysis (33%). Other signs and symptoms include diarrhea (50%), nausea and vomiting (25%), headache, confusion, hallucinations, seizures, hyponatremia and hypophosphatemia (50%), and leukocytosis. One third of affected patients require assisted mechanical ventilation, and 10% of patients develop acute renal failure. Interstitial fibrosis may develop as a late sequela of infection.

Pathology

GROSS

- Focal, lobular, and multilobar lung involvement
- Small abscesses may be present in some cases.

MICROSCOPIC

- One third of cases demonstrate predominantly neutrophilic infiltration.
- One third of cases demonstrate predominantly monocytic and macrophage infiltration.
- One third of cases demonstrate a mixed combination of macrophages and neutrophils.
- Intra-alveolar fibrin deposition, hemorrhage, and vasculitis (30%)

Imaging Findings

RADIOGRAPHY

- Patchy, peripheral, nonsegmental consolidation initially unilateral and confined to one lobe (**Fig. 56A**)
- Common rapid contiguous and noncontiguous lobar progression and bilateral lung involvement (**Figs. 56A** and **56B**)
- Nodular and mass-like consolidations
- Cavitation and lymphadenopathy are unusual.
- Pleural effusion (50–66%)

Treatment

- Macrolides (e.g., azithromycin) and quinolones

Prognosis

- Rapid response to antibiotic therapy
- 5–25% mortality rate

PEARL_____

- Radiographic improvement lags far behind clinical improvement. The mean time for radiographic resolution is 5 weeks.

Suggested Readings

Fraser RS, Müller NL, Colman N, Paré PD. Pulmonary infection. In: Fraser RS, Müller NL, Colman N, Paré PD, eds. Fraser and Paré's Diagnosis of Diseases of the Chest, 4th ed. Philadelphia: Saunders, 1999:770–775

Tan MJ, Tan JS, Hamor RH, File TM Jr, Breiman RF. The radiologic manifestations of Legionnaire's disease: the Ohio community-based pneumonia incidence study group. Chest 2000;117:398–403

Travis WD, Colby TV, Koss MN, Rosado-de-Christenson ML, Müller NL, King TE Jr. Lung infections. In: King DW, ed. Atlas of Nontumor Pathology: Non-Neoplastic Disorders of the Lower Respiratory Tract, first series, fascicle 2. Washington, DC: American Registry of Pathology; 2002:553–556

CASE 57 Pulmonary Nocardiosis

Clinical Presentation

A 46-year-old man with cough and night sweats for several weeks

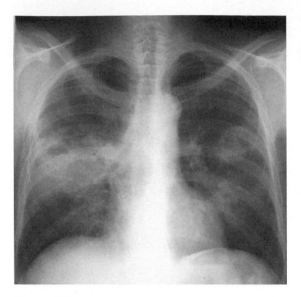

Figure 57A

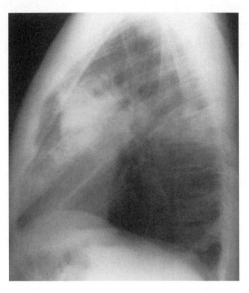

Figure 57B

Radiologic Findings

PA (**Fig. 57A**) and lateral (**Fig. 57B**) chest radiographs reveal a mass-like consolidation with associated cavitation in the anterior segment of the right upper lobe. Ill-defined cavitary masses are also present in the left upper and lower lobes.

Diagnosis

Pulmonary nocardiosis

Differential Diagnosis

- *Actinomyces* sp. pneumonia
- Atypical mycobacterial pulmonary infection
- Various fungal pneumonias

Discussion

Background

Pulmonary infection with *Nocardia asteroides* (nocardiosis) is usually acquired through inhalation of saprophytic organisms. Person-to-person transmission and blood-borne infection from infected catheters are rare. The primary risk factor for pulmonary nocardiosis is immunodeficiency (e.g., lymphoreticular malignancy). Other risk factors include chronic obstructive pulmonary disease (COPD), Cushing disease, acquired immunodeficiency syndrome (AIDS), patients with systemic lupus erythematosus receiving methotrexate or corticosteroids, and alveolar lipoproteinosis.

Etiology

Nocardiosis is caused by the aerobic, gram-positive, weakly acid-fast bacillus *Nocardia* sp. *Nocardia asteroides* accounts for 80% of pulmonary and disseminated infections. The bacterium is ubiquitous, found in soil and decaying vegetable matter throughout the world.

Clinical Findings

Immunocompetent patients have a subacute presentation lasting several days to weeks. Symptoms may wax and wane, delaying diagnosis. Common symptoms include fatigue, low-grade fever, weight loss, and productive cough. Less often, patients experience dyspnea, pleuritic chest pain, and hemoptysis. Most patients have a moderate leukocytosis with neutrophilia. Immunocompromised patients may have a more acute presentation. Fifty percent of patients with pulmonary nocardiosis have disseminated infection to the brain, kidneys, skin, and bone. Pulmonary infection may be complicated by empyema and chest wall involvement.

Pathology

GROSS

- Multiple confluent pus-containing abscesses

MICROSCOPIC

- Extensive suppuration and necrosis
- Numerous neutrophils associated with variable numbers of macrophages

Imaging Findings

RADIOGRAPHY

- Homogeneous, nonsegmental parenchymal consolidation, often peripheral multilobar, and abutting pleural surfaces (**Figs. 57A** and **57B**)
- Less often, multifocal peripheral nodules or masses with irregular borders
- Cavitation in approximately one third of the nodules, masses, or areas of consolidation (**Figs. 57A** and **57B**).
- Pleural effusion in up to 50% of cases
- Rarely chest wall involvement

CT

- Multifocal consolidations
- Localized areas of low attenuation with peripheral rim enhancement in areas of consolidation
- Variable-sized pulmonary nodules
- Pleural effusion, empyema, or pleural thickening
- Lymphadenopathy uncommon

Treatment

- Sulfonamides
- Empyema drainage

Prognosis

- Immunocompetent patient: less than 5% mortality rate
- Immunocompromised patient: 40% fatality rate
- Worse prognosis in patients with COPD, HIV infection, and disseminated disease (e.g., brain abscess)

PEARL_____

- Although the imaging findings of pulmonary nocardiosis resemble those of actinomycosis, the former is more likely to occur in immunocompromised patients and to disseminate hematogenously.

Suggested Readings

Fraser RS, Müller NL, Colman N, Paré PD. Pulmonary infection. In: Fraser RS, Müller NL, Colman N, Paré PD, eds. Fraser and Paré's Diagnosis of Diseases of the Chest, 4th ed. Philadelphia: Saunders, 1999:957–958

Mari B, Monton C, Mariscal D, Lujan M, Sala M, Domingo C. Pulmonary nocardiosis: clinical experience in ten cases. Respiration 2001;68:382–388

Travis WD, Colby TV, Koss MN, Rosado-de-Christenson ML, Müller NL, King TE Jr. Lung infections. In: King DW, ed. Atlas of Nontumor Pathology: Non-Neoplastic Disorders of the Lower Respiratory Tract, first series, fascicle 2. Washington, DC: American Registry of Pathology; 2002:557–560

CASE 58 Pulmonary Actinomycosis

Clinical Presentation

A 39-year-old man with fever, cough, sputum production, and left-sided chest pain

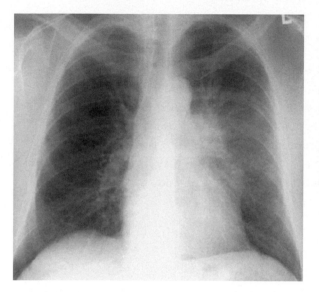

Figure 58A

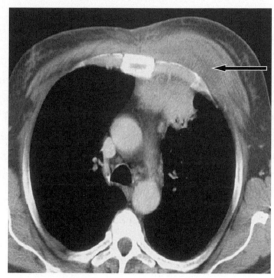

Figure 58B

Radiologic Findings

PA chest radiograph (**Fig. 58A**) reveals ill-defined left perihilar and upper lobe opacity without air bronchograms. Contrast-enhanced chest CT (mediastinal window) (**Fig. 58B**) shows a mass-like region of consolidation in the medial anterior segment of the left upper lobe extending into the anterior mediastinum and invading the left anterior chest wall and pectoralis musculature (arrow).

Diagnosis

Actinomyces pneumonia with chest wall invasion

Differential Diagnosis

- Pulmonary nocardiosis
- *Mycobacterium tuberculosis* pulmonary infection
- *Blastomyces dermatitides* pulmonary infection
- *Cryptococcus neoformans* pulmonary infection
- Primary lung cancer

Discussion

Background

Pulmonary infection with *Actinomyces* results from aspiration of oropharyngeal secretions or by extension from a subphrenic or liver abscess. Suppuration, sulfur granules, abscesses, and sinus tracts

237

characterize actinomycosis. The diagnosis is established by the detection of yellow sulfur granules (i.e., aggregates of mycelial fragments).

Etiology

Actinomycosis is caused by the anaerobic bacteria *Actinomyces* sp., and the usual pulmonary pathogen is *Actinomyces israelii*. *Actinomyces* sp. bacteria normally inhabit the oropharynx.

Clinical Findings

Actinomycosis most often manifests with cervicofascial infection following dental extraction. The incidence of pulmonary disease has markedly declined in most developed countries following the introduction of antibiotics. Most infections occur in immunocompetent individuals. Patients may present with productive cough, fever, weight loss, occasional hemoptysis, and pleuritic chest pain. Leukocytosis and anemia are common. Complications include rupture of abscesses into the pleura with subsequent empyema or bronchopleural fistula. Chronic lung involvement may result in pulmonary fibrosis. Infection may extend into the adjacent mediastinum or chest wall. Endobronchial infection may cause hemoptysis.

Pathology

GROSS

- Multiple abscesses interconnected by sinus tracts and surrounded by variable amounts of fibrous tissue
- Frequent pleural fibrosis and adhesions

MICROSCOPIC

- Abscesses composed of an outer rim of granulation tissue surrounding polymorphonuclear leukocytes; may contain sulfur granules
- True granulomas formation rare

Imaging Findings

RADIOGRAPHY

- Peripheral, nonsegmental airspace consolidation (**Fig. 58A**)
- Predilection for the lower lobes
- Associated abscess formation and cavitation may be identified.
- Focal mass with or without associated cavitation; may mimic primary lung cancer
- Less common radiographic presentations include lobar atelectasis or segmental opacities (e.g., localized endobronchial disease); miliary nodules, multiple nodules, and bilateral apical opacities (**Fig. 58B**).
- Isolated pleural effusion usually indicates empyema.

CT

- Consolidation: may cross interlobar fissures and other anatomic boundaries (**Fig. 58B**)
- Consolidation may be complicated by cavitation.
- Parenchymal mass or nodule with low attenuation center and peripheral rim enhancement (38%)
- Pleural thickening adjacent to the region of parenchymal consolidation
- Chest wall involvement (e.g., soft tissue mass, rib abnormalities)

- Characteristic "wavy" periosteal reaction involving one or several contiguous ribs in the absence of empyema or lung consolidation
- Frank rib or vertebral body destruction
- Small pleural effusions (seen in up to 62% of cases)
- Hilar and/or mediastinal lymphadenopathy (75%)
- Mediastinal and/or pericardial involvement (uncommon) (**Fig. 58B**)

Treatment

- Penicillin; antibiotic of choice

Prognosis

- 90% cure rate with appropriate antibiotic therapy

PEARLS_____

- Actinomycosis manifests in a variety of forms and may mimic other infections or neoplasms.
- A clinical pattern of remission and exacerbation of symptoms occurring in parallel with initiation and cessation of antibiotic therapy is a helpful diagnostic clue.

Suggested Readings

Cheon JE. IM JG, Kim MY, Lee JS, Choi GM, Yeon KM. Thoracic actinomycosis: CT findings. Radiology 1998;209:229–233

Fraser RS, Müller NL, Colman N, Paré PD. Pulmonary infection. In: Fraser RS, Müller NL, Colman N, Paré PD, eds. Fraser and Paré's Diagnosis of Diseases of the Chest, 4th ed. Philadelphia: Saunders, 1999:953–957

Travis WD, Colby TV, Koss MN, Rosado-de-Christenson ML, Müller NL, King TE Jr. Lung infections. In: King DW, ed. Atlas of Nontumor Pathology: Non-Neoplastic Disorders of the Lower Respiratory Tract, first series, fascicle 2. Washington, DC: American Registry of Pathology; 2002:560–563

CASE 59 *Rhodococcus* Pneumonia

Clinical Presentation

A 33-year-old man with AIDS employed as a horse breeder, with a CD4 count < 10, complains of fever, malaise, cough, and pleuritic chest pain.

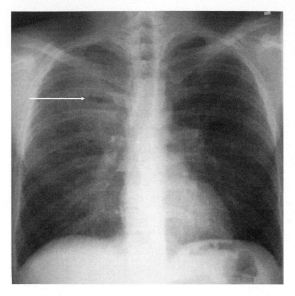

Figure 59A

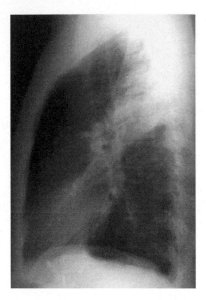

Figure 59B

Radiologic Findings

PA (**Fig. 59A**) and lateral (**Fig. 59B**) chest radiographs show a mass-like consolidation with associated cavitation (arrow) in the posterior segment of the right upper lobe. Note the absence of volume loss, air bronchograms, and pleural effusion.

Diagnosis

Rhodococcus equi pneumonia

Differential Diagnosis

• Postprimary tuberculosis pulmonary infection
• Other community-acquired pneumonias
• Various fungal pulmonary infections
• Primary and secondary lung cancer

Discussion

Background

Human infection with *Rhodococcus equi* results from inhalation of contaminated aerosols. Pulmonary infection usually occurs in immunocompromised persons, especially those with acquired immunodeficiency syndrome (AIDS) and a CD4 count of less than 200 cells/mm^3.

240

Etiology

Pulmonary infection is caused by the aerobic, gram-positive or gram-variable, pleomorphic, weakly acid-fast coccobacillus *R. equi*, which is found worldwide in the soil and feces of some animals, especially horses. Thirty percent of infected patients have a history of exposure to animals, particularly horses.

Clinical Findings

Pulmonary manifestations of infection include cough, fever, dyspnea, and chest pain. Extrapulmonary infection occurs in 7% of affected individuals and may manifest with brain abscess, endophthalmitis, prostatic abscess, lymphadenitis, bacteremia, and psoas abscess. Extrapulmonary relapse occurs in 13% of patients with *R. equi* pneumonia. Although the diagnosis may be established from analysis of sputum, blood cultures, bronchial lavage fluid, or other infected tissue the organism may be inadvertently dismissed as a contaminant if the laboratory is not notified in advance of the suspicion of *Rhodococcus* pulmonary infection. Complications of *R. equi* pulmonary infection include pulmonary malakoplakia and abscess formation.

Pathology

GROSS

- Large areas of consolidation with or without cavitation
- Lung abscesses may reach 8 cm in diameter.

MICROSCOPIC

- Malakoplakia associated with abscesses
- Abscess with central neutrophils and necrosis
- Tissue surrounding abscess infiltrated with histiocytes
- Peripheral organizing pneumonia

Imaging Findings

RADIOGRAPHY

- Dense parenchymal consolidation with an upper lobe predilection (**Figs. 59A** and **59B**)
- Thick-walled cavitation following appropriate antibiotic therapy (**Fig. 59A**)
- Uncommon tracheobronchial dissemination (e.g., multifocal pulmonary opacities paralleling the bronchi)
- Mediastinal lymphadenopathy not uncommon
- Pleural effusion (occurs in up to 20% of cases)

Treatment

- Frequent resistance to penicillins and cephalosporins
- Immunocompetent patients: extended spectrum macrolide or fluoroquinolone
- Immunocompromised patients: two or more agents able to penetrate macrophages
- Prolonged medical therapy (at least 2 to 6 months) due to tendency to relapse
- Surgical resection of nodular or cavitary lesions in refractory or resistant cases

Prognosis

- Immunocompetent patients: 11% mortality rate

- Immunocompromised patients without HIV infection: 20 to 25% mortality rate
- Immunocompromised patients with HIV infection: 50 to 55% mortality rate

Suggested Readings

Kedlaya I, Ing MB, Wong SS. *Rhodococcus equi* infections in immunocompetent hosts: case report and review. Clin Infect Dis 2001;32:E39–E46

Patel S, Wolf T. Cavitary lung lesions due to coinfection of *Rhodococcus equi* and *Mycobacterium kansasii* in a patient with acquired immunodeficiency syndrome. Am J Med 2002;112:678–680

Stiles BM, Isaacs RB, Daniel TM, Jones DR. Role of surgery in *Rhodococcus equi* pulmonary infections. J Infect 2002;45:59–61

Travis WD, Colby TV, Koss MN, Rosado-de-Christenson ML, Müller NL, King TE Jr. Lung infections. In: King DW, ed. Atlas of Nontumor Pathology: Non-Neoplastic Disorders of the Lower Respiratory Tract, first series, fascicle 2. Washington, DC: American Registry of Pathology; 2002:569–571

Weinstock DM, Brown AE. *Rhodococcus equi*: an emerging pathogen. Clin Infect Dis 2002;34:1379–1385

CASE 60 *Mycobacterium tuberculosis* Pulmonary Infection

Clinical Presentation

A 55-year-old man with a history of alcohol and drug abuse and chronic cough, low-grade fever, and weight loss

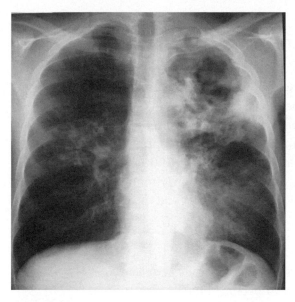

Figure 60A

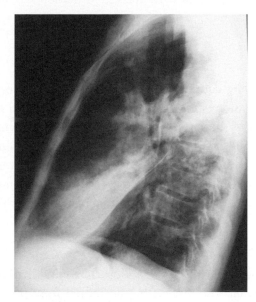

Figure 60B

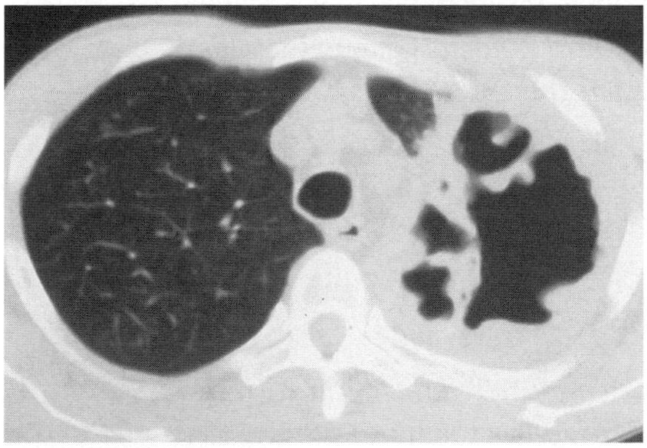

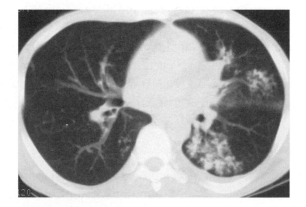

Figure 60C

Figure 60D

Radiologic Findings

PA (**Fig. 60A**) and lateral (**Fig. 60B**) chest radiographs demonstrate a large left upper lobe cavity with irregular nodular borders and adjacent pleural thickening. Note right lower lobe, lingular, and left lower lobe consolidations. Unenhanced chest CT (lung window) (**Figs. 60C** and **60D**) demonstrates the irregular left upper lobe cavity (**Fig. 60C**) and tree-in-bud and centrilobular opacities in the lingula, left lower, and right lower lobes (**Fig. 60D**) consistent with tracheobronchial dissemination of infection.

Diagnosis

Tuberculosis

Differential Diagnosis

- Other infectious granulomatous diseases (fungi and atypical organisms)
- Multifocal bacterial pneumonia with abscess formation

Discussion

Background

Tuberculosis is the leading cause of death from infectious disease worldwide. Approximately one third of the world population is infected, with over eight million new cases and three million deaths reported annually, most of these (95%) occurring in developing countries. The highest disease prevalences are reported in Southeast Asia and sub-Saharan Africa. In the United States, approximately 15 million individuals are infected, with a prevalence of approximately 6 cases per 100,000 persons. Individuals at risk in the United States include those in ethnically diverse populations, immigrants, minorities, the homeless, the immunocompromised (particularly HIV-infected patients), and the elderly.

Etiology

Tuberculosis is caused by organisms in the *Mycobacterium tuberculosis* complex, typically *M. tuberculosis, M. bovis,* and *M. africanum.* The disease is transmitted from person to person through inhalation of droplets (1–5 μm) containing tubercle bacilli. The organisms are deposited in the middle and lower lung zones, multiply within macrophages, and disseminate via lymphatic and hematogenous routes. Cell-mediated immunity develops up to 10 weeks after initial infection. Most patients contain their disease, but approximately 10% develop active tuberculosis, typically within the first 2 years after initial exposure. Remote infection may also occur through reactivation of organisms that survive in areas of high oxygen tension or via exogenous infection. Progression to active infection is more common in HIV-infected individuals, occurring in 50% of patients within the first 2 years after initial infection.

Clinical Findings

Latent tuberculosis refers to the development of conversion to a positive tuberculin skin test (purified protein derivative, PPD) in an asymptomatic individual without active tuberculosis disease. Patients with active tuberculosis have clinical, radiologic, and/or laboratory signs of infection. Primary tuberculosis refers to disease at the site of initial deposition of bacteria and may manifest as severe cavitary pneumonia (progressive primary tuberculosis). Postprimary tuberculosis is caused by reactivation of dormant organisms (or exogenous reinfection) typically in areas of high oxygen tension. Pulmonary symptoms include cough, hemoptysis, pleuritic pain, and rarely dyspnea. Constitutional symptoms include fever, night sweats, anorexia, weight loss, weakness, and malaise. Patients with primary or postprimary tuberculosis may be asymptomatic.

Pathology

GROSS

- Primary tuberculosis
  - Ghon focus: round centrally necrotic nodule up to 2 cm in diameter; heals with fibrosis and/or calcification

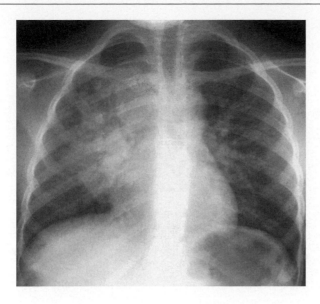

Figure 60E PA chest radiograph of a child with primary tuberculosis demonstrates a coalescent perihilar right lung consolidation with ipsilateral hilar and mediastinal lymphadenopathy.

- Ranke complex: Ghon focus in association with ipsilateral hilar and/or mediastinal lymphadenopathy
- Progressive: necrotizing cavitary consolidation
- Postprimary tuberculosis
  - Cavitary disease in the apical upper lobe or superior segments of the lower lobes with central (caseous) necrosis
- Complications
  - Miliary disease: 1 to 4 mm well-defined nodules
  - Caseous necrosis and cavitation with vascular, pleural, and/or chest wall involvement
  - Chronic cavities with saprophytic fungal growth; mycetoma formation

MICROSCOPIC

- Thin, curved acid-fast bacilli (in sputum or tissue); stain optimally with Ziehl-Neelsen
- Necrotizing (caseating) granulomas; central necrosis surrounded by epithelioid histiocytes and multinucleated giant cells; may progress to fibrosis and calcification

Imaging Findings

RADIOGRAPHY

- Primary tuberculosis
  - Consolidation: usually right-sided (**Fig. 60E**), dense, homogeneous; segmental, lobar, or multifocal; may be associated with ipsilateral lymphadenopathy (**Fig. 60E**); cavitary consolidation in progressive primary tuberculosis
  - Lymphadenopathy: typically unilateral, usually right hilar and/or right paratracheal, most common in children (**Fig. 60E**)
  - Atelectasis: usually lobar and right-sided (30% of affected children)
  - Self-limited unilateral or bilateral pleural effusion, most common in adults
  - Calcification of Ranke complex (lung lesion and ipsilateral lymph nodes)
- Postprimary tuberculosis
  - Consolidation: apical and posterior segments of upper lobes (85%), superior segments of lower lobes (14%), ill-defined borders, satellite nodules
  - Cavitation (45%); thin or thick walls (**Figs. 60A** and **60B**), focal or multifocal, air-fluid levels

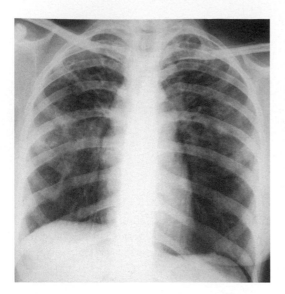

Figure 60F PA chest radiograph of a middle-aged woman with active tuberculosis, chronic cough, and fatigue demonstrates bilateral upper lobe reticular-nodular opacities, bronchiectasis, volume loss, and hilar retraction.

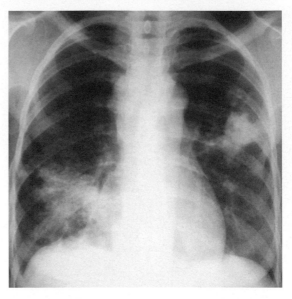

Figure 60G PA chest radiograph of a 27-year-old woman with AIDS and recently diagnosed active tuberculosis demonstrates bilateral multifocal nodular consolidations with associated mediastinal lymphadenopathy.

- • Perihilar nodular and/or linear opacities, volume loss (**Fig. 60F**)
- • Multifocal ill-defined 5 to 10 mm airspace nodular opacities (**Figs. 60A** and **60B**)
- • Tuberculoma; solitary (or multiple) pulmonary nodule, variable size, well-defined or ill-defined margins; may exhibit calcification
- • Pleural involvement: unilateral loculated pleural effusion; may exhibit calcifications; may remain stable for years
- • HIV-infected patients (**Fig. 60G**)
  - • Lymphadenopathy; may be bilateral
  - • Lymphadenopathy with consolidation
  - • Lower frequency of cavitation
  - • Miliary nodules

CT/HRCT

- • Peripheral rim enhancement surrounding enlarged lymph nodes (over 50%)
- • Visualization of subtle cavitation (**Figs. 60C** and **60H**)
- • Centrilobular nodules (2–4 mm) with linear branching opacities (tree-in-bud) (**Figs. 60D** and **60H**)
- • Ill-defined nodules (4–8 mm), lobular consolidations, thickened interlobular septa
- • Tuberculoma: rim enhancement, calcification in 30%, satellite lesions in 80%
- • Bronchial narrowing (bronchostenosis) with mural thickening, bronchiectasis
- • HIV-infected patients:
  - • Lymphadenopathy: right paratracheal/hilar, subcarinal, or bilateral
  - • Consolidations, nodules, tuberculomas
- • Complications:
  - • Empyema: pleural calcification (e.g., calcific pleuritis), bronchopleural fistula, empyema necessitatis
  - • End-stage lung disease

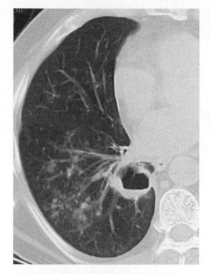

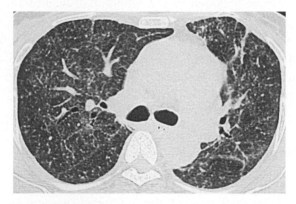

Figure 60H Unenhanced chest CT (lung window, coned to the right lung) of an asymptomatic 45-year-old man with active tuberculosis demonstrates a right lower lobe thin-walled cavity with an air-fluid level and surrounding tree-in-bud centrilobular opacities consistent with tracheobronchial dissemination of infection.

Figure 60I HRCT (lung window) of a 56-year-old woman with miliary tuberculosis shows multifocal well-defined tiny nodular opacities randomly distributed throughout the lungs.

- Mycetoma formation in chronic cavities (see Case 65)
- Miliary disease; 1 to 3 mm noncalcified nodules with random distribution, nodular thickened interlobular septa (**Fig. 60I**)
- Bronchostenosis

ANGIOGRAPHY

- Evaluation and treatment of patients with significant hemoptysis
  - Identification of hypertrophied bronchial arteries and embolization
  - Identification of Rasmussen (pulmonary artery) aneurysm and embolization

Treatment

- First-line drugs: isoniazid, rifampin, streptomycin, ethambutol, and pyrazinamide
- Typically isoniazid, rifampin, and pyrazinamide for 8 weeks, followed by isoniazid and rifampin for 16 weeks (unless resistance develops)
- Latent tuberculosis infection: 6 to 12 months of isoniazid (occasionally rifampin and pyrazinamide) in selected patients in the United States
- Directly observed therapy short course (DOTS): improved compliance and prevention of drug resistance in endemic areas and selected U.S. populations

Prognosis

- Adequate therapy; excellent prognosis, prevention of disease transmission

PEARLS_____

- Patients with active tuberculosis disease who fail to improve after 3 months of therapy may be infected with drug-resistant organisms.
- Tuberculosis must be included in the differential diagnosis of patients with AIDS who exhibit intrathoracic lymphadenopathy (**Fig. 60G**).
- Imaging findings in patients with delayed diagnosis of tuberculosis include normal chest radiograph, nodule or mass, parenchymal abnormalities attributed to inactive disease, isolated pleural effusion, isolated lymphadenopathy, and parenchymal abnormalities in unusual locations.

Suggested Readings

American Thoracic Society and the Centers for Disease Control and Prevention. Diagnostic standards and classification of tuberculosis in adults and children. Am J Respir Crit Care Med 2000;161: 1376–1395. This official statement of the American Thoracic Society and the Centers for Disease Control and Prevention was adopted by the ATS Board of Directors, July 1999. This statement was endorsed by the Council of the Infectious Disease Society of America, September 1999.

Fraser RS, Müller NL, Colman N, Paré PD. Mycobacteria. In: Fraser RS, Müller NL, Colman N, Paré PD, eds. Fraser and Paré's Diagnosis of Diseases of the Chest, 4th ed. Philadelphia: Saunders, 1999: 798–873

Leung AN. Pulmonary tuberculosis: the essentials. Radiology 1999;210:307–322

Small PM, Fujiwara PI. Management of tuberculosis. N Engl J Med 2001;345:189–200

Travis WD, Colby TV, Koss MN, Rosado-de-Christenson ML, Müller NL, King TE Jr. Lung infections. In: King DW, ed. Atlas of Nontumor Pathology: Non-Neoplastic Disorders of the Lower Respiratory Tract, first series, fascicle 2. Washington, DC: American Registry of Pathology;2002:539–727

CASE 61 Nontuberculous Mycobacteria Pulmonary Infection

Clinical Presentation

An elderly man with cough and weight loss

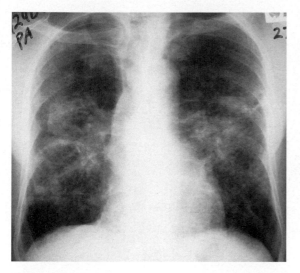

Figure 61A

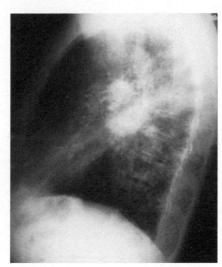

Figure 61B

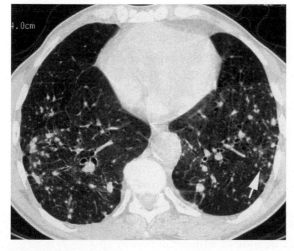

Figure 61C

(Figs. 61A, 61B, and 61C courtesy of Diane C. Strollo, M.D., University of Pittsburgh Medical Center, Pittsburgh, Pennsylvania.)

Radiologic Findings

PA (**Fig. 61A**) and lateral (**Fig. 61B**) chest radiographs demonstrate bilateral confluent perihilar consolidations and scattered small nodular opacities. Unenhanced chest CT (lung window) (**Fig. 61C**) demonstrates multifocal small nodules of various sizes, centrilobular and branching opacities (tree-in-bud) (arrow), and architectural distortion.

Diagnosis

Mycobacterium avium-intracellulare infection

Differential Diagnosis

- *Mycobacterium tuberculosis* pulmonary infection
- Bronchopneumonia
- Infectious bronchiolitis
- Asian panbronchiolitis

Discussion

Background

Mycobacteria other than *M. tuberculosis* may cause pulmonary and systemic infection in immunocompetent and immunocompromised individuals. These organisms occur ubiquitously in the environment (soil, water, plants, and animals).

Etiology

Nontuberculous mycobacterial infections are produced by a variety of organisms including *M. avium*, *M. intracellulare* [*M. avium-intracellulare* (MAI) or *M. avium* complex], *M. kansasii,* and *M. fortuitum*. It is thought that infection occurs from environmental exposures, as there are no documented cases of person-to-person transmission. Infection may occur through inhalation or via the gastrointestinal tract.

Clinical Findings

There are strict diagnostic criteria generally based on clinical and imaging evidence of infection with repeated isolation of atypical mycobacteria in sputum, bronchial washings, and/or transbronchial or open lung biopsies. Affected immunocompetent patients include elderly white men with chronic obstructive pulmonary disease or interstitial fibrosis and middle-aged and elderly white women without underlying pulmonary disease. Symptoms are insidious and include cough, hemoptysis, and weight loss. Immunocompromised patients at risk for developing nontuberculous mycobacterial infections include patients with AIDS, alcoholism, and diabetes mellitus.

Pathology

GROSS

- Upper lobe cavitary lung disease indistinguishable from tuberculosis
- Consolidation
- Bronchiectasis

MICROSCOPIC

- Acid-fast bacilli morphologically indistinguishable from *M. tuberculosis*
- Granulomatous inflammation: noncaseating, less commonly caseating
- Patients with AIDS; numerous intracellular acid-fast bacilli, absence of well-formed granulomas

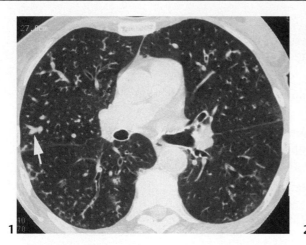
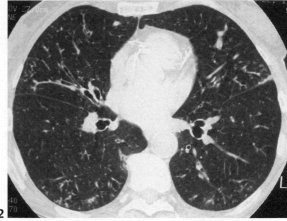

Figure 61D (1,2) Unenhanced chest CT (lung window) of an elderly woman with *M. avium* complex pulmonary infection demonstrates bronchiectasis and multifocal small pulmonary nodules. Note the mucus-filled dilated bronchi (arrow). (Courtesy of Diane C. Strollo, M.D., University of Pittsburgh Medical Center, Pittsburgh, Pennsylvania.)

Imaging Findings

RADIOGRAPHY

- May be indistinguishable from imaging findings of *M. tuberculosis* pulmonary infection: consolidation, linear and/or nodular opacities, in apical and posterior segments of upper lobes
- Cavitation (90%)
- Pleural thickening (40%)
- Solitary or multiple nodules (**Figs. 61A** and **61B**)
- Patients with AIDS
  - Normal radiographs
  - Mediastinal/hilar lymphadenopathy
  - Consolidations, nodular opacities
  - Miliary nodules

CT/HRCT

- Multifocal nodular opacities or patchy airspace consolidation
- Bronchiectasis, particularly in the middle lobe and lingula (**Fig. 61D**)
- Centrilobular nodules and linear branching opacities (tree-in-bud) (**Fig. 61C**)
- Thick- or thin-walled cavitation; associated centrilobular nodules suggest endobronchial dissemination
- Scarring and volume loss
- Pleural effusion and/or thickening
- Lymphadenopathy

Treatment

- Antimycobacterial drug therapy

Prognosis

- Progression of untreated disease
- Clinical stability in some colonized patients with repeated positive cultures
- Poor prognosis with severe underlying lung disease and disseminated infection in immunocompromised patients

252 PULMONARY INFECTIONS AND ASPIRATION PNEUMONIA: LESS BACTERIAL PNEUMONIAS

Suggested Readings

Fraser RS, Müller NL, Colman N, Paré PD. Mycobacteria. In: Fraser RS, Müller NL, Colman N, Paré PD, eds. Fraser and Paré's Diagnosis of Diseases of the Chest, 4th ed. Philadelphia: Saunders, 1999: 798–873

Goo JM, Im J-G. CT of tuberculosis and nontuberculous mycobacterial infections. Radiol Clin North Am 2002;40:73–87

Travis WD, Colby TV, Koss MN, Rosado-de-Christenson ML, Müller NL, King TE Jr. Lung infections. In: King DW, ed. Atlas of Nontumor Pathology: Non-Neoplastic Disorders of the Lower Respiratory Tract, first series, fascicle 2. Washington, DC: American Registry of Pathology; 2002:539–727

Webb WR, Müller NL, Naidich DP. Diseases characterized primarily by nodular or reticulo-nodular opacities. In: Webb WR, Müller NL, Naidich DP, eds. High-resolution CT of the Lung, 3rd ed. Philadelphia: Lippincott Williams & Wilkins, 2001;259–353

CASE 62 Histoplasmosis

Clinical Presentation

An asymptomatic adult woman evaluated for an enlarging lung nodule

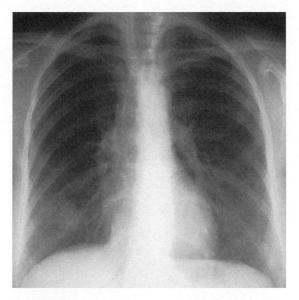

Figure 62A

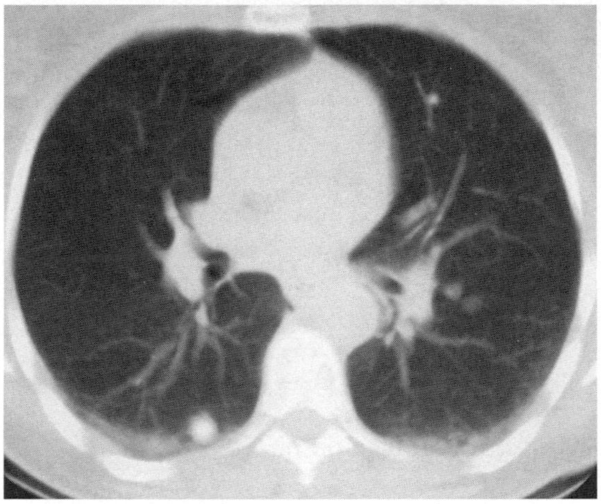

Figure 62B

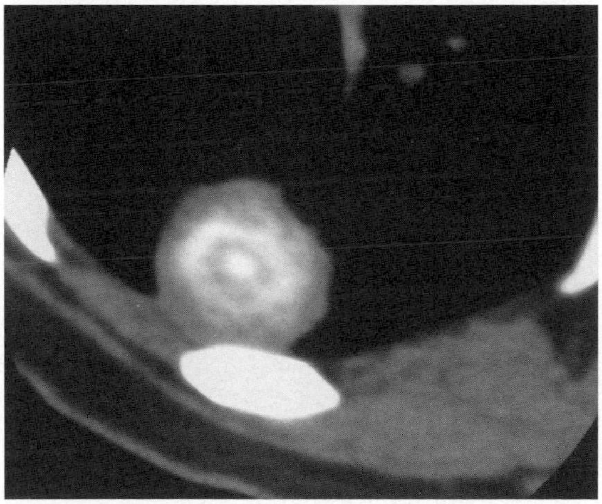

Figure 62C

Radiologic Findings

PA chest radiograph (**Fig. 62A**) demonstrates a well-defined 3 cm right lower lobe mass. Unenhanced chest CT (lung window) (**Fig. 62B**) demonstrates multiple bilateral dense pulmonary nodules of various sizes. Unenhanced HRCT (mediastinal window) (**Fig. 62C**) demonstrates laminar concentric calcification within the right lower lobe mass.

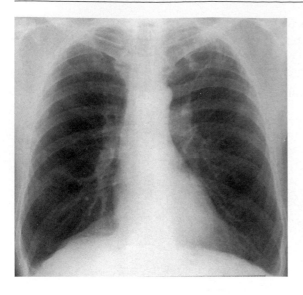

Figure 62D PA chest radiograph of a 42-year-old man with chronic histoplasmosis and hemoptysis demonstrates bilateral apical nodular opacities, a left upper lobe cavity, and left upper lobe volume loss.

Diagnosis

Pulmonary histoplasmosis, histoplasmoma

Differential Diagnosis

- Granulomas; other fungal infections
- Granulomas; tuberculosis

Discussion

Background

Histoplasmosis is a fungal infection endemic to the south-central United States, especially the Mississippi River and Ohio River valleys.

Etiology

Histoplasmosis is caused by *Histoplasma capsulatum*, a dimorphic fungus transmitted through inhalation of airborne spores typically released from infected soil enriched by bird droppings or guano. Inhaled organisms multiply within macrophages and undergo lymphatic and hematogenous dissemination. Cellular immunity develops within 2 weeks with subsequent healing.

Clinical Findings

The vast majority of histoplasmosis infections are self-limited and do not produce symptoms. A small percentage of affected individuals experience an intense point-source exposure and present with fever, headache, myalgia, chest pain, and cough. Severe illness resembling the acute respiratory distress syndrome may also occur. Chronic histoplasmosis typically affects middle-aged white men with a history of cigarette smoking and emphysema who present with cough, dyspnea, night sweats, and/or hemoptysis. Disseminated histoplasmosis affects immunocompromised patients who develop fever, weight loss, anorexia, malaise, cough, and organomegaly.

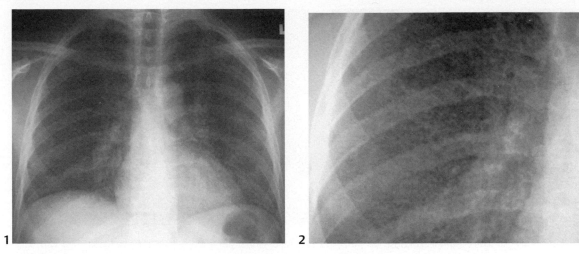

Figure 62E (1,2) PA **(1)** and coned-down PA **(2)** chest radiographs of a 28-year-old man with AIDS, chills, fever, and disseminated histoplasmosis demonstrate profuse bilateral miliary nodules.

Pathology

GROSS

- Granulomas: spherical nodules or masses with concentric laminating fibrosis

MICROSCOPIC

- Yeast-like spherical (2–4 μm) organisms with narrow-based budding, best identified with Gomori methenamine silver (GMS) stain
- Acute fibrinous pneumonia; may progress to granulomatous inflammation
- Chronic infection: necrotizing granulomas; prone to calcification
- Disseminated disease: profuse tissue infiltration by *H. capsulatum*

Imaging Findings

RADIOGRAPHY

- Acute histoplasmosis
  - Focal or multifocal ill-defined consolidation
  - Lymphadenopathy
  - Diffuse bilateral opacities with heavy exposures; may heal with calcification
- Histoplasmoma (**Fig. 62A**)
  - Single or multiple well-defined pulmonary nodules (0.5–3 cm)
  - Central or diffuse calcification
  - Ipsilateral calcified hilar and/or mediastinal lymph nodes
- Chronic histoplasmosis (**Fig. 62D**)
  - Segmental or subsegmental apical consolidations
  - Nodular or linear opacities
  - Thick-walled apical bullae
  - Upper lobe volume loss
- Disseminated histoplasmosis (**Fig. 62E**)
  - Miliary nodules
  - Irregular linear opacities
  - Airspace opacities; may progress to diffuse consolidation

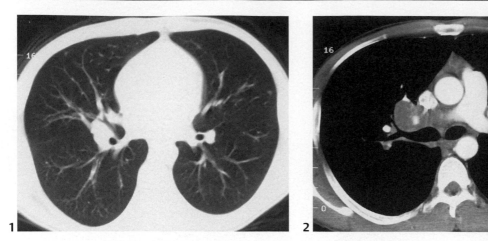

Figure 62F (1,2) Contrast-enhanced chest CT [lung **(1)** and mediastinal **(2)** window] of a 27-year-old man with fever, dyspnea and histoplasmosis demonstrates bilateral small lung nodules and low-attenuation right-sided hilar and mediastinal lymphadenopathy.

CT

- Demonstration of subtle parenchymal involvement (**Figs. 62F1** and **62B**)
- Histoplasmoma (**Figs. 62B** and **62C**)
  - Central, diffuse, laminated calcification (**Fig. 62C**)
  - Peripheral juxtapleural location, typically in posterior lower lobes (**Figs. 62B** and **62C**)
- Lymphadenopathy (**Fig. 62F2**)
  - Identification of calcification
  - Broncholithiasis: endobronchial erosion of adjacent calcified lymph nodes with resultant atelectasis or consolidation

Treatment

- Antifungal therapy for chronic and disseminated histoplasmosis

Prognosis

- Good prognosis in self-limited infections
- Guarded prognosis in disseminated and progressive chronic disease
- Progression to mediastinal fibrosis (see Section XII)

Suggested Readings

Fraser RS, Müller NL, Colman N, Paré PD. Fungi and actinomyces. In: Fraser RS, Müller NL, Colman N, Paré PD, eds. Fraser and Paré's Diagnosis of Diseases of the Chest, 4th ed. Philadelphia: Saunders, 1999:875–978

Gurney JW, Conces DJ Jr. Pulmonary histoplasmosis. Radiology 1996;199:297–306

Travis WD, Colby TV, Koss MN, Rosado-de-Christenson ML, Müller NL, King TE Jr. Lung infections. In: King DW, ed. Atlas of Nontumor Pathology: Non-Neoplastic Disorders of the Lower Respiratory Tract, first series, fascicle 2. Washington, DC: American Registry of Pathology; 2002:539–727

CASE 63 Pulmonary Coccidioidomycosis

Clinical Presentation

A 78-year-old man from Arizona with cough, myalgias, and headache

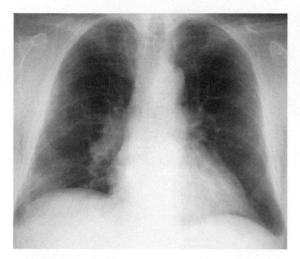

Figure 63A

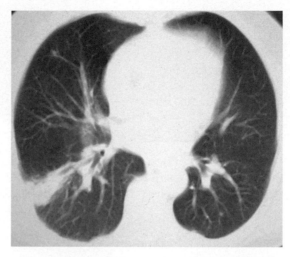

Figure 63B

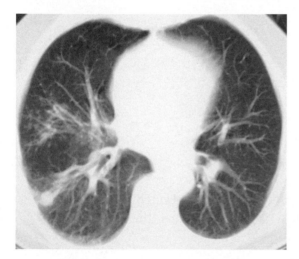

Figure 63C

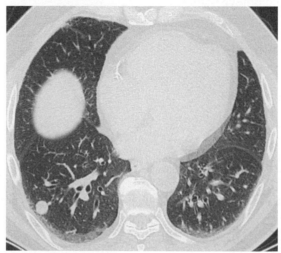

Figure 63D

Radiologic Findings

PA chest radiograph (**Fig. 63A**) demonstrates ill-defined nodular opacities in the right middle and lower lung zones. Unenhanced chest CT (lung window) (**Fig. 63B**) demonstrates a wedge-shaped right lower lobe consolidation and bilateral small pulmonary nodules. Unenhanced chest CT (lung window) (**Fig. 63C**) obtained 6 months after presentation demonstrates improvement of the right lower lobe consolidation with a residual pulmonary nodule as well as multiple right middle lobe centrilobular nodules. HRCT (lung window) (**Fig. 63D**) obtained 1 year after presentation demonstrates a well-defined right lower lobe solitary pulmonary nodule.

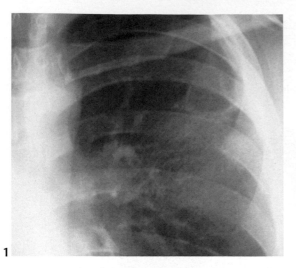
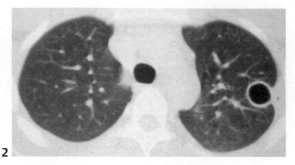

Figure 63E (1,2) PA chest radiograph **(1)**, coned to the left upper lobe, of a 22-year-old man with chronic coccidioidomycosis demonstrates a thin-walled cavity. Unenhanced chest CT (lung window) **(2)** demonstrates the thin-walled cavity and adjacent pleural thickening. This patient later developed a left spontaneous pneumothorax.

Diagnosis

Pulmonary coccidioidomycosis

Differential Diagnosis

- Granuloma; other fungal infection
- Granuloma; tuberculosis

Discussion

Background

Coccidioidomycosis is a highly infectious fungal disease endemic in the southwestern United States, northern and central Mexico, and Central and South America. It is estimated that there are 100,000 new cases of coccidioidomycosis each year in the United States.

Etiology

Coccidioidomycosis is caused by *Coccidioides immitis*, a multimorphic fungus transmitted through inhalation of infected soil, typically in dry, hot climates.

Clinical Findings

Most patients (80%) with primary coccidioidomycosis are asymptomatic. Symptomatic patients with primary infection present with nonspecific symptoms including fever, cough, chest pain, and headache. Valley fever occurs in up to 20% of patients with symptomatic coccidioidomycosis and manifests with erythema nodosum, erythema multiforme, arthralgia, and occasional eosinophilia. Patients with chronic coccidioidomycosis have a prolonged symptomatic course with cough, weight loss, fever, and hemoptysis. Disseminated disease preferentially affects African Americans, Filipinos, pregnant women, and immunosuppressed patients (particularly those with AIDS). These patients may

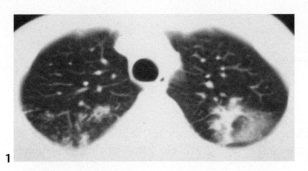
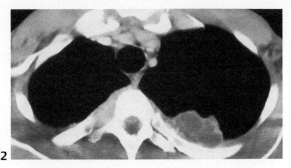

Figure 63F (1,2) Contrast-enhanced chest CT [lung **(1)** and mediastinal **(2)** window] of an immunocompromised patient with disseminated coccidioidomycosis demonstrates a left upper lobe mass-like consolidation with central low attenuation, right upper lobe nodular and centrilobular opacities **(1)**, and low-attenuation chest wall abscesses with peripheral enhancement **(2)**.

develop a severe pulmonary illness as well as skin, osseous, renal, and/or central nervous system involvement.

Pathology

GROSS

- Consolidations, masses, nodules
- Central necrosis, cavitation

MICROSCOPIC

- Identification of round, thick-walled spherules (30–100 μm) containing multiple endospores
- Neutrophilic pneumonitis, progression to necrotizing granulomatous inflammation

Imaging Findings

- Primary coccidioidomycosis
  - Focal or multifocal, unilateral lower lobe consolidation (**Figs. 63A, 63B,** and **63C**)
  - Lymphadenopathy in 20%
  - Healing with formation of a pulmonary nodule (granuloma) (**Fig. 63D**) or chronic thin-walled ("grape skin") cavity (may change size over time) (**Fig. 63E**)
- Chronic coccidioidomycosis
  - Upper lobe involvement
  - Small nodular or linear opacities
  - Single or multiple cavities
  - Volume loss
- Disseminated coccidioidomycosis (**Fig. 63F**)
  - Multifocal nodules or reticular opacities
  - Miliary nodules

Treatment

- Oral antifungal agents
- Amphotericin B for disseminated disease and immunocompromised patients
- Surgical excision of chronic cavitary lesions, particularly with hemoptysis or pleuropulmonary involvement

Prognosis

- Favorable prognosis in self-limited infection
- Poor prognosis in disseminated disease and impaired host immunity

Suggested Readings

Fraser RS, Müller NL, Colman N, Paré PD. Fungi and actinomyces. In: Fraser RS, Müller NL, Colman N, Paré PD, eds. Fraser and Paré's Diagnosis of Diseases of the Chest, 4th ed. Philadelphia: Saunders, 1999:875–978

Travis WD, Colby TV, Koss MN, Rosado-de-Christenson ML, Müller NL, King TE Jr. Lung infections. In: King DW, ed. Atlas of Nontumor Pathology: Non-Neoplastic Disorders of the Lower Respiratory Tract, first series, fascicle 2. Washington, DC: American Registry of Pathology; 2002:539–727

CASE 64 Pulmonary Blastomycosis

Clinical Presentation

A 24-year-old man with cough, fever, chills, and hemoptysis

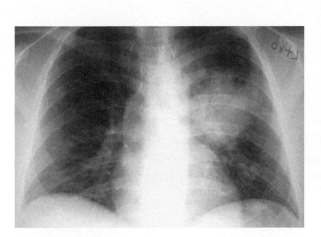

Figure 64A

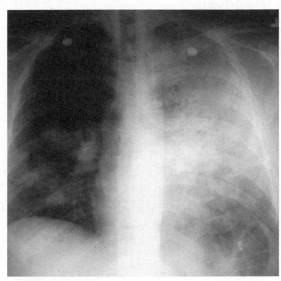

Figure 64B

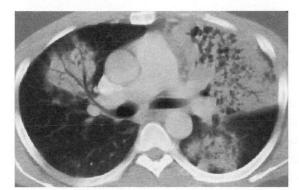

Figure 64C

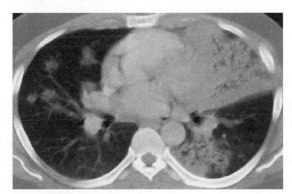

Figure 64D

(Figs. 64A, 64B, 64C, and 64D courtesy of Helen T. Winer-Muram, M.D., Indiana University Medical Center, Indianapolis, Indiana.)

Radiologic Findings

PA chest radiograph (**Fig. 64A**) demonstrates a left perihilar mass-like consolidation. PA chest radiograph obtained several days after failure to respond to antibiotic therapy (**Fig. 64B**) demonstrates diffuse left lung consolidation and multifocal nodular opacities in the right lung. Contrast-enhanced chest CT (lung window) (**Figs. 64C** and **64D**) demonstrates a large left upper lobe consolidation, mass-like consolidations in the left lower and right upper lobes, and multifocal airspace nodules in the right upper and middle lobes. Note air bronchograms within virtually all parenchymal consolidations and early cavitation (**Fig. 64C**) in the left upper lobe.

Diagnosis

Pulmonary blastomycosis

Differential Diagnosis

- Primary (multifocal) lung cancer or lymphoma
- Multifocal pulmonary infection
- Vasculitis

Discussion

Background

Blastomycosis is a fungal infection that is endemic in the Mississippi, Missouri, and Ohio River valleys, northern Wisconsin and Minnesota, and the adjacent Canadian provinces, as well as in other regions of the Americas, Europe, and Asia. The fungus grows in nitrogen-rich soil near streams, rivers, and lakes.

Etiology

Blastomycosis is caused by *Blastomyces dermatitides*, a fungus acquired by inhalation of infected soil. Many outbreaks occur near recreational water.

Clinical Findings

Sporadic cases of blastomycosis are most common in men who engage in outdoor activities, but patients of all ages may become infected in highly endemic areas. Most affected patients present with a subacute or chronic illness with low-grade fever, cough, night sweats, and/or weight loss. Patients may also present acutely with signs and symptoms resembling bacterial pneumonia: fever, cough, and pleuritic pain. Less frequently, affected patients present with a self-limited flu-like illness or with fulminant infection resulting in acute respiratory distress syndrome with high fever and hypoxemia. Infected individuals may be entirely asymptomatic. Late reactivation of disease may result in skin and osseous involvement.

Pathology

GROSS

- Focal or coalescent consolidations
- Pulmonary masses
- Pulmonary fibrosis and cavitary disease

MICROSCOPIC

- Spherical or ovoid, yeast-like, thick-walled multinucleated fungal forms (2 to 15 μm) with single broad-based budding, best visualized with Gomori methenamine silver (GMS) and periodic acid-Schiff (PAS) stains
- Neutrophilic response and abscess formation; progression to granulomatous inflammation with neutrophilic microabscesses

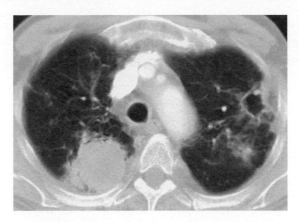

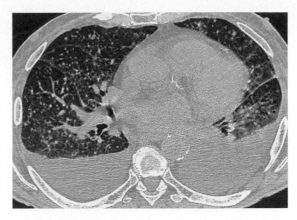

Figure 64E Contrast-enhanced chest CT (lung window) of a middle-aged man with blastomycosis demonstrates multifocal parenchymal opacities and a cavitary lesion in the left upper lobe. Note the well-defined right upper lobe mass that mimics a neoplasm.

Figure 64F Unenhanced HRCT (lung window) of a young patient with disseminated blastomycosis demonstrates bilateral pleural effusions and multifocal bilateral miliary nodules. (Courtesy of Helen T. Winer-Muram, M.D., Indiana University Medical Center, Indianapolis, Indiana.)

Imaging Findings

RADIOGRAPHY

- Consolidation: focal (**Fig. 64A**), multifocal (**Fig. 64B**), patchy, or confluent; may be diffuse and slowly progressing (**Fig. 64B**); may exhibit air bronchograms and/or satellite lesions (**Fig. 64B**)
- Mass or nodule: focal, multifocal; when solitary may mimic lung cancer (**Figs. 64A** and **64B**)
- Cavitation (15%)
- Interstitial nodular or micronodular opacities, miliary nodules
- Pleural thickening common, pleural effusion (10–15%)
- Rarely calcification or lymphadenopathy

CT

- Focal or multifocal mass (**Figs. 64C, 64D,** and **64E**)
- Focal/multifocal consolidations (**Figs. 64C** and **64D**)
- Perihilar distribution (**Figs. 64C** and **64D**)
- Air bronchograms (88%) (**Figs. 64C** and **64D**)
- Nodules (**Fig. 64F**), satellite lesions (**Figs. 64C** and **64D**)
- May demonstrate calcification in lymph nodes and pulmonary lesions
- Uncommon cavitation (**64E**) and hilar and/or mediastinal lymphadenopathy
- Pleural effusion and/or thickening (**Fig. 64F**)

Treatment

- Oral itraconazole in most affected patients
- Patients with severe acute presentation: amphotericin B

Prognosis

- Favorable prognosis in patients with mild or self-limited infection even without therapy
- 90% cure rates in treated patients
- Poor prognosis with overwhelming infection, systemic dissemination, and/or immune compromise

PITFALL_____

- Slow radiographic and clinical improvement, absence of change, and/or progression should prompt exclusion of infectious granulomatous disease in patients undergoing treatment for presumed bacterial pneumonia.

Suggested Readings

Davies SF, Sarosi GA. Epidemiological and clinical features of pulmonary blastomycosis. Semin Respir Infect 1997;12:206–218

Fraser RS, Müller NL, Colman N, Paré PD. Fungi and actinomyces. In: Fraser RS, Müller NL, Colman N, Paré PD, eds. Fraser and Paré's Diagnosis of Diseases of the Chest, 4th ed. Philadelphia: Saunders, 1999:875–978

Kuzo RS, Goodman LR. Blastomycosis. Semin Roentgenol 1996;31:45–51

Travis WD, Colby TV, Koss MN, Rosado-de-Christenson ML, Müller NL, King TE Jr. Lung infections. In: King DW, ed. Atlas of Nontumor Pathology: Non-Neoplastic Disorders of the Lower Respiratory Tract, first series, fascicle 2. Washington, DC: American Registry of Pathology; 22002:539–727

Winer-Muram HT, Beals DH, Cole FH Jr. Blastomycosis of the lung: CT features. Radiology 1992; 182:829–832

CASE 65 Pulmonary Aspergillosis

Clinical Presentation

A 67-year-old man with weight loss and prior tuberculosis

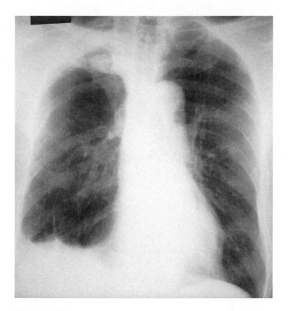

Figure 65A

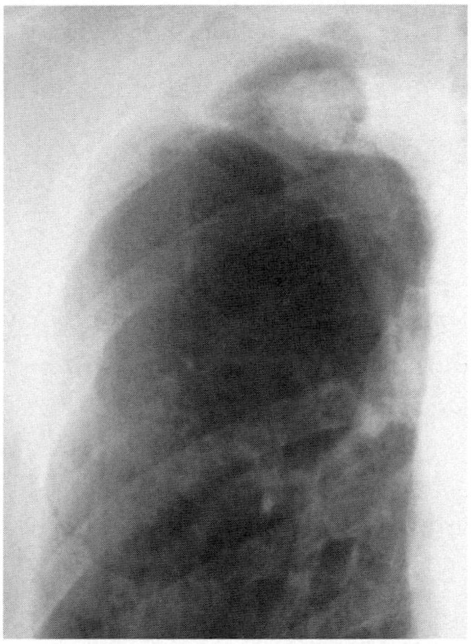

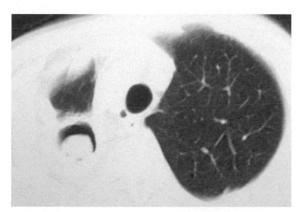

Figure 65B

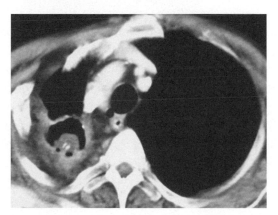

Figure 65C

Figure 65D

(Figs. 65A, 65B, 65C, and 65D courtesy of Wanda M. Kirejczyk, M.D., New Britain General Hospital, New Britain, Connecticut.)

Radiologic Findings

PA (**Fig. 65A**) and coned-down (**Fig. 65B**) chest radiographs demonstrate a right upper lobe cavity with adjacent pleural thickening and right upper lobe volume loss. A soft tissue mass is located in the dependent portion of the cavity. Contrast-enhanced chest CT [lung (**Fig. 65C**) and mediastinal (**Fig. 65D**) window] demonstrates the mass in the dependent portion of the cavity. Note adjacent pleural thickening and punctate calcification within the mass and the wall of the cavity.

Diagnosis

Aspergillosis, mycetoma within a chronic tuberculous cavity

Differential Diagnosis

- Mycetoma secondary to other fungi
- Chronic necrotizing aspergillosis
- Cavitary lung cancer with necrotic lung or mycetoma formation

Discussion

Background

The fungi classified as *Aspergillus* sp. occur worldwide and may produce disease through colonization of abnormal lung tissue or through vascular and tissue invasion in immunocompromised individuals.

Etiology

Aspergillosis is typically caused by three major species of fungi: *Aspergillus fumigatus, A. flavus,* and *A. niger.*

Clinical Findings

Patients with saprophytic aspergilloma (mycetoma, fungus ball) usually have a normal immunity and abnormal lung parenchyma, typically cavitary lung disease. These patients may be entirely asymptomatic. However, patients with mycetoma may present with hemoptysis, which may be massive. Angioinvasive aspergillosis typically occurs in patients with severe neutropenia (absolute neutrophil counts < 500 × 10^3/mL) who present with fever, dyspnea, cough, and chest pain. Chronic necrotizing (semi-invasive) aspergillosis affects patients with severe underlying lung disease who present with fever, productive cough, and dyspnea. Aspergillus may produce necrotizing pseudomembranous tracheobronchitis in a small percentage of immunocompromised patients who present with dyspnea, wheezing, and cough.

Pathology

GROSS

- Mycetoma: friable brown-to-red mass in dependent aspect of a thick-walled lung cavity
- Angioinvasive aspergillosis: nodular pulmonary infarct within crescent-shaped cavity with surrounding pulmonary hemorrhage
- Chronic necrotizing aspergillosis: consolidation and bronchiectatic cavities
- Necrotizing pseudomembranous tracheobronchitis: fungal pseudomembrane along tracheal and bronchial luminal surface with epithelial erosion

MICROSCOPIC

- Septated hyphae with 45-degree branching best seen with Gomori methenamine silver (GMS) or periodic acid-Schiff (PAS) stains
- Mycetoma: mass composed of concentric layers of mycelia
- Angioinvasive aspergillosis: vascular invasion and occlusion by fungus, with resultant pulmonary infarction

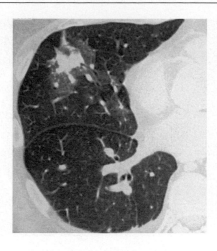

Figure 65E HRCT (lung window) targeted to the right lung of a neutropenic man with invasive aspergillosis demonstrates an irregular pulmonary nodule surrounded by ground-glass opacity (CT "halo sign"). Reproduced with permission from Bazan C, McCarthy MJ, Rosado de Christenson ML, Chintapalli K. Radiology of fungal infections. In: Anaissie EJ, McGinnis MR, Pfaller MA. Clinical Mycology. New York: Churchill Livingstone, 2003; 96–156.

- Chronic necrotizing aspergillosis: necrotizing granulomatous pneumonia, mycetomas within bronchiectatic cavities, and local invasion of surrounding tissues
- Necrotizing pseudomembranous tracheobronchitis: exudate of necrotic material, mucus, inflammatory cells, and fungal organisms

Imaging Findings

RADIOGRAPHY

- Mycetoma (**Figs. 65A** and **65B**)
  - Gravity-dependent soft tissue nodule or mass within preexisting cavity
  - Air-crescent sign: crescent of air in the nondependent aspect of cavity surrounding the mycetoma
  - Thin-walled cavities; with focal mural thickening or air-fluid levels
- Angioinvasive aspergillosis
  - Normal radiographs in early disease
  - Focal or multifocal pulmonary nodules or masses with ill-defined borders; may progress to coalescence
  - Segmental or lobar consolidation
  - Cavitation during recovery from chemotherapy-induced neutropenia, intracavitary soft tissue mass (necrotic lung) surrounded by an air crescent
- Chronic necrotizing aspergillosis
  - Upper lobe consolidation with slowly progressive cavitation
  - Intracavitary soft tissue mass, adjacent pleural thickening

CT/HRCT

- Mycetoma (**Figs. 65C** and **65D**)
  - Early lesions; focal or multifocal thickening of cavity wall
  - Mobility within lung cavity or adherence to cavity wall
  - Heterogeneous attenuation from calcification or air trapped within interstices in mycetoma
  - Complete obliteration of cavity space by intracavitary fungal mass
- Angioinvasive aspergillosis
  - Focal or multifocal nodules, masses, or consolidations with ill-defined borders (**Figs. 65E** and **65F**)
  - "Halo sign": ground-glass attenuation surrounding nodules or consolidations (**Fig. 65E**)

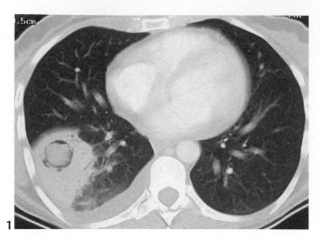 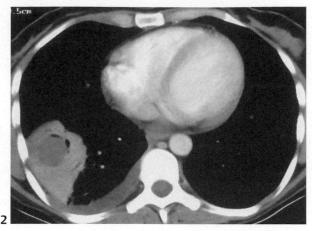

Figure 65F (1,2) Contrast-enhanced chest CT [lung **(1)** and mediastinal **(2)** window] of a 43-year-old woman with leukemia and invasive aspergillosis demonstrates a wedge-shaped consolidation in the right lower lobe with peripheral air bronchograms, central cavitation, an intracavitary mass, and an ipsilateral pleural effusion. Note that the intracavitary mass (representing necrotic lung) fails to enhance with contrast **(1)**.

- Cavitation with air crescent around homogeneous intracavitary soft tissue mass (necrotic lung); occurs during recovery from neutropenia (**Fig. 65F**)
- Pleural effusion (**Fig. 65F**)
- Pleural, chest wall, mediastinal invasion
- Chronic necrotizing aspergillosis
  - Lobar or segmental consolidation, ground-glass opacity
  - Pleural thickening
  - Multifocal pulmonary nodules with peripheral ground-glass opacity
  - Multiple cavities

Treatment

- Mycetoma: surgical excision, bronchial artery embolization to control hemoptysis, intracavitary instillation of antifungal agents
- Angioinvasive and chronic aspergillosis: intravenous amphotericin B, excision of residual nodular lesions after recovery from neutropenia

Prognosis

- Mycetoma: good prognosis in symptomatic and treated patients; rarely death from massive hemoptysis
- Chronic necrotizing aspergillosis: indolent course
- Angioinvasive aspergillosis: generally poor prognosis, but recovery reported with early diagnosis, reversal of immunosuppression, and antifungal therapy

PEARL_____

- Angioinvasive aspergillosis should be considered in the setting of severe neutropenia, signs and symptoms of infection, and new pulmonary nodules, masses or consolidations.

PITFALL_____

- The CT "halo sign" (**Fig. 65E**) is not pathognomonic for angioinvasive fungal infection and has been described in other infections, vasculitides, neoplasms, and lymphoproliferative disorders.

Suggested Readings

Franquet T, Müller NL, Giménez A, Domingo P, Plaza V, Bordes R. Semiinvasive pulmonary aspergillosis in chronic obstructive pulmonary disease: radiologic and pathologic findings in nine patients. AJR Am J Roentgenol 2000;174:51–56

Fraser RS, Müller NL, Colman N, Paré PD. Fungi and actinomyces. In: Fraser RS, Müller NL, Colman N, Paré PD, eds. Fraser and Paré's Diagnosis of Diseases of the Chest, 4th ed. Philadelphia: WB Saunders, 1999;875–978

Gaeta M, Blandino A, Scribano E, Minutoli F, Volta S, Pandolfo I. Computed tomography halo sign in pulmonary nodules: frequency and diagnostic value. J Thorac Imaging 1999;14:109–113

Travis WD, Colby TV, Koss MN, Rosado-de-Christenson ML, Müller NL, King TE Jr. Lung infections. In: King DW, ed. Atlas of Nontumor Pathology: Non-Neoplastic Disorders of the Lower Respiratory Tract, first series, fascicle 2. Washington, DC: American Registry of Pathology and Armed Forces Institute of Pathology, 2002:539–727

Won HJ, Lee KS, Cheon J-E, et al. Invasive pulmonary aspergillosis: prediction at thin-section CT in patients with neutropenia—a prospective study. Radiology 1998;208:777–782

CASE 66 *Pneumocystis* Pneumonia

Clinical Presentation

A 40-year-old man with acquired immunodeficiency syndrome (AIDS), CD4 count 160 cells/μL, and nonproductive cough, fever, dyspnea, and hypoxemia

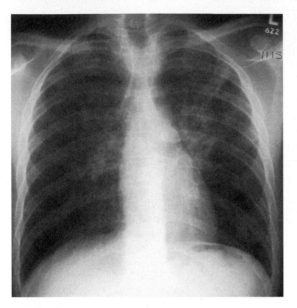

Figure 66A

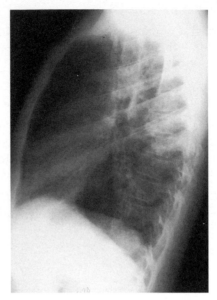

Figure 66B

Radiologic Findings

PA (**Fig. 66A**) and lateral (**Fig. 66B**) chest radiographs reveal patchy, bilateral perihilar and upper lobe ground-glass and nodular opacities without lymphadenopathy or pleural effusions.

Diagnosis

Pneumocystis jiroveci pneumonia

Differential Diagnosis

- *Histoplasma capsulatum* pulmonary infection
- *Torulopsis glabrata* pulmonary infection
- *Cryptococcus neoformans* pulmonary infection

Discussion

Background

Infection from Pneumocystis has a worldwide distribution. The organism that causes human pulmonary infection, formerly known as *Pneumocystis carinii* pneumonia, is now named *Pneumocystis jiroveci* (pronounced yee-row-vet-zee), in honor of the Czech parasitologist Otto Jirovec. The organism is now considered a fungus, based on nucleic acid and biochemical analysis. Pneumocystis is likely acquired through inhalation of airborne respiratory secretions. Risk factors for pulmonary infection include congenital or acquired disorders affecting cell-mediated immunity, organ transplantation, chemotherapy for hematologic or lymphoreticular malignancy, and AIDS. *Pneumocystis jiroveci* is the second most common cause of pneumonia in patients with AIDS and affects up to 80% of patients at some time during the course of their illness.

Etiology

Pneumocystis jiroveci pneumonia (or PCP for Pneumocystis pneumonia) causes subclinical infection in most persons during childhood. Latent infection develops into opportunistic pneumonia when an individual becomes immunosuppressed.

Clinical Findings

The clinical presentation of affected patients is variable. Signs and symptoms may be mild, but disease may be fulminant and may rapidly progress to respiratory failure. Patients with AIDS tend to have a more indolent course. A nonproductive cough, dyspnea, and fever are common symptoms and signs. Hypoxemia occurs in 80 to 95% of affected patients, and the diffusing capacity for carbon monoxide (DLCO) is invariably diminished. Ninety percent of HIV-infected patients have an elevated lactate dehydrogenase (LDH) level, with a mean value of 375 ± 23 IU/L. Complications include secondary spontaneous pneumothoraces, which complicate approximately 12% of infections and are a poor prognostic sign. Cytomegalovirus pneumonia is the most common associated concomitant infection.

Complications

Pathology

GROSS

- May resemble confluent bronchopneumonia or extensive airspace pneumonia
- Usually involves several lobes and both lungs
- Cysts especially in the upper lobes
- Rarely endobronchial mass

MICROSCOPIC

- Alveolar interstitial inflammation
- Proliferation of type II alveolar epithelial cells
- Finely vacuolated eosinophilic exudate in the alveolar spaces (e.g., cysts, trophozoites, surfactant, fibrin, immunoglobulins, proteins)
- Frequent variability in histologic findings

Imaging Findings

RADIOGRAPHY

- Normal (10% of proven pulmonary infections)
- Typically bilateral, symmetric ground-glass or reticular opacities with a diffuse, perihilar, or lower lung zone predominance (**Figs. 66A** and **66B**)

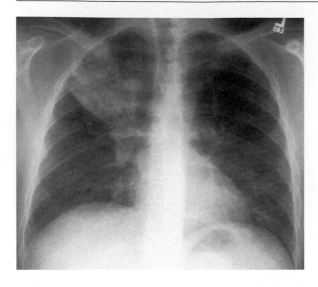

Figure 66C PA chest radiograph of a 39-year-old man with AIDS, endobronchial *Pneumocystis jiroveci* infection and postobstructive pneumonia demonstrates focal consolidation in the posterior segment of the right upper lobe and diffuse bilateral reticular opacities. Bronchoscopy revealed a right upper lobe endobronchial mass secondary to *Pneumocystis jiroveci*.

- Less often upper lung zone predominance (**Figs. 66A** and **66B**)
- Ground-glass opacities with progression to diffuse airspace consolidation
- Air-filled cysts or pneumatoceles (5–35%); more common in upper lung zones; ranging between 1 and 10 cm in diameter, with walls less than 1 mm in thickness
- Pneumothorax (12%); may be recurrent
- Less frequent manifestations: focal lobar consolidation (**Fig. 66C**); solitary pulmonary nodule or mass; miliary nodules; cavitation; mediastinal or hilar lymphadenopathy; pleural effusion; lymph node and visceral calcification

HRCT

- Symmetric, bilateral ground-glass opacities (92%) with a diffuse, perihilar, or patchy distribution and intervening areas of normal lung parenchyma
- Airspace consolidation (38%)
- Cysts (33%)
- Small nodules (25%)
- Irregular linear opacities or thickened interlobular septa (17%)
- Hilar or mediastinal lymphadenopathy (identified in up to 25% of cases)
- Pleural effusion (identified in up to 17% of cases)

Treatment

- Preferred prophylaxis: Trimethoprim-sulfamethoxazole
- Trimethoprim-sulfamethoxazole and intravenous pentamidine for acute infection
- Early administration of glucocorticoids within hours of beginning pharmacotherapy reduces risk of respiratory failure and death by more than 50% in hypoxic patients.

Prognosis

- Usually favorable, with 50 to 95% survival rate if appropriately treated
- Poor prognosis with rising LDH level despite appropriate therapy
- Relapses in 50 to 75% of patients with AIDS and 10 to 20% of immunosuppressed patients unless given additional therapy

PEARL

- HIV-infected patients with CD4 counts < 200 cells/μL are five times more likely to develop *Pneumocystis jiroveci* pneumonia than patients with CD4 counts > 200 cells/μL.

Suggested Readings

Fraser RS, Müller NL, Colman N, Paré PD. Pulmonary infection. In: Fraser and Paré's Diagnosis of Diseases of the Chest, 4th ed. Philadelphia: Saunders, 1999:1656–1670

Lee KH, Lee JS, Lynch DA, Song KS, Lim TH. The radiologic differential diagnosis of diffuse lung diseases characterized by multiple cysts or cavities. J Comput Assist Tomogr 2002;26:5–12

Travis WD, Colby TV, Koss MN, Rosado-de-Christenson ML, Müller NL, King TE Jr. Lung infections. In: King DW, ed. Atlas of Nontumor Pathology: Non-Neoplastic Disorders of the Lower Respiratory Tract, first series, fascicle 2. Washington, DC: American Registry of Pathology; 2002:668–680.

CASE 67 Cytomegalovirus Pneumonia

Clinical Presentation

Two cases: A 33-year-old woman with AIDS and new onset of cough and fever (**Figs. 67A** and **67B**); a 28-year-old woman with acute myelogenous leukemia, neutropenia, and recent nonproductive cough, fever, and headache following bone marrow transplantation (**Figs. 67C** and **67D**)

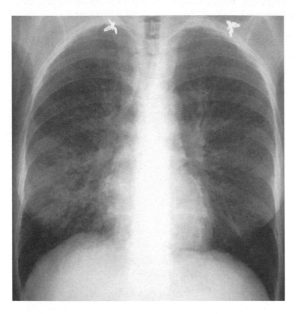

Figure 67A

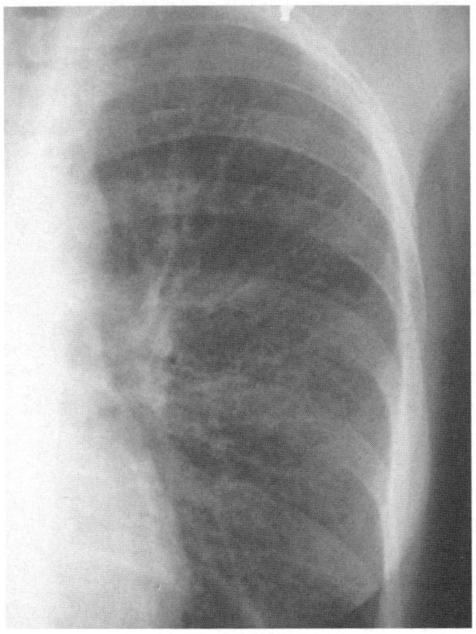

Figure 67B

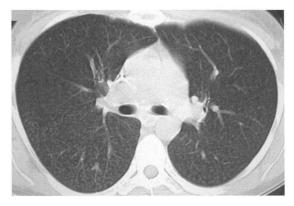

Figure 67C

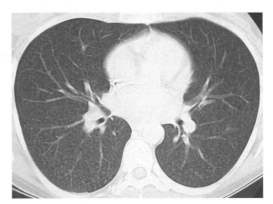

Figure 67D

(Figs. 67C and 67D courtesy of Diane C. Strollo, M.D., University of Pittsburgh, Pittsburgh, Pennsylvania.)

Radiologic Findings

PA (**Fig. 67A**) and coned-down (**Fig. 67B**) chest radiographs demonstrate profuse bilateral perihilar nodular and reticular opacities worse in the right lung. HRCT (lung window) (**Figs. 67C** and **67D**) demonstrates profuse bilateral centrilobular ground-glass micronodules.

274

Diagnosis

Cytomegalovirus pneumonia

Differential Diagnosis

- Other opportunistic pneumonias (fungal, viral)
- Secondary malignant neoplasia
- Extrinsic allergic alveolitis

Discussion

Background

Based on antibody titers, the prevalence of infection by cytomegalovirus (CMV) ranges from 40 to 100% in adults worldwide and approximates 100% for HIV-infected homosexual men and 80% for intravenous drug users. Disease is very rarely documented in immunocompetent individuals.

Etiology

Cytomegalovirus pneumonia is caused by CMV, a herpes virus with a double-stranded DNA.

Clinical Findings

Cytomegalovirus produces opportunistic infections that typically affect allogeneic bone marrow and lung transplant recipients. CMV pneumonia usually occurs between 60 days and 6 months after transplantation. Other clinical settings in which CMV infections occur include treatment with immunosuppressive drugs, the acquired immune deficiency syndrome (AIDS), and other immunodeficiency states. While commonly isolated from the lungs of patients with AIDS, the presence of CMV does not always correlate with clinical disease. Presenting symptoms include fever, cough, dyspnea, and hypoxemia. Extrapulmonary manifestations include retinitis and gastrointestinal involvement.

Pathology

- CMV nuclear and/or cytoplasmic inclusions associated with miliary nodules, diffuse interstitial pneumonia, alveolar hemorrhage, or diffuse alveolar damage

Imaging Findings

RADIOGRAPHY

- Bilateral reticular opacities (**Figs. 67A** and **67B**)
- Bilateral small (**Figs. 67A** and **67B**) and large nodular opacities
- Bilateral diffuse airspace consolidations and/or ground-glass opacities
- Less commonly lobar consolidation

CT/HRCT

- Bilateral small nodules and/or micronodules (**Figs. 67C** and **67D**)
- Nonsegmental consolidation

- Ground-glass opacities
- Linear opacities
- Rarely pleural effusion, mediastinal lymphadenopathy

Treatment

- Antiviral therapy with ganciclovir
- Prophylactic therapy with ganciclovir

Prognosis

- High mortality in cases of severe immunosuppression

Suggested Readings

Kang E-Y, Patz EF, Müller NL. Cytomegalovirus pneumonia in transplant patients: CT findings. J Comput Assist Tomogr 1996;20:295–299

Salomon N, Perlman DC. Cytomegalovirus pneumonia. Semin Respir Infect 1999;14:353–358

Travis WD, Colby TV, Koss MN, Rosado-de-Christenson ML, Müller NL, King TE Jr. Pulmonary infections. In: King DW, ed. Atlas of Nontumor Pathology: Non-Neoplastic Disorders of the Lower Respiratory Tract, first series, fascicle 2. Washington, DC: American Registry of Pathology and Armed Forces Institute of Pathology, 2002: 539–727

Winer-Muram HT, Gurney JW, Bozeman PM, Krance RA. Pulmonary complications after bone marrow transplantation. Radiol Clin North Am 1996;34:97–117

CASE 68 Varicella (Chickenpox) Pneumonia

Clinical Presentation

A 25-year-old pregnant woman with a 5-day history of vesicular skin rash followed by progressive dyspnea, cough, pleuritic chest pain, tachypnea, and respiratory failure necessitating intubation and mechanical ventilation

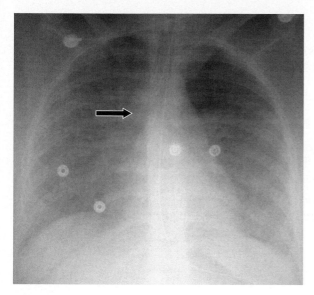

Figure 68A

Radiologic Findings

AP chest radiograph (**Fig. 68A**) shows extensive bilateral airspace disease characterized by multiple 5 to 10 mm nodular opacities most heavily concentrated in the perihilar regions and lower lobes. Note the right paratracheal lymphadenopathy (arrow).

Diagnosis

Varicella (chickenpox) pneumonia

Differential Diagnosis

- Disseminated fungal pulmonary infection
- Miliary tuberculosis pulmonary infection
- Metastatic disease

Discussion

Background

The overall incidence of varicella pneumonia is 15%. Most cases occur in young adults. Patients with lymphoma and leukemia are at risk. Varicella pneumonia occurs in up to 45% of bone marrow

277

transplant recipients and in up to 33% of patients with acute leukemia. Ten percent of pregnant women with varicella infection develop pneumonia, which can be severe and is often life threatening. Predisposing factors include immunodeficiency, leukemia, and lymphoma. Zoster is usually a localized cutaneous eruption that occurs most often in the elderly. It is most severe in patients with lymphoreticular neoplasms and in patients receiving immunosuppressive or radiation therapy. Dissemination of infection beyond the affected dermatome (e.g., pneumonitis) occurs in a minority of patients.

Etiology

Herpes varicella-zoster pneumonia is caused by the herpes varicella-zoster virus (VZV). Infection with VZV has two clinical manifestations: varicella (chickenpox) and herpes zoster (shingles). Pneumonia may complicate either, but it occurs more often with varicella.

Clinical Findings

Acute varicella pneumonia usually develops 1 to 6 days after the skin rash. Signs and symptoms include cough, dyspnea, tachypnea, chest pain, cyanosis, and rarely hemoptysis. Zoster pneumonia has similar signs and symptoms. Complications of varicella pneumonia include respiratory failure and pulmonary infarction. Disseminated zoster may be complicated by hepatitis, meningoencephalitis, and uveitis.

Pathology

GROSS

- Vesicles in the trachea, larger bronchi, and on the pleural surface
- Diffuse multicentric hemorrhage and necrosis

MICROSCOPIC

- Interstitial mononuclear inflammatory infiltrate
- Intraalveolar proteinaceous exudate, edema, hemorrhage, hyaline membranes

Imaging Findings

RADIOGRAPHY

- Multiple 5 to 10 mm nodular opacities that tend to coalesce in the perihilar regions and lower lung zones (**Fig. 68A**)
- Rapidly progressive airspace consolidation
- Less often small nodules or miliary-like nodules
- Hilar and/or paratracheal lymphadenopathy without calcification (**Fig. 68A**)
- Uncommon pleural effusion
- Unique manifestation: widespread 2 to 3 mm calcified nodules in both lungs with lower lobe predilection (< 2%) (**Fig. 68B**)

HRCT

- Nodules
- Nodules with subsequent coalescence
- Nodules with surrounding ground-glass attenuation
- Patchy ground-glass attenuation

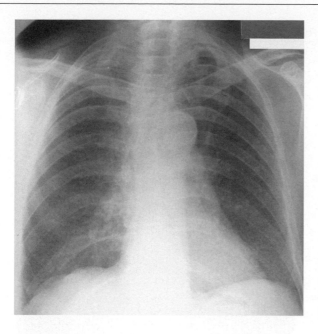

Figure 68B PA chest radiograph of a 35-year-old man with previous varicella pneumonia demonstrates diffuse bilateral 2 to 3 mm calcified nodules with a perihilar and lower lobe distribution.

Treatment

- Intravenous Acyclovir
- Possible steroids
- Isolation procedures to control spread of this highly contagious infection

Prognosis

- 10% mortality rate

PEARL

- Clinical improvement precedes radiographic clearing by several weeks or longer

Suggested Readings

Fraser RS, Müller NL, Colman N, Paré PD. Pulmonary infection. In: Fraser RS, Müller NL, Colman N, Paré PD, eds. Fraser and Paré's Diagnosis of Diseases of the Chest, 4th ed. Philadelphia: Saunders, 1999:999–1004

Kim JS, Ryu CW, Lee SI, Sung DW, Park CK. High-resolution CT findings of varicella-zoster pneumonia. AJR Am J Roentgenol 1999;172:113–116

Travis WD, Colby TV, Koss MN, Rosado-de-Christenson ML, Müller NL, King TE Jr. Lung infections. In: King DW, ed. Atlas of Nontumor Pathology: Non-Neoplastic Disorders of the Lower Respiratory Tract, first series, fascicle 2. Washington, DC: American Registry of Pathology; 2002:646–6648.

CASE 69 Influenza Pneumonia

Clinical Presentation

A 33-year-old man with acute onset of fever, chills, and headache

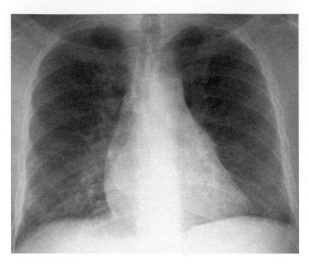

Figure 69A

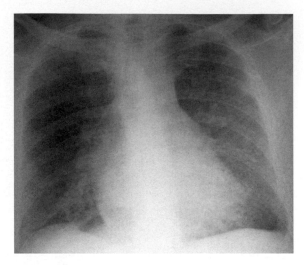

Figure 69B

Radiologic Findings

PA chest radiograph (**Fig. 69A**) demonstrates bilateral reticular opacities. PA chest radiograph obtained 10 days later (**Fig. 69B**) demonstrates progression of reticular opacities, new patchy ground-glass opacities, and small bilateral pleural effusions.

Diagnosis

Influenza pneumonia

Differential Diagnosis

- Other viral pneumonias
- Various atypical pneumonias

Discussion

Background

The influenza virus is a leading respiratory pathogen that affects persons of all ages and is responsible for annual epidemics worldwide.

Etiology

Influenza pneumonia is caused by the influenza virus, an RNA virus. Three types (A, B, and C) are identified based on antigenic differences in internal proteins. Variations in surface glycoproteins result in evasion of preexisting host immunity (antigenic drift) and in the emergence of viruses to which there is no preexisting immunity (antigenic shift). Antigenic drift is responsible for annual winter outbreaks of influenza, and antigenic shift is responsible for influenza pandemics. The virus is transmitted from person to person via inhalation of infected airborne secretions.

Clinical Findings

Affected patients have an acute presentation with fever, chills, myalgias, arthralgias, cough, sore throat, and rhinorrhea. The acute phase lasts approximately 5 days, and the infection typically follows a self-limited course. Adults with chronic underlying diseases, women in the third trimester of pregnancy, and immunosuppressed patients may develop a severe life-threatening pneumonia that may be complicated by secondary bacterial infection. Systemic complications including Guillain-Barré syndrome, toxic shock syndrome, and Reye's syndrome may occur.

Pathology

- Bronchiolitis with necrosis of the bronchial epithelium and neutrophilic exudates in the bronchial lumen
- Airspace and/or interstitial edema and fibrin deposition
- Progression to hyaline membrane deposition and acute alveolar damage
- Chronic interstitial fibrosis

Imaging Findings

- Poorly defined lower lobe segmental consolidation
- Perihilar reticular nodular opacities (**Fig. 69A**)
- Progression to more confluent airspace disease on serial radiography (**Fig. 69B**)

Treatment

- Prevention through annual vaccination with inactivated influenza virus vaccine, particularly for elderly patients and those with chronic disease
- Supportive therapy with bed rest, antipyretics, hydration, and antitussives
- Antiviral drugs in high-risk individuals

Prognosis

- Generally favorable
- Increased likelihood of bacterial superinfection and fatal course in immunocompromised patients and patients in developing countries

PEARL

- Superimposed associated bacterial pneumonia must be excluded.

Suggested Readings

Fraser RS, Müller NL, Colman N, Paré PD. Viruses, mycoplasmas, chlamydiae, and rickettsiae. In: Fraser RS, Müller NL, Colman N, Paré PD, eds. Fraser and Paré's Diagnosis of Diseases of the Chest, 4th ed. Philadelphia: WB Saunders, 1999;979–1032

Piedra PA. Influenza virus pneumonia: pathogenesis, treatment, and prevention. Semin Respir Infect 1995;10:216–223

Travis WD, Colby TV, Koss MN, Rosado-de-Christenson ML, Müller NL, King TE Jr. Lung infections. In: King DW, ed. Atlas of Nontumor Pathology: Non-Neoplastic Disorders of the Lower Respiratory Tract, first series, fascicle 2. Washington, DC: American Registry of Pathology and Armed Forces Institute of Pathology, 2002:539–727

CASE 70 *Mycoplasma* Pneumonia

Clinical Presentation

A 60-year-old woman with malaise and dyspnea

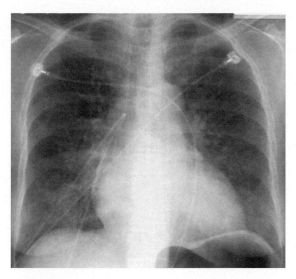

Figure 70A

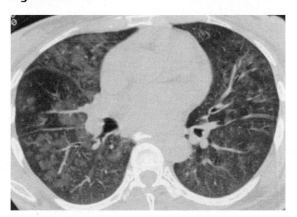

Figure 70B

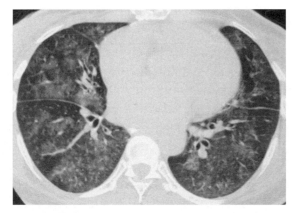

Figure 70C

(Figs. 70A, 70B, and 70C courtesy of Rosita M. Shah, M.D., University of Pennsylvania Medical Center, Philadelphia, Pennsylvania.)

Radiologic Findings

AP chest radiograph (**Fig. 70A**) demonstrates bilateral patchy ground-glass opacities. Unenhanced chest CT (lung window) (**Figs. 70B** and **70C**) demonstrates bilateral widespread ill-defined centrilobular nodules and ground-glass lobular opacities.

Diagnosis

Mycoplasma pneumonia

Differential Diagnosis

- Typical bacterial pneumonia
- Viral pulmonary infection
- Extrinsic allergic alveolitis

Discussion

Background

Mycoplasma is considered an "atypical" bacterium that lacks a cell wall and produces human pulmonary infection through extracellular growth and interference with ciliary function. It is a common cause of community-acquired pneumonia and is probably responsible for approximately 20 to 30% of the pneumonias that affect the general population. Infections occur year-round, but typically in the fall and winter months.

Etiology

Mycoplasma pneumonia is caused by the organism *Mycoplasma pneumoniae*. The disease is transmitted through close contact with infected individuals and inhalation of infected respiratory droplets.

Clinical Findings

Mycoplasma pneumonia typically occurs in children, adolescents, and young adults, although approximately 15% of affected patients are over the age of 40 years. After an incubation period of several days, patients develop symptoms of pharyngitis. Constitutional symptoms may follow, typically fever, chills, myalgias, headache, and malaise. Cough is usually dry, but may be productive of mucoid sputum. Extrapulmonary manifestations include lymphadenopathy, skin rash, and pharyngeal, conjunctival, gastrointestinal, central nervous system, and cardiac involvement. Rarely, affected patients may develop acute respiratory distress syndrome. The diagnosis is usually made based on clinical presentation, normal white blood cell count, and elevated titers of serum cold agglutinins.

Pathology

- Bronchiolitis; neutrophilic luminal infiltrate, chronic bronchial wall inflammation
- Inflammation of alveolar interstitium

Imaging Findings

RADIOGRAPHY

- Unilateral or bilateral patchy airspace consolidation or ground-glass opacity (**Fig. 70A**)
- Segmental or lobar consolidation, may exhibit air bronchograms.
- Reticular and nodular interstitial opacities (**Fig. 70A**)
- Bronchial wall thickening
- Lower lobe predominance
- Pleural effusion (20% of cases)
- Hilar lymphadenopathy in children

CT/HRCT

- Poorly defined centrilobular nodules (**Figs. 70B** and **70C**)
- Patchy lobular consolidation or ground-glass opacity (**Figs. 70B** and **70C**)
- Thickening of bronchovascular interstitium

Treatment

- Antibiotic therapy with doxycycline or erythromycin

Prognosis

- Good; typically with complete recovery and radiographic resolution in approximately 8 weeks
- Rarely, residual bronchiectasis, interstitial fibrosis, constrictive bronchiolitis

PEARL_____

- Delayed resolution of radiologic abnormalities in patients treated for *mycoplasma* pneumonia suggests superinfection with other bacteria.

Suggested Readings

Corley DE, Winterbauer RH. Infectious diseases that result in slowly resolving and chronic pneumonia. Semin Respir Infect 1993;8:3–13

Fraser RS, Müller NL, Colman N, Paré PD. Viruses, mycoplasmas, chlamydiae, and rickettsiae. In: Fraser RS, Müller NL, Colman N, Paré PD, eds. Fraser and Paré's Diagnosis of Diseases of the Chest, 4th ed. Philadelphia: Saunders, 1999; 979–1032

Reittner P, Müller NL, Heyneman L, et al. Mycoplasma pneumoniae pneumonia: radiographic and high-resolution CT features in 28 patients. AJR Am J Roentgenol 2000;174:37–41

Travis WD, Colby TV, Koss MN, Rosado-de-Christenson ML, Müller NL, King TE Jr. Pulmonary infections. In: King DW, ed. Atlas of Nontumor Pathology: Non-Neoplastic Disorders of the Lower Respiratory Tract, first series, fascicle 2. Washington, DC: American Registry of Pathology and Armed Forces Institute of Pathology, 2002:539–727

CASE 71 Aspiration Pneumonia: Mendelson Syndrome

Clinical Presentation

A 44-year-old woman admitted with variceal bleeding and witnessed aspiration following endoscopy

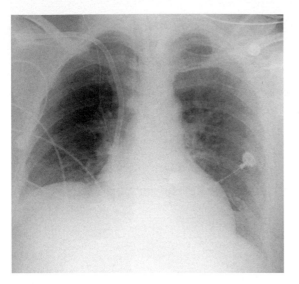

Figure 71A

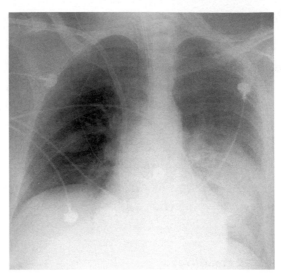

Figure 71B

Radiologic Findings

AP chest radiograph (**Fig. 71A**) before endoscopy shows appropriately positioned life support tubes and lines, an elevated right diaphragm, and clear lungs. AP chest radiograph (**Fig. 71B**) following endoscopy and witnessed aspiration reveals a new large, ill-defined consolidation in the left perihilar region and a smaller consolidation in the right mid-lung.

Diagnosis

Aspiration chemical pneumonitis; Mendelson's syndrome

Differential Diagnosis

None

Discussion

Background

Risk factors for aspiration include altered consciousness (e.g., drugs, alcohol, anesthesia, postictal states, cerebral vascular accidents, head trauma), upper gastrointestinal tract abnormalities (e.g., reflux, dysmotility syndromes), glottic closure disruption (e.g., endotracheal intubation or tracheostomy; endoscopic procedures), and recumbent positioning.

286

Etiology

Aspiration results from inhalation of particulate matter, fluids, or secretions from the stomach and/or oropharynx into the lungs. Small-volume aspirates are common and readily handled by normal defense mechanisms (e.g., glottic closure, cough reflex) without ill sequelae. Aspiration pneumonia occurs when these mechanisms fail and the aspirate is toxic to the lungs (chemical pneumonitis), contains pathogens that induce an inflammatory response (bacterial anaerobic or mixed aerobic-anaerobic infection), or the aspirated material blocks the airway (airway obstruction). Classic chemical pneumonitis occurs following aspiration of a large volume of toxic gastric acid.

Clinical Findings

Patients with aspiration may present acutely with dyspnea, tachypnea, and tachycardia. Other signs and symptoms include fever, bronchospasm, hypoxemia, cyanosis, and pink frothy sputum. Complications include pulmonary edema, hemorrhage, and acute lung injury that may progress to respiratory failure (12%). Secondary bacterial infection may also complicate aspiration.

Pathology

GROSS

- Parenchymal edema, hemorrhage, and acute or organizing bronchopneumonia
- Mucopurulent exudate in the airways
- Nonspecific pulmonary fibrosis in cases of chronic aspiration

MICROSCOPIC

- Extensive acid-induced epithelial damage, edema, hemorrhage, hyaline membranes

Imaging Findings

- Focal or multifocal airspace disease (**Fig. 71B**)
  - Dependent on volume of aspirate, composition of aspirate (pure gastric acid vs admixed with food), and patient position at the time of aspiration
  - Aspiration in the supine position: consolidation with preferential involvement of the posterior segments of the upper lobes and superior segments of the lower lobes (**Fig. 71B**)
  - Aspiration of pure gastric acid with a low pH; patchy perihilar bilateral airspace consolidation, which worsens over several days, and then either improves or progresses to ARDS
- Resolution in 7 to 10 days in survivors

Treatment

- Supportive care with intubation and mechanical ventilation
- Tracheal suctioning to remove particulate matter in cases of witnessed aspiration
- Antibiotics if secondary infection is suspected or develops

Prognosis

- Acute aspiration of gastric acid; 30 to 50% mortality rate
- 62% of patients: rapid radiographic clearing
- 25% of patients: initial rapid clinical improvement followed by new or expanding radiographic opacities (differential diagnosis includes secondary bacterial infection and pulmonary embolus)

PEARLS_____

- Aspiration of material admixed with food usually follows a segmental distribution, affecting one of the posterior segments of the upper or lower lobes, and may resemble bronchopneumonia. There is usually some degree of concomitant atelectasis.
- In cases of repeated aspiration bronchiectasis and pulmonary fibrosis may occur.

Suggested Readings

Franquet T, Gimenez A, Roson N, Torrubia S, Sabate JM, Perez C. Aspiration diseases: findings, pitfalls, and differential diagnosis. Radiographics 2000;20:673–685

Fraser RS, Müller NL, Colman N, Paré PD. Pulmonary infection. In: Fraser and Paré's Diagnosis of Diseases of the Chest, 4th ed. Philadelphia: Saunders, 1999:2485–2500

Travis WD, Colby TV, Koss MN, Rosado-de-Christenson ML, Müller NL, King TE Jr. Lung infections. In: King DW, ed. Atlas of Nontumor Pathology: Non-Neoplastic Disorders of the Lower Respiratory Tract, first series, fascicle 2. Washington, DC: American Registry of Pathology; 2002:187–196

SECTION VI
Neoplastic Diseases

CASE 72 Lung Cancer: Adenocarcinoma

Clinical Presentation

A 65-year-old man with cough and chest pain

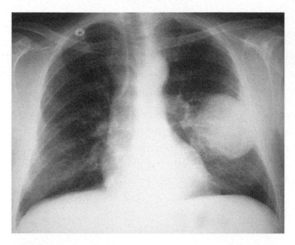

Figure 72A

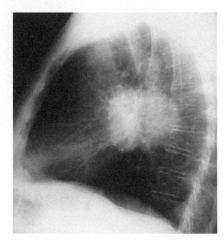

Figure 72B

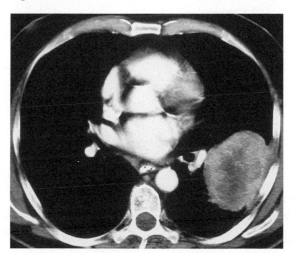

Figure 72C

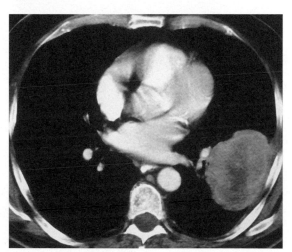

Figure 72D

Radiologic Findings

PA (**Fig. 72A**) and lateral (**Fig. 72B**) chest radiographs demonstrate a spherical mass with lobular contours in the left mid-lung. Contrast-enhanced chest CT (mediastinal window) (**Figs. 72C** and **72D**) demonstrates a heterogeneously enhancing mass with irregular central low attenuation related to necrosis. The mass abuts lobar and segmental bronchi medially (**Fig. 72D**) and the adjacent pleura laterally, and local invasion cannot be excluded.

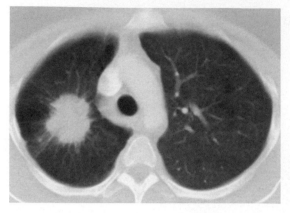

Figure 72E Unenhanced chest CT (lung window) of a middle-aged woman with adenocarcinoma shows a spiculated right upper lobe mass. Note that some tumor spicules extend to the pleural surface, producing "pleural tails" and focal retraction.

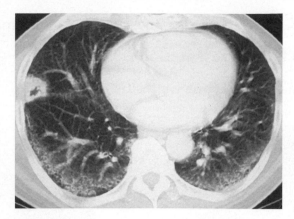

Figure 72F Unenhanced chest CT (lung window) of a 66-year-old man with idiopathic pulmonary fibrosis shows a peripheral right middle lobe cavitary mass, which represented an adenocarcinoma. Note the spiculated lesion borders and the thick nodular cavity wall.

Diagnosis

Lung cancer: adenocarcinoma

Differential Diagnosis

- Lung cancer, other cell type
- Other primary malignant neoplasm
- Lung abscess
- Solitary metastasis (rare)

Discussion

Background

Lung cancer is a primary malignant epithelial neoplasm and the most common fatal malignancy of men and women in North America. Four principal cell types (adenocarcinoma, squamous cell carcinoma, small cell carcinoma, and large cell carcinoma) are recognized, but multidifferentiated tumors also occur. Adenocarcinoma is the most frequently diagnosed cell type of lung cancer in the United States. It is characterized by its slow local growth and early metastases.

Etiology

Lung cancer is strongly associated with exposure to inhaled carcinogens, particularly cigarette smoke. While all cell types are related to cigarette smoking, adenocarcinoma exhibits a weak association with cigarette smoking and is the most common cell type diagnosed in nonsmokers and in women. Lung cancer is also associated with exposure to occupational and environmental agents such as asbestos and radon. Conditions characterized by pulmonary fibrosis (such as usual interstitial pneumonitis and progressive systemic sclerosis) are associated with an increased incidence of lung cancer, particularly adenocarcinoma. Atypical adenomatous hyperplasia is the postulated preinvasive or precursor lesion of adenocarcinoma. It is most common in women and is found most frequently in cancer-bearing lungs, particularly in association with adenocarcinoma.

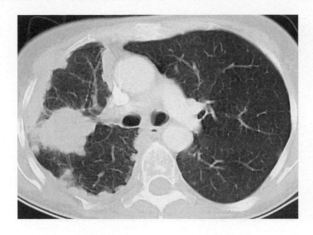

Figure 72G Contrast-ehanced chest CT (lung window) of a 43-year-old woman with adenocarcinoma demonstrates a lobular right upper lobe mass and circumferential nodular pleural thickening with encasement and volume loss of the right lung. The imaging findings mimic those of malignant pleural mesothelioma.

Clinical Findings

Over 90% of patients with lung cancer are symptomatic at presentation. Large masses may produce cough, dyspnea, and/or chest discomfort. Pleural and chest wall invasion results in pleuritic or localized chest pain. Central adenocarcinomas may produce symptoms of bronchial obstruction. Paraneoplastic syndromes such as thrombophlebitis and nonbacterial thrombotic endocarditis may occur in association with adenocarcinoma. A minority of affected patients are asymptomatic and diagnosed incidentally because of abnormal chest radiographs.

Pathology

GROSS

- Peripheral, juxtapleural mass; frequent central fibrosis, pleural puckering, spiculated borders
- Isolated peripheral mass (50%); peripheral mass with lymphadenopathy; central mass (50%)
- Variable size; small nodule to large mass that may replace an entire lung
- Contiguous pleural invasion; progression to circumferential pleural involvement mimicking malignant pleural mesothelioma

MICROSCOPIC

- Glandular differentiation, mucin production
- Acinar, papillary, bronchioloalveolar, and solid growth patterns
- Histologic heterogeneity; coexistence of several growth patterns in a single lesion

Imaging Findings

RADIOGRAPHY

- Solitary pulmonary nodule or mass of variable border characteristics; ill-defined, spiculated, or well-defined lobular contours (**Figs. 72A** and **72B**)
- Associated hilar and/or mediastinal lymphadenopathy

CT

- Peripheral nodule or mass with lobular or spiculated borders (**Figs. 72C, 72D, 72E, 72F, 72G,** and **72H1**)
- Cavitation (in up to 15% of lung cancers) (**Fig. 72F**) and calcification (usually eccentric, in up to 10% of lung cancers), more common in large tumors
- Contrast enhancement (**Figs. 72C** and **72D**)

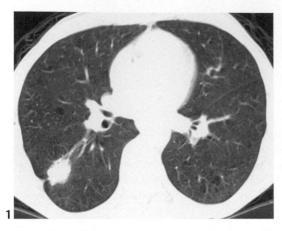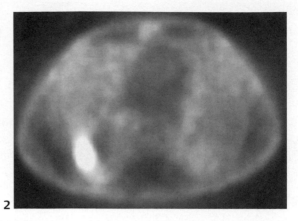

Figure 72H (1,2) Unenhanced chest CT (lung window) **(1)** of a 67-year-old woman with adenocarcinoma demonstrates a right lower lobe mass with spiculated borders with a pleural tail and focal pleural retraction. Axial PET image **(2)** demonstrates intense FDG uptake in the mass. (Courtesy of Diane C. Strollo, M.D., University of Pittsburgh, Pittsburgh, Pennsylvania.)

- Pleural effusion, pleural masses, or both in cases with pleural involvement (**Fig. 72G**)
- Osseous destruction indicates chest wall involvement.
- Lesion characterization, staging, and biopsy/resection planning; evaluation of adjacent structures [pleura (**Fig. 72G**), chest wall, mediastinum] to exclude invasion

MR

- More sensitive than CT for demonstration of chest wall involvement
- Demonstration of hilar/mediastinal lymphadenopathy, particularly if contraindication for intravenous administration of iodinated contrast

POSITRON EMISSION TOMOGRAPHY (PET)

- Noninvasive evaluation of patients with lung cancer; imaging after intravenous administration of 2-(fluorine-18)-fluoro-2-deoxy-D-glucose (18-FDG); FDG accumulation from increased glucose utilization by malignant cells (**Fig. 72H2**)
- High sensitivity (**Fig. 72H2**) and negative predictive value in nodules over 1 cm in diameter

Treatment

- See Cases 77, 78, 79, 80, and 81

Prognosis

- See Cases 77, 78, 79, 80, and 81

PEARLS_____

- All cell types of lung cancer exhibit a predilection for the upper lobes.
- The doubling time (time required for doubling of tumor volume) of adenocarcinomas ranges between 7 and 465 days. Size stability of a pulmonary nodule for 2 years is a reliable criterion for benignity.
- Tumor size does not allow distinction between benign and malignant pulmonary nodules, but large masses (> 3 cm) are more likely to be malignant (**Figs. 72A, 72B, 72C,** and **72D**).

- While irregular spiculated lesion borders are suggestive of malignancy (**Figs. 72E, 72F,** and **72H1**), they are also described in benign conditions. However, lung cancer may also manifest as a well-defined nonlobular pulmonary nodule.
- The "tail sign" refers to a linear opacity that extends from a peripheral mass to the adjacent pleura with associated focal pleural retraction (**Figs. 72E** and **72H1**). It is seen in up to 80% of peripheral lung cancers imaged with high-resolution computed tomography (HRCT) and is most commonly associated with adenocarcinoma.
- Absence of contrast enhancement or enhancement of less than 15 Hounsfield units (HU) on CT in a homogeneous solitary pulmonary nodule (up to 30 mm in diameter) virtually excludes lung cancer.
- Patients with pulmonary fibrosis have a higher incidence of lung cancer, typically adenocarcinoma. These tumors exhibit a predilection for the lower lobes and the lung periphery (**Fig. 72F**).
- Malignant pleural mesothelioma typically manifests with circumferential nodular pleural thickening. However, peripheral adenocarcinoma may diffusely involve the pleura and manifest with identical imaging findings (**Fig. 72G**).

Suggested Readings

Beckles MA, Spiro SG, Colice GL, Rudd RM. Initial evaluation of the patient with lung cancer: symptoms, signs, laboratory tests, and paraneoplastic syndromes. Chest 2003;123:97S–104S

Colby T, Koss M, Travis WD. Adenocarcinoma of the lung (excluding bronchioloalveolar carcinoma). In: Rosai J, Sobin LH, eds. Atlas of Tumor Pathology: Tumors of the Lower Respiratory Tract, fascicle 13, series 3. Washington, DC: Armed Forces Institute of Pathology, 1995:179–202

Fraser RS, Müller NL, Colman N, Paré PD. Pulmonary carcinoma. In: Fraser RS, Müller NL, Colman N, Paré PD, eds. Fraser and Paré's Diagnosis of Diseases of the Chest, 4th ed. Philadelphia: Saunders, 1999:1069–1228

Travis WD, Colby TV, Corrin B, et al. Histological Typing of Lung and Pleural Tumours: International Histological Classification of Tumours, 3rd ed. Berlin: Springer-Verlag, 1999

CASE 73 Lung Cancer: Bronchioloalveolar Carcinoma

Clinical Presentation

Asymptomatic 71-year-old woman imaged prior to breast surgery

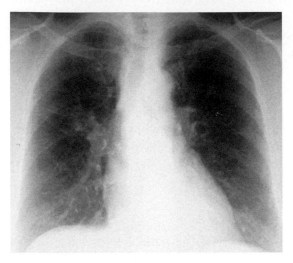

Figure 73A

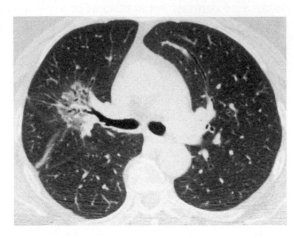

Figure 73B

Radiologic Findings

PA (**Fig. 73A**) chest radiograph demonstrates an ill-defined right upper lobe nodular opacity. Unenhanced chest CT (**Fig. 73B**) (lung window) demonstrates a heterogeneous 3 cm pulmonary nodule that surrounds the right upper lobe bronchus. Note the lesion's heterogeneous attenuation, irregular margins, pleural tails, internal patent bronchi, and air bronchiolograms.

Diagnosis

Lung cancer: bronchioloalveolar carcinoma

Differential Diagnosis

- Pneumonia
- Pulmonary lymphoma

Discussion

Background

- Bronchioloalveolar carcinoma is a subtype of adenocarcinoma with distinctive morphologic and prognostic features. It represents approximately 5% of lung cancers.

296

Etiology

- Bronchioloalveolar carcinoma (BAC) strongly resembles atypical adenomatous hyperplasia (AAH), the postulated precursor lesion of adenocarcinoma. Studies suggest that BAC is either closely associated with AAH or develops from the latter.

Clinical Findings

Approximately 50% of BACs are diagnosed in asymptomatic patients with incidentally discovered solitary pulmonary nodules. Patients with BAC that manifests with consolidation, or multifocal nodules, masses, and consolidations, may present with cough and fever. Mucin-producing BACs with extensive lung involvement may result in bronchorrhea (cough productive of copious amounts of sputum). Profound bronchorrhea may be complicated by hypovolemia and electrolyte imbalance.

Pathology

GROSS

- Arises beyond a recognizable bronchus
- Solitary peripheral pulmonary nodule without local invasion or lymphadenopathy
- Focal consolidation, multifocal nodules, masses, or consolidations

MICROSCOPIC

- Neoplastic cells line airspaces and respect underlying pulmonary interstitium (lepidic growth)
- Mucinous and nonmucinous cell types
- No stromal, vascular, or pleural invasion
  - Reliable diagnosis cannot be made on small fine-needle aspiration biopsies
  - Invasive adenocarcinoma may exhibit a bronchioloalveolar growth pattern
- Tracheobronchial dissemination; multifocal lung involvement

Imaging Findings

RADIOGRAPHY

- Peripheral solitary pulmonary nodule or mass (**Fig. 73A**)
- Less frequently, focal consolidation, multifocal nodules, masses, and/or consolidations

CT

- Heterogeneous attenuation including ground-glass opacity, air bronchograms/bronchiolograms, and intratumoral "bubble-like" cystic airspaces (**Figs. 73B** and **73C**)
- Irregular or ill-defined margins, pleural tails (**Figs. 73B** and **73C**)
- Focal nodule or mass (**Figs. 73B** and **73C**) or consolidation (**Fig. 73D1**)
- Multifocal ground-glass opacities, consolidations (**Fig. 73D2**), and/or nodules; centrilobular nodules
- CT angiogram sign (visualization of contrast-enhanced vessels within a mass) described in mucinous BACs
- CT bronchus sign (visualization of a patent bronchus within a lesion) described in several cell types of lung cancer, typically BACs (**Fig. 73B**)
- Documentation of multifocal lung involvement; may represent tracheobronchial dissemination (**Fig. 73D2**)

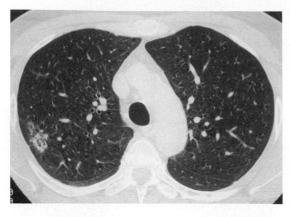

Figure 73C Unenhanced chest CT (lung window) of an asymptomatic patient with BAC demonstrates a 3 cm peripheral nodule of heterogeneous attenuation. Note the lesion's irregular contours, pleural tail, peripheral ground-glass opacity, and internal air lucencies.

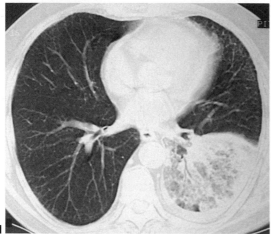

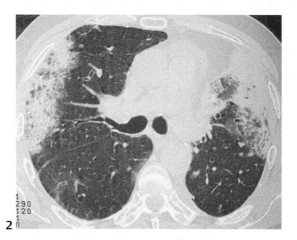

Figure 73D (1) Unenhanced chest CT (lung window) of a 74-year-old man with cough, fever, and BAC demonstrates a left lower lobe consolidation and a small ipsilateral pleural effusion. **(2)** Unenhanced chest CT (lung window) performed several months after left lower lobectomy demonstrates multifocal peripheral consolidations and ground-glass opacities affecting all the visualized pulmonary lobes, which represented multifocal BAC (likely resulting from tracheobronchial dissemination).

Treatment

- See Cases 77, 78, 79, 80, and 81

Prognosis

- Small resected lesions (< 2 cm); excellent prognosis: 5-year survival near 100%
- See Cases 77, 78, 79, 80, and 81

PEARLS_____

- Visualization of air bronchograms/bronchiolograms in a pulmonary nodule suggests malignancy (**Figs. 73B** and **73C**).
- Cavitation, local invasion, lymph node, pleural and extrathoracic metastases are not typical of BAC and suggest an invasive carcinoma.
- BAC demonstrate less 2-(fluorine-18)-fluoro-2-deoxy-D-glucose (18-FDG) activity than other cell types of lung cancer and may result in negative PET scans.

Suggested Readings

Akira M, Atagi S, Kawahara M, Iuchi K, Johkoh T. High-resolution CT findings of diffuse bronchioloalveolar carcinoma in 38 patients. AJR Am J Roentgenol 1999;173:1623–1629

Colby T, Koss M, Travis WD. Bronchioloalveolar carcinoma. In: Rosai J, Sobin LH, eds. Atlas of Tumor Pathology: Tumors of the Lower Respiratory Tract, fascicle 13, series 3. Washington, DC: Armed Forces Institute of Pathology, 1995:202–234

Marom EM, Sarvis S, Herndon JE II, Patz EF Jr. T1 lung cancers: sensitivity of diagnosis with fluorodeoxyglucose PET. Radiology 2002;223:453–459

Mihara N, Ichikado K, Johkoh T, et al. The subtypes of localized bronchioloalveolar carcinoma: CT-pathologic correlation in 18 cases. AJR Am J Roentgenol 1999;173:75–79

Travis WD, Colby TV, Corrin B, et al. Histological Typing of Lung and Pleural Tumours: International Histological Classification of Tumours, 3rd ed. Berlin: Springer-Verlag, 1999

CASE 74 Lung Cancer: Squamous Cell Carcinoma

Clinical Presentation

A 57-year-old woman with cough, hemoptysis, and weight loss

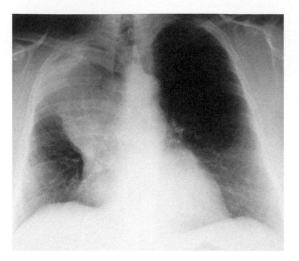

Figure 74A

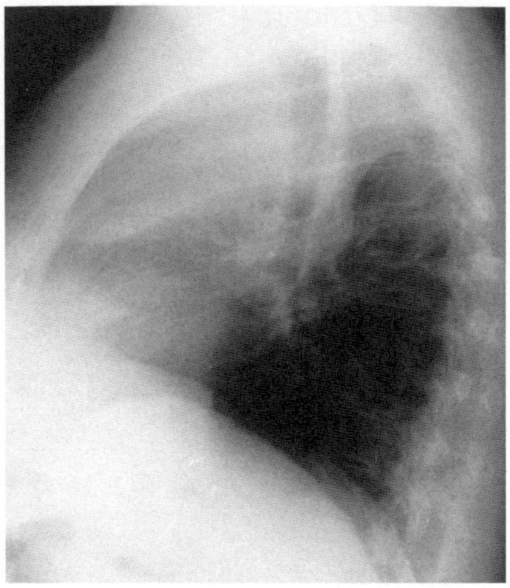

Figure 74B

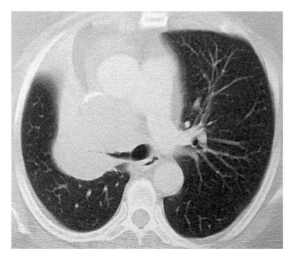

Figure 74C

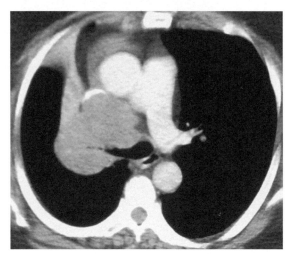

Figure 74D

Radiologic Findings

PA (**Fig. 74A**) and lateral (**Fig. 74B**) chest radiographs demonstrate a large right hilar mass with associated right upper lobe volume loss. Note the reverse-S shape produced by the concave outline of the lateral aspect of the minor fissure and the convex outline of the central mass (**Fig. 74A**), the so-called S sign of Golden. Contrast-enhanced chest CT (lung and mediastinal window) (**Figs. 74C** and **74D**) demonstrates a large central mass, which produces severe irregular narrowing of the right mainstem bronchus (**Fig. 74C**), atelectasis of the right upper lobe (**Fig. 74D**), and deformity and narrowing of the superior vena cava consistent with local invasion (**Fig. 74D**).

Diagnosis

Lung cancer: squamous cell carcinoma

Differential Diagnosis

- Lung cancer, other cell type
- Other primary malignant neoplasm
- Pulmonary lymphoma
- Mediastinal metastases

Discussion

Background

Squamous cell carcinoma, a subtype of lung cancer, accounts for approximately 30% of all lung carcinomas. It is characterized by the rapid local growth of the primary neoplasm and the relatively late occurrence of distant metastases.

Etiology

Squamous cell carcinoma has a strong association with cigarette smoking and exposure to other inhaled carcinogens, and is particularly associated with occupational exposure to nickel.

Clinical Findings

Squamous cell carcinomas are rapidly growing neoplasms with a predilection for the central airways. Affected patients usually exhibit early signs and symptoms of airway obstruction including cough, hemoptysis, wheezing, and obstructive pneumonia. Some patients present with paraneoplastic syndromes, such as hypercalcemia resulting from a parathyroid hormone–related peptide produced by the tumor. Digital clubbing and hypertrophic osteoarthropathy are most frequently associated with squamous cell carcinoma and adenocarcinoma. Hypertrophic osteoarthropathy is observed in less than 5% of patients with non–small cell lung cancer and typically manifests as painful bilateral arthropathy of the ankles, knees, and wrists and periosteal new bone formation of the distal aspects of the long bones of the extremities.

Pathology

GROSS

- Central irregular exophytic endoluminal polypoid mass of the main, segmental, or subsegmental bronchi, with frequent invasion of the bronchial wall and adjacent lung
- Peripheral squamous cell carcinomas increasingly recognized
- Atelectasis and pneumonia in association with central obstructing tumors
- Necrosis and hemorrhage in up to one third of cases
- May exhibit cavitation and secondary infection

MICROSCOPIC

- Individual cell keratinization; keratin pearls in well-differentiated tumors
- Intercellular bridges between adjacent tumor cells

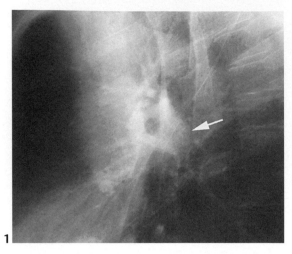
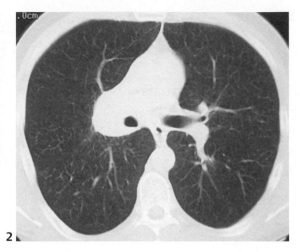

Figure 74E (1,2) Coned-down lateral chest radiograph **(1)** of a 41-year-old man with a central squamous cell carcinoma demonstrates thickening of the posterior wall of the bronchus intermedius with a nodular posterior contour (arrow), suggestive of malignancy and lymphadenopathy. Unenhanced chest CT **(2)** (lung window) demonstrates a right central mass and adjacent bronchial wall thickening.

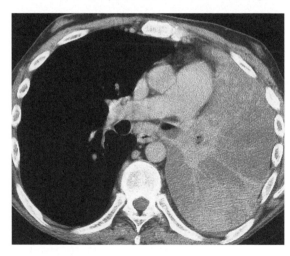

Figure 74F Unenhanced chest CT (mediastinal window) demonstrates a central spiculated soft tissue mass encasing the left mainstem bronchus surrounded by low attenuation "drowned" lung. Note the absence of air bronchograms and the subcarinal (station 7 ATS) lymphadenopathy.

Imaging Findings

RADIOGRAPHY

- Frequent secondary atelectasis (absent air bronchograms) (**Figs. 74A** and **74B**), obstructive pneumonia, and/or mucoid impaction; may be dominant radiologic abnormalities
- Central mass (**Figs. 74A, 74B,** and **74E1**)
- Wall thickening of anterior segmental bronchi of right and left upper lobes and superior segmental left upper lobe bronchus
- Thickened (> 3 mm) posterior wall of bronchus intermedius (lateral radiography) (**Fig. 74E1**)
- Peripheral lung nodule or mass
- Cavitation
- Lymphadenopathy (**Fig. 74E1**)

CT

- Bronchial wall thickening (**Figs. 74C, 74D,** and **74E2**)
- Irregular central mass with abrupt obstruction of bronchial lumen (**Figs. 74C, 74D, 74F,** and **74G1**)

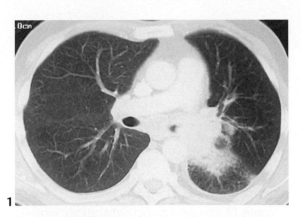 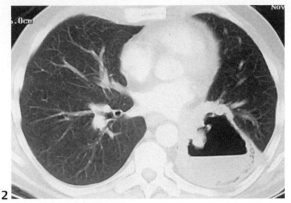

Figure 74G (1,2) Contrast-enhanced chest CT (lung window) of a 58-year-old man with a central squamous cell carcinoma demonstrates an irregular soft tissue mass obstructing the left lower lobe bronchus **(1)** with distal lower lobe consolidation and cavitation **(2)**.

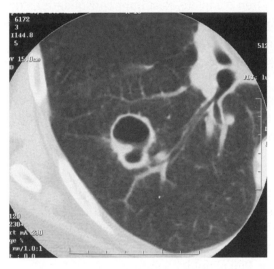

Figure 74H High-resolution computed tomography (HRCT) (lung window) targeted to the right lung of an asymptomatic 50-year-old man with squamous cell carcinoma demonstrates a 2.8 cm cavitary nodule in the right lower lobe. Note the irregular nodular cavity wall.

- Postobstructive consolidation (**Figs. 74F** and **74G**), atelectasis (**Figs. 74C** and **74D**); intravenous contrast administration may help differentiate tumor from adjacent consolidation/atelectasis, as tumor typically enhances less than atelectatic lung
- Peripheral mass or nodule (**Fig. 74H**)
- Cavitation; central or eccentric, irregular inner surface (**Figs. 74G2** and **74H**)
- Mediastinal (**Figs. 74C** and **74D**), osseous or soft tissue invasion
- Lymphadenopathy (**Figs. 74C, 74D, 74E2,** and **74F**)

MR

- More sensitive than CT for demonstration of chest wall involvement
- Distinction of tumor from surrounding atelectasis/consolidation
- Demonstration of hilar/mediastinal lymphadenopathy, particularly if contraindication for administration of intravenous iodinated contrast

PET

- Noninvasive evaluation of patients with lung cancer; imaging after intravenous administration of 2-(fluorine-18)-fluoro-2-deoxy-D-glucose (18-FDG); FDG accumulation from increased glucose utilization by malignant cells
- High sensitivity and negative predictive value in tumors over 1 cm in diameter

Treatment

• See Cases 77, 78, 79, 80, and 81

Prognosis

• See Cases 77, 78, 79, 80, and 81

PEARLS_____

• The S sign of Golden refers to lobar collapse associated with a central obstructing mass, which produces a convex contour medial to the concave contour of the atelectatic right upper lobe on frontal radiography (resulting in a reverse-S shape) (**Fig. 74A**). Similar contour abnormalities are seen on other lobes and on lateral radiography. This finding is highly suggestive of malignancy.

• Airway obstruction from a central lung carcinoma is often complete. Resultant consolidations do not typically exhibit air bronchograms and are characterized by volume loss. However, obstructive pneumonitis with consolidation may limit loss of volume, and airspaces may fill with fluid, a finding known as "drowned lung" (**Fig. 74F**). Long-standing obstruction may also result in infection and abscess formation (**Fig. 74G2**).

• Squamous cell carcinoma is the most frequent cell type of lung cancer to exhibit cavitation. Most cavitary cancers exhibit irregular nodular inner cavity walls between 0.5 and 3.0 cm thick (**Fig. 74H**), but thin, smooth cavity walls (that may mimic benign conditions) are also described.

Suggested Readings

Colby T, Koss M, Travis WD. Squamous cell carcinoma and variants. In: Rosai J, Sobin LH, eds. Atlas of Tumor Pathology: Tumors of the Lower Respiratory Tract, fascicle 13, series 3. Washington, DC: Armed Forces Institute of Pathology, 1995:157–178

Felson B. The lobes. In: Felson B, ed. Chest Roentgenology. Philadelphia: Saunders, 1973:71–142

Fraser RS, Müller NL, Colman N, Paré PD. Atelectasis. In: Fraser RS, Müller NL, Colman N, Paré PD, eds. Fraser and Paré's Diagnosis of Diseases of the Chest, 4th ed. Philadelphia: Saunders, 1999:513–562

Fraser RS, Müller NL, Colman N, Paré PD. Pulmonary carcinoma. In: Fraser RS, Müller NL, Colman N, Paré PD, eds. Fraser and Paré's Diagnosis of Diseases of the Chest, 4th ed. Philadelphia: Saunders, 1999:1069–1228

Travis WD, Colby TV, Corrin B, et al. Histological Typing of Lung and Pleural Tumours: International Histological Classification of Tumours, 3rd ed. Berlin: Springer-Verlag, 1999

CASE 75 Lung Cancer: Small Cell Carcinoma

Clinical Presentation

A 60-year-old woman with facial swelling and weight loss

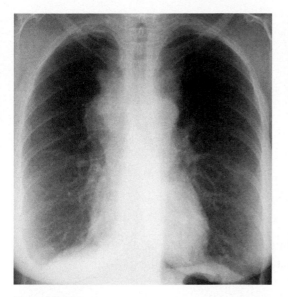

Figure 75A

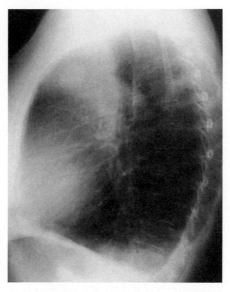

Figure 75B

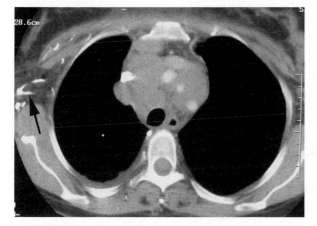

Figure 75C

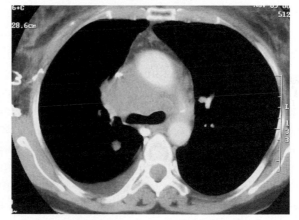

Figure 75D

Radiologic Findings

PA (**Fig. 75A**) and lateral (**Fig. 75B**) chest radiographs demonstrate a mediastinal mass of lobular borders that extends to both sides of midline and is predominantly located in the anterior mediastinum (**Fig. 75B**). Note the small right pleural effusion. Contrast-enhanced chest CT (mediastinal window) (**Figs. 75C** and **75D**) demonstrates extensive mediastinal lymphadenopathy encasing the great vessels and a small right pleural effusion. Note almost complete obliteration of the lumen of the superior vena cava (**Fig. 75D**), enhancing chest wall collateral vessels (arrow), and intense enhancement of the azygos vein consistent with superior vena cava obstruction.

Diagnosis

Lung cancer: small cell carcinoma

Differential Diagnosis

- Lung cancer, other cell type
- Pulmonary lymphoma
- Mediastinal metastases

Discussion

Background

Small cell carcinoma is a highly aggressive cell type of lung cancer that accounts for approximately 13.8 to 20% of all lung carcinomas. It is characterized by rapid local tumor growth and frequent metastases at presentation.

Etiology

All cell types of lung cancer are associated with cigarette smoking, but small cell carcinoma demonstrates the strongest association. This cell type is also strongly associated with occupational exposure to chloromethyl ether and radon gas.

Clinical Findings

Patients with small cell carcinoma are typically elderly men with a significant history of cigarette smoking. Symptoms such as cough and dyspnea often relate to central airway obstruction. Locally invasive tumors may grow into the mediastinum with resultant retrosternal pain. Small cell carcinoma is the most common cause of the superior vena cava syndrome, characterized by facial and upper extremity swelling, headache, and dizziness. Patients with small cell carcinoma may also present with signs and symptoms related to metastatic disease such as anorexia, malaise, fever, and weight loss. Secretion of peptide hormones may result in paraneoplastic syndromes related to excessive production of adrenocorticotropic hormone (ACTH) or antidiuretic hormone (ADH). Small cell carcinoma may also be associated with paraneoplastic autoimmune neurologic syndromes such as Lambert-Eaton myasthenic syndrome, peripheral neuropathy, and cortical cerebellar degeneration.

Pathology

GROSS

- Central mass near major bronchi; submucosal tumor with rare mucosal or endoluminal growth
- Bronchial encasement with extrinsic stenosis/obstruction
- Vascular invasion/encasement
- Peripheral nodule or mass (approximately 5% of cases)
- Lymphadenopathy

MICROSCOPIC

- Small, round to oval neoplastic cells with scant cytoplasm, ill-defined borders, granular nuclear chromatin, and absent or inconspicuous nucleoli
- High mitotic rates; average of 60 to 70 mitoses per 2 mm^2 (or 10 high power fields)
- Frequent and extensive necrosis

- Neuroendocrine features
- Frequent lymph node metastases

Imaging Findings

RADIOGRAPHY

- Large central mass with hilar or mediastinal lymphadenopathy (**Figs. 75A** and **75B**)
- Hilar or mediastinal lymphadenopathy as dominant finding without visualization of primary tumor (**Figs. 75A** and **75B**)
- Rarely peripheral nodule/mass with or without lymphadenopathy

CT

- Primary tumor assessment, demonstration of local invasion (**Figs. 75C** and **75D**)
- Identification of lymphadenopathy (**Figs. 75C** and **75D**)
- Demonstration of superior vena cava obstruction on contrast-enhanced CT; nonvisualization of superior vena cava lumen, enhancement of chest wall/mediastinal collateral vessels (**Figs. 75C** and **75D**)
- Identification of liver, adrenal gland, or chest wall metastases

MR

- May be superior to CT in demonstrating mediastinal invasion; multiplanar imaging assessment of vascular/pericardial invasion without need for intravenous contrast

Treatment

- Platinum-based chemotherapy
- Consideration of concurrent radiotherapy for patients with limited-stage small cell lung cancer
- Surgical excision with combination chemotherapy for rare patients with very limited-stage disease (T1/T2 and N0)
- Prophylactic cranial irradiation in patients with complete remission
- Endovascular stenting for patients with superior vena cava syndrome with prompt relief of symptoms and return to normal hemodynamics

Prognosis

- Poor prognosis; 5-year survival of 1 to 5%
- Median survival without treatment of 2 to 4 months
- Response to chemotherapy frequent but of short duration (4 months for patients with extensive-stage disease; 12 months for patients with limited-stage disease)

PEARL_____

- Patients with small cell lung cancer are generally staged using a two-stage system. Those with limited-stage disease have tumor involvement restricted to the ipsilateral hemithorax within one radiation therapy port, and those with extensive-stage disease have extensive metastases.

Suggested Readings

Fraser RS, Müller NL, Colman N, Paré PD. Pulmonary carcinoma. In: Fraser RS, Müller NL, Colman N, Paré PD, eds. Fraser and Paré's Diagnosis of Diseases of the Chest, 4th ed. Philadelphia: Saunders, 1999:1069–1228

Lanciego C, Chacón JL, Julián A, et al. Stenting as first option for endovascular treatment of malignant superior vena cava syndrome. AJR Am J Roentgenol 2001;177:585–593

Simon GR, Wagner H. Small cell lung cancer. Chest 2003;123:259S–271S

Travis WD, Colby TV, Corrin B, et al. Histological Typing of Lung and Pleural Tumours: International Histological Classification of Tumours, 3rd ed. Berlin: Springer-Verlag, 1999

Zakowski MF. Pathology of small cell carcinoma of the lung. Semin Oncol 2003;30:3–8

CASE 76 Lung Cancer: Large Cell Carcinoma

Clinical Presentation

A 70-year-old woman with right chest wall pain

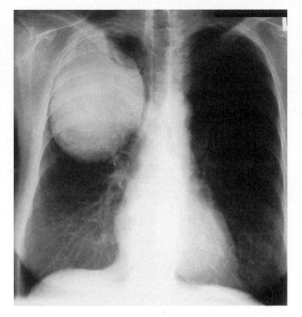

Figure 76A

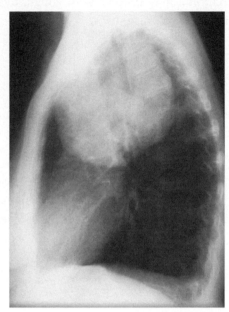

Figure 76B

Radiologic Findings

PA (**Fig. 76A**) and lateral (**Fig. 76B**) chest radiographs demonstrate a large ovoid right upper lobe mass of lobular contours with adjacent right apical pleural thickening and possible destruction of the anterolateral portions of the second and third right ribs.

Diagnosis

Lung cancer, large cell carcinoma

Differential Diagnosis

- Lung cancer, other cell type
- Pulmonary lymphoma
- Lung abscess

Discussion

Background

Large cell carcinoma is an aggressive cell type of lung cancer that accounts for up to 15% of all lung carcinomas. These neoplasms typically exhibit rapid growth and are frequently metastatic at presentation.

Etiology

Large cell carcinomas, like other cell types of lung cancer, are associated with cigarette smoking.

Clinical Findings

Patients with large cell carcinoma may present with cough, dyspnea, and/or chest pain related to tumor size, obstruction, and/or local invasion.

Pathology

GROSS

- Large, typically peripheral tumors; often measure over 3 cm at presentation
- Frequent necrosis, uncommon cavitation

MICROSCOPIC

- Diagnosis of exclusion; no features of glandular (adeno), squamous, or small cell differentiation
- Large cells, moderate cytoplasm, large nuclei, and prominent nucleoli
- Frequent mitoses, average of 75 per 2 mm^2 (or 10 high power fields)
- Frequent necrosis

Imaging Findings

RADIOGRAPHY

- Large peripheral lung mass (**Figs. 76A** and **76B**)
- Large central mass
- Mass with associated hilar and/or mediastinal lymphadenopathy

CT

- Large mass
- Frequent heterogeneous attenuation, particularly after intravenous contrast administration
- Frequent lymphadenopathy
- Assessment of local invasion

MR

- Superior to CT for visualization of chest wall/mediastinal invasion

Treatment

- See Cases 77, 78, 79, 80, and 81.

Prognosis

- See Cases 77, 78, 79, 80, and 81.

Suggested Readings

Fraser RS, Müller NL, Colman N, Paré PD. Pulmonary carcinoma. In: Fraser RS, Müller NL, Colman N, Paré PD, eds. Fraser and Paré's Diagnosis of Diseases of the Chest, 4th ed. Philadelphia: Saunders, 1999:1069–1228

Travis WD, Colby TV, Corrin B, et al. Histological Typing of Lung and Pleural Tumours: International Histological Classification of Tumours, 3rd ed. Berlin: Springer-Verlag, 1999

CASE 77 Lung Cancer: Stage I

Clinical Presentation

Asymptomatic 49-year-old man with a history of cigarette smoking

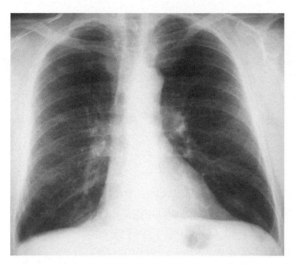

Figure 77A

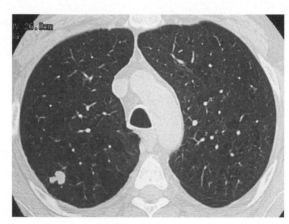

Figure 77B

Stage I

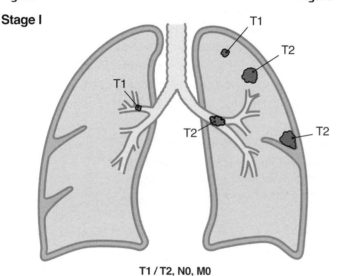

T1 / T2, N0, M0

Figure 77C

Radiologic Findings

PA (**Fig. 77A**) chest radiograph demonstrates a right upper lobe solitary pulmonary nodule that projects over the fifth posterior rib and the fourth intercostal space. Unenhanced HRCT (lung window) (**Fig. 77B**) demonstrates a well-defined lobular 1 cm right upper lobe nodule and proximal acinar emphysema. **Fig. 77C** depicts the spectrum of lesions categorized as stage I lung cancers; these are peripheral pulmonary nodules/masses that may exhibit focal involvement of the adjacent visceral pleura and central lesions located at least 2 cm distal to the carina without metastases to lymph nodes or distant sites.

311

Diagnosis

Lung cancer, adenocarcinoma: stage I

Differential Diagnosis

- Lung cancer, other cell types
- Bronchial carcinoid
- Benign solitary pulmonary nodule (such as granuloma or hamartoma)

Discussion

Background

Pathologists classify lung cancers according to the histologic cell types outlined by the World Health Organization (WHO) Histological Typing of Lung and Pleural Tumours. However, for the purposes of patient management, it is usually sufficient to determine whether a given lung cancer exhibits small cell or non–small cell histology. In general, only non–small cell lung cancers are considered for surgical treatment. T1 lung cancers are completely intrapulmonary lesions and measure 3 cm or less or are endobronchial lesions located distal to the orifice of a lobar bronchus (**Fig. 77C**). T2 lung cancers measure more than 3 cm in size and may focally involve the adjacent visceral pleura (**Fig. 77C**). Lung cancers located within the mainstem bronchi at least 2 cm from the carina are also considered T2 lesions, and associated atelectasis/consolidation may extend to the hilum but does not involve the entire lung (**Fig. 77C**). T1 and T2 lung cancers without local lymph node metastases (N0) and without metastases to distant lymph nodes or other organs (M0) are classified as stage I lung cancers. Stage IA refers to T1N0M0 lesions, and stage IB refers to T2N0M0 lesions (**Table 77–1**).

Clinical stage refers to the best estimation of the extent of disease prior to surgery. Surgical-pathologic stage refers to the actual stage of disease found on exploration/excision and final microscopic evaluation. Thus, staging of lung cancer using imaging studies is a form of clinical staging.

Table 77-1   Stage I Lung Cancer

	T1	T2
N0, M0	Stage IA	Stage IB

Clinical Findings

Patients with peripheral stage I lung cancers are often asymptomatic. Patients with central stage I lung cancers may have symptoms related to bronchial obstruction such as cough, hemoptysis, and/or wheezing.

Pathology

- All cell types of lung cancer may manifest as stage I lung cancers, particularly adenocarcinomas and squamous cell carcinomas.
- See Cases 72, 73, 74, 75, and 76.

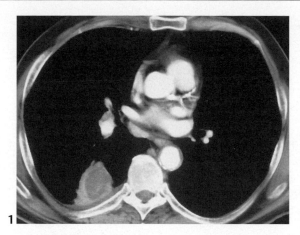
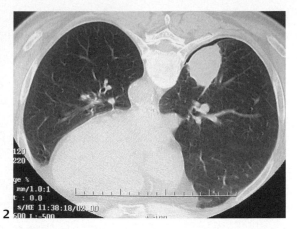

Figure 77D (1,2) Contrast-enhanced chest CT (mediastinal window) **(1)** of a 63-year-old man with non–small cell lung cancer demonstrates a peripheral heterogeneous right lower lobe mass with adjacent pleural thickening. Parietal pleural invasion cannot be excluded. Unenhanced prone chest CT (lung window) **(2)** obtained following lung biopsy (complicated by pneumothorax) shows that the tumor "falls away" from the parietal pleura, excluding local invasion. While the presence of visceral pleural invasion cannot be established, this is a T2 lesion based on its size. In the absence of lymphadenopathy or metastatic disease, it represents stage IB lung cancer.

Imaging Findings

RADIOGRAPHY

- Solitary pulmonary nodule/mass (**Fig. 77A**)
- Central (endobronchial) nodule/mass, at least 2 cm distal to carina, with or without associated atelectasis and/or consolidation not involving an entire lung
- Absence of lymphadenopathy (**Fig. 77A**)
- Absence of pleural effusion (**Fig. 77A**)

CT

- Characterization of lesion size and location
- Solitary pulmonary nodule/mass (**Figs. 77B** and **77D**)
- Central (endobronchial) nodule/mass, at least 2 cm distal to carina (**Fig. 77E1**); may be associated with atelectasis or consolidation not involving an entire lung (**Fig. 77E2**)

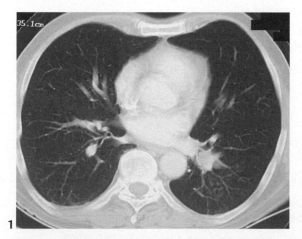
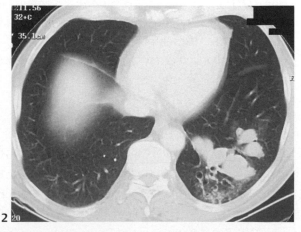

Figure 77E (1,2) Contrast-enhanced chest CT (lung window) of a 67-year-old man with squamous cell carcinoma demonstrates an irregular endobronchial mass **(1)** in the left lower lobe posterior segmental bronchus with distal mucoid impaction and bronchiectasis **(2).** This is a T1 lesion, and in the absence of metastases to lymph nodes or distant organs, represents a stage IA lung cancer.

- Evaluation of adjacent structures (mediastinum, pleura, chest wall); exclusion of pleural effusion and invasion of the chest wall/mediastinum (**Fig. 77D**)

MR

- Characterization of lesion size and location
- Evaluation of hilar/mediastinal lymph nodes, distinction of neoplasm from adjacent vascular structures
- Evaluation of chest wall/mediastinum for exclusion of local invasion

PET

- Absence of activity in hilar/mediastinal lymph nodes (see Case 72, **Fig. 72H(2)**)
- Absence of activity in extrathoracic lymph nodes and other organs (see Case 72, **Fig. 72H(2)**)

Treatment

- Complete surgical resection (lobectomy, bilobectomy, pneumonectomy with clear margins); sublobar resection in selected patients who cannot tolerate more extensive lung resection
- Consideration of additional local therapy in patients with positive resection margins (re-resection or radiation)
- Intraoperative systematic mediastinal lymph node dissection for accurate surgical/pathologic staging
- Radiation therapy for patients who are not surgical candidates

Prognosis

- 67% 5-year survivals for patients with surgical-pathologic stage IA lung cancers
- 57% 5-year survivals for patients with surgical-pathologic stage IB lung cancers

PEARLS_____

- CT is useful in demonstrating calcification within granulomatous hilar and mediastinal lymph nodes, which virtually excludes neoplastic involvement.
- Lesions that abut the pleura on CT or MR may represent T2 (visceral pleural involvement) (**Fig. 77D**) or T3 (parietal pleural involvement) lung cancers.
- Lymph node metastases may manifest as normal (short axis under 1 cm) lymph nodes.
- MR facilitates distinction of lymph nodes from adjacent vascular structures in patients in whom contrast-enhanced chest CT is contraindicated because of sensitivity to iodinated contrast material.

Suggested Readings

Farrell MA, McAdams HP, Herndon JE II, Patz EF Jr. Non-small cell lung cancer: FDG PET for nodal staging in patients with stage I disease. Radiology 2000;215:886–890

Mountain CF. Revisions in the international system for staging lung cancer. Chest 1997;111:1710–1717

Silvestri GA, Tanoue LT, Margolis ML, Barker J, Detterbeck F. The noninvasive staging of non-small cell lung cancer. The guidelines. Chest 2003;123:147S–156S

Smythe WR. Treatment of stage I non-small cell lung carcinoma. Chest 2003;123:181S–187S

CASE 78 Lung Cancer: Stage II

Clinical Presentation

A 79-year-old woman with chest pain, cough, and hemoptysis

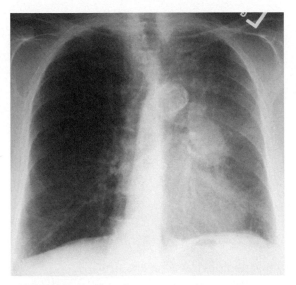

Figure 78A

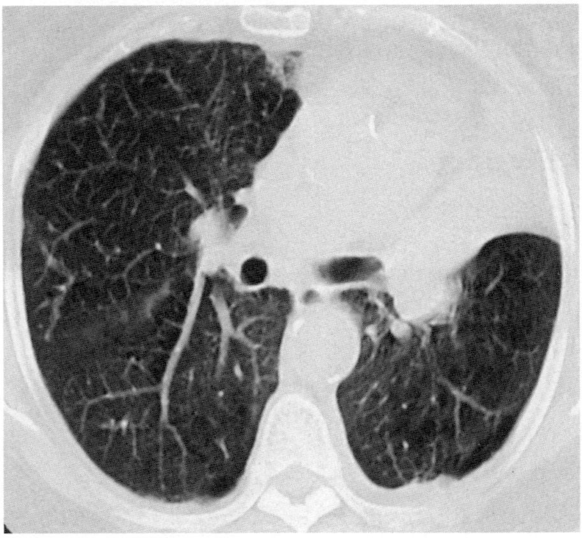

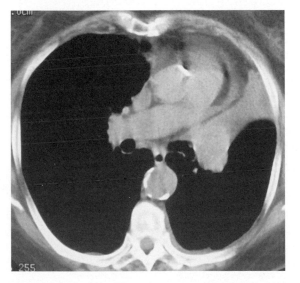

Figure 78C

Figure 78B

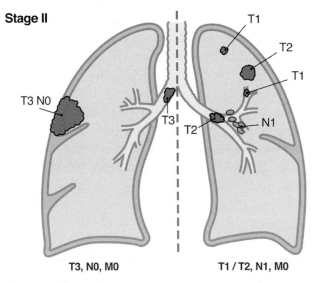

Figure 78D

Radiologic Findings

PA (**Fig. 78A**) chest radiograph demonstrates a left hilar mass with ipsilateral volume loss. Unenhanced chest CT (lung and mediastinal window) (**Figs. 78B** and **78C**) demonstrates an ovoid mass that obstructs the left upper lobe bronchus with resultant left upper lobe atelectasis. Involvement of left hilar lymph nodes was confirmed at surgery. **Fig. 78D** depicts the spectrum of lesions categorized as stage II lung cancers: T1 or T2 lesions with neoplastic involvement of ipsilateral peribronchial/hilar lymph nodes and T3 lesions without intrathoracic lymph node involvement, in the absence of metastases to mediastinal or contralateral intrathoracic lymph nodes, distant lymph node sites, or extrapulmonary organs.

Diagnosis

Lung cancer, squamous cell carcinoma: stage IIB

Differential Diagnosis

- Lung cancer, other cell type
- Bronchial carcinoid
- Pulmonary lymphoma

Discussion

Background

T1 and T2 lung cancers are discussed in Case 77. T3 lung cancers may invade nonvital adjacent structures, which typically can be excised en bloc with the primary tumor, such as the parietal pleura, chest wall (including superior sulcus tumors), diaphragm, and parietal pericardium (**Fig. 78D**). The T3 descriptor is also used for central lung cancers (in the mainstem bronchus) located within 2 cm from the carina (but not involving the carina); associated atelectasis/consolidation does not involve the entire lung. N1 lymph node involvement refers to neoplastic involvement of ipsilateral lymph nodes, which lie within the visceral pleura (hilar [ATS station 10], interlobar [ATS station 11], lobar [ATS station 12], segmental [ATS station 13], subsegmental [ATS station 14]) either by lymphatic metastases or direct neoplastic extension (**Fig. 78D**). T1 and T2 lesions with N1 lymph node involvement and T3 lesions without intrathoracic lymph node involvement (N0) are classified as stage II lesions provided there are no distant metastases (M0). Stage IIA refers to T1N1M0 lesions, and stage IIB refers to T2N1M0 and T3N0M0 lesions (**Table 78–1**).

Table 78-1   Stage II Lung Cancer

	T1	T2	T3
N0, M0	Stage IA	Stage IB	Stage IIB
N1, M0	**Stage IIA**	**Stage IIB**	**Stage IIIA**

Clinical Findings

Patients with stage II lung cancer are often symptomatic. Central lesions may produce cough and/or hemoptysis from endobronchial obstruction. Peripheral lesions with parietal pleura and/or chest wall involvement may manifest with local pain.

Pathology

- All cell types of lung cancer may manifest as stage II lesions.
- See Cases 72, 73, 74, 75, and 76.

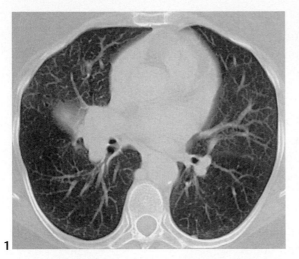 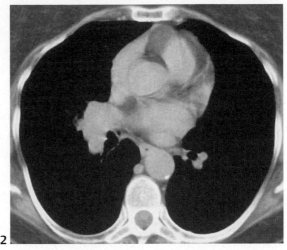

Figure 78E (1,2) Unenhanced chest CT [lung **(1)** and mediastinal **(2)** window] of a 69-year-old woman with cough and right middle lobe atelectasis demonstrates a lobular right hilar mass at the origin of the right middle lobe bronchus. At surgery, a 3 cm squamous cell carcinoma with ipsilateral hilar lymph node metastases was diagnosed.

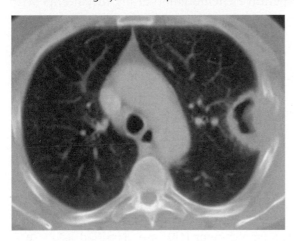

Figure 78F Contrast-enhanced chest CT (lung window) of a 58-year-old man with left chest pain and hemoptysis demonstrates a peripheral cavitary spiculated left upper lobe mass that invades the adjacent chest wall with resultant rib destruction. Small mediastinal lymph nodes were negative for tumor at mediastinoscopy. A left upper lobectomy with en bloc chest wall resection demonstrated a stage IIB squamous cell carcinoma.

Imaging Findings

RADIOGRAPHY

- Solitary peripheral pulmonary nodule (T1)/mass (T2); ipsilateral hilar lymphadenopathy
- Central nodule/mass located at least 2 cm from the carina (T2) (**Fig. 78A**); associated atelectasis/consolidation not involving an entire lung (**Fig. 78A**); ipsilateral hilar lymphadenopathy
- Central nodule/mass located within 2 cm from the carina, not involving the carina (T3); associated atelectasis consolidation not involving an entire lung; no lymphadenopathy
- Peripheral nodule/mass with adjacent chest wall invasion (T3); no lymphadenopathy

CT

- Characterization of lesion size and location; evaluation of intrathoracic lymph nodes
- Peripheral lung nodule/mass; ipsilateral hilar lymphadenopathy
- Central mass at least 2 cm from the carina (T1); with or without atelectasis/consolidation; with ipsilateral hilar lymphadenopathy (**Figs. 78B, 78C,** and **78E**)
- Central mass within 2 cm from the carina without carinal involvement (T3); atelectasis/consolidation not involving the entire lung; without lymphadenopathy
- Peripheral nodule/mass with chest wall (**Fig. 78F**), focal pleural, diaphragmatic, or parietal pericardial invasion; without lymphadenopathy

MR

- Evaluation of central lesions for size, location, and exclusion of carinal involvement
- Evaluation of peripheral lesions to exclude invasion of mediastinum, chest wall, or diaphragm
- Evaluation of hilar lymph nodes; distinction from vascular structures

PET

- Activity in ipsilateral hilar lymph nodes in association with T1/T2 lesions
- Absence of activity in thoracic lymph nodes in association with T3 lesions
- Absence of activity in mediastinal, contralateral, or distant lymph nodes or distant organs

Treatment

- Complete surgical excision (lobectomy, bilobectomy, pneumonectomy with clear margins)
- Resection of ipsilateral intrapulmonary (N1) lymph nodes
- Mediastinal lymph node dissection for accurate surgical-pathologic staging
- En bloc resection of adjacent involved structure (chest wall, mediastinal pleura, or fat) for patients with T3 disease; consideration of preoperative chemoradiotherapy in patients with potentially resectable Pancoast tumors (without lymph node metastases, vascular or vertebral body invasion)
- Consideration of postoperative radiation therapy in completely resected patients with stage II lung cancer (decreases local recurrence but does not affect survival) and in patients with incompletely resected T3 lesions
- Consideration of sleeve lobectomy over pneumonectomy for patients with N1 disease

Prognosis

- 55% 5-year survivals in patients with surgical-pathologic stage IIA lung cancers
- 38 to 39% 5-year survivals in patients with surgical-pathologic stage IIB lung cancers

PEARLS_____

- Stage IIA lung cancers are rare and represent approximately 5% of all cases. Stage IIB cancers represent approximately 15 to 25% of resected lesions.
- Lung cancers that abut the adjacent pleura on CT/MR may represent T2 (visceral pleural involvement) (**Fig. 77D**) or T3 (parietal pleural/chest wall involvement) (**Fig. 78F**) lesions.
- CT criteria that suggest resectability of lung cancers that abut the mediastinum include less than 3 cm of contact with the mediastinum, less than 90 degrees of circumferential contact with the aorta, and presence of a fatty plane between the mass and the mediastinum. MR may be slightly more accurate than CT in the assessment of mediastinal invasion and is superior to CT in the assessment of pericardial invasion.

Suggested Readings

Detterbeck FC, Jones DR, Kernstine KH, Naunheim KS. Special treatment issues. Chest 2003;123: 244S–258S

Fraser RS, Müller NL, Colman N, Paré PD. Pulmonary carcinoma. In: Fraser RS, Müller NL, Colman N, Paré PD, eds. Fraser and Paré's Diagnosis of Diseases of the Chest, 4th ed. Philadelphia: Saunders, 1999:1069–1228

Mountain CF. Revisions in the international system for staging lung cancer. Chest 1997;111: 1710–1717

Scott WJ, Howington J, Movsas B. Treatment of stage II non-small cell lung cancer. Chest 2003;123: 188S–201S

Silvestri GA, Tanoue LT, Margolis ML, Barker J, Detterbeck F. The noninvasive staging of non-small cell lung cancer: the guidelines. Chest 2003;123:147S–156S

CASE 79 Lung Cancer: Stage IIIA

Clinical Presentation

A 44-year-old man with cough

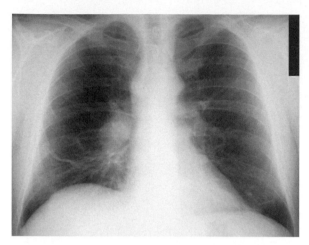

Figure 79A

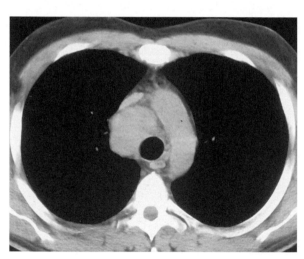

Figure 79C

Stage IIIA

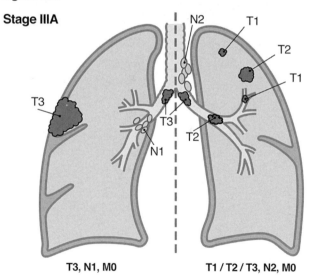

Figure 79D

Radiologic Findings

PA chest radiograph (**Fig. 79A**) demonstrates a right hilar mass with associated ipsilateral volume loss and right paratracheal lymphadenopathy. Unenhanced chest CT (lung and mediastinal window) (**Figs. 79B** and **79C**) demonstrates a large soft tissue mass that obstructs the right middle lobe bronchus and produces right middle lobe atelectasis. Note the subcarinal (ATS station 7) (**Fig. 79B**) and right paratracheal (ATS station 4R) lymphadenopathy (**Fig. 79C**). Normal-sized contralateral para-tracheal (ATS station 4L) lymph nodes are also present. Diagram (**Fig. 79D**) depicts the spectrum of lesions categorized as stage IIIA lung cancers: T1, T2, or T3 lesions with neoplastic involvement of ipsilateral mediastinal lymph nodes (N2), and T3 lesions with neoplastic involvement of ipsilateral hilar lymph nodes (N1), in the absence of metastases to contralateral intrathoracic lymph nodes, extrathoracic lymph nodes, or distant organs.

Diagnosis

Lung cancer, non-small cell carcinoma: stage IIIA

Differential Diagnosis

- Lung cancer, other cell type
- Bronchial carcinoid
- Pulmonary lymphoma

Discussion

Background

T1 and T2 lung cancers are discussed in Case 77. T3 lung cancers and N1 lymph node involvement are discussed in Case 78. N2 lymph node involvement refers to neoplastic involvement of mediastinal lymph nodes ipsilateral to the primary tumor, including highest mediastinal (ATS station 1), upper (ATS station 2) and lower (ATS station 4) paratracheal, prevascular (ATS station 3A), retrotracheal (ATS station 3P), subaortic (ATS station 5), paraaortic (ATS station 6), subcarinal (ATS station 7), paraesophageal (ATS station 8), and pulmonary ligament (ATS station 9) lymph nodes (**Fig. 79D**). T1, T2, and T3 lung cancers with N2 lymph node involvement and T3 lesions with N1 lymph node involvement are classified as stage IIIA lesions provided there are no distant metastases (M0) (**Table 79–1, Fig. 79D**). Stage IIIA lung cancers are considered advanced but potentially operable tumors.

Table 79-1   Stage IIIA Lung Cancer

	T1	T2	T3
N0, M0	Stage IA	Stage IB	Stage IIB
N1, M0	Stage IIA	Stage IIB	Stage IIIA
N2, M0	**Stage IIIA**	**Stage IIIA**	**Stage IIIA**

Pathology

- All cell types of lung cancer may manifest as stage IIIA lesions.
- See Cases 72, 73, 74, 75, and 76.

Clinical Findings

- Patients with stage IIIA lung cancers are often symptomatic from bronchial obstruction by central tumors or because of symptoms related to local invasion by T3 lesions.

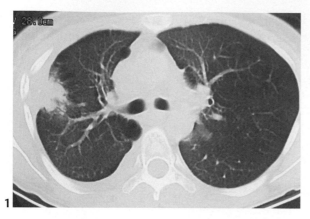
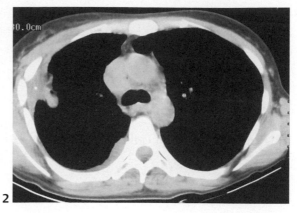

Figure 79E (1,2) Unenhanced chest CT [lung **(1)** and mediastinal **(2)** window] of a 38-year-old woman who presented with right chest wall pain secondary to a locally invasive adenocarcinoma demonstrates a peripheral lung mass that exhibits lobular borders **(1)** and focal internal punctate calcification **(2).** Note ipsilateral pleural thickening and/or fluid, local chest wall invasion, and ipsilateral mediastinal lymph node enlargement (ATS station 4R and station 6) (N2) **(2).** Exclusion of malignant pleural effusion is necessary to rule out a T4 lesion.

Imaging Findings

RADIOGRAPHY

- Peripheral or central (not involving the carina) nodule/mass with ipsilateral mediastinal lymphadenopathy (**Fig. 79A**)
- Peripheral nodule/mass with adjacent chest wall invasion associated with ipsilateral hilar and/or ipsilateral mediastinal lymphadenopathy

CT

- Peripheral lung nodule/mass with ipsilateral mediastinal lymphadenopathy (**Fig. 79E**)
- Peripheral mass with chest wall, pericardial, or diaphragmatic invasion, and ipsilateral hilar or mediastinal lymphadenopathy (**Fig. 79E**)
- Central mass at least 2 cm from the carina (T1, T2); with or without atelectasis/consolidation; with ipsilateral mediastinal lymphadenopathy (**Figs. 79B** and **79C**)
- Central mass within 2 cm from the carina without carinal involvement (T3) with or without atelectasis/consolidation and ipsilateral hilar/mediastinal lymphadenopathy

MR

- Evaluation of central lesions for size, location, and exclusion of carinal involvement
- Evaluation of mediastinal lymph nodes, distinction from vascular structures
- Evaluation of apical lung masses to determine extent of invasion, exclude invasion of adjacent vertebral bodies, great vessels, and/or aerodigestive tract
- Evaluation of pericardial/diaphragmatic involvement with multiplanar imaging

PET

- Demonstration of activity in ipsilateral mediastinal lymph nodes for T1, T2, and T3 lesions
- Demonstration of activity in ipsilateral hilar lymph nodes for T3 lesions
- Absent activity in contralateral intrathoracic lymph nodes, extrathoracic lymph nodes, and distant organs

Treatment

- Treatment recommendations for patients with T3N1, stage IIIA lung cancer are the same as for patients with stage II lung cancer (see Case 78).

- Complete surgical excision (lobectomy, bilobectomy, pneumonectomy with clear margins) and systematic mediastinal lymph node sampling/dissection for accurate surgical-pathologic staging
- Patients with single-station mediastinal lymph node metastases recognized at thoracotomy (occult)—lung resection if feasible and mediastinal lymphadenectomy
  - Consideration of adjuvant postoperative radiotherapy for fully resected lesions; no improvement in survival, but significant decrease in local recurrence
  - Consideration of adjuvant postoperative chemotherapy for fully resected lesions in the setting of a clinical trial
- Consideration of induction (neoadjuvant therapy) in patients with presurgical stage IIIA disease in the setting of a clinical trial
- Postoperative radiotherapy in patients with incomplete resection and those with residual lymph node disease
- Combination chemotherapy and radiotherapy in patients with unresectable stage IIIA disease

Prognosis

- Poor
- 23 to 25% 5-year survivals in patients with surgical-pathologic stage IIIA lung cancers

PEARLS_____

- Approximately 10% of patients with lung cancer have stage IIIA disease with ipsilateral mediastinal (N2) lymph node metastases at presentation.
- CT may demonstrate tumor-free enlarged mediastinal lymph nodes, and mediastinal metastases may manifest with normal-sized (short axis < 1 cm) lymph nodes. The sensitivity and specificity of CT for mediastinal lymph node staging are 60 and 81%, respectively, with overall positive and negative predictive values of 53 and 82%, respectively. Approximately 40% of lymph nodes considered malignant at CT (based on size criteria) are benign.
- MR imaging is complementary to CT for staging lung cancer. The disadvantages of MR in mediastinal evaluation include its low sensitivity to calcium and the potential of characterizing a cluster of normal-sized lymph nodes as lymph node enlargement. MR facilitates distinction of lymph nodes from vascular structures in patients in whom contrast-enhanced chest CT is contraindicated because of sensitivity to iodinated contrast.
- Abnormal uptake on a PET scan is defined as a standard uptake value of greater than 2.5 or uptake greater than background mediastinal activity. The sensitivity and specificity of PET imaging for mediastinal staging are 85 and 88%, respectively, with overall positive and negative predictive values of 78 and 93%, respectively. In general, patients with a negative PET scan do not require mediastinoscopy. Those patients with a positive PET study require further tissue sampling as inflammatory and granulomatous lesions may result in a positive PET scan.

Suggested Readings

Mountain CF. Revisions in the international system for staging lung cancer. Chest 1997;111:1710–1717

Robinson LA, Wagner H Jr, Ruckdeschel JC. Treatment of stage IIIA non-small cell lung cancer. Chest 2003;123:202S–220S

Silvestri GA, Tanoue LT, Margolis ML, Barker J, Detterbeck F. The noninvasive staging of non-small cell lung cancer: the guidelines. Chest 2003;123:147S–156S

CASE 80 Lung Cancer: Stage IIIB

Clinical Presentation

An elderly man with cough, dysphagia, recent hoarseness, and neck vein distention

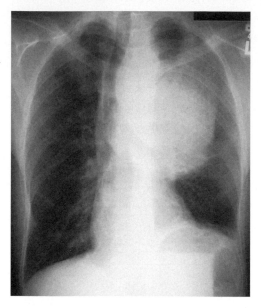

Figure 80A

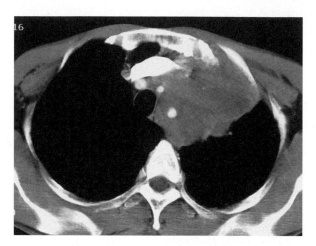

Figure 80B

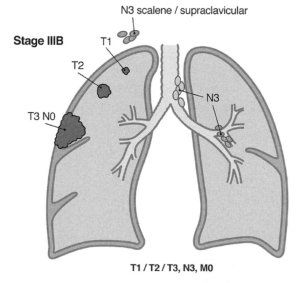

Figure 80C

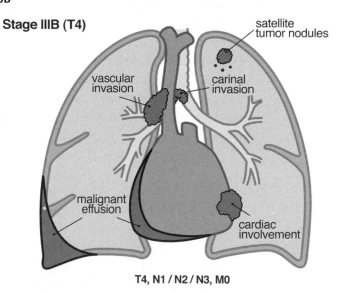

Figure 80D

Radiologic Findings

PA chest radiograph (**Fig. 80A**) demonstrates a large left superior mediastinal mass of lobular contours, which produces mass effect on the trachea. Note the associated ipsilateral volume loss and diaphragmatic elevation. Contrast-enhanced chest CT (mediastinal window) (**Fig. 80B**) demonstrates

324

a large heterogeneous mass that invades the mediastinum and encases the mediastinal great vessels (**Fig. 80C**). **Fig. 80D** depicts the spectrum of lesions categorized as stage IIIB lung cancers; T1, T2, or T3 lesions with neoplastic involvement of contralateral, scalene, and/or supraclavicular lymph nodes (N3) (**Fig. 80C**), and T4 (**Fig. 80D**) lesions with or without neoplastic involvement of ipsilateral hilar lymph nodes (N1), ipsilateral mediastinal lymph nodes (N2), and/or extensive intrathoracic lymph node metastases (N3), in the absence of metastases to extrathoracic lymph nodes or distant organs. Note: Associated N1, N2, and N3 lymph node involvement was not illustrated in **Fig. 80D** to clearly depict the many manifestations of T4 lung cancer.

Diagnosis

Lung cancer, non–small cell carcinoma: stage IIIB

Differential Diagnosis

- Lung cancer, small cell carcinoma
- Pulmonary lymphoma
- Germ cell neoplasm, malignant
- Thymoma, invasive

Discussion

Background

T1 and T2 lung cancers are discussed in Case 77. T3 lung cancers and N1 lymph node involvement are discussed in Case 78. N2 lymph node involvement is discussed in Case 79. T4 lung cancers generally invade vital mediastinal structures such as the heart, esophagus, trachea, and great vessels (**Fig. 80D**). Central lung cancers that invade the carina are also classified as T4 lesions as well as those that invade a vertebral body, produce malignant pleural and/or pericardial effusions, or exhibit satellite tumor nodules within the primary tumor lobe (**Fig. 80D**). T4 lung cancers are generally considered unresectable. N3 lymph node involvement refers to metastases to mediastinal lymph nodes contralateral to the primary tumor as well as metastases to ipsilateral or contralateral scalene or supraclavicular lymph nodes (**Fig. 80C**). T1, T2, T3, and T4 lesions with N3 lymph node involvement (**Fig. 80C**) and T4 lesions with N0, N1, N2, or N3 lymph node involvement (**Fig. 80D**) are classified as stage IIIB lung cancers (**Table 80-1**), provided there are no metastases to distant extrathoracic lymph nodes or other organs (M0). Stage IIIB lung cancers are considered advanced inoperable tumors. Some patients with stage IIIB lung cancers may be candidates for multimodality therapies, including surgical resection.

Table 80-1 Stage IIIB Lung Cancer

	T1	T2	T3	T4
N0, M0	Stage IA	Stage IB	Stage IIB	**Stage IIIB**
N1, M0	Stage IIA	Stage IIB	Stage IIIA	**Stage IIIB**
N2, M0	Stage IIIA	Stage IIIA	Stage IIIA	**Stage IIIB**
N3, M0	**Stage IIIB**	**Stage IIIB**	**Stage IIIB**	**Stage IIIB**

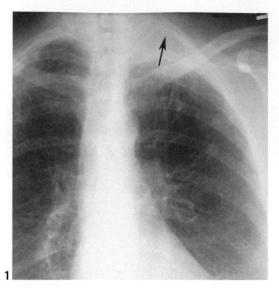 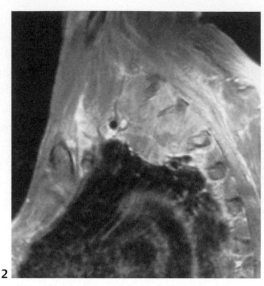

Figure 80E (1,2) Coned-down PA chest radiograph **(1)** of a 56-year-old woman who presented with left upper extremity pain demonstrates a left apical lung mass with spiculated borders, associated focal pleural thickening, and destruction of the left posterior second rib (arrow). Gadolinium-enhanced sagittal T1-weighted MR image **(2)** demonstrates a large chest wall soft tissue mass that invades an adjacent vertebral body and encases the left subclavian and left vertebral arteries.

Clinical Findings

Patients with T4 lung cancer have advanced local disease and may present with symptoms related to the primary tumor (cough, dyspnea, hemoptysis, and chest discomfort) with or without superimposed symptoms related to intrathoracic tumor spread. Hoarseness may result from recurrent laryngeal nerve palsy and is more common in left-sided tumors. Pancoast tumors (apical lung neoplasm that invades adjacent chest wall structures) may result in ipsilateral upper extremity pain and Horner syndrome (unilateral enophthalmos, ptosis, myosis, and anhydrosis from involvement of the sympathetic chain and stellate ganglion). Superior vena cava obstruction may result in facial swelling, visible venous distention, headache, and dizziness (see Case 75). Dysphagia and dyspnea may relate to invasion of the esophagus or trachea.

Imaging Findings

RADIOGRAPHY

- Central mass with mediastinal widening; mediastinal mass (**Fig. 80A**)
- Nodule/mass with contralateral lymphadenopathy
- Nodule/mass with ipsilateral or contralateral (malignant) pleural effusion
- Apical lung mass in association with adjacent chest wall involvement (**Fig. 80E**) and clinical syndrome indicating T4 disease

CT

- Demonstration of mediastinal invasion or vascular encasement (**Figs. 75C** and **75D** in Case 75, and **Fig. 80B**)
- Demonstration of carinal involvement (**Fig. 80F1**)
- Demonstration of tracheal, esophageal, or cardiac invasion (**Fig. 80F2**)
- Demonstration of satellite tumor nodules in primary tumor lobe

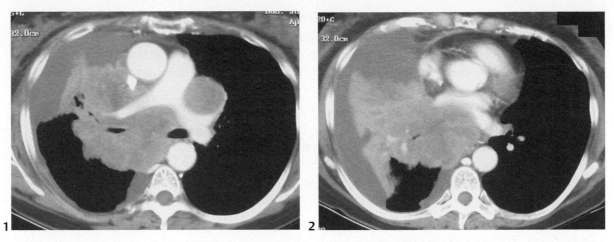

Figure 80F (1,2) Contrast-enhanced chest CT (mediastinal window) of a 61-year-old woman with weight loss and dyspnea demonstrates an advanced (T4) central lung cancer that invades the carina, esophagus **(1)** and heart **(2)** and encases the superior vena cava and the right pulmonary artery **(1)**. Note the large loculated (cytologically proven malignant) right pleural effusion **(1,2)** and contralateral mediastinal lymphadenopathy (N3) **(1)**.

- Demonstration of contralateral hilar/mediastinal (**Fig. 80F1**) and/or ipsilateral or contralateral scalene or supraclavicular lymphadenopathy
- Demonstration of (malignant) pleural effusion or pleural masses (**Fig. 72G** in Case 72 and **Fig. 80F**)

MR

- Demonstration of mediastinal invasion or vascular encasement (**Fig. 80E2**)
- Demonstration of carinal involvement
- Demonstration of tracheal, esophageal, or cardiac invasion
- Demonstration of contralateral hilar/mediastinal and/or ipsilateral or contralateral scalene or supraclavicular lymphadenopathy without need for intravenous contrast administration
- Demonstration of (malignant) pleural effusion or pleural masses
- Multiplanar imaging of apical lung lesions with demonstration of vertebral invasion and assessment of resectability (exclusion of brachial plexus/vertebral body involvement) (**Fig. 80E2**)

Treatment

- Consideration of surgical resection for patients with T4 disease characterized by satellite tumor nodules in the primary tumor lobe and for patients with carinal involvement
- Combined chemoradiotherapy in patients with good performance scores and without malignant pleural effusion

Prognosis

- Dismal
- 3 to 7% 5-year survivals in patients with surgical-pathologic stage IIIB lung cancers

PEARLS

- Approximately 10 to 15% of patients with lung cancer have stage IIIB disease at presentation.

- MR may be more sensitive than CT in the detection of mediastinal invasion and is considered superior in visualization of the pericardium, the cardiac chambers, and the great vessels.
- Tumors that abut the mediastinum are not considered unresectable, although those that have greater than 3 cm contact with the mediastinum may prove to be unresectable.

Suggested Readings

Beckles MA, Spiro SG, Colice GL, Rudd RM. Initial evaluation of the patient with lung cancer: symptoms, signs, laboratory tests, and paraneoplastic syndromes. Chest 2003;123:97S–104S

Detterbeck FC, Jones DR, Kernstine KH, Naunheim KS. Special treatment issues. Chest 2003; 123:244S–258S

Jett JR, Scott WJ, Rivera MP, Sause WT. Guidelines on treatment of stage IIIB non-small cell lung cancer. Chest 2003;123:221S–225S

Mountain CF. Revisions in the international system for staging lung cancer. Chest 1997;111:1710–1717

Silvestri GA, Tanoue LT, Margolis ML, Barker J, Detterbeck F. The noninvasive staging of non-small cell lung cancer: the guidelines. Chest 2003;123:147S–156S

CASE 81 Lung Cancer: Stage IV

Clinical Presentation

A 66-year-old man with cough and weight loss

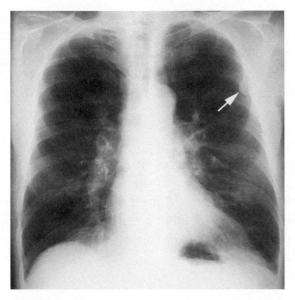

Figure 81A

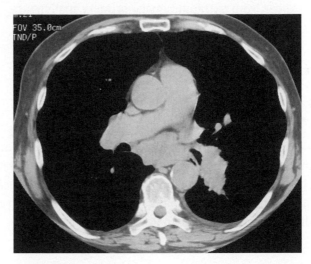

Figure 81B

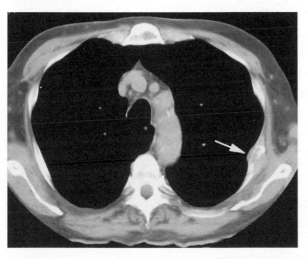

Figure 81C

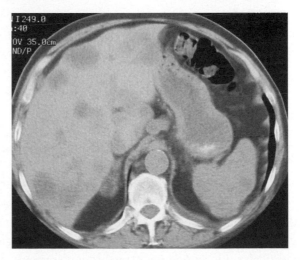

Figure 81D

Radiologic Findings

PA chest radiograph (**Fig. 81A**) demonstrates a left hilar mass and an extrapulmonary nodule of the left superolateral hemithorax (arrow). Unenhanced chest CT (mediastinal window) (**Figs. 81B** and **81C**) demonstrates a central left lower lobe mass with associated subcarinal (ATS station 7) lymphadenopathy (N2) (**Fig. 81B**) and a left rib metastasis (**Fig. 81C**) with associated osseous destruction (arrow). Unenhanced CT of the upper abdomen (soft tissue window) (**Fig. 81D**) demonstrates multifocal low-attenuation hepatic lesions and enlargement of the right adrenal gland consistent with metastases.

329

Diagnosis

Lung cancer, poorly differentiated non–small cell carcinoma: stage IV

Differential Diagnosis

- Metastatic small cell lung cancer
- Metastatic cancer from extrapulmonary primary malignancy

Discussion

Background

Stage IV lung cancers are inoperable neoplasms and are characterized by the presence of distant metastases to extrathoracic lymph nodes and extrapulmonary organs. Common sites of metastatic involvement include the liver, bone, adrenal gland, kidney, and brain. These tumors are given an M1 designation. The M1 descriptor also applies to primary lung cancers with satellite tumor nodules in an ipsilateral nonprimary tumor pulmonary lobe. Metastatic lung cancer (M1) is classified as stage IV disease regardless of its T or N designation.

Clinical Findings

Patients with stage IV lung cancer may present because of symptoms related to the primary tumor, but approximately one third present with symptoms related to distant metastases, such as constitutional symptoms and signs that may include malaise, anorexia, weight loss, and fatigue. Affected patients may present because of central nervous system or skeletal complaints (bone pain) related to metastatic disease. Patients with skeletal metastases may present with hypercalcemia. Hepatic metastases may manifest with epigastric pain and jaundice.

Imaging Findings

RADIOGRAPHY

- May only show evidence of the primary tumor or of thoracic lymph node metastases
- May demonstrate metastatic involvement of chest wall, soft tissue, or skeletal structures (**Fig. 81A**)
- May show evidence of a pleural effusion (requires cytologic proof of malignancy)
- May show multifocal lung nodules (synchronous primary cancers vs pulmonary metastases)

CT

- May reveal satellite tumor nodules (**Fig. 81E**)
- May reveal unsuspected pleural effusion (requires cytologic proof of malignancy)
- May reveal evidence of clinically unsuspected liver, adrenal, and/or skeletal metastases (**Figs. 81C, 81D,** and **81F2**)

MR

- May reveal evidence of clinically unsuspected liver, adrenal, or skeletal metastases

PET

- Increased activity on whole-body imaging corresponding to suspected or unsuspected metastases (**Figs. 81F3** and **81F4**)

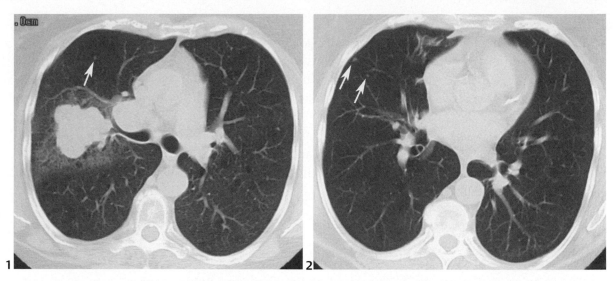

Figure 81E (1,2) Unenhanced chest CT (lung window) of a 59-year old woman with cough and non–small cell lung cancer demonstrates a lobular right perihilar mass with ipsilateral hilar (ATS station 10R) lymphadenopathy. The multiple small pulmonary nodules (arrows) in the ipsilateral right middle **(1,2)** and lower lobes (not shown) represented satellite neoplastic lesions (M1) and characterize this lesion as a stage IV lung cancer.

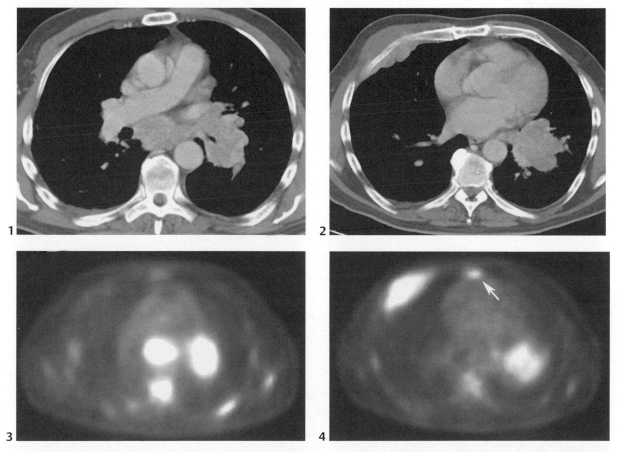

Figure 81F (1–4) Unenhanced chest CT (mediastinal window) of a 42-year-old man with advanced adenocarcinoma demonstrates a left hilar mass with associated subcarinal (ATS station 7) lymphadenopathy (N2) **(1)** as well as a right chest wall mass **(2)** consistent with metastatic disease (M1). **(3,4)** Axial PET images demonstrate intense FDG uptake in the mass, the subcarinal lymph nodes, and the chest wall lesion as well as an unsuspected focus of abnormal FDG uptake (arrow) in the anterior mediastinum **(4).** (Courtesy of Diane C. Strollo, M.D., University of Pittsburgh, Pittsburgh, Pennsylvania.)

Treatment

- Combination chemotherapy for patients with good performance status
- Consideration of resection in selected patients with T4N0 or T4N1 lung cancers; lobectomy in patients with satellite nodules in the primary tumor lobe
- Consideration of curative resection of both lesions in patients with two synchronous (primary) lung cancers
- Consideration of resection or radiosurgical ablation of solitary brain metastases in patients with potentially resectable (N0, N1) primary lung cancer
- Consideration of resection of solitary adrenal metastases in patients with potentially resectable (N0, N1) primary lung cancer

Prognosis

- Dismal
- 1% 5-year survival in patients with surgical-pathological stage IV lung cancers

PEARLS_____

- Adrenal adenomas are present in up to 9% of the population, and adrenal abnormalities are a common finding in the setting of lung cancer. Adrenal adenomas predominate in patients with T1N0 non–small cell lung cancers. Adrenal metastases are associated with large metastatic lung cancers. MR imaging may be useful in distinguishing benign from malignant adrenal lesions, but tissue confirmation may ultimately be required.
- Most liver lesions represent hepatic cysts or hemangiomas. Contrast administration, MRI, ultrasonography, and ultimately biopsy may be required to exclude metastatic disease.
- Clinical evaluation must guide extrathoracic imaging for exclusion of metastatic disease in patients with suspected stage I or stage II lung cancers. Patients with stage IIIA and stage IIIB lung cancers should undergo routine imaging for exclusion of extrathoracic metastases (head CT/MR, bone scan, abdominal CT, PET).

Suggested Readings

Detterbeck FC, Jones DR, Kernstine KH, Naunheim KS. Special treatment issues. Chest 2003;123: 244S–258S

Fraser RS, Müller NL, Colman N, Paré PD. Pulmonary carcinoma. In: Fraser RS, Müller NL, Colman N, Paré PD, eds. Fraser and Paré's Diagnosis of Diseases of the Chest, 4th ed. Philadelphia: Saunders, 1999:1069–1228

Mountain CF. Revisions in the international system for staging lung cancer. Chest 1997;111:1710–1717

Silvestri GA, Tanoue LT, Margolis ML, Barker J, Detterbeck F. The noninvasive staging of non-small cell lung cancer: the guidelines. Chest 2003;123:147S–156S

Socinski MA, Morris DE, Masters GA, Lilenbaum R. Chemotherapeutic management of stage IV non-small cell lung cancer. Chest 2003;123:226S–243S

CASE 82 Pulmonary Metastases

Clinical Presentation

A 50-year-old woman status post-hysterectomy for uterine cancer

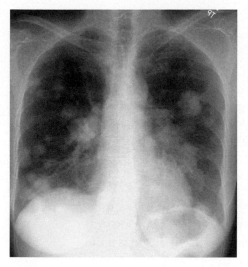

Figure 82A

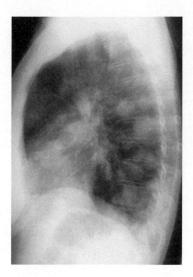

Figure 82B

Radiologic Findings

PA (**Fig. 82A**) and lateral (**Fig. 82B**) chest radiographs demonstrate multiple bilateral well-defined spherical pulmonary nodules and masses most numerous in the lower lobes.

Diagnosis

Pulmonary metastases

Differential Diagnosis

- Primary pulmonary lymphoma
- Multifocal lung cancer (bronchioloalveolar carcinoma, adenocarcinoma)
- Hematogenous infection
- Pulmonary angiitis and granulomatosis

Discussion

Background

The term *metastasis* is generally defined as the transfer of disease from one organ to another that is not in direct contiguity. In the setting of neoplasia, metastases are characteristic of malignancy. Pulmonary metastases represent the most frequent pulmonary neoplasm. Depending on the location of the primary tumor, lung metastases may represent early or late neoplastic dissemination. Secondary lung neoplasia may occur via hematogenous, lymphatic, and/or tracheobronchial routes.

333

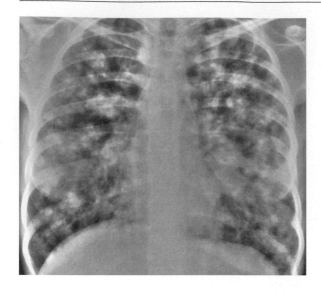

Figure 82C PA chest radiograph of a young woman with metastatic choriocarcinoma demonstrates multifocal bilateral nodular opacities with ill-defined borders that mimic diffuse multifocal airspace disease.

Etiology

Pulmonary metastases typically result from hematogenous dissemination of malignancy. The neoplastic cells are transported to the lung and arrive at the capillary bed. Thus, most primary neoplasms that produce lung metastases have a rich vascular supply and a venous drainage into the systemic circulation (vena cava). Pulmonary metastases may in turn metastasize and produce disseminated malignancy.

Clinical Findings

Patients with pulmonary metastases may be entirely asymptomatic. When metastases are numerous, large, or involve the airways and pleura, affected patients may experience dyspnea, cough, chest pain, and/or respiratory failure. Patients with lymphangitic carcinomatosis typically present with dyspnea. Patients with metastatic sarcoma may present because of a spontaneous pneumothorax. Most patients with pulmonary metastases have a known history of malignancy. Rarely, patients may present with pulmonary metastases from an unknown primary malignant neoplasm.

Pathology

GROSS

- Focal or multifocal nodules/masses; typically well-defined, spherical, peripheral, basilar
- Ill-defined borders in hemorrhagic metastases
- Variable size
- Interstitial thickening in lymphangitic carcinomatosis (see Case 132)

MICROSCOPIC

- Homogeneous cell population consistent with primary neoplasm
- Adjacent to peripheral pulmonary arteries, intravascular tumor emboli, pulmonary or bronchial artery supply
- Interstitial tumor, edema, and desmoplasia in lymphangitic carcinomatosis (see Case 132)

Imaging Findings

RADIOGRAPHY

- Bilateral multifocal well-defined nodules/masses; spherical morphology (**Figs. 82A** and **82B**)
- Variable size (range from miliary nodules to large "cannonball" masses)

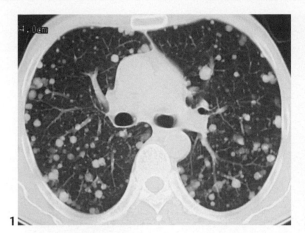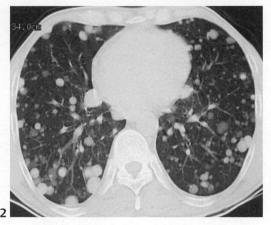

Figure 82D (1,2) Unenhanced chest CT (lung window) of a 58-year-old man with metastatic salivary gland carcinoma demonstrates multiple bilateral well-defined pulmonary nodules and masses. Note the spherical morphology of the lesions, their angiocentric distribution, and the preferential involvement of the lung periphery and the lower lobes.

- Multifocal opacities with ill-defined borders; may mimic airspace disease (**Fig. 82C**)
- Most numerous in the lower lobes (**Figs. 82A** and **82B**)
- May exhibit associated hilar/mediastinal lymphadenopathy
- May exhibit associated pleural effusion(s)
- Rarely
  - Cavitation
    - Most frequent in metastases from squamous cell carcinomas
    - Also described in adenocarcinomas and sarcomas
  - Calcification
  - Solitary nodule/mass
  - Endobronchial lesion; may exhibit atelectasis/consolidation
  - Lymphangitic carcinomatosis (see Case 132)

CT

- Multifocal well-defined spherical pulmonary nodules/masses (**Fig. 82D**)
- Most numerous in lung bases and lung periphery (**Fig. 82D**)
- May exhibit associated lymphadenopathy and/or pleural effusion
- Angiocentric distribution; pulmonary vessel coursing to medial aspect of metastasis (**Fig. 82D**)
- Rarely
  - Cavitation (**Fig. 82E**)
  - Calcification
  - Solitary nodule/mass (**Fig. 82F**)
  - Lymphangitic carcinomatosis (see Case 132)

Treatment

- Chemotherapy
- Surgical excision of solitary or limited pulmonary metastases (when lung is the only affected site) with continued surveillance and possible additional metastasectomies

Prognosis

- Poor
- Better prognosis in patients with limited metastases who are candidates for metastasectomy

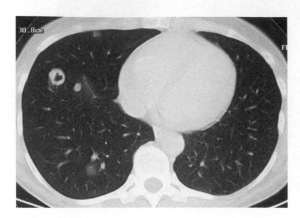

Figure 82E Contrast-enhanced chest CT (lung window) of a middle-aged woman with metastatic ovarian carcinoma demonstrates several right lung metastases, one of which exhibits cavitation. Note the nodular morphology and irregular thickness of the cavity wall.

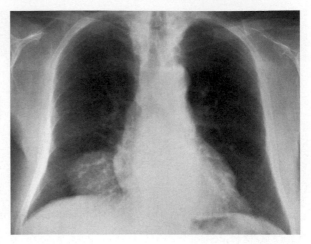

Figure 82F PA chest radiograph of a middle-aged woman with metastatic melanoma demonstrates a large right lower lobe mass that represented a solitary metastasis.

PEARLS

- CT is more sensitive than radiography in detecting pulmonary metastases, particularly for small nodules (3 mm). However, it is also less specific as it detects unrelated benign, previously unsuspected pulmonary nodules. The likelihood of benign disease increases when pulmonary nodules are only detected on CT.
- Solitary pulmonary metastases are rare. Thus, lung cancer must always be included in the differential diagnosis of a patient with known malignancy who presents with a new pulmonary nodule or mass. Solitary metastases typically result from sarcomas, melanoma (**Fig. 82F**), colon, breast, and genitourinary cancers. A new solitary nodule in a patient with known invasive melanoma (**Fig. 82F**) or skeletal sarcoma is more likely to represent a metastasis. A new solitary nodule in a patient with known squamous cell carcinoma or lymphoma is more likely to represent a new primary lung cancer.
- Patients with endobronchial metastases may exhibit findings of bronchial obstruction (pneumonia, atelectasis) that mimic the presenting manifestations of central lung cancer.

Suggested Readings

Coppage L, Shaw C, Curtis AM. Metastatic disease to the chest in patients with extrathoracic malignancy. J Thorac Imaging 1987;2:24–37

Fraser RS, Müller NL, Colman N, Paré PD. Secondary neoplasms. In: Fraser RS, Müller NL, Colman N, Paré PD, eds. Fraser and Paré's Diagnosis of Diseases of the Chest, 4th ed. Philadelphia: Saunders, 1999:1381–1417

Reiner B, Siegel E, Sawyer R, Brocato RM, Maroney M, Hooper F. The impact of routine CT of the chest on the diagnosis and management of newly diagnosed squamous cell carcinoma of the head and neck. AJR Am J Roentgenol 1997;169:667–671

Seo JB, Im JG, Goo JM, Chung MJ, Kim MY. Atypical pulmonary metastases: spectrum of radiologic findings. Radiographics 2001;21:403–417

CASE 83 Bronchial Carcinoid

Clinical Presentation

An 18-year-old woman with cough and hemoptysis

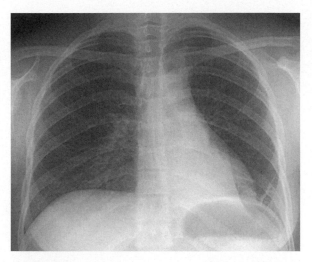

Figure 83A

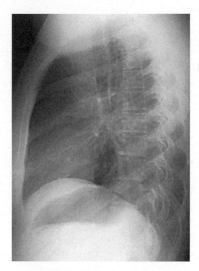

Figure 83B

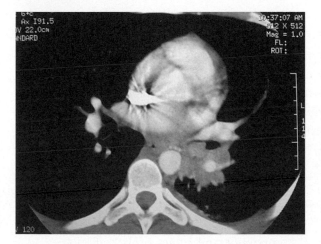

Figure 83C

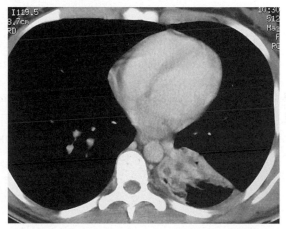

Figure 83D

Radiologic Findings

PA (**Fig. 83A**) and lateral (**Fig. 83B**) chest radiographs demonstrate left lower lobe atelectasis. Contrast-enhanced chest CT (mediastinal window) (**Figs. 83C** and **83D**) demonstrates a small lobular-enhancing, partially endobronchial lesion (**Fig. 83C**) that obstructs the left lower lobe bronchus with resultant volume loss and bronchiectasis (**Fig. 83D**).

Diagnosis

Bronchial carcinoid

Differential Diagnosis

- Mucoepidermoid carcinoma
- Adenoid cystic carcinoma
- Benign mesenchymal neoplasm
- Central lung cancer (rare in adolescents and young adults)

Discussion

Background

Bronchial carcinoid is a malignant primary pulmonary neoplasm of neuroendocrine differentiation. It is a rare lung malignancy that represents approximately 2% of all lung tumors.

Etiology

Bronchial carcinoids are thought to derive from the neuroendocrine cells of the bronchial epithelium. There is no documented association with cigarette smoking or other carcinogens.

Clinical Findings

Carcinoid typically affects adult men and women, with an average age of 45 years and a wide age range. Carcinoid is the most common primary lung neoplasm of children, and most pediatric patients are adolescents. Affected patients are typically symptomatic and present with cough and recurrent pulmonary infection. Hemoptysis, chest pain, wheezing, and/or dyspnea may also occur. Some patients are asymptomatic and are diagnosed incidentally. Rarely, patients with bronchial carcinoid present with symptoms related to ectopic adrenocorticotropic hormone (ACTH) production by the lesion.

Pathology

GROSS

- Well-circumscribed nodule/mass with frequent endoluminal component and intact bronchial mucosa over the lesion; large central bronchi most frequently affected
- Completely endobronchial, partially endobronchial, abutting bronchial wall
- Frequent bronchial wall invasion
- Frequent bronchial obstruction with pneumonia, atelectasis, or bronchiectasis
- Peripheral solitary pulmonary nodule/mass

MICROSCOPIC

- Polygonal cells with eosinophilic cytoplasm, and round nuclei with fine stippled chromatin and inconspicuous nucleoli
- Organoid pattern within a rich fibrovascular stroma; cells arranged in nests or solid sheets
- Typical bronchial carcinoid; less than two mitoses per 2 mm^2 (or 10 high power fields), absent necrosis
- Atypical bronchial carcinoid (10–20% of pulmonary carcinoids); two or more mitoses per 2 mm^2 (or 10 high power fields)

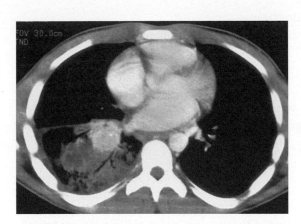

Figure 83E Contrast-enhanced chest CT (mediastinal window) of a young man with recurrent right lower lobe pneumonia and hemoptysis secondary to a typical bronchial carcinoid demonstrates a lobular-enhancing central mass with a small focus of calcification and distal consolidation and bronchiectasis.

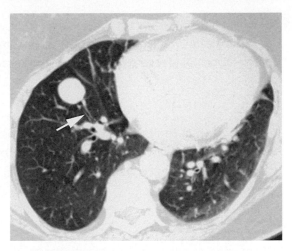

Figure 83F Unenhanced chest CT (lung window) of an asymptomatic 61-year-old woman status post-bilateral lumpectomies for breast carcinoma and an incidentally found bronchial carcinoid demonstrates a well-defined spherical lobular right lower lobe soft tissue mass. Note the bronchus (arrow) that courses toward the lesion.

Imaging Findings

RADIOGRAPHY

- Well-defined hilar or perihilar mass
- Well-defined endobronchial nodule or mass
- Atelectasis, consolidation, mucoid impaction (may be dominant findings and may obscure central mass) (**Figs. 83A** and **83B**)
- Size ranges from 2 to 5 cm; atypical carcinoids usually larger
- Peripheral well-defined solitary pulmonary nodule/mass

CT

- Spherical/ovoid, well-defined lobular nodule/mass within or near central bronchi (**Figs. 83C** and **83E**)
- Intralesional calcification (diffuse or punctate) in approximately 30% (**Fig. 83E**)
- Marked enhancement on contrast-enhanced chest CT (**Figs. 83C** and **83E**)
- Visualization of endoluminal tumor or bronchial relationship (**Figs. 83C, 83E,** and **83F**)
- Evaluation of distal lung parenchyma; volume loss, air trapping, consolidation, bronchiectasis (**Figs. 83D** and **83E**)
- Lymphadenopathy; up to 50% of patients with atypical carcinoid

MR

- Well-defined spherical/ovoid mass; high signal intensity on T1- and T2-weighted images
- Demonstration of contrast enhancement

SCINTIGRAPHY

- Octreotide uptake in hormonally active and occult carcinoid tumors; correlation with cross-sectional imaging for localization of abnormal activity

Treatment

- Surgical excision; typically lobectomy or pneumonectomy
- Tracheobronchial sleeve resection for central carcinoids with normal distal lung parenchyma

Prognosis

- Typical bronchial carcinoid; excellent prognosis, with 92% 5-year survivals
- Atypical bronchial carcinoid; less favorable prognosis, with 69% 5-year survivals and increased risk for local recurrence, particularly with local lymph node metastases

PEARL_____

- PET imaging is not useful in the diagnosis of carcinoid tumors, as many exhibit low metabolic activity.

Suggested Readings

Rosado de Christenson ML, Abbott GF, Kirejczyk WM, Galvin JR, Travis WD. Thoracic carcinoids: radiologic-pathologic correlation. Radiographics 1999;19:707–736

Travis WD, Colby TV, Corrin B, et al. Histological Typing of Lung and Pleural Tumours: International Histological Classification of Tumours, 3rd ed. Berlin: Springer-Verlag, 1999

CASE 84 Pulmonary Lymphoma

Clinical Presentation

Asymptomatic 71-year-old man evaluated because of an abnormal chest radiograph

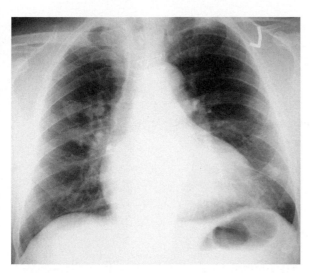

Figure 84A

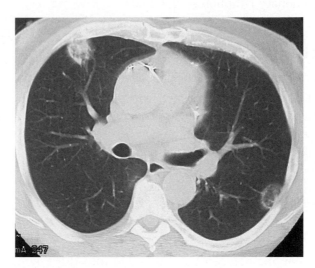

Figure 84B

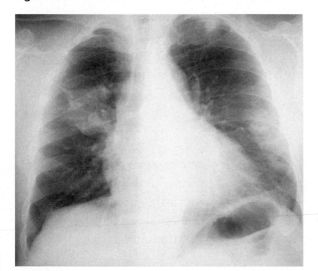

Figure 84C

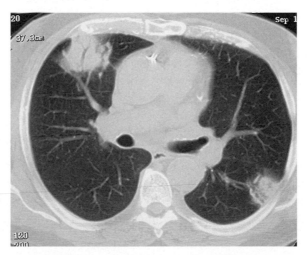

Figure 84D

Radiologic Findings

PA chest radiograph (**Fig. 84A**) demonstrates multifocal bilateral nodular opacities without associated lymphadenopathy or pleural effusion. Unenhanced chest CT (lung window) (**Fig. 84B**) demonstrates multifocal juxtapleural nodular opacities of heterogeneous attenuation. Biopsy confirmed the diagnosis of primary pulmonary lymphoma of bronchus-associated lymphoid tissue (BALT). Follow-up PA chest radiograph (**Fig. 84C**) obtained 3 years later demonstrates interval growth and coalescence of multifocal bilateral nodular opacities. Unenhanced chest CT (lung window) (**Fig. 84D**) confirms the interval growth of the lesions and demonstrates internal air bronchograms.

Diagnosis

Primary pulmonary lymphoma, low grade

Differential Diagnosis

- Multifocal lung cancer (bronchioloalveolar carcinoma)
- Pulmonary metastases
- Pneumonia (including chronic organizing pneumonia) or other multifocal infection
- Cryptogenic organizing pneumonia
- Pulmonary angiitis and granulomatosis

Discussion

Background

Pulmonary lymphomas can be subdivided into those lymphomas limited to the lung (primary) and those in which the lung is affected secondarily. Primary pulmonary lymphoma is defined as extranodal pulmonary lymphoma (with or without involvement of regional lymph nodes) without evidence of extrathoracic disease for a time period of at least 3 months. It is a rare lung malignancy and comprises approximately 0.3% of all primary lung neoplasms. Secondary pulmonary lymphoma is much more frequent and occurs in approximately 40% of patients with lymphoma.

Etiology

Primary pulmonary lymphomas are typically non-Hodgkin's lymphomas thought to arise from mucosa-associated lymphoid tissue (MALT), which in the lung is called bronchus-associated lymphoid tissue (BALT). BALT is thought to develop as a response to long-term exposure to various antigens such as cigarette smoke, pulmonary infections, and autoimmune disorders. Secondary pulmonary lymphoma represents hematogenous or lymphatic dissemination of extrapulmonary lymphoma.

Clinical Findings

While patients with high-grade pulmonary lymphoma and those with pulmonary involvement by disseminated lymphoma may be asymptomatic, many present with pulmonary or systemic complaints. Patients with low-grade pulmonary lymphoma are often asymptomatic (50%) and are diagnosed incidentally because of an abnormal chest radiograph. Symptoms of cough, chest pain, and dyspnea may also occur. Patients with primary pulmonary lymphoma are typically in the sixth and seventh decades of life, and women may be more frequently affected. Affected individuals frequently exhibit immunologic abnormalities, including Sjögren syndrome, Hashimoto thyroiditis, systemic lupus erythematosus, and human immunodeficiency virus (HIV) infection.

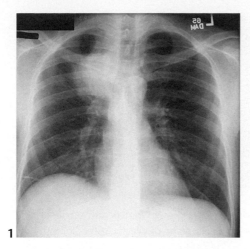
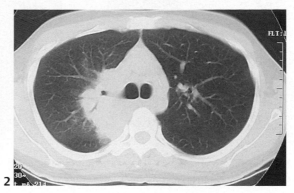

Figure 84E (1,2) PA chest radiograph **(1)** of a 37-year-old man with HIV infection, cough, and chest pain shows a large right upper lobe mass, which abuts the right superior mediastinum. Unenhanced chest CT (lung window) **(2)** demonstrates a large right upper lobe consolidation of irregular borders with internal air bronchograms. There was no lymphadenopathy. At surgery, primary pulmonary lymphoma was diagnosed.

Pathology

GROSS

- Focal nodule, mass, or consolidation
- Multifocal nodules, masses, or consolidations
- Perilymphatic, peribronchial, plaque-like pleural infiltration

MICROSCOPIC

- Low-grade primary pulmonary lymphoma
  - Small lymphocytes, plasma cells, centrocyte-like cells, monoclonal B cells, and ill-formed granulomas
  - Rare mitoses; may form germinal centers
  - Distinction from other nonneoplastic lymphoid proliferations
- High-grade primary pulmonary lymphoma
  - Large B cell non-Hodgkin lymphoma with atypia, mitotic features, and necrosis

Imaging Findings

RADIOGRAPHY

- Low-grade primary pulmonary lymphoma
  - Focal nodule, mass, or consolidation
  - Multifocal pulmonary nodules, masses, or consolidations (**Figs. 84A** and **84C**)
  - Frequent air bronchograms (**Fig. 84C**)
  - Common indolent course with slow growth over months to years (**Figs. 84A** and **84C**)
- High-grade primary pulmonary lymphoma
  - Focal nodule, mass, or consolidation (**Fig. 84E1**)
  - Multifocal consolidation
  - Diffuse interstitial opacities
  - May exhibit rapid progression

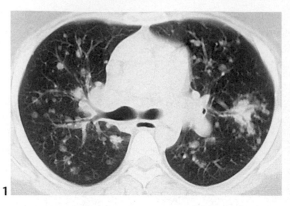
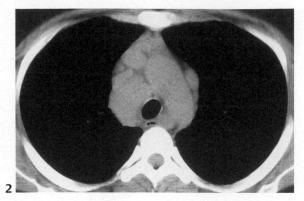

Figure 84F (1,2) Unenhanced chest CT [lung **(1)** and mediastinal **(2)** window] of a young woman with secondary pulmonary involvement by Hodgkin lymphoma shows multifocal pulmonary nodules, some of which cluster along the airways **(1)** and mediastinal lymphadenopathy **(2)**.

CT

- Low-grade primary pulmonary lymphoma
  - Focal or multifocal nodules, masses, or consolidations (**Figs. 84B** and **84D**)
  - Ground-glass opacities (**Fig. 84B**), CT halo sign
  - Air bronchograms (90%) (**Figs. 84B** and **84D**); bronchial stretching, narrowing, or dilatation
  - Bubble-like lucencies
  - Pleural effusion in up to 10% of cases
  - Lymphadenopathy in 5 to 30% of cases
- High-grade primary pulmonary lymphoma
  - Focal nodule, mass, or consolidation (**Fig. 84E2**)
  - Multifocal consolidations, masses, or reticular opacities

Treatment

- Surgical excision in patients with focal primary pulmonary lymphoma
- Surgical excision or adjuvant chemotherapy in patients with bulky or multifocal lymphoma

Prognosis

- Excellent in low-grade primary pulmonary lymphoma; most cured by excision, 80 to 90% 5-year survivals and 50 to 70% 10-year survivals
- Local recurrence in as many as 50% of patients
- Poor in high-grade primary pulmonary lymphoma; up to 30% 5-year survivals

PEARLS

- Low-grade lymphomas represent approximately 90% of all primary pulmonary lymphomas.
- Mediastinal Hodgkin lymphoma is common and may progress to secondary pulmonary involvement manifesting with coarse perihilar reticular opacities, multifocal nodular opacities, or subpleural nodules or masses (**Fig. 84F**). Air bronchograms may be seen. Primary pulmonary Hodgkin's lymphoma is rare.
- Lymphomatoid granulomatosis is a type of pulmonary lymphoma characterized by polymorphous angiocentric lymphoid infiltrates with necrosis and vascular infiltration. It manifests radiologically as solitary or multiple pulmonary nodules/masses that may exhibit cavitation.

Suggested Readings

Bazot M, Cadranel J, Benayoun S, Tassart M, Bigot JM, Carette MF. Primary pulmonary AIDS-related lymphoma: radiographic and CT findings. Chest 1999;116:1282–1286

Ferraro P, Trastek VF, Adlakha H, Deschamps C, Allen MS, Pairolero PC. Primary non-Hodgkin's lymphoma of the lung. Ann Thorac Surg 2000;69:993–997

Kurtin PJ, Myers JL, Adlakha H, et al. Pathologic and clinical features of primary pulmonary extranodal marginal zone B-cell lymphoma of MALT type. Am J Surg Pathol 2001;25:997–1008

Lee DK, Im JG, Lee KS, et al. B-cell lymphoma of bronchus-associated lymphoid tissue (BALT): CT features in 10 patients. J Comput Assist Tomogr 2000;24:30–34

O'Donnell PG, Jackson SA, Tung KT, Hassan B, Wilkins B, Mead GM. Radiological appearances of lymphomas arising from mucosa-associated lymphoid tissue (MALT) in the lung. Clin Radiol 1998; 53:258–263

Travis WD, Colby TV, Corrin B, et al. Histological Typing of Lung and Pleural Tumours: International Histological Classification of Tumours, 3rd ed. Berlin: Springer-Verlag, 1999

CASE 85 Hamartoma

Clinical Presentation

A 40-year-old man with hemoptysis

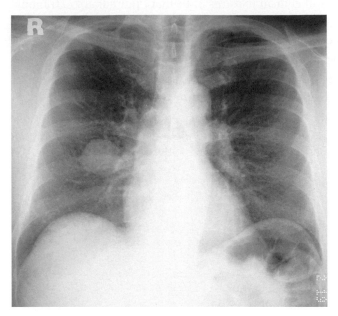

Figure 85A

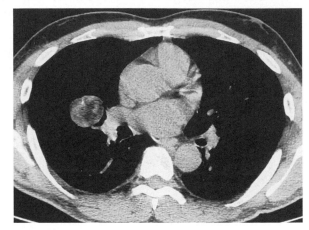

Figure 85B

Radiologic Findings

PA (**Fig. 85A**) chest radiograph demonstrates a well-defined 3 cm mass of lobular borders in the right mid-lung. Unenhanced chest CT (mediastinal window) (**Fig. 85B**) shows areas of fat and soft tissue attenuation within the lesion as well as a small focus of punctate calcification.

Diagnosis

Hamartoma

Differential Diagnosis

None

Discussion

Background

Pulmonary hamartoma was previously considered a nonneoplastic lesion characterized as an abnormal mixture of tissues or an abnormal proportion of a single tissue element normally present in the lung. Today, hamartoma is classified as a benign pulmonary neoplasm. It accounts for approximately 8% of lung neoplasms, is considered the most common benign tumor of the lung, and represents approximately 77% of all benign lung neoplasms.

346

Etiology

Pulmonary hamartoma is thought to arise from peribronchial mesenchymal tissues, but its etiology remains unknown.

Clinical Findings

Pulmonary hamartomas typically affect asymptomatic patients who are diagnosed incidentally because of an abnormal chest radiograph. Males are more commonly affected than females, with a male-to-female ratio of 2–3:1. Most patients with hamartoma are older than 40 years, and the peak incidence of occurrence is in the sixth to seventh decades of life. Patients with pulmonary hamartoma may present with symptoms, which are usually related to endobronchial lesions or extrinsic airway involvement. Most hamartomas occur as solitary lung nodules or masses. Rare cases of multifocal pulmonary chondromas are reported in association with gastric smooth muscle neoplasms and functioning extra-adrenal paragangliomas (Carney's triad).

Pathology

GROSS

- Well-circumscribed white or gray solitary lung nodule or mass
- Cartilaginous consistency
- Size range from 0.2 to 6 cm; mean size of 1.5 cm
- Broad-based endobronchial nodule in 1.4 to 19.5% of cases; may produce obstructive changes

MICROSCOPIC

- Cartilage, connective tissue, adipose tissue, bone, and smooth muscle
- Peripheral epithelial-lined cleft-like spaces; may represent entrapped respiratory epithelium

Imaging Findings

RADIOGRAPHY

- Well-defined solitary pulmonary nodule/mass (**Figs. 85A** and **85C1**)
- Rare visualization of cartilaginous ("popcorn") calcification; increased frequency with increasing lesion size
- Obstructive pneumonia or atelectasis in cases of endobronchial hamartoma

CT

- CT diagnostic criteria:
  - Well-defined borders (**Figs. 85B** and **85C2**)
  - Diameter of 2.5 cm or less (**Fig. 85C2**)
  - Internal foci of fat attenuation or fat alternating with foci of calcification (**Figs. 85B** and **85D**)
- Thin-section CT more sensitive in detecting small foci of fat or calcification
- May manifest as a noncalcified lesion without fat attenuation
- Internal enhancing septa on contrast-enhanced CT
- Endobronchial hamartoma; foci of fat and/or calcification within endoluminal well-defined nodule/mass; bronchial obstruction (**Fig. 85D**)

MR

- Lobular nodule/mass of intermediate signal intensity on T1-weighted images and high signal intensity on T2-weighted images

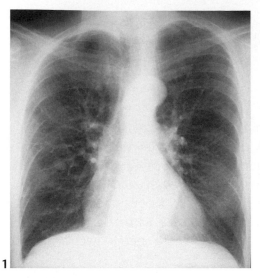 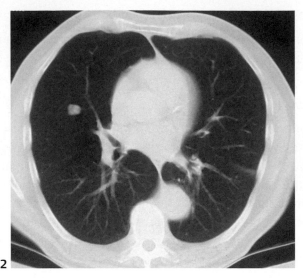

Figure 85C (1,2) PA chest radiograph **(1)** of an asymptomatic elderly man with a long history of cigarette smoking and an incidentally discovered pulmonary hamartoma demonstrates a well-defined soft tissue nodule in the right middle lobe. Unenhanced chest CT (lung window) **(2)** demonstrates a lobular, well-defined solitary pulmonary nodule of heterogeneous attenuation with internal low-attenuation foci.

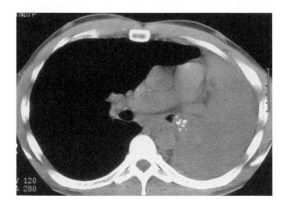

Figure 85D Unenhanced chest CT (mediastinal window) of a man who presented with cough demonstrates left lung atelectasis secondary to left mainstem bronchus obstruction by an endoluminal mass. Note multiple foci of punctate calcification within the lesion. At surgery, an endobronchial hamartoma was found.

- Demonstration of internal fat signal
- Enhancing intralesional tissue septa

Treatment

- Surgical excision; wedge resection, or enucleation, easily "shelled out" from surrounding lung
- Sleeve excision, lobectomy, pneumonectomy for central lesions

Prognosis

- Excellent
- Excision curative; rare recurrences, no reports of malignant transformation

PEARLS

- Hamartomas exhibit slow growth over time, ranging from 1 to 10 mm per year.
- Transthoracic needle biopsy of pulmonary hamartoma yields an 85% diagnostic accuracy.

Suggested Readings

Colby T, Koss M, Travis WD. Hamartoma. In: Rosai J, Sobin LH, eds. Atlas of Tumor Pathology: Tumors of the Lower Respiratory Tract, fascicle 13, series 3. Washington, DC: Armed Forces Institute of Pathology, 1995:319–325

Gjevre JA, Myers JL, Prakash UBS. Pulmonary hamartomas. Mayo Clin Proc 1996;71:14–20

Myers CA, White CS. Cartilaginous disorders of the chest. RadioGraphics 1998;18:1109–1123.

Siegelman SS, Khouri NF, Scott WW Jr, et al. Pulmonary hamartoma: CT findings. Radiology 1986;160:313–317

Travis WD, Colby TV, Corrin B, et al. Histological Typing of Lung and Pleural Tumours: International Histological Classification of Tumours, 3rd ed. Berlin: Springer-Verlag, 1999

SECTION VII
Trauma

CASE 86 Hemomediastinum: Acute Traumatic Aortic Injury

Clinical Presentation

A young man involved in a high-speed motor vehicle collision

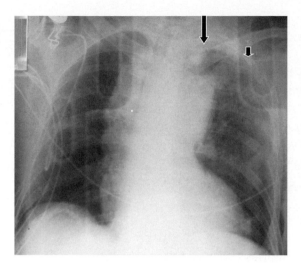

Figure 86A

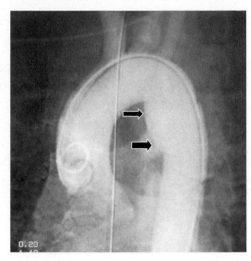

Figure 86B

Radiologic Findings

AP chest radiograph (**Fig. 86A**) reveals marked widening of the superior mediastinum and poor delineation of the descending thoracic aortic interface and left paraspinal line. The right paratracheal stripe is wide, the trachea is deviated to the right, and the left mainstem bronchus is displaced inferiorly. There is a left apical cap of extrapleural blood (long arrow). The left first rib and scapula (short arrow) are fractured. Multiple additional left ribs are also fractured. Subcutaneous air dissects along the left chest wall and into the neck. Left anterior oblique aortogram (**Fig. 86B**) shows a large pseudoaneurysm at the aortic isthmus (arrows).

Diagnosis

Hemomediastinum with acute traumatic aortic injury

Differential Diagnosis

None

Discussion

Background

Blunt chest trauma accounts for 100,000 hospital admissions and 25,000 deaths a year, in the United States alone. Chest injuries are the third most frequent type of injury sustained during high-speed motor vehicle collisions, and alone or in combination with other injuries, they account for more than 50% of all traumatic deaths. Acute traumatic aortic injury (ATAI) is a life-threatening sequela of severe closed chest trauma. Some 80 to 90% of acute aortic injuries occur in the setting of severe motor vehicle collisions, and 5 to 10% of injuries are associated with motor vehicle–pedestrian collisions. ATAI is responsible for 16% of all deaths from motor vehicle collisions. An additional 5 to 10% of acute aortic injuries are associated with falls, usually greater than 30 feet.

Etiology

Acute traumatic aortic injuries occur most commonly at the aortic isthmus immediately distal to the left subclavian artery (80–85%). The second most common site is the ascending aorta (5–9%), followed by the distal descending aorta at the diaphragmatic hiatus (1–3%). Multiple lacerations develop in 6 to 18% of cases. Mechanisms of injury include *shearing forces* (the rate of deceleration of the mobile aortic arch differs from the fixed descending aorta), *bending stresses* (the aorta is flexed over the left pulmonary artery and left mainstem bronchus), and the *osseous pinch* (the aorta is squeezed between the manubrium, clavicle, and first rib anteriorly, and the thoracic spine posteriorly).

Clinical Findings

There may be few, if any, clinical signs or symptoms. Associated injuries (fractured ribs, sternum, pelvis, and ruptures of the diaphragm and spleen) are common and may produce symptoms. An incomplete aortic tear (intact adventitial layer) may convert to a complete rupture (involving all three vessel layers), which is rapidly fatal.

Pathology

GROSS

- Mediastinal hematoma and/or hemorrhage
- Pseudoaneurysm of the thoracic aorta at the site of injury
- Fatal cardiac injuries found in 25% of patients at autopsy

MICROSCOPIC

- Aortic tear is usually transversely oriented and involves the layers of the aorta to varying degrees.
- Complete tear: involves all three layers: intima, media, and adventitia.
- Incomplete tear: traumatic pseudoaneurysm contained by adventitia and mediastinal structures

Imaging Findings

RADIOGRAPHY

- Signs of hemomediastinum and indirect signs of possible ATAI
  - Superior mediastinal widening at the transverse aorta (**Fig. 86A**)
  - Abnormal aortic contour or poor definition of transverse aorta (**Fig. 86A**)
  - Opacification of the aorticopulmonary window
  - Rightward deviation of the trachea or endotracheal tube (**Fig. 86A**)
  - Nasogastric tube deviation to the right of the T4 spinous process
  - Thickened or poorly defined left paraspinal line
  - Poor definition of the descending thoracic aortic interface
  - Widened right paratracheal stripe (more than 5 mm) (**Fig. 86A**)

- Displacement of left mainstem bronchus more than 40 degrees from the horizontal (**Fig. 86A**)
- Left hemothorax and/or a left apical cap (**Fig. 86A**)
- Fractures of the left first and second ribs (**Fig. 86A**)
- Nonspecific signs; may be seen with a variety of other mediastinal and chest wall injuries (e.g., nonaortic vascular injuries, fractures of sternum and thoracic spine)
- Mediastinal widening (sensitivity 92%; specificity 10%) and poor definition of the transverse aorta most sensitive signs of potential ATAI
- Negative predictive value of normal chest radiograph is 98%.

TRANSCATHETER AORTOGRAPHY (SENSITIVITY APPROACHES 100%; SPECIFICITY 99–100%)

- Intimal irregularity or intraluminal filling defect (i.e., intimal flap) (**Fig. 86B**)
- Contrast outside the projected aortic lumen (i.e., pseudoaneurysm) (**Fig. 86B**)
- Atypical or equivocal findings (1–5%)
  - Anatomic variants (e.g., ductus diverticulum, aortic spindle, infundibulum of the third intercostal or bronchial artery)
  - Atheromatous plaques
  - Artifacts (e.g., respiratory motion, digital subtraction, physiologic mixing of contrast)

Treatment

- Nonoperative management with pulse pressure reduction (i.e., β-blockers) and endovascular stent-grafts
- Operative excision of the tear and placement of a Dacron graft
  - Partial cardiopulmonary bypass without systemic heparinization
  - Cardiopulmonary bypass with systemic heparinization

Prognosis

- Eighty to 85% of patients die at the accident scene from complete aortic tears.
- Fifteen percent of survivors (incomplete aortic tears) are at risk for developing complete tears.
  - Thirty percent die within 6 hours.
  - Forty to 50% die within 24 hours.
  - Ninety percent die within 4 months without treatment.
  - Only 2% survive long-term without intervention (**Fig. 86C**).

PEARLS_____

- One must be able to mentally draw out the margins of the right paratracheal stripe and transverse and descending thoracic aorta on every blunt trauma chest radiograph. If one cannot do so, the mediastinum is not normal and warrants further imaging to exclude an acute traumatic aortic injury (e.g., better chest radiograph, CT, aortography).
- The most common diagnostic challenge is to differentiate a traumatic aortic isthmus pseudoaneurysm from a normal ductus diverticulum. The ductus diverticulum is the remnant of the ductus arteriosus. The aortic isthmus is located anteromedially, just distal to the origin of the left subclavian artery. This is the most common site of acute aortic injury. This is also the location of the ductus diverticulum, a smooth anteromedial outpouching of the aortic isthmus that is a normal finding and should not be confused with a pseudoaneurysm, which often appears more angulated or irregular.

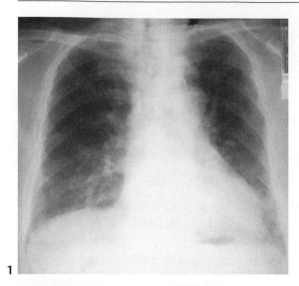

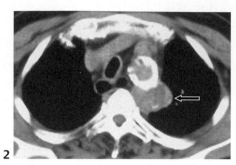

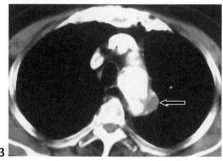

Figure 86C (1–3) PA chest radiograph **(1)** of a 72-year-old man who was involved in a nearly fatal car collision 40 years ago shows an abnormal contour of the transverse aorta which exhibits peripheral mural calcifications. Noncontrasted (mediastinal window) **(2)** and contrast-enhanced (mediastinal window) **(3)** chest CT confirms a chronic pseudoaneurysm (arrow) from a remote unrecognized traumatic aortic injury.

- Goodman et al classified the contour of the isthmus as follows:
  - Type I: a concave isthmus contour.
  - Type II: mild straightening or convexity without a discrete bulge.
  - Type III: a discrete focal bulge of the aortic isthmus called the ductus diverticulum.

Suggested Readings

Czermak BV, Waldenberger P, Perkmann R, et al. Placement of endovascular stent-grafts for emergency treatment of acute disease of the descending thoracic aorta. AJR Am J Roentgenol 2002;179:337–345

Goodman PC, Jeffrey RB, Minagi H, et al. Angiographic evaluation of the ductus diverticulum. Cardiovasc Intervent Radiol 1982;5(1):1–4

Holmes JH IV, Bloch RD, Hall RA, Carter YM, Karmy-Jones RC. Natural history of traumatic rupture of the thoracic aorta managed nonoperatively: a longitudinal analysis. Ann Thorac Surg 2002;73: 1149–1154

Mirvis SE, Bidwell JK, Buddemeyer EU, et al. Value of chest radiography in excluding traumatic aortic rupture. Radiology 1987;163:487–493

Mirvis SE, Shanmuganathan K, Buell J, Rodriguez A. Use of spiral computed tomography for the assessment of blunt trauma patients with potential aortic injury. J Trauma 1998;45:922–930

Parmley LF, Mattingly TW, Manion WC, Jahnke EJ Jr. Non-penetrating traumatic injury of the aorta. Circulation 1958;17:1086–1101

CASE 87 Acute Traumatic Aortic Injury: CT

Clinical Presentation

A 26-year-old woman involved in a high-speed motor vehicle collision with an abnormal AP chest radiograph (not illustrated) that could not be cleared for potential mediastinal trauma

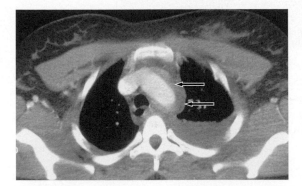

Figure 87A

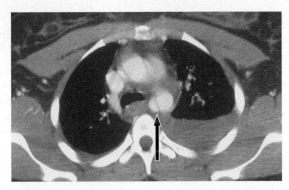

Figure 87B

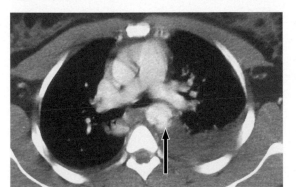

Figure 87C

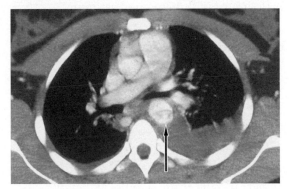

Figure 87D

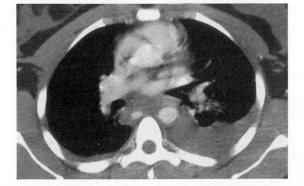

Figure 87E

Radiologic Findings

Contrast-enhanced chest CT (**Figs. 87A** to **87E**) (mediastinal window) demonstrates classic findings of an acute traumatic aortic injury (ATAI). Middle mediastinal blood surrounds the transverse aorta (**Fig. 87A,** arrows), which exhibits a contour abnormality and pseudoaneurysm in the proximal and (**Fig. 87B,** arrow) descending thoracic aorta (**Fig. 87C,** arrow). Intraluminal debris (**Fig. 87D,** arrow) and a marked caliber change (pseudocoarctation) are also seen in the descending thoracic aorta (**Fig. 87E**). Note the ipsilateral hemothorax.

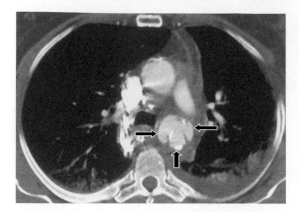

Figure 87F Contrast-enhanced chest CT (mediastinal window) of a 75-year-old woman involved in a motor vehicle collision demonstrates a posttraumatic pseudoaneurysm in the proximal descending thoracic aorta (arrows).

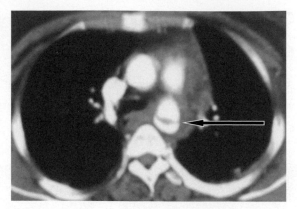

Figure 87G Contrast-enhanced chest CT (mediastinal window) of a trauma victim with an abnormal mediastinum on initial chest radiography demonstrates an intimal flap (arrow), a posttraumatic pseudoaneurysm at the aortic isthmus, and a hemomediastinum.

Diagnosis

Acute traumatic aortic injury with hemomediastinum

Differential Diagnosis

None

Discussion

Background

Traumatic thoracic aortic injuries are not infrequent in high-speed motor vehicle collisions with deceleration on impact, in falls from significant heights (e.g., greater than 30 feet), and in blast injuries. Only 15% of patients with acute thoracic aortic injuries survive to reach the hospital. Without emergent intervention, these patients are at high risk for rupture and sudden hypovolemic shock and death, due to exsanguination into the chest cavity.

Clinical Findings

There may be few, if any, clinical signs or symptoms. Potential signs of acute thoracic aorta and/or great vessel injury include (1) external evidence of significant chest trauma (e.g., steering wheel impression, palpable fractures of the sternum or thoracic spine, left flail chest), (2) hypotension and/or hypovolemia, (3) elevated central venous pressure, (4) an expanding hematoma at the thoracic inlet, (5) diminished or absent upper extremity pulses, (6) upper extremity hypertension, (7) and an interscapular murmur on auscultation.

Pathology

GROSS

- Mediastinal hematoma and/or hemorrhage
- Pseudoaneurysm of the thoracic aorta at the site of injury
- Fatal cardiac injuries found in 25% of patients at autopsy

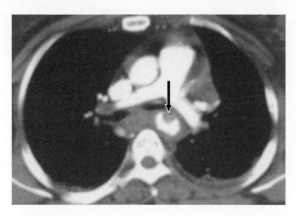

Figure 87H Contrast-enhanced chest CT (mediastinal window) of a high-speed motor vehicle accident victim demonstrates intraluminal debris in a disrupted thoracic aorta (arrow).

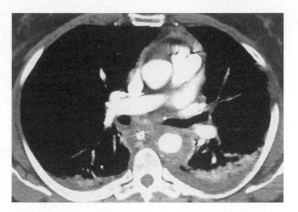

Figure 87I Contrast-enhanced chest CT (mediastinal window) of a motor vehicle accident victim demonstrates periaortic blood. An occult tear at the aortic isthmus was seen at aortography (not illustrated) and surgically repaired.

MICROSCOPIC

- Aortic tear is usually transversely oriented and involves the layers of the aorta to varying degrees.
- Complete tear involves all three layers: intima, media, and adventitia.
- Incomplete tear: traumatic pseudoaneurysm contained by adventitia and mediastinal structures

Imaging Findings

DIRECT CT SIGNS OF ATAI (SENSITIVITY 90–100%; SPECIFICITY 82–99%)

- Critical importance of evaluating aorta at level of left main pulmonary artery
  - Pseudoaneurysm (**Fig. 87F**)
  - Intraluminal filling defect; intimal flap (**Fig. 87G**) or dissection
  - Intraluminal debris (**Fig. 87H**) or irregular aortic contour
  - Pseudocoarctation (aorta narrows at site of tear) (**Fig. 87E**)

INDIRECT CT SIGNS OF ATAI (SENSITIVITY 100%; SPECIFICITY 87%)

- Mediastinal hematoma contiguous with aorta (i.e., periaortic) (**Fig. 87I**)
- In ≤ 17% of aortic injuries—isolated aortic contour or luminal irregularities may occur without significant periaortic blood or hemomediastinum

FALSE CT SCAN RESULTS

- Suboptimal contrast bolus
- Left arm injections with beam hardening artifacts and branch vessel origin obscuration
- Respiratory motion and aortic pulsations
- Partial volume averaging with pulmonary artery or unopacified brachiocephalic vein
- Prominent periaortic mediastinal vessels
- Atheromatous plaque
- Normal thymic tissue
- Periaortic atelectasis and pleural fluid
- Normal variants (ductus bump, infundibulum of third intercostal or bronchial artery)

Treatment

- Nonoperative management with pulse pressure reduction (i.e., β-blockers) and endovascular stent-grafts
- Operative excision of the tear and placement of a Dacron graft

Prognosis

- Death at scene of accident from complete aortic tears in 80 to 85% of patients
- Risk of developing complete tears in 15% of survivors (with incomplete aortic tears)

PEARLS

- Thin collimated images (i.e., minimum 5 mm reconstructed at 2–3 mm) are mandatory for studying the thoracic aorta and branch vessels. Multiplanar reformatted (MPR) and maximum intensity projection (MIP) images are helpful for branch vessel evaluation and surgical planning.
- Misleading artifacts can be minimized with right arm injections, moving ECG leads to the shoulders for the scan, and removal of nasogastric tubes when feasible.
- There is no relationship between isolated anterior mediastinal hematoma and ATAI.
- When in doubt about any CT finding related to the thoracic aorta or branch vessels, the finding should be further evaluated with a repeat CT or aortography. Transesophageal echosonography may prove helpful in selected cases.

Suggested Readings

Gavant ML, Flick P, Mendke P, Gold RE. CT Aortography of thoracic aortic rupture. AJR Am J Roentgenol 1996;166:955–961

Kwon CC, Gill IS, Fallon WF, et al. Delayed operative intervention in the management of traumatic descending thoracic aortic rupture. Ann Thorac Surg 2002;74:S1888–S1898

Mirvis SE, Shanmuganathan K, Buell J, Rodriguez A. Use of spiral computed tomography for the assessment of blunt trauma patients with potential aortic injury. J Trauma 1998;45:922–930

Mirvis SE, Shanmuganathan K, Miller BH, White CS, Turney SZ. Traumatic aortic injury: diagnosis with contrast-enhanced thoracic CT—five year experience at a major trauma center. Radiology 1996; 200:413–422

Parker MS, Matheson TL, Rao AV. et. al. Making the transition: the role of helical CT in the evaluation of potentially acute thoracic aortic injuries. AJR Am J Roentgenol 2001;176:1267–1272

CASE 88 Acute Traumatic Brachiocephalic Artery Transection

Clinical Presentation

Young woman involved in a high-speed motor vehicle collision

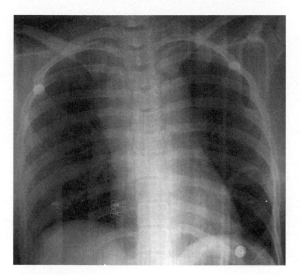

Figure 88A

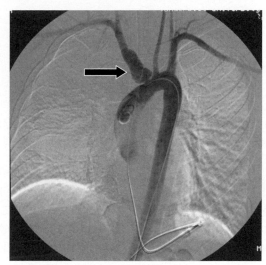

Figure 88B

Radiologic Findings

Anteroposterior (AP) chest radiograph (**Fig. 88A**) demonstrates a grossly widened superior mediastinum. The right and left paratracheal stripes are widened, there is poor definition of the aortic knob, and there is opacification of the aorticopulmonary window. Aortogram (**Fig. 88B**) reveals a traumatic injury involving the origin of the brachiocephalic artery with extension into the right subclavian artery. Notice the large irregular brachiocephalic artery pseudoaneurysm (arrow).

Diagnosis

Acute traumatic brachiocephalic artery transection

Differential Diagnosis

None

Discussion

Background

Blunt trauma can produce lacerations of the thoracic great vessels. The majority involve the left subclavian artery, a few involve the base of the brachiocephalic artery, and the left carotid is injured least often. Isolated blunt brachiocephalic, carotid, and subclavian artery injuries are uncommon (1–3%) but often-lethal complications of severe deceleration trauma. These injuries are associated with concomitant injuries of the thoracic aorta and usually occur at their origin off the arch. Other associated injuries are usually severe and include sternal-manubrial fractures (10%), left posterior sternoclavicular joint dislocations (10%), and scapulothoracic dissociation.

Clinical Findings

Clinical signs, such as a blood pressure gradient between the upper extremities, are highly suggestive but are not usually present.

Pathology

GROSS

- Mediastinal hematoma and/or hemorrhage
- Posttraumatic pseudoaneurysm of the brachiocephalic artery at the site of injury
- Concomitant injury of the thoracic aorta may be present

MICROSCOPIC

- Intimal tear is usually transversely oriented and involves the layers of the brachiocephalic artery to varying degrees
- Complete tear involves all three layers: intima, media, and adventitia
- Incomplete tear: traumatic pseudoaneurysm contained by adventitia and mediastinal structures

Imaging Findings

RADIOGRAPHY

- Superior mediastinal widening at the transverse aorta (**Fig. 88A;** see Case 86, **Fig. 86A**)
- Abnormal aortic contour or poor definition of transverse aorta (**Fig. 86A**)
- Opacification of the aorticopulmonary window
- Rightward deviation of the trachea or endotracheal tube (**Fig. 86A**)
- Nasogastric tube deviation to the right of the T4 spinous process
- Thickened or poorly defined left paraspinal line
- Poor definition of the descending thoracic aortic interface
- Widened right paratracheal stripe (more than 5 mm) (**Fig. 88A;** see Case 86, **Fig. 86A**)
- Displacement of left mainstem bronchus more than 40 degrees from the horizontal (**Fig. 86A**)
- Left hemothorax and/or a left apical cap (**Fig. 86A**)
- Fractures of the left first and second ribs (**Fig. 86A**)

CT

- MPR and MIP coronal and oblique sagittal images very useful for branch vessel evaluation.
- Superior and/or middle mediastinal hematoma (see Case 87)
- Peribranch vessel hematoma
- Affected branch vessels fail to opacify with contrast media.
- Extravasation of contrast from lacerated branch vessel
- Abnormal contour and/or caliber of affected branch vessel
- Pseudoaneurysm or intimal tear
- Concomitant thoracic aortic injury

ANGIOGRAPHY

- Intimal tear (**Fig. 88B**)
- Extravasation of contrast
- Dissection with an intimal flap

- Pseudoaneurysm (**Fig. 88B**)
- Pseudocoarctation

Treatment

- Temporary arterial balloon occlusion
- Median sternotomy with cervical extension if necessary
- Repair with polyester patch, Gore-Tex graft, blood vessel reconstruction, or transplantation of the great saphenous vein

Prognosis

- Low preoperative and intraoperative survival rates
- Death from acute bleeding, cerebral ischemia, or concomitant injuries

Suggested Readings

Anastasiadis K, Channon KM, Ratnatunga C. Traumatic innominate artery transection. J Cardiovasc Surg (Torino) 2002;43:697–700

Desai M, Baxter AB, Karmy-Jones R, Borsa JJ. Potentially life-saving role for temporary endovascular balloon occlusion in atypical mediastinal hematoma. AJR Am J Roentgenol 2002;178:1180

Fishman JE. Imaging of blunt aortic and great vessel trauma. J Thorac Imaging 2000;15:97–103

Letsou G, Gertler JP, Baker CC, Hammond GL. Blunt innominate injury: a report of three cases. J Trauma 1989;29:104–108

Poole GV. Fracture of the upper ribs and injury to the great vessels. Surg Gynecol Obstet 1989; 169:275–282

CASE 89 Vena Cava Injury

Clinical Presentation

Young woman involved in a serious motor vehicle collision

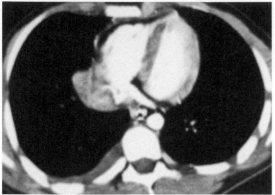

Figure 89A

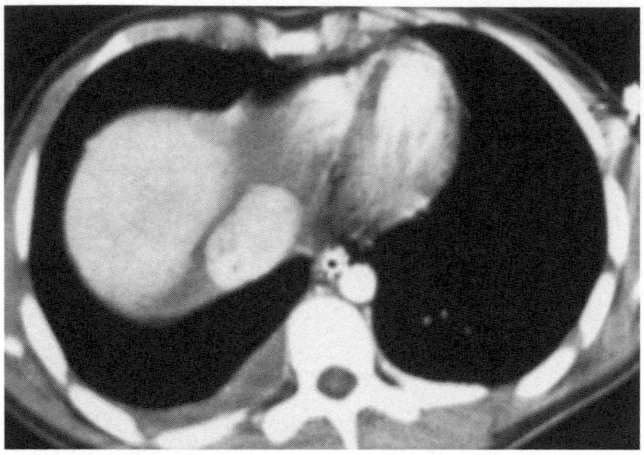

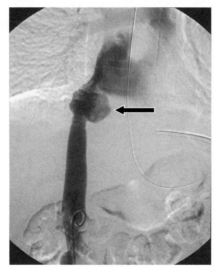

Figure 89B

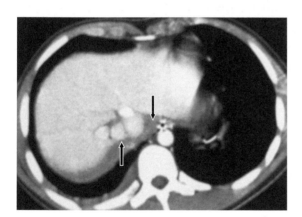

Figure 89C

Figure 89D

Radiologic Findings

Contrast-enhanced chest CT (**Figs. 89A** to **89C**) (mediastinal window) reveals marked enlargement of the suprahepatic inferior vena cava immediately inferior to the right atrium. Notice the small pericardial effusion, right hemothorax, and free fluid surrounding the proximal hepatic veins (arrows). Contrast vena cavagram (**Fig. 89D**) shows aneurysmal dilatation of the supradiaphragmatic inferior vena cava just proximal to the right atrium (arrow), without evidence of gross extravasation.

Diagnosis

Traumatic pseudoaneurysm of supradiaphragmatic inferior vena cava

Differential Diagnosis

None

Discussion

Background

Injury to the inferior vena cava carries a very high mortality, ranging from 57 to 95%. The usual cause of death in such cases is hypovolemic shock or renal failure. Gunshot wounds are the most frequent cause of inferior vena cava injuries, and 55% of such patients have circulatory instability on admission. Iatrogenic injury to the inferior vena cava may also occur during operative procedures in its vicinity. Blunt injuries limited to the major veins of the thorax are rare. These patients usually present with associated injuries to the other major thoracic vascular structures.

Clinical Findings

The clinical history, including mechanism of injury, and physical examination is similar to that seen in the setting of acute traumatic aortic and great vessel arterial injuries. Approximately 33% of patients with a traumatic injury of the vena cava die before reaching the hospital. The mortality is reported to be as high as 50% in those who survive to reach medical care. Death is commonly caused by intraoperative exsanguination during attempted intraoperative repair of the injured inferior vena cava. Venous complications in survivors are not infrequent and include venous hypertension, inferior vena cava thrombosis, inferior vena cava syndrome, and fatal pulmonary embolism.

Pathology

GROSS

- Retroperitoneal hemorrhage
- Hemoperitoneum may be present.
- Pseudoaneurysm of the vena cava with or without a contained hematoma

MICROSCOPIC

- Venous tear involves the layers of the cava to varying degrees.
- Complete tear involves all three layers: intima, media, and adventitia.
- Incomplete tear: traumatic pseudoaneurysm contained by adventitia and mediastinal structures

Imaging Findings

CT

- Hemopericardium (with intrapericardial caval disruption) and/or right-sided hemothorax (**Figs. 89A, 89B,** and **89C**)
- Irregular or amorphous appearing inferior vena cava; pseudoaneurysm (**Figs. 89A, 89B,** and **89C**)
- Contrast extravasation from lacerated vena cava
- Hemoperitoneum, liver laceration, and/or free fluid around the hepatic veins (**Fig. 89C**)
- Retrohepatic or retroperitoneal hematoma

VENOGRAPHY

- Inferior vena cava pseudoaneurysm (**Fig. 89D**)
- Vena cava luminal filling defect
- Contrast extravasation

Treatment

- Management of hypovolemic shock and blood transfusion
- Placement of intravenous lines below the level of the diaphragm
- Primary venorrhaphy, ligation, or prosthetic grafting
- Preservation of a luminal diameter at least 25% of normal in suprarenal vena cava repairs
- Fenestrated stent-grafts in select cases

Prognosis

- Lowest survival for patients arriving in shock and failing to respond to initial resuscitative measures, those actively bleeding at laparotomy, and those with retrohepatic vena cava injuries
- High mortality in cases of retrohepatic and subdiaphragmatic inferior vena cava injury

PEARLS_____

- The site of injury and hemodynamic status on admission are the principal factors related to morbidity and mortality for patients with inferior vena cava injuries.
- Concomitant injuries to the thoracic and/or abdominal aorta, liver, and bowel are not infrequent.

Suggested Readings

Buckman RF, Pathak AS, Badellino MM, Bradley KM. Injuries of the inferior vena cava. Surg Clin North Am 2001;81:1431–1447

Carr JA, Kralovich KA, Patton JH, Horst HM. Primary venorrhaphy for traumatic inferior vena cava injuries. Am Surg 2001;67:207–214

Cunningham PR, Foil MB. The ripped cava. J Natl Med Assoc 1995;87:305–307

Ombrellaro MP, Freeman MB, Stevens SL, Diamond DL, Goldman MH. Predictors of survival after inferior vena cava injuries. Am Surg 1997;63:178–183

Porter JM, Ivatury RR, Islamk SZ, Vinzons A, Stahl WM. Inferior vena cava injuries: non-invasive follow-up of venorrhaphy. J Trauma 1997;42:913–918

Sullivan VV, Voris TK, Borlaza GS, Lampman RM, Sood M, Shanley CJ. Incidental discovery of an inferior vena cava aneurysm. Ann Vasc Surg 2002;16:513–515

Watarida S, Nishi T, Furukawa A, et al. Fenestrated stent-graft for traumatic juxtahepatic inferior vena cava injury. J Endovasc Ther 2002;9:134–137

CASE 90 Lung Contusion

Clinical Presentation

A young man involved in a motorcycle collision

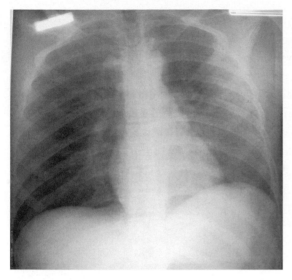

Figure 90A

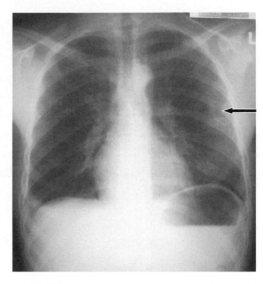

Figure 90B

Radiologic Findings

Initial AP chest radiograph (**Fig. 90A**) shows an ill-defined, nonsegmental, consolidation in the axillary portion of the left upper lobe. AP chest radiograph (**Fig. 90B**) obtained 3 days later reveals an underlying pulmonary laceration with posttraumatic pneumatocele (arrow) initially masked by the consolidation.

Diagnosis

Lung contusion with underlying lung laceration

Differential Diagnosis

• Atypical airspace edema
• Aspiration pneumonia

Discussion

Background

Lung contusions are among the most common traumatic lung injuries, seen in 30 to 70% of victims of blunt chest trauma, even in the absence of rib fractures. Lung contusions may also occur in penetrating and blast injuries.

367

Etiology

Contusions result from loss of vessel wall integrity leading to subsequent intraparenchymal and alveolar hemorrhage. The accumulation of blood in the affected areas increases during the first 6 to 8 hours, and usually recedes within 7 to 10 days. The degree of capillary leak into contused lung may be accentuated by aggressive fluid resuscitation.

Clinical Findings

Contusions may be occult and mild or severe, widespread, and associated with respiratory failure. They may exist despite normal chest radiography and absence of external signs of chest wall trauma. The onset of signs and symptoms may be slow and may progress over 24 hours. Signs and symptoms include dyspnea, hypoxemia, tachycardia, absent breath sounds, and cyanosis. Approximately 87 percent of patients with pulmonary contusion have associated extrathoracic injuries. Although underestimated on initial radiographic and clinical examinations, an accurate estimate of the extent of contusion is clinically significant because of its associations with post-traumatic respiratory insufficiency.

Pathology

GROSS

- Parenchymal contusion with hemorrhage into lung tissue
- Edema
- Atelectasis

MICROSCOPIC

- Hemorrhage into pulmonary interstitium and alveoli

Imaging Findings

RADIOGRAPHY

- Inconspicuous findings in up to one fourth of lung contusions involving up to one third of the lung
- Patchy, nonsegmental, ill-defined, peripheral airspace opacities often situated adjacent to solid structures (e.g., ribs, vertebrae, heart, liver) (**Fig. 90A**)
- May be obscured by coexisting hemothorax, aspiration, or atelectasis
- Coup and contracoup contusions described

CT

- Higher sensitivity for detection of contusion when compared to radiography, but similar morphologic features (**Fig. 90C**)
- Demonstration of air-bronchograms within consolidations; may not be appreciated on radiography

Treatment

- Pain control, pulmonary toilet, and supplemental oxygen are the primary therapies for pulmonary contusion
- Large and/or multifocal lung contusions often characterized by shunting and dead space ventilation, necessitating endotracheal intubation and mechanical ventilation
- Judicious fluid management

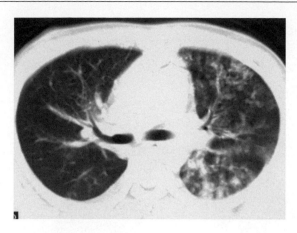

Figure 90C Contrast-enhanced chest CT (lung window) of a blunt trauma victim with lung contusion shows ill-defined, nonsegmental, ground-glass opacities in the peripheral left upper and lower lobes.

Prognosis

- Forty to 57% of patients with pulmonary contusion require mechanical ventilation.
- Up to 31% mortality reported in patients with massive contusions.

PEARLS

- Radiographic opacities that develop more than 24 hours following the initial injury are unlikely to represent contusions and more likely represent aspiration, superimposed infection, or infarction.
- Opacities that fail to resolve within 10 to 14 days likely represent postlaceration hematoma, nosocomial pneumonia, aspiration, atelectasis, or acute respiratory distress syndrome (ARDS).
- Basilar contusions associated with rib fractures should alert the radiologist to the possibility of subdiaphragmatic visceral trauma.
- Cases of severe trauma with complicating long bone injuries and airspace opacities developing in the first few days also raise the specter of fat embolism syndrome.

Suggested Readings

Miller PR, Croce MA, Bee TK, et al. ARDS after pulmonary contusion: accurate measurement of contusion volume identifies high-risk patients. J Trauma 2001;51:223–228

Miller PR, Croce MA, Kilgo PD, Scott J, Fabian TC. Acute respiratory distress syndrome in blunt trauma: identification of independent risk factors. Am Surg 2002;68:845–850

Parker MS, Matheson TL, Rao AV, et al. Spiral CT in blunt thoracic trauma: detection of "unsuspected" concomitant injuries. The Radiologist 2000;7:137–146

Van Hise ML, Primack SL, Israel RS, Müller NL. CT in blunt chest trauma: indications and limitations. Radiographics 1998;18:1071–1084

CASE 91 Lung Contusion and Laceration

Clinical Presentation

An 18-year-old man involved in a motorcycle accident

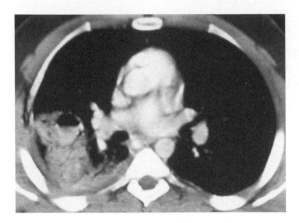

Figure 91A

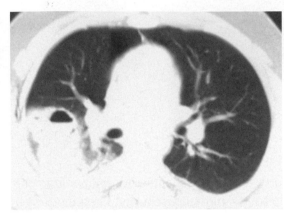

Figure 91B

Radiologic Findings

Contrast-enhanced chest CT (**Fig. 91A,** mediastinal window, and **Fig. 91B,** lung window) demonstrates extensive consolidation in the posterior segment of the right upper lobe with an associated 2 cm rounded lesion containing an air-fluid level.

Diagnosis

Pulmonary contusion with complicating laceration

Differential Diagnosis

None

Discussion

Background

Pulmonary laceration, or traumatic pneumatocoele, is often present in association with pulmonary contusion. Pulmonary laceration can be difficult to recognize on chest radiography, often obscured by the contusion or hemothorax. CT is more sensitive. Lacerations usually appear as oval or round cavities and may contain an air-fluid level due to hemorrhage into the cavity, or a crescent sign due to air outlining a lung hematoma. Pulmonary lacerations occur in both blunt and penetrating trauma. Lacerations may be superficial and juxtapleural or may occur deep in the lung parenchyma.

Etiology

There are four mechanisms by which pulmonary lacerations occur. The most common is *compression rupture* of lung tissue. *Compression shears* are vertically oriented and paravertebral in location.

370

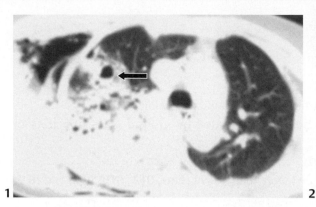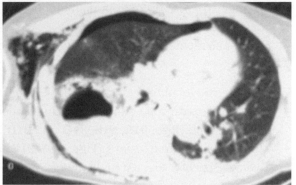

Figure 91C (1) Contrast-enhanced chest CT (lung window) of a severe blunt chest trauma victim reveals multiple variable-sized lucencies, at least one with an air-fluid level (arrow), in a densely consolidated, contused right upper lung, consistent with pulverized lung. **(2)** Contrast-enhanced chest CT (lung window) shows a 5 cm laceration within a densely consolidated, contused right lower lobe. Note the ipsilateral pneumothorax.

Parenchymal penetrations are small and result from injuries such as displaced rib fractures and bullet and knife wounds. Rarely, *tearing* of preexistent *adhesions* results in parenchymal lacerations. If the laceration fills with blood (i.e., from associated vascular tears), a spherical *pulmonary hematoma* forms. If it fills with air (i.e., from associated tears in bronchi or bronchioles), an air-containing *posttraumatic pneumatocele* or *air cyst* forms. If both blood and air are present, an air-fluid level may be seen. *Pulverized lung* may occur in severe blunt chest trauma, is best appreciated on CT (**Fig. 91C1**), and is characterized by multiple small 5 to 10 mm lucencies in a region of dense consolidation.

Clinical Findings

The signs and symptoms of pulmonary contusion depend on the extent of the injury. Patients may present with varying degrees of respiratory difficulty. Physical examination often demonstrates decreased breath sounds over the affected area. An overlying chest wall injury is frequently present. Pulmonary lacerations may be associated with persistent hemothorax and pneumothorax (**Fig. 91C2**) secondary to concomitant tears in the bronchi, vessels, and visceral pleura. These parenchymal injuries may become secondarily infected, and are often associated with persistent clinical air-leaks and the need for prolonged chest tube drainage due to the development of bronchopleural fistula(s).

Pathology

- Oval or round cavity(ies) that may be associated with pulmonary contusion
- Pseudomembrane, a few millimeters in thickness

Imaging Findings

RADIOGRAPHY

- Although present immediately, often overlooked or obscured on initial studies by adjacent contusion, hemothorax, or pneumothorax
- Faint linear opacity corresponding to the air-filled pneumatocele, earliest finding
- Usually round or oval, but may take several days to develop classic morphology
- May be isolated or multiple

- Average size of 2 to 5 cm in diameter
- May contain air-fluid levels
- Rapid enlargement of pneumatoceles in patients receiving positive pressure ventilation

CT

- Most sensitive and specific modality for identification and characterization
- Spherical or variable-shaped air-fluid collection(s) surrounded by ground-glass opacities or consolidation (**Figs. 91A, 91B, 91C,** and **91D**)
- Isolated or multiple lesions (**Figs. 91A, 91B, 91C,** and **91D**)
- Average size of 2 to 5 cm in diameter; but can be larger than 10 cm (**Figs. 91A, 91B, 91C,** and **91D**)

Treatment

- Supportive
- Evacuation of the pleural space where appropriate

Prognosis

- In the absence of complications or pulverized lung, isolated lacerations are an indicator of injury severity, but otherwise have little clinical significance.

PEARL_____

- Organized hematomas may persist for months following the injury and may be misdiagnosed as lung abscesses or neoplasms in the absence of clinical history. Evaluation of serial chest radiographs is necessary to make the appropriate diagnosis.

Suggested Readings

Kang EY, Müller NL. CT in blunt chest trauma: pulmonary, tracheobronchial, and diaphragmatic injuries. Semin Ultrasound CT MR 1996;17:114–118

Kuhlman JE, Pozniak MA, Collins J, Knisely BL. Radiographic and CT findings of blunt chest trauma: aortic injuries and looking beyond them. Radiographics 1998;18:1085–1108

Shanmuganathan K, Mirvis SE. Imaging diagnosis of nonaortic thoracic injury. Radiol Clin North Am 1999;37:533–551

Wagner RB, Crawford WO Jr, Schimpf PP. Classification of parenchymal injuries of the lung. Radiology 1988;167:77–82

Zinck SE, Primack SL. Radiographic and CT findings in blunt chest trauma. J Thorac Imaging 2000;15: 87–96

CASE 92 Post-Traumatic Pneumothorax: Deep Sulcus Sign

Clinical Presentation

Young man involved in a motor vehicle collision

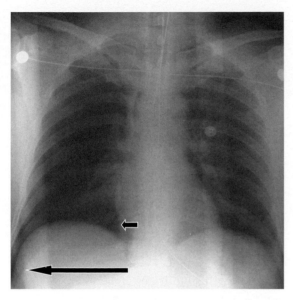

Figure 92A

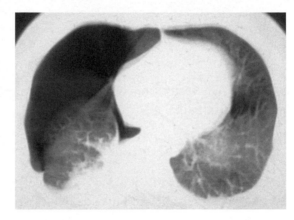

Figure 92B

Radiologic Findings

AP supine chest radiograph (**Fig. 92A**) demonstrates a relatively hyperlucent right hemithorax and hemidiaphragm. The right cardiophrenic angle is also lucent (short arrow) and the lateral sulcus unusually deep (long arrow). Contrast-enhanced chest CT (**Fig. 92B;** lung window), reveals a large right pneumothorax.

Diagnosis

Posttraumatic pneumothorax; "deep sulcus" sign

Differential Diagnosis

None

Discussion

Background

Pneumothorax is the second most common chest injury. Simple pneumothoraces occur in 15 to 38% of blunt, and 18 to 19% of penetrating, chest trauma victims.

373

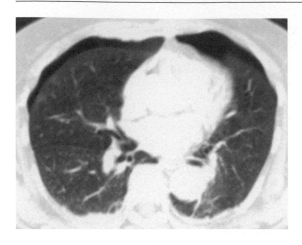

Figure 92C Contrast-enhanced chest CT (lung window) of a 77-year-old woman involved in a motor vehicle collision reveals unsuspected bilateral pneumothoraces.

Etiology

Traumatic pneumothoraces may result from alveolar compression, parenchymal laceration, tracheo-bronchial disruption, and barotrauma.

Clinical Findings

Patients with traumatic pneumothorax may complain of pleuritic chest pain or dyspnea and pain at the site of rib fractures. Physical examination may demonstrate decreased breath sounds and hyper-resonance to percussion over the affected hemithorax. Not infrequently, patients with traumatic pneumothoraces also have some element of hemorrhage producing a hemopneumothorax. On imaging studies, free pleural air rises to the most nondependent portion of the pleural space. In erect patients, air rises to the apex. Most trauma patients are imaged in the supine position, in which case the nondependent aspect of the pleural space is at the lung base along the diaphragm. Posttraumatic pneumothoraces are often bilateral (**Fig. 92C**), and often associated with hemothorax. The significance of a pneumothorax depends not on its absolute size but on its physiologic effect. The underlying respiratory reserve largely affects the latter. All pneumothoraces in trauma victims are potentially significant regardless of size, because even seemingly inconsequential pneumothoraces may rapidly become life threatening under the influence of general anesthesia or positive-pressure ventilation.

Pathology

- Laceration in the pleura that may be associated with a tear in the lung parenchyma
- Hemorrhage
- Edema

Imaging Findings

SUPINE CHEST RADIOGRAPHY (SENSITIVITY 36%; SPECIFICITY 100%)

- Hyperlucent lung base (**Fig. 92A**)
- Unusually clear definition of the diaphragm, cardiac apex, and/or cardiophrenic angle (**Fig. 92A**)
- Deep costophrenic (i.e., lateral) sulcus (**Fig. 92A**)

ULTRASOUND (SENSITIVITY 100%; SPECIFICITY 94%)

- More sensitive than supine chest radiography and as sensitive as CT
- Diagnostic findings: horizontal artifacts and absence of lung sliding
- Exclusion of pneumothorax by detection of the "comet tail" artifact at the anterior chest wall

CT

- Air in the nondependent aspect of the pleural space (**Figs. 92B** and **92C**)
- Identifies twice as many pneumothoraces as chest radiography (**Fig. 92C**)

Treatment

- Pain control and pulmonary toilet
- Small to moderate radiographically occult pneumothoraces managed without chest tubes in patients not requiring positive-pressure ventilation
- Anterolateral pneumothoraces best managed with pleural drainage
- Videothoracoscopy and small wedge resections for diagnosis and treatment of persistent posttraumatic pneumothoraces secondary to lung lacerations

Prognosis

- Good if recognized and managed appropriately

PEARLS

- The presence of subcutaneous air on imaging studies should alert the radiologist to a possible occult pneumothorax.
- Limited images through the lung bases in trauma patients undergoing head or abdominal CT can quickly reveal the presence or absence of radiographically inconspicuous pneumothorax.

Suggested Readings

Gordon R. The deep sulcus sign. Radiology 1980;136:25–27

Karaaslan T, Meuli R, Androux R, Duvoisin B, Hessler C, Schnyder P. Traumatic chest lesions in patients with severe head trauma: a comparative study with computed tomography and conventional chest roentgenograms. J Trauma 1995;39:1081–1086

Parker MS, Matheson TL, Rao AV, et al. Spiral CT in blunt thoracic trauma: detection of "unsuspected" concomitant injuries. The Radiologist 2000;7:137–146

Rowan KR, Kirkpatrick AW, Liu D, Forkheim KE, Mayo JR, Nicolaou S. Traumatic pneumothorax detection with thoracic US: correlation with chest radiography and CT—initial experience. Radiology 2002;225:210–214

Wolfman NT, Myers WS, Glauser SJ, Meredith JW, Chen MY. Validity of CT classification on management of occult pneumothorax: a prospective study. AJR Am J Roentgenol 1998;171:1317–1320

CASE 93 Hemothorax

Clinical Presentation

A 57-year-old man involved in a boating accident with hypotension on admission

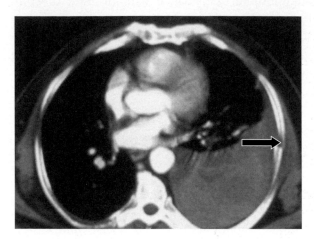

Figure 93A

Radiologic Findings

Contrast-enhanced chest CT (mediastinal window) (**Fig. 93A**) demonstrates a large mixed attenuation left pleural fluid collection. Note the displaced left rib fractures (arrow).

Diagnosis

Traumatic hemothorax

Differential Diagnosis

None

Discussion

Background

Acute hemothorax occurs in 23 to 51% of blunt, and 64 to 82% of penetrating, chest trauma victims. It frequently accompanies pulmonary contusion and laceration, and is often bilateral.

Etiology

Hemothorax results from such injuries as intercostal vessel lacerations, mediastinal contusions, aortic tears, disruptions in the diaphragm and tracheobronchial tree, and iatrogenic line insertions.

Clinical Findings

Patients complain of pain and shortness of breath. Physical examination findings vary with the extent of the hemothorax. Most hemothoraces are associated with diminished breath sounds and dullness to percussion over the affected area. Massive hemothoraces are due to major vascular injuries and manifest with the aforementioned physical findings and shock. Hemothorax is the most common cause of shock in blunt chest trauma victims. Each hemithorax can accommodate 30 to 40% of the patient's total blood volume. If hemorrhage is severe, hypovolemic shock occurs. Respiratory distress may occur when the volume of the hemothorax significantly compresses adjacent lung parenchyma.

Pathology

- Accumulation of blood in the pleural space
- Intercostal vein and/or artery laceration or avulsion
- Internal mammary vein and/or artery laceration or avulsion
- Edema
- Atelectasis of adjacent lung
- Lung contusion may be present

Imaging Findings

RADIOGRAPHY

- Limited role
- Enlarging pleural fluid collection
- Progressive thoracic opacification
- Ipsilateral lung collapse
- Deviation of mediastinum toward the unaffected side
- May exhibit displaced or nondisplaced rib fractures

CT

- High or mixed attenuation pleural fluid collection with adjacent relaxation atelectasis (**Fig. 93A**)
- Isolated or multiple rib fractures (**Fig. 93A**)
- May be associated with pulmonary contusion, laceration, and pneumothorax
- Visualization of extravasation of contrast media from disrupted vessels

Treatment

- None for spontaneously subsiding bleeding
- Simple tube thoracostomy
- Closed drainage for hemothorax with volumes of 500 to 1500 mL that stops bleeding after thoracostomy tube placement
- Thoracotomy for hemothorax with volumes of > 1500 to 2000 mL or continued bleeding > 200 to 300 mL/hour (10–15% patients)
- Early evacuation by video thoracoscopy or thoracotomy of clotted hemothorax to improve pulmonary function, prevent empyema (e.g., *Staphylococcus* sp.), and delay fibrothorax; ideally within 3 days of admission

Prognosis

- Poor with systolic blood pressure < 80 mm Hg on arrival at the hospital, and blood loss of > 1000 mL through the chest tube within the first 2 hours after arrival

PEARLS

- Significant prolonged bloody pleural drainage indicates serious lung or mediastinal injury.
- Persistent accumulation of pleural fluid may also result from thoracic duct tears.

Suggested Readings

Ambrogi MC, Lucchi M, Dini P, Mussi A, Angeletti CA. Videothoracoscopy for evaluation and treatment of hemothorax. J Cardiovasc Surg (Torino) 2002;43:109–112

Parker MS, Matheson TL, Rao AV, et al. Spiral CT in blunt thoracic trauma: detection of "unsuspected" concomitant injuries. The Radiologist 2000;7:137–146

CASE 94 Tracheobronchial Injuries

Clinical Presentation

A 17-year-old involved in a motorcycle collision sustained clavicle and femur fractures, and was readmitted 2 weeks after discharge with dyspnea and chest pain. A chest radiograph revealed a total left pneumothorax (not illustrated) treated with chest tube placement.

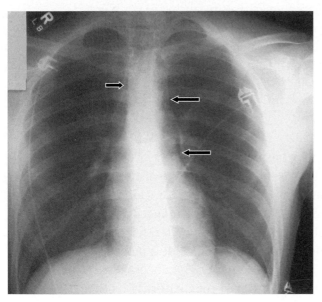

Figure 94A

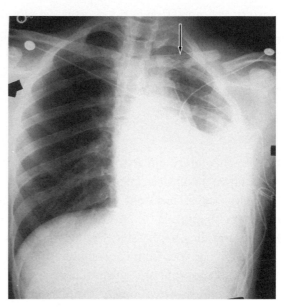

Figure 94B

Radiologic Findings

Initial AP chest radiograph (**Fig. 94A**) shows a displaced left midclavicular fracture and pneumomediastinum (arrows). AP chest radiograph obtained on readmission after chest tube placement (**Fig. 94B**) reveals a persistent left pneumothorax (arrow), left lower lobe collapse, and mediastinal shift.

Diagnosis

Missed left mainstem bronchial fracture, confirmed on bronchoscopy.

Differential Diagnosis

None

Discussion

Background

Rupture of the trachea and/or major bronchi occurs in approximately 1.5% of blunt chest trauma victims with mortality rates as high as 50%. Approximately 80% of bronchial ruptures occur within 2.5 cm of the carina.

Etiology

Rapid anteroposterior compression of the chest is the most common mechanism causing major blunt tracheobronchial injuries. Tracheobronchial injuries may also occur following penetrating trauma to the thorax. Iatrogenic injury may rarely follow over distention of the endotracheal tube cuff or instrumentation of the tracheobronchial tree. Fractures of the bronchi are more common than those of the trachea. The right side is affected more often than the left.

Clinical Findings

Many patients with this injury die at the accident scene due to inadequate ventilation or associated injuries before definitive therapy can be provided. Surviving patients are often in respiratory distress and present with physical signs consistent with a massive pneumothorax. Ipsilateral breath sounds are severely diminished or absent, and the affected hemithorax is hyperresonant to percussion. Subcutaneous air may be present and may be massive. Hemodynamic instability may be caused by tension pneumothorax or massive blood loss from concomitant injuries. Additional signs may include a persistent pneumothorax despite appropriate chest tube placement, dyspnea, hemoptysis, subcutaneous/mediastinal air, and cyanosis. Occasionally, overdistention of the endotracheal tube cuff may be the only sign of tracheal injury. Injuries are often unrecognized on initial exams, and delayed diagnosis is common. Only one third of affected patients are diagnosed in the first 24 hours, and only half within the first month. Definitive diagnosis requires fiberoptic bronchoscopy. Sequelae of unrecognized bronchial tears include airway stenosis, bronchomalacia, recurrent lobar atelectasis, and pneumonia.

Pathology

- Fractures parallel the cartilaginous rings; bronchial injuries
- Fractures usually simple and horizontally oriented; intrathoracic tracheal injuries
- Longitudinal or complex tears; minority of intrathoracic tracheal injuries
- Disruption of the peribronchial connective tissue
- Varying degrees of bleeding and inflammation

Imaging Findings

RADIOGRAPHY

- Persistent pneumothorax (50%) despite appropriate chest tube placement (**Fig. 94B**)
- Increasing subcutaneous air, pneumomediastinum/pneumothorax (**Fig. 94A**)
- Abnormal appearance or position of endotracheal (ET) tube
  - Overdistention of cuff (> 30 mm)
  - Tube protrusion beyond expected margins of tracheal lumen
  - Extraluminal tube tip position
- Associated fractures of the upper thoracic skeleton (e.g., first three ribs, clavicle, sternum, scapula) (40%) (**Fig. 94A**)

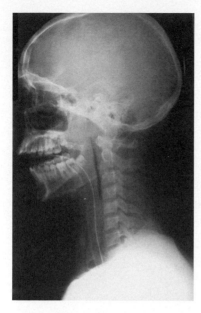

Figure 94C Lateral cervical spine radiograph of a young trauma victim with a near-complete tracheal fracture reveals a large amount of prevertebral and paratracheal air dissecting into the retropharyngeal space.

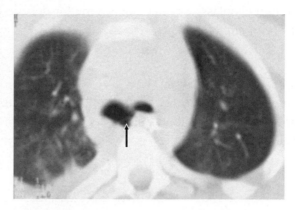

Figure 94D Contrast-enhanced chest CT (lung window) of a young motor vehicle collision victim with a near-complete right mainstem bronchus tear demonstrates asymmetric dilatation of the right mainstem bronchus. Notice the irregular posterior bronchial wall and peribronchial collection of air (arrow).

- Fallen lung sign (i.e., affected lung collapses peripherally rather than centrally) (**Fig. 94B**)
- Elevation of the hyoid bone above the C3 vertebral body (i.e., neck trauma with proximal tracheal injury)
- Cervical air on lateral cervical radiographs (**Fig. 94C**)

CT

- Abnormal course of a mainstem bronchus
- Discontinuity of the affected bronchus
- Focal narrowing of the affected bronchus
- Irregularity of the bronchial wall (**Fig. 94D**)
- Focal peribronchial collections of air or blood (**Fig. 94D**)
- Fallen lung sign
- Atelectasis, pulmonary contusion, and/or laceration
- Pneumomediastinum
- Thoracic skeletal injuries
    - Clavicle
    - Sternum
    - Ribs; usually first or second (2–91%)
    - Scapula
- Traumatic pseudoaneurysm of the pulmonary artery; rare

Treatment

- Antibiotics and intubation with the cuff inflated distal to the tear for localized short lacerations not involving the full thickness of the tracheal wall

- Early surgical repair in all other cases
  - Ipsilateral thoracotomy on the affected side after single-lung ventilation is established on the uninjured side
  - Jet-insufflation may be required in some patients.
  - Operative repair consists of debridement of the injury and a primary end-to-end anastomosis.
- Consideration of bronchoplasty or pneumonectomy for delayed strictures from incomplete tears or lobar collapse from complete tears

Prognosis

- Early recognition is important in this otherwise life-threatening injury.
- Associated injuries also have a significant impact on morbidity and mortality.
- Approximately 19% surgical morbidity

PEARLS_____

- The possibility of tracheobronchial fracture must be considered in patients with severe blunt chest trauma with associated pneumothorax that does not respond to chest tube drainage, pneumothorax and pneumomediastinum in the absence of pleural effusion, and/or mediastinal and deep cervical air in a patient not receiving positive-pressure ventilation.
- Atelectasis may be a late manifestation of a missed tracheobronchial injury, occurring weeks or months after the fracture.

Suggested Readings

Balci AE, Eren N, Eren S, Ulku R. Surgical treatment of post-traumatic tracheobronchial injuries: 14-year experience. Eur J Cardiothorac Surg 2002;22:984–989

Gabor S, Renner H, Pinter H, et al. Indications for surgery in tracheobronchial ruptures. Eur J Cardiothorac Surg 2001;20:399–404

Kang EY, Müller NL. CT in blunt chest trauma: pulmonary, tracheobronchial, and diaphragmatic injuries. Semin Ultrasound CT MR 1996;17:114–118

Kunisch-Hoppe M, Hoppe M, Rauber K, Popella C, Rau WS. Tracheal rupture caused by blunt chest trauma: radiological and clinical features. Eur Radiol 2000;10:480–483

Wintermark M, Schnyder P, Wicky S. Blunt traumatic rupture of a mainstem bronchus: spiral CT demonstration of the "fallen lung" sign. Eur Radiol 2001;11:409–411

CASE 95 Traumatic Rupture Left Hemidiaphragm

Clinical Presentation

An unrestrained driver involved in a serious motor vehicle collision had diminished breath sounds on the left and an unstable pelvic fracture.

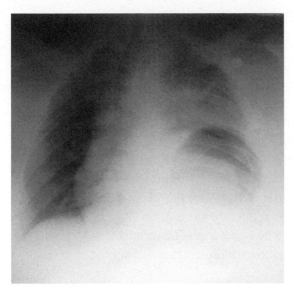

Figure 95A

Radiologic Findings

AP chest radiograph (**Fig. 95A**) demonstrates marked rightward mediastinal shift. A large hyperlucent "bubble" occupies the mid- and lower left thorax. The nasogastric tube follows an anomalous broad U-shaped course into the stomach. Numerous left rib fractures and a left apical pleural cap are present.

Diagnosis

Traumatic rupture of the left hemidiaphragm

Differential Diagnosis

• Eventration or elevation of the diaphragm
• Diaphragmatic paralysis

Discussion

Background

Diaphragmatic injuries occur in 0.8 to 8.0% of blunt trauma victims. More injuries are diagnosed on the left (77–90%) as compared to the right side. Most tears are radial, more than 10 cm in length, and posterolateral. Approximately 15% of stab wounds and 45% of gunshot wounds to the lower chest are complicated by diaphragmatic injuries. Diaphragmatic injuries should be suspected in any

383

penetrating trauma victim with wounds below the 4th anterior, the 6th lateral, and the 8th posterior intercostal spaces.

Etiology

A sudden increase in intrathoracic or intraabdominal pressure against a fixed diaphragm accounts for most blunt diaphragmatic injuries. Other postulated mechanisms of injury include shearing stress on a stretched diaphragm and avulsion of the diaphragm from its points of attachment.

Clinical Findings

An acute diaphragmatic injury should be considered in patients who sustain significant thoracoabdominal trauma and present with dyspnea or respiratory distress. Because of the very high incidence of associated injuries (e.g., lacerations of the liver (16%) and/or spleen (48%)), hypovolemic shock is not uncommon. Additional associated injuries include rib fractures (52%), pelvic fractures (52%), and closed head injuries (32%). Left-sided diaphragmatic injuries are associated with herniation of subdiaphragmatic viscera into the chest. The stomach and colon are the most common organs to herniate into the thorax. Three fourths of patients have herniation of other intraabdominal organs (e.g., omentum, spleen, kidney, and pancreas). Acute herniation may be associated with life-threatening tension effects on ventilation. Delayed herniation may be complicated by bowel strangulation. Splenosis may manifest as imaging abnormalities decades later and should not be confused with malignant disease.

Pathology

- Roughly equal incidence of left-sided and right-sided injuries at autopsy
- Tears usually located in the posterolateral diaphragm
- Radial orientation
- Often large, more than 10 cm
- Associated hematoma and/or contusion

Imaging Findings

CHEST RADIOGRAPHY

- May appear normal initially
- Elevated asymmetric, poorly visualized, or irregular-appearing diaphragm (**Figs. 95A** and **95B**)
- Herniation of bowel or abdominal organs into the thorax (**Figs. 95A** and **95B**)
- Abnormal U-shaped course of the nasogastric tube (**Figs. 95A** and **95B**)
- Contralateral mediastinal shift in the absence of a pneumothorax or large effusion (**Figs. 95A** and **95B**)
- Persistent contralateral mediastinal shift despite the presence of a thoracostomy tube (**Fig. 95B**)
- Skeletal thoracic trauma (e.g., rib fractures) (**Figs. 95A** and **95B**)

ULTRASONOGRAPHY

- Permits direct visualization of the hemidiaphragm
- Focal disruption or interruption of diaphragmatic echoes at the site of injury
- More useful in evaluation of the right hemidiaphragm
- Stomach/colon gas limits evaluation of the left hemidiaphragm.

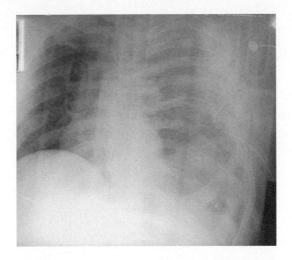

Figure 95B AP chest radiograph of a 50-year-old motor vehicle accident victim with a left diaphragmatic rupture shows complete left hemithorax opacification, a poorly defined left diaphragm, marked rightward mediastinal shift despite a left chest tube, and a flail left thorax. The nasogastric tube follows an anomalous broad U-shaped course. Intrathoracic herniation of the stomach, spleen, and pancreatic tail was found intraoperatively.

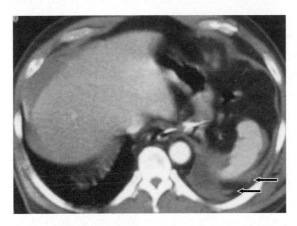

Figure 95C Contrast-enhanced chest CT (mediastinal window) of a blunt trauma victim reveals an abrupt discontinuity of the left posterolateral diaphragm (arrows). Note the perisplenic hematoma and free fluid about the liver. Primary repair of the diaphragmatic tear was subsequently performed via open laparotomy.

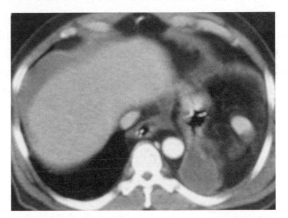

Figure 95D Contrast-enhanced chest CT (mediastinal window) of a 64-year-old man involved in a motor vehicle collision shows hemoperitoneum about the liver edge, as well as herniation of the stomach into the chest through the ruptured diaphragm (CT collar sign). (From Parker MS, Matheson TL, Rao AV, et al. Etiology of the widened mediastinum: blunt thoracic trauma. *The Radiologist* 2001;8(1):23–32, with permission.)

CT (SENSITIVITY 50–100%; SPECIFICITY 86–100%)

- Use of single breath hold and thin collimation (3 mm) with reconstructions every 2 mm and sagittal and coronal reformations and maximum intensity projection (MIP) images to aid in the diagnosis
- Left hemidiaphragmatic injuries
    - Abrupt discontinuity of the diaphragm (73–82%) with or without herniation of the stomach or other viscera into the thorax (**Fig. 95C**)
    - "Absent diaphragm" sign (i.e., nonvisualization of diaphragm in an area where it does not contact another organ and should otherwise be seen)
    - "Collar" sign (i.e., focal constriction of herniated viscera, stomach, or bowel) (**Fig. 95D**)
    - Visualization of peritoneal fat, bowel, or viscera lateral to the lung or diaphragm or posterior to the diaphragmatic crus

- Right hemidiaphragmatic injuries
  - Focal indentation of the liver
  - Mushroom-like mass in the right hemithorax where herniated liver is constricted by the tear
- Additional findings
  - Diaphragmatic thickening is highly suggestive of blunt diaphragmatic rupture in the absence of retroperitoneal contusion, but does not distinguish between injury requiring surgical repair and partial-thickness diaphragmatic rupture.
  - Concomitant injuries of the liver and/or spleen
  - Rib fractures
  - Pelvic fractures
  - Active arterial extravasation of contrast material at level of the diaphragm

MR

- Primary role in nonacute or difficult cases
- Utility of coronal and sagittal T1-weighted images to trace the course of the diaphragm from its insertions to the dome
- Helpful in differentiating traumatic injuries from eventration or simple elevation
- Coronal T1-weighted images for optimal visualization of low tears involving the crus
- Identification of normal diaphragm as a decreased signal intensity (SI) band outlined by higher signal intensity abdominal and mediastinal fat on the left, and the liver on the right

Treatment

- General supportive measures
- Most injuries can be repaired primarily.
- Posterolateral injury of the right hemidiaphragm
  - Injury best approached through the chest because the liver obscures the abdominal approach.
- Centrally located injuries
  - Most easily repaired
- Lateral injuries near the chest wall
  - May require reattachment of the diaphragm to the chest wall by encirclement of the ribs with suture during the repair
- Laparoscopy as an alternative to open repair of small traumatic diaphragmatic lacerations
- Open laparotomy for large (> 10 cm) tears adjacent to or including the esophageal hiatus
- Synthetic mesh (e.g., polypropylene, Dacron) is occasionally needed to repair large defects.

Prognosis

- Overall mortality of approximately 34% secondary to delayed herniation of abdominal viscera, bowel strangulation, and associated abdominal and thoracic injuries

PEARLS_____

- Diaphragmatic injuries may not be appreciated if patients are intubated, as positive pressure ventilation may prevent herniation of abdominal contents until weaning.
- Associated atelectasis or pleural effusions may obscure or mimic diaphragmatic tears.
- Normal discontinuities in the posterior diaphragm are seen in 6 to 11% of nontrauma patients (i.e., congenital Bochdalek defects) and in up to 35% of elderly patients.

Suggested Readings

Iochum S, Ludig T, Walter F, Sebbag H, Grosdidier G, Blum AG. Imaging of diaphragmatic injury: a diagnostic challenge? Radiographics 2002;22:S103–S118

Karmy-Jones R, Carter Y, Stern E. The impact of positive pressure ventilation on the diagnosis of traumatic diaphragmatic injury. Am Surg 2002;68:167–172

Killeen KL, Shanmuganathan K, Mirvis SE. Imaging of traumatic diaphragmatic injuries. Semin Ultrasound CT MR 2002;23:184–192

Larici AR, Gotway MB, Litt HI, et al. Helical CT with sagittal and coronal reconstructions: accuracy for detection of diaphragmatic injury. AJR Am J Roentgenol 2002;179:451–457

Shanmuganathan K, Killeen K, Mirvis SE, White CS. Imaging of diaphragmatic injuries. J Thorac Imaging 2000;15:104–111

CASE 96 Isolated Sternal Fracture

Clinical Presentation

A 59-year-old man who was wearing a seat belt rear-ended a stationary tractor-trailer at 35 mph and complains of localized pain and tenderness over the midchest.

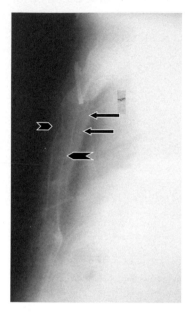

Figure 96A

Radiologic Findings

Lateral sternal radiograph (**Fig. 96A**) reveals a displaced sternal fracture (arrowheads) approximately 4 cm below the sternomanubrial joint. Retrosternal hematoma and fat create the opacity behind the sternum (arrows). AP chest radiograph (not illustrated) was grossly unremarkable.

Diagnosis

Isolated sternal fracture

Differential Diagnosis

None

Discussion

Background

Sternal fractures occur in approximately 3% of patients injured in motor vehicle collisions. The prevalence is higher in restrained front-seat occupants involved in frontal collisions, and the frequency increases with age.

Etiology

The majority of sternal fractures are caused by motor vehicle collisions. The upper and middle thirds of the sternum are most commonly affected. Most fractures occur within 2 cm of the manubrial-sternal junction.

Clinical Findings

Patients with sternal fractures complain of localized inspiratory pain around the injured area or dyspnea. Physical examination reveals local tenderness, swelling, and ecchymosis over the injury. A palpable defect or fracture-related crepitus may also be present. Associated injuries occur in 55 to 70% of patients with sternal fractures. The most common associated injuries are rib fractures, long bone fractures, and closed head injuries.

Simple isolated fractures are usually benign and unassociated with myocardial contusion. Depressed, segmental, and manubrial fractures are often associated with myocardial contusion-laceration, hemopericardium, great vessel injuries, thoracic spine and rib fractures, and head trauma. The latter patients often require further evaluation with ECG, cardiac enzymes, and multiple gated acquistion (MUGA) nuclear scintigraphy.

Imaging Findings

RADIOGRAPHY

- Usually not evident on frontal chest radiographs
- May demonstrate mediastinal widening
- May be difficult to appreciate on oblique sternal radiographs
- Usually well delineated on lateral chest or dedicated lateral sternal radiographs (**Fig. 96A**)

ULTRASOUND

- Utility as a diagnostic and triage tool in patients with complicated sternal fractures associated with other injuries
- Superior to lateral radiography for diagnosing sternal fractures but not as accurate in the assessment of degree of fracture fragment displacement
- Hematoma; hypoechoic area over the sternum
- Disruption of cortical bone or a step in the bone outline
- Identification of fragment dislocation

CT

- Direct fracture visualization and assessment of degree of displacement; optimal with MPR and MIP sagital reformations allow for optimal direct fracture visualization and the degree of displacement (**Fig. 96B**)
- Indirect evidence of fracture: soft tissue, parasternal, or retrosternal hematoma (**Fig. 96C**)
- Preservation of fat plane between hematoma and aorta; suggests that hematoma is not related to aortic or great vessel injury

Treatment

- Rest and pain control with analgesics for isolated sternal fractures
- Minimize activities involving use of pectoral and shoulder girdle muscles
- Surgical stabilization for displaced or unstable sternal fractures
  - Open reduction and internal fixation
  - Wire suturing and placement of plates and screws

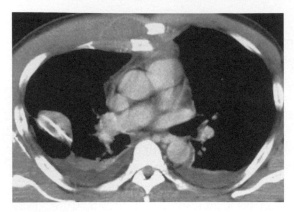

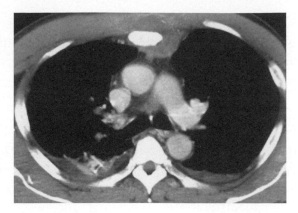

Figure 96B Contrast-enhanced chest CT (mediastinal window) shows a depressed sternal fracture. Notice its proximity to the mediastinal great vessels, the large retrosternal and chest wall hematomas, and bilateral effusions.

Figure 96C Contrast-enhanced chest CT (mediastinal window) reveals an eccentric retro- and parasternal hematoma. A fracture was not identified.

Prognosis

- Good outcome for patients with isolated sternal fractures and a normal ECG

PEARL

- Patients with complex sternal fracture require careful evaluation for associated flexion spine injuries

Suggested Readings

Engin G, Yekeler E, Guloglu R, Acunas B, Acunas G. US versus conventional radiography in the diagnosis of sternal fractures. Acta Radiol 2000;41:296–299

Hills MW, Delprado AM, Deane SA. Sternal fractures: associated injuries and management. J Trauma 1993;35:55–60

Parker MS, Matheson TL, Rao AV, et al. Spiral CT in blunt thoracic trauma: detection of "unsuspected" concomitant injuries. The Radiologist 2000;7:137–146

Rashid MA, Ortenwall P, Wikstrom T. Cardiovascular injuries associated with sternal fractures. Eur J Surg 2001;167:243–248

Wiener Y, Achildiev B, Karni T, Halevi A. Echocardiogram in sternal fracture. Am J Emerg Med 2001; 19:403–405

CASE 97 Posterior Clavicular Head Dislocation

Clinical Presentation

A 15-year-old fell off his dirt bike while attempting to jump over an embankment.

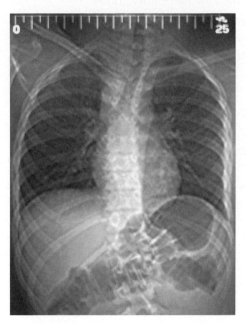

Figure 97A

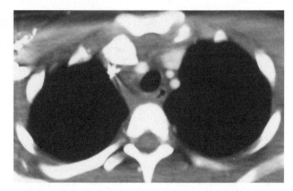

Figure 97B

Radiologic Findings

Frontal chest CT scout (**Fig. 97A**) shows asymmetric alignment of the clavicles; the right clavicle lies lower than the left. A right paratracheal opacity is also present. Contrast-enhanced chest CT (**Fig. 97B**) (mediastinal window) reveals posterior displacement of the right clavicular head at the sternoclavicular joint with the medial edge abutting the brachiocephalic artery. Note the right paratracheal hematoma.

Diagnosis

Posterior dislocation of the right sternoclavicular joint

Differential Diagnosis

None

Discussion

Background

Posterior sternoclavicular subluxations and dislocations are relatively rare, representing approximately 1% of all orthopedic dislocations. Such dislocations can be difficult to diagnose clinically and on radiography.

391

Etiology

Strong lateral compressive forces against the shoulder cause dislocation of the sternoclavicular joint.

Clinical Findings

Anterior dislocation of the sternoclavicular joint is more common than posterior dislocation. Anterior dislocations are easily diagnosed on physical examination by noting a palpable focal mass at the site of injury. Posterior dislocations are a more difficult clinical challenge. Occassionally, an indentation may be noted adjacent to the sternum. Patients with sternoclavicular dislocations often complain of pain with arm motion or when a compressive force is applied against their shoulder. Posterior sternoclavicular joint dislocations must be recognized and treated as soon as possible. Although some patients may be asymptomatic, others may complain of pain around the clavicle, have symptoms related to aerodigestive tract compression, exhibit hypotension, or experience brachial plexopathy. Unrecognized dislocations may lead to severe life- or limb-threatening injuries resulting from concomitant injury to the trachea, esophagus, pleura (e.g., pneumothorax), great vessels, and brachial plexus.

Imaging Findings

RADIOGRAPHY

- Limited role
- Patient must be neutrally positioned.
- Apparent asymmetry in clavicular head height (**Fig. 97A**)
- Lateral displacement of the proximal end of the clavicle (**Fig. 97A**)

CT

- Imaging modality of choice
- Retrosternal dislocation readily appreciated (**Fig. 97B**)
- Perijoint space and/or mediastinal hematoma (**Fig. 97B**)
- Pneumomediastinum and/or pneumothorax may be present
- Exclusion of associated injuries

Treatment

- Anterior dislocation
  - Manual reduction with local anesthesia and sedatives; affected arm is abducted and extended while lateral traction is applied to the extremity; direct pressure is exerted over the medial clavicle
- Posterior dislocation
  - Pain control, possibly including general anesthesia
  - Open reduction and surgical stabilization if closed reduction fails
- Treatment of concomitant injuries

Prognosis

- Significant morbidity and mortality secondary to concomitant aerodigestive tract and great vessel injuries

Suggested Readings

Ferrera PC, Wheeling HM. Sternoclavicular joint injuries. Am J Emerg Med 2000;18:58–61

McCulloch P, Henley BM, Linnau KF. Radiographic clues for high-energy trauma: three cases of sternoclavicular dislocation. AJR Am J Roentgenol 2001;176:1534

Parker MS, Matheson TL, Rao AV, et al. Spiral CT in blunt thoracic trauma: detection of "unsuspected" concomitant injuries. The Radiologist 2000;7:137–146

Rajaratnam S, Kermis M, Apthorp L. Posterior dislocation of the sternoclavicular joint: a case report and review of the clinical anatomy of the region. Clin Anat 2002;15:108–111

CASE 98 Bilateral Flail Chest

Clinical Presentation

A 40-year-old man involved in a motor vehicle collision, ejected from the vehicle, and in unstable condition

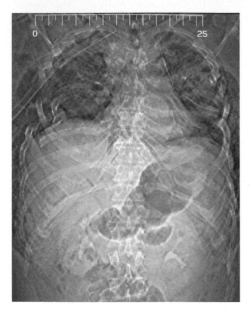

Figure 98A

Radiologic Findings

Frontal chest CT scout (**Fig. 98A**) shows multiple bilateral displaced rib fractures, many with marked angulation. The mediastinum is widened with poor definition of normal lines, stripes, and interfaces. Extensive subcutaneous air is present.

Diagnosis

Bilateral flail chest with acute traumatic aortic injury (ATAI) (latter not illustrated)

Differential Diagnosis

None

Discussion

Background

Flail chest is the most serious blunt chest wall injury. It is present when there are five or more contiguous rib fractures, or three or more ribs fractured in two or more locations. These fractures create an abnormally mobile, free floating, unstable segment of the chest wall that moves paradoxically during the respiratory cycle. That is, the chest wall moves inward with inspiration, and outward with expiration. The traumatic separation of the ribs from their costochondral cartilages may also result in a flail segment. Associated intrathoracic injuries include pulmonary contusion (46%) and pneumothorax or hemothorax, or both (70%). The incidence of great vessel, tracheobronchial, and diaphragmatic injuries is not greater than that of trauma patients without flail chest.

Etiology

Traumatic flail chest results from severe sudden anteroposterior compression of the thorax and is most often a complication of high-speed motor vehicle collisions and blast or crushing injuries.

Clinical Findings

The majority of patients with flail chest complain of severe pain, shortness of breath, and require prolonged ventilator support. Respiratory failure results primarily from underlying lung injury (e.g., pulmonary contusion and/or laceration); however, pendelluft (i.e., contralateral movement of dead space gas from the flail to the nonflail side) may contribute in some cases. Twenty-seven percent of patients with flail chest develop acute respiratory distress syndrome (ARDS).

Imaging Findings

- Multiple contiguous rib fractures with marked fracture fragment angulation (**Fig. 98A**)
- Pneumothorax/hemothorax/hemopneumothorax
- Pulmonary laceration and/or atelectasis
- Subcutaneous and/or mediastinal air (**Fig. 98A**)

Treatment

- Pain control
  - Oral and/or parenteral analgesics
  - Epidural analgesics
  - Intercostal nerve blocks
- Operative chest wall stabilization (e.g., external fixation devices; pins and/or plates for internal fixation) for improvement of gas exchange and early extubation in patients with flail chest and respiratory insufficiency without pulmonary contusion
- Supportive care for patients with flail chest and pulmonary contusion; no benefit from chest wall stabilization

Prognosis

- Morbidity and mortality range from 3 to 60%; depend on the extent of intrathoracic injury, extent of associated nonthoracic injuries, and the patient's age.

PEARL_____

- Flail chest wall injuries may be clinically unrecognized if the affected segment is "fixed" in place by a large chest wall hematoma.

Suggested Readings

Ciraulo DL, Elliott D, Mitchell KA, Rodriquez A. Flail chest as a marker for significant injuries. J Am Coll Surg 1994;178:466–470

Lardinois D, Krueger T, Dusmet M, Ghisletta N, Gugger M, Ris HB. Pulmonary function testing after operative stabilization of the chest wall for flail chest. Eur J Cardiothorac Surg 2001;20:496–501

Voggenreiter G, Neudeck F, Aufmkolk M, Obertacke U, Schmit-Neuerburg KP. Operative chest wall stabilization in flail chest—outcomes of patients with or without pulmonary contusion. J Am Coll Surg 1998;187:130–138

Weyant MJ, Bleier JI, Naama H, et al. Severe crushed chest injury with large flail segment: computed tomographic three-dimensional reconstruction. J Trauma 2002;52:605

CASE 99 Vertebral Compression Fracture

Clinical Presentation

A 38-year-old restrained driver involved in a motor vehicle collision

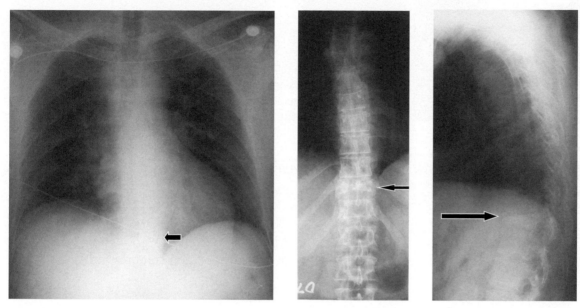

Figure 99A **Figure 99B** **Figure 99C**

Radiologic Findings

AP chest radiograph (**Fig. 99A**) shows a subtle bulge in the left paraspinal line (short arrow). This prompted acquiring dedicated AP (**Fig. 99B**) and lateral (**Fig. 99C**) thoracic spine radiographs showing marked compression deformity of T11 (long arrow).

Diagnosis

Acute compression fracture of T11 vertebral body with paraspinal hematoma

Differential Diagnosis

None

Discussion

Background

Compression fractures are the most common injury (52%) in the thoracic spine. Thoracic spine fractures occur in 3% of blunt chest trauma victims and account for 16 to 30% of all spine fractures. Most fractures involve the "functional" thoracolumbar spine (i.e., T9–T11). These spinal fractures

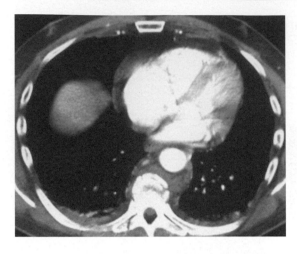

Figure 99D Contrast-enhanced chest CT (mediastinal window) of a 60-year-old man thrown through the windshield during a motor vehicle collision shows a paravertebral-posterior mediastinal hematoma and compression fracture at T9. Similar findings were present at T7 and T8 (not illustrated).

are often radiographically occult; only 51% of thoracic spine fractures are identified on initial chest radiography.

Etiology

Thoracic spine vertebral compression fractures typically result from hyperflexion and compression injuries of the chest.

Clinical Findings

Fracture-dislocation injuries of the thoracic spine are frequently clinically devastating. The prevalence of neurologic deficits in patients with thoracic spine fractures is as high as 62%, far greater than those occurring with injuries to the cervical spine (32%) or the lumbar spine (2%). Chylothorax may rarely complicate thoracic spine fracture-dislocations. Only 12% of patients with fracture-dislocations of the thoracic spine are neurologically intact at presentation; 62% of patients have "complete" neurologic deficits, and over 20% have multilevel injuries. These injuries may be noncontiguous in up to 27% of cases.

Imaging Findings

RADIOGRAPHY

- Mediastinal widening and/or widening of the paraspinal lines (**Figs. 99A** and **99B**)
- Left apical pleural cap
- Deviation of the nasogastric tube
- Loss of vertebral body height and/or poor definition of pedicle(s) (**Figs. 99B** and **99C**)

CT

- Paraspinal hematoma (**Fig. 99D**)
- Mediastinal hematoma confined to the paravertebral compartment (**Fig. 99D**)
- Spinous process, transverse process, pedicle, or vertebral body fractures (**Fig. 99D**)
- Use of reformatted coronal and sagittal images, lateral CT scout, maximum intensity projection (MIP) images to aid in diagnosis
- Dedicated thoracic spine CT performed to assess for retropulsion
- Pneumorachis
- Thoracic spine MR for further evaluation as clinically indicated

Treatment

- Early surgical stabilization and fixation (within 3 days of injury) in patients with thoracic spine fractures to allow earlier mobilization and reduces the incidence of pneumonia
- Conservative management of associated traumatic chylothorax for at least 4 weeks before surgical intervention is considered

Prognosis

- "Complete" neurologic deficits in up to two thirds of patients

PEARLS_____

- As chest CT often reveals unsuspected fracture-dislocations of the thoracic spine, it is imperative to inspect the skeleton and soft tissues of all blunt chest trauma victims undergoing CT imaging.
- Sternal fractures are often associated with thoracic spine fractures.

Suggested Readings

Croce MA, Bee TK, Pritchard E, Miller PR, Fabian TC. Does optimal timing for spine fracture fixation exist? Ann Surg 2001;233:851–858

Holmes JF, Miller PQ, Panacek EA, Lin S. Horne NS, Mower WR. Epidemiology of thoracolumbar spine injury in blunt trauma. Acad Emerg Med 2001;8:866–872

Ikonomidis JS, Boulanger BR, Brenneman FD. Chylothorax after blunt chest trauma: a report of 2 cases. Can J Surg 1997;40:135–138

Parker MS, Matheson TL, Rao AV, et al. Spiral CT in blunt thoracic trauma: detection of "unsuspected" concomitant injuries. The Radiologist 2000;7:137–146

Robertson A, Branfoot T, Barlow IF, Giannoudis PV. Spine injury patterns resulting from car and motorcycle accidents. Spine 2002;27:2825–2830

CASE 100 ARPS: Ventilator-induced Barotrauma

Clinical Presentation

A 51-year-old woman with acute respiratory distress syndrome (ARDS) and progressive hypoxemia

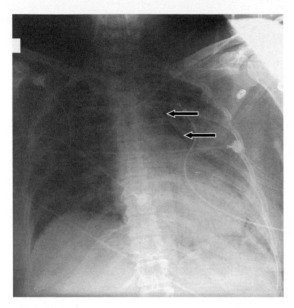

Figure 100A

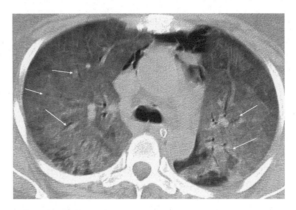

Figure 100B

Radiologic Findings

AP chest radiograph (**Fig. 100A**) shows bilateral perihilar ground-glass opacities consistent with ARDS. Pneumomediastinum parallels the left heart border (arrows). Subtle spherical and tubular lucencies parallel the bronchovascular bundles in a right perihilar and left upper lobe distribution. Contrast-enhanced chest CT (**Fig. 100B**) (lung window) reveals diffuse ground-glass opacities, pneumomediastinum, interlobular air, and subtle perivascular air (long arrows).

Diagnosis

ARDS with ventilator-induced barotrauma

Differential Diagnosis

None

Discussion

Background

Barotrauma is a sequela of ventilator-induced lung injury. The spectrum of injuries includes pulmonary interstitial air, pneumomediastinum, subcutaneous air, pneumoretroperitoneum, and

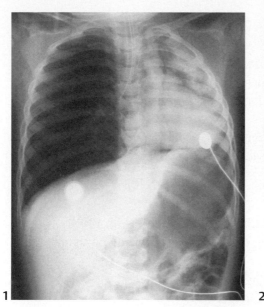 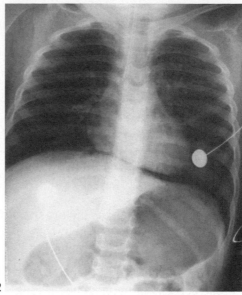

Figure 100C (1) AP chest radiograph of a pediatric burn victim shows right mainstem bronchus intubation, left lower lobe collapse, and pneumomediastinum. **(2)** Follow-up AP chest radiograph again reveals a low-lying endotracheal (ET) tube. Note the "continuous diaphragm" sign reflecting barotrauma-induced lung injury and pneumomediastinum from delivery of excess tidal volume to the right lung. The left lower lobe has reexpanded.

spontaneous pneumothorax. It is estimated that barotrauma affects 10 to 65% of all patients requiring mechanical ventilation. High-risk patients include those with chronic obstructive lung disease and ARDS.

Etiology

Inappropriate gas delivery for the available lung volume results in alveolar overdistention and rupture (e.g., high peak pressures, mainstem bronchial intubations) (**Figs. 100C** and **100D**). Compression of a thorax filled with a volume of gas that exceeds its new thoracic volume (e.g., crushing injury to the chest, a concussive wave from a closed-space explosion) is another potential cause of barotrauma.

Clinical Findings

Excessive tidal volume and/or end-inspiratory lung volume is the main determinant of ventilator-induced lung injury. Clinical signs of ventilator-induced barotrauma include agitation, tachypnea, hypoxemia, and either high-pressure or high-tidal volume alarm. Patients with barotrauma may develop potentially life-threatening tension pneumothorax

Pathology

- Rupture of alveoli with dissection of gas along the interlobular septa and perivascular bundles (i.e., pulmonary interstitial air)
- Interstitial air rupture into the mediastinum (i.e., pneumomediastinum) and/or the pleural cavity (i.e., pneumothorax)

Imaging Findings

RADIOGRAPHY

- Hyperinflated lungs (lung length $\geq$ 24.7 cm; 6th anterior rib intersection with the diaphragm)
- Spherical and/or tubular lucencies paralleling the bronchovascular bundles (**Fig. 100A**)
- Large juxtapleural cysts without definable walls, along the mediastinal and diaphragmatic borders, compressing the adjacent lung
- Concomitant pneumothorax, pneumomediastinum ("continuous diaphragm" sign), subcutaneous air, pneumoretroperitoneum, and/or rarely pneumopericardium (**Fig. 100C**)

CT

- Hyperinflated lungs
- Spherical and/or tubular lucencies paralleling the bronchovascular bundles (**Fig. 100B**)
- Large juxtapleural cysts without definable walls, along the mediastinal and diaphragmatic borders, compressing the adjacent lung
- Perivascular air and/or air within interlobular septa (**Fig. 100B**)
- Air cysts and bronchiectasis in nondependent lung
- Pneumomediastinum (**Fig. 100B**)
- Pneumothorax
- Subcutaneous air

Treatment

- Medical: sedation to reduce agitation, bronchodilation to reduce airway resistance, diuretics to eliminate extravascular lung fluid, and clearing secretions
- Surgical: may entail placement of one or more chest tubes
- Perfluorocarbon (PFC) partial liquid ventilation may reduce ventilator-induced lung injury and may have a greater clinical role in the future.
- Prone ventilation in select patients

Prognosis

- Morbidity and mortality rates for patients with ARDS are approximately 40 to 50%. The rates associated with barotrauma depend on the form it takes (i.e., no increased rate with subcutaneous air vs 100% mortality rate for unrecognized tension pneumothorax).

Suggested Readings

Eisner MD, Thompson BT, Schoenfeld D, Anzueto A, Matthay MA. Airways pressures and early barotrauma in patients with acute lung injury and acute respiratory distress syndrome. Am J Respir Crit Care Med 2002;165:978–982

Johnson MM, Ely EW, Chiles C, et al. Radiographic assessment of hyperinflation: correlation with objective chest radiographic measurements and mechanical ventilator parameters. Chest 1998;113:1698–1704

Ricard JD, Lemaire F. Liquid ventilation. Curr Opin Crit Care 2001;7:8–14

Treggiari MM, Romand JA, Martin JB, Sutter PM. Air cysts and bronchiectasis prevail in nondependent areas in severe acute respiratory distress syndrome: a computed tomographic study of ventilator-associated changes. Crit Care Med 2002;30:1747–1752

SECTION VIII

Life Support Tubes, Lines, and Monitoring Devices

CASE 101 Esophageal Intubation

Clinical Presentation

A young man involved in a motor vehicle collision had a prolonged extrication, was intubated in the field, but did not respond to resuscitation efforts.

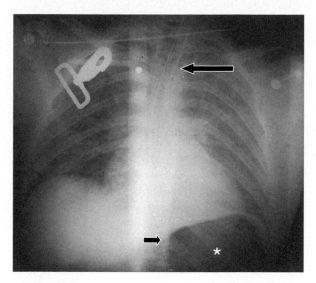

Figure 101A

Radiologic Findings

AP chest radiograph (**Fig. 101A**) shows a nasogastric tube coursing to the stomach. The side port terminates above the esophagogastric junction (short arrow). Note the marked gastric distention (*). The endotracheal tube (long arrows) parallels the course of the nasogastric tube and does not overlie the tracheal air column.

Diagnosis

Esophageal intubation

Differential Diagnosis

None

Discussion

Background

Esophageal intubation complicates approximately 8% of attempted endotracheal intubations in critically ill patients. The incidence is as high as 67% when intubation is performed in the field under less than optimal conditions, as confirming successful placement can be difficult.

405

Clinical Findings

Physical examination is often unreliable in confirming appropriate endotracheal tube placement. Direct visualization of the vocal cords can be limited by inadequate lighting, the presence of blood and vomitus, and altered anatomy secondary to trauma. Auscultation can be difficult in noisy environments, and transmitted breath sounds can be misleading. Fogging of the endotracheal tube may be observed in over 50% of esophageal intubations. Capnographic determination of end-tidal CO_2 ($E_T CO_2$) levels via a colorimetric device is becoming a standard of care in prehospital and emergency settings, but can be unreliable in the settings of cardiac arrest, ongoing cardiopulmonary resuscitation, and low cardiac output states, all of which are characterized by low expired CO_2 concentrations. An esophageal detector device is also gaining popularity. Appropriate endotracheal tube placement requires radiographic confirmation in all cases.

Imaging Findings

- Borders of the endotracheal tube visualized lateral to the tracheal air column (**Fig. 101A**)
- Gaseous distention of the distal esophagus or stomach (**Fig. 101A**)
- Tracheal deviation by an overinflated endotracheal balloon cuff

Treatment

- Prompt correction of tube position

Prognosis

- Good if recognized and rapidly corrected
- Anoxic brain injury when unrecognized

PEARL_____

- Because the trachea and esophagus are often superimposed in the AP plane, radiographic recognition of esophageal intubation can sometimes be difficult. Right posterior oblique chest radiographs and cross-table lateral soft tissue neck radiographs can be helpful in problematic cases.

Suggested Readings

Coontz DA, Gratton M. Endotracheal rules of engagement: how to reduce the incidence of unrecognized esophageal intubations. JEMS 2002;27:44–50, 52–54, 56–59

Gremec S. Comparison of three different methods to confirm tracheal tube placement in emergency intubation. Intensive Care Med 2002;28:701–704

Katz SH, Falk JL. Misplaced endotracheal tube by paramedics in an urban medical services system. Ann Emerg Med 2001;37:32–37

Maleck WH. Distinguishing endotracheal and esophageal intubation. Anesthesiology 2001;94: 539–540

CASE 102 Right Mainstem Bronchus Intubation

Clinical Presentation

A young boy struck by a car had initial endotracheal tube placement complicated by esophageal intubation.

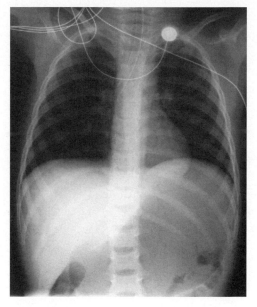

Figure 102A

Radiologic Findings

AP chest radiograph (**Fig. 102A**) was obtained following repositioning of the endotracheal tube. The ET tube courses down the right mainstem bronchus and needs to be retracted 4 to 5 cm. Notice the gastric distention from the preceding esophageal intubation.

Diagnosis

Right mainstem bronchus intubation

Differential Diagnosis

None

Discussion

Background

In children under 12 years of age, the right and left mainstem bronchi come off the trachea at approximately the same angle, and neither bronchus is more prone to inadvertent intubation. In adults, the right mainstem bronchus comes off at a 25-degree angle, whereas the left mainstem bronchus comes off at a 45-degree angle. Thus, the right mainstem bronchus is more prone to inadvertent intubation in adults. Approximately 15% of initial ET tube placements are incorrect. The incidence of mainstem

407

bronchial intubation is even higher when patients are intubated in the field. Women also have a greater risk for suboptimal ET tube placement following emergent intubation.

Clinical Findings

Confirmation of successful ET tube placement by physical exam alone is unreliable. Auscultation can reveal equal breath sounds in up to 60% of right mainstem bronchial intubations.

Imaging Findings

- Endotracheal tube within bronchial lumen (**Fig. 102A**)
- Overinflation of affected hemithorax
- Resorption atelectasis of contralateral hemithorax
- Manifestations of barotrauma may be visualized.
- Optimal ET tube tip position
  - Tip 5.0 ± 2.0 cm above the carina with head in neutral position; chin position and vertebral body attitude used as clues to determine head position
  - ET tube descent of up to 2.0 cm with head and neck flexion, ascent of up to 2.0 cm with head and neck extension, migration of 1.0 cm with head and neck rotation
  - Optimal ET tube width of one half to two thirds the width of the tracheal lumen

Treatment

- Prompt correction of tube position

Prognosis

- Contralateral atelectasis, ipsilateral barotrauma, and spontaneous pneumothorax when uncorrected
- Right upper lobe collapse with ET tube extension into bronchus intermedius

Suggested Readings

Schwartz DE, Lieberman JA, Cohen NH. Women are at a greater risk than men for malpositioning of the endotracheal tube following emergent intubation. Crit Care Med 1995;23:1306–1308

Tocino I. Chest imaging in the intensive care unit. Eur J Radiol 1996;23:46–57

CASE 103 Malpositioned Endotracheal Tube and Cuff Overinflation

Clinical Presentation

A young woman involved in a motor vehicle collision several days earlier had recent repositioning of endotracheal (ET) tube.

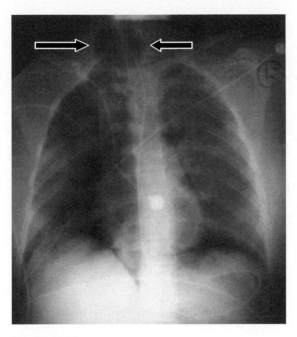

Figure 103A

Radiologic Findings

AP chest radiograph (**Fig. 103A**) demonstrates a high-riding ET tube and gross overinflation of the balloon cuff (arrows). The lower margin of the cuff is 1.5 cm from the tip of the ET tube. Note the pneumomediastinum and subcutaneous air not present on radiographs obtained before the ET tube manipulation.

Diagnosis

Malpositioned ET tube and overinflated balloon cuff complicated by tracheal laceration and pneumomediastinum

Differential Diagnosis

None

Discussion

Background

Malpositioned ET tubes may injure the airway. Injuries to the larynx, hypopharynx, trachea, and pyriform sinuses may follow traumatic intubations, high-riding ET tube placements, and balloon cuff overinflation.

Clinical Findings

Traumatic airway intubations may result in pneumomediastinum, spontaneous pneumothorax, and subcutaneous air. The latter may be recognized by crepitus along the neck, axilla, and anterior chest wall.

Imaging Findings

- High ET tube position (**Fig. 103A**)
- The ET balloon cuff should never distend the tracheal lumen (**Fig. 103A**).
- Inflation of the cuff > 2.8 cm is abnormal (normal 2.0–2.5 cm) (**Fig. 103A**).
- Lower margin of the cuff < 1.3 cm from the tube tip (normal distance 2.5 cm)
- Pneumothorax may be present
- Pneumomediastinum may be identified
- Subcutaneous air may be visualized (**Fig. 103A**)

Treatment

- Maintain the airway.
- Airway injury may be self-limited or may require surgical repair.

Prognosis

- Dependent on the extent of the airway injury and its early recognition

PEARLS_____

- If one encounters resistance during inflation of the balloon cuff, the location of the ET tube should be reassessed.
- High-riding ET tubes are more prone to inadvertent extubation and may damage the vocal cords.
- Persistent overinflation of the balloon cuff may result in mucosal ischemia and necrosis and potential perforation or stricture formation. (e.g., tracheal stenosis, tracheomalacia) (see Case 16)

Suggested Reading

Tocino I. Chest imaging in the intensive care unit. Eur J Radiol 1996;23:46–57

CASE 104 Complications of Tracheostomy Tube Placement

Clinical Presentation

A 73-year-old man recently diagnosed with head and neck carcinoma had a recent tracheostomy, and continues to ooze blood from his stoma.

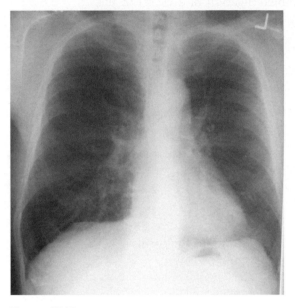

Figure 104A

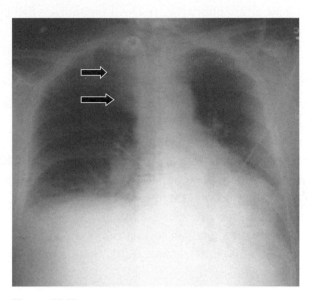

Figure 104B

Radiologic Findings

Preoperative PA chest radiograph (**Fig. 104A**) reveals underlying obstructive lung disease, but a normal-appearing mediastinum. First postoperative AP portable chest radiograph (**Fig. 104B**) shows a large eccentric right-sided superior mediastinal mass (arrows) and bibasilar airspace disease. The tracheostomy device is slightly rotated.

Diagnosis

Superior mediastinal hematoma complicating tracheostomy placement and bibasilar aspiration of blood

Differential Diagnosis

None

Discussion

Background

Portable chest radiographs are obtained following tracheostomy tube placement to assess for tube position and possible procedure-related complications. The latter include pneumothorax (1–2%), pneumomediastinum (Hamman's disease), mediastinal hematoma, subcutaneous air, aspiration secondary to aspirated blood, and tracheoesophageal fistula (see Case 19).

411

Clinical Findings

Bleeding may complicate tracheostomy tube placement by either percutaneous or open techniques. Minor bleeding occurs in 3 to 20% of percutaneous tracheostomy tube placements, and in 1 to 80% of open procedures. A small amount of bleeding may occur from the tracheostomy stoma during the first few postoperative days and usually diminishes over 24 to 48 hours. Major bleeding complicates up to 10% of tracheostomy placements by either technique. It may manifest as continuous bleeding or bright red blood from the stoma. This indicates incomplete ligation of a vessel or possible brachiocephalic artery injury (i.e., tracheal-innominate fistula). The latter complicates 0.4 to 4.5% of tracheostomy tube placements.

Imaging Findings

- Large amounts of subcutaneous air; suggest traumatic tube placement with potential aerodigestive tract injury
- Pneumomediastinum and/or pneumothorax
- Lower lobe consolidations from aspiration of blood (**Fig. 104B**)
- Mediastinal hematoma from traumatic venous or arterial injury (**Fig. 104B**)
- Expected findings in uncomplicated cases:
  - Midline tube position
  - Tube tip terminating one half to two thirds the distance from the stoma to the carina
  - Tube width of approximately two thirds the width of the tracheal lumen

Treatment

- Maintain the airway
- Petroleum gauze placed around the tracheostomy and packed into the wound
- Ligation of the bleeding vessel

Prognosis

- Good when bleeding is recognized early and treated promptly

Suggested Readings

Goodman RG, Kuzo RS, eds. Intensive care radiology [review]. Radiol Clin North Am 1996;34:1–190

McCarroll KA, ed. Imaging in the intensive care unit. Crit Care Clin 1994;10(2)

Tocino I. Chest imaging in the intensive care unit. Eur J Radiol 1996;23:46–57

CASE 105 Left Subclavian Line: Persistent Left SVC

Clinical Presentation

A 28-year-old man who recently had a new central venous line placed

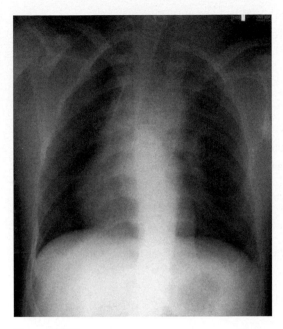

Figure 105A

Radiologic Findings

AP chest radiograph (**Fig. 105A**) demonstrates a right internal jugular central venous catheter coursing into the superior vena cava and a left subclavian central venous catheter coursing into the coronary sinus via a persistent left superior vena cava. Note the vertically oriented opacity in the left superior mediastinum and paratracheal region.

Diagnosis

Left subclavian line placed in a persistent left superior vena cava (SVC)

Differential Diagnosis

- Left internal thoracic vein
- Left superior intercostal vein
- Pericardiophrenic vein

Discussion

Background

A persistent left-sided SVC is the most common thoracic venous anomaly. It occurs in 0.5% of the general population and in 5 to 10% of patients with congenital heart disease. The left SVC persists when the caudal portion of the left anterior cardinal vein fails to regress (see Case 8). The left-sided

413

SVC courses lateral to the transverse aorta and left hilum and drains into the right atrium via an enlarged coronary sinus in over 90% of cases. Rarely, it may drain directly into the left atrium, creating a right-to-left shunt. It is associated with an absent right-sided SVC in 20% cases.

Clinical Findings

Persistence of the left SVC is usually an incidental finding. In patients with congenital heart disease, it may be associated with septal defects, partial anomalous venous return, and azygos continuation of the inferior vena cava.

Imaging Findings

RADIOGRAPHY

- Prominent left paratracheal stripe or left superior mediastinal vascular opacity (**Fig. 105A**)
- Abnormal left paramediastinal course of central venous catheters and leads (**Fig. 105A**)

CT/MR

- Absent or small left brachiocephalic vein (65%)
- Absent right SVC (20%)
- Tubular opacity paralleling the transverse aorta, coursing over the left hilum, and draining into an enlarged coronary sinus

Treatment

- None; patients are usually asymptomatic without physiologic abnormalities.

Prognosis

- Good

PEARLS_____

- Recognition of persistent left superior vena cava may be relevant during implantation of pacemaker leads, radiofrequency ablation, cardiac surgery for placement of a retrograde coronary sinus cardioplegia catheter, superior vena cava filter placements, and transjugular intrahepatic portosystemic shunt (TIPS) placement.
- Inadvertent cannulation of the pericardiophrenic vein may result in fatal cardiac tamponade.

Suggested Readings

Fisher KL, Leung AN. Radiographic appearance of central venous catheters. AJR Am J Roentgenol 1996; 166:329–337

Gerber TC, Kuzo RS. Images in cardiovascular medicine: persistent left superior vena cava demonstrated with multislice spiral computed tomography. Circulation 2002;105:79

Meijboom WB, Vanderheyden M. Biventricular pacing and persistent left superior vena cava: case report and review of the literature. Acta Cardiol 2002;57:287–290

Ricketts RR. Central venous catheterization via persistent left superior vena cava. Am Surg 1996;62:517

Sarodia BD, Stoller JK. Persistent left superior vena cava: case report and literature review. Respir Care 2000;45:411–416

CASE 106 Venous Catheter Cannulation of the Azygos Arch

Clinical Presentation

A 35-year-old man who had an intravenous port catheter placed for chemotherapy

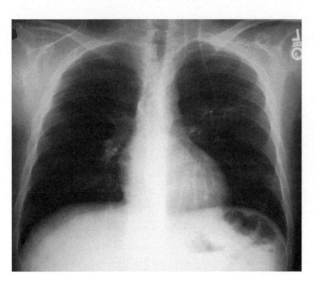

Figure 106A

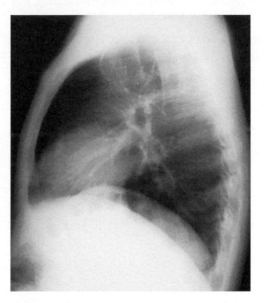

Figure 106B

Radiologic Findings

PA (**Fig. 106A**) and lateral (**Fig. 106B**) chest radiographs demonstrate the intravenous port catheter introduced via a left internal jugular approach. It follows an unusual course and lies medial, inferior, and posterior to the superior vena cava system.

Diagnosis

Venous catheter cannulation of the azygos arch

Differential Diagnosis

None

Discussion

Background

Malpositioning of central venous catheters in the azygos arch is seen in 1.2% of postprocedural radiographic examinations; 69% of such malpositioned lines are introduced via a left subclavian approach, 19% via a left internal jugular approach, and 12% via the right subclavian vein. No cases of inadvertent azygos cannulation via the right internal jugular vein have been reported.

415

Clinical Findings

Complications occur in 19% of inadvertent azygos arch cannulations. Most consist of venous perforation, but also include azygos arch venous obstruction, thrombosis, and stenosis.

Imaging Findings

- Catheter coursing medial to the bronchus intermedius and subcarinal region on frontal radiograph (**Fig. 106A**)
- Reverse-S–shaped course of catheter; terminating posterior to the posterior wall of the bronchus intermedius at the T5–T6 level on the lateral radiograph (**Fig. 106B**)
- Catheter within azygos arch on CT studies

Treatment

- Catheter removal

Prognosis

- Good if recognized early and the venous line is replaced

PEARL_____

- The risk of azygos arch cannulation is increased if catheters are inserted via left-sided veins.

Suggested Readings

Bankier AA, Mallek R, Weismayr MN. Azygos arch cannulation by central venous catheters: radiographic detection of malposition and subsequent complications. J Thorac Imaging 1997;12:64–69

Fisher KL, Leung AN. Radiographic appearance of central venous catheters. AJR Am J Roentgenol 1996; 166:329–337

CASE 107 Malpositioned Central Venous Catheter

Clinical Presentation

A 28-year-old man who has had a new central line placed

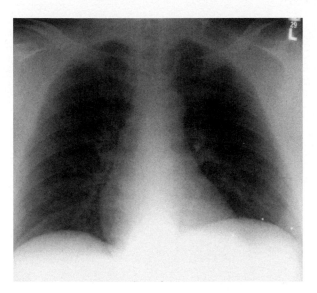

Figure 107A

Radiologic Findings

AP chest radiograph (**Fig. 107A**) demonstrates that the new left internal jugular catheter follows an anomalous course into the ipsilateral subclavian and axillary venous system.

Diagnosis

Malpositioned central venous catheter

Differential Diagnosis

None

Discussion

Background

Five million central venous catheters are placed annually in the United States. Such catheters are routinely used in critically ill patients for venous access and to monitor central venous pressures. Central venous catheters may be introduced via the subclavian, internal jugular, or femoral venous systems.

Clinical Findings

Early complications associated with central venous catheter placement include pneumothorax (1–5%); hydrothorax; hemothorax; chylothorax; arterial puncture; hematoma; nerve injury; catheter,

417

wire, or air embolism; and malposition. Up to 40% of catheters are malpositioned on the initial postprocedural radiograph.

Imaging Findings

- Radiographic demonstration of catheter malposition (**Fig. 107A**)
- CT demonstration of catheter malposition
- Optimal location of catheter tip in the distal superior vena cava, approximately 3 cm proximal to the superior vena cava–right atrial junction

Treatment

- Repositioning or replacement of malpositioned catheters
- Complications addressed appropriately (e.g., pneumothorax, hematoma)

Prognosis

- Good if recognized and addressed early

PEARLS_____

- Catheters in the brachiocephalic system produce inaccurate central venous pressure readings.
- Catheters in the right atrium are associated with an increased risk of perforation and arrhythmias.
- Every postprocedural radiograph should be inspected for potential complications related to central line placement or attempted placement. The opposite hemithorax must also be carefully assessed as bilateral punctures may have been attempted.

Suggested Readings

Bahk JH. The optimal location of central venous catheters. Anesth Analg 2002;94:1372–1373

Keenan SP. Use of ultrasound to pace central lines. J Crit Care 2002;17:126–137

Miller AH, Roth BA, Mills TJ, Woody JR, Longmoor CE, Foster B. Ultrasound guidance versus the landmark technique for the placement of central venous catheters in the emergency department. Acad Emerg Med 2002;9:800–805

Polderman KH, Girbes AJ. Central venous catheter use. Part 1: mechanical complications. Intensive Care Med 2002;28:1–17

Ruesch S, Walder B, Tramer MR. Complications of central venous catheters: internal jugular versus subclavian access—a systemic review. Crit Care Med 2002;30:454–460

CASE 108 Central Venous Catheter Malpositioned in the Left Subclavian Artery

Clinical Presentation

A 21-year-old trauma victim who recently had a new central venous catheter placed

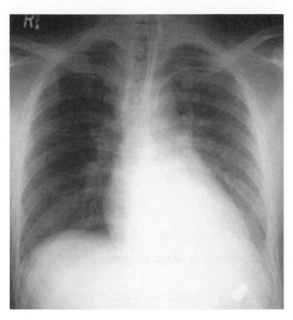

Figure 108A

Radiologic Findings

AP chest radiograph (**Fig. 108A**) demonstrates the recently placed left subclavian line following an anomalous course vertically behind the transverse aorta. Note the collapsed left lower lobe and the retained bullet in the left upper quadrant.

Diagnosis

Central venous catheter malpositioned in the left subclavian artery

Differential Diagnosis

- Extravascular catheter
- Left internal thoracic artery or vein cannulation

Discussion

Background

Accidental arterial puncture and/or cannulation complicate the placement of approximately 1 to 5% of internal jugular, 1% of subclavian, and 5 to 10% of femoral venous line attempts.

419

Clinical Findings

Arterial entry may be recognized at the time of the attempted venipuncture via the return of bright red or pulsatile blood. However, this is not always reliable. In problematic cases, a transducer or manometer may be helpful. One can also obtain an arterial blood gas analysis of the returned blood.

Imaging Findings

- Arterial catheter course (**Fig. 108A**)
- Apical opacity and/or mediastinal widening from extrapleural hematoma

Treatment

- Carotid punctures: prompt catheter removal, application of pressure for several minutes and airway monitoring
- Subclavian artery punctures: may be complicated by life-threatening hemorrhage and pseudoaneurysm formation; may require collagen plugs, embolization, surgical closure devices, and oversewing of the injury

Prognosis

- Dependent on the punctured artery and the extent of the vascular injury
- Good for small extrapleural hematomas; self-limited and gradually resorb over days to weeks, depending on their size
- Consideration of surgical evacuation of large hematomas that are prone to secondary infection, especially with *Staphylococcus* sp.

PEARL_____

- Ultrasound guidance reduces the incidence of arterial punctures and should be used in potentially problematic cases (e.g., large body habitus, altered anatomy secondary to congenital musculoskeletal deformities and surgery, burns, or trauma).

Suggested Readings

Baldwin RT, Kieta DR, Gallagher MW. Complicated right subclavian artery pseudoaneurysm after central venipuncture. Ann Thorac Surg 1996;62:581–582

Dowling K, Herr A, Siskin G, Sansivero GE, Stainken B. Use of a collagen plug device to seal a subclavian artery puncture secondary to intra-arterial dialysis catheter placement. J Vasc Intervent Radiol 1999;10:33–35

Fisher KL, Leung AN. Radiographic appearance of central venous catheters. AJR Am J Roentgenol 1996;166:329–337

Keenan SP. Use of ultrasound to pace central lines. J Crit Care 2002;17:126–137

Miller AH, Roth BA, Mills TJ, Woody JR, Longmoor CE, Foster B. Ultrasound guidance versus the landmark technique for the placement of central venous catheters in the emergency department. Acad Emerg Med 2002;9:800–805

Ruesch S, Walder B, Tramer MR. Complications of central venous catheters: internal jugular versus subclavian access—a systemic review. Crit Care Med 2002;30:454–460

CASE 109 Venous Access Line Fracture and Embolization

Clinical Presentation

A 42-year-old woman who is receiving chemotherapy

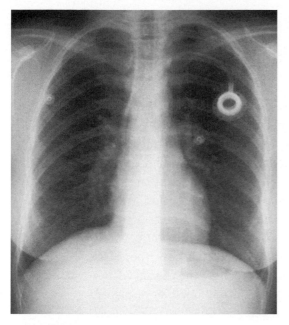

Figure 109A

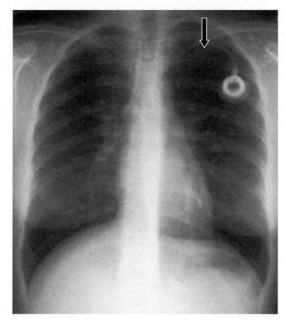

Figure 109B

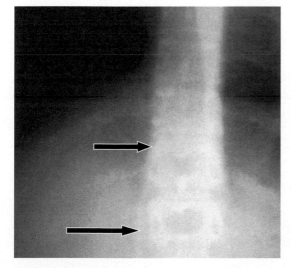

Figure 109C

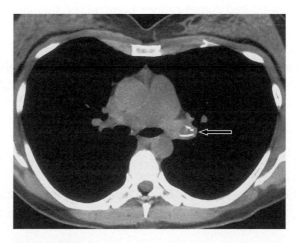

Figure 109D

Radiologic Findings

PA (**Fig. 109A**) chest radiograph demonstrates a well-positioned venous access port introduced via the left subclavian vein. Follow-up PA chest radiograph 2 months later (**Fig. 109B**) demonstrates foreshortening of the preexistent catheter at the level of the left first rib and clavicle (arrow). The distal 10 cm of the fractured catheter has embolized to the inferior vena cava (**Fig. 109C**; cropped PA chest radiograph; arrows). Unenhanced chest CT (mediastinal window) (**Fig. 109D**) of another patient following unsuccessful removal of her peripherally inserted central catheter (PICC) line shows the embolized distal PICC line redundantly coiled in the left interlobar pulmonary artery (arrow).

Diagnosis

Venous access line fracture and embolization

Differential Diagnosis

None

Discussion

Background

The increased use of interventional procedures, monitoring devices, central venous catheters, and long-term implanted venous access ports for chemotherapeutic infusion has led to the increased occurrence of intravascular foreign bodies. Although catheter fragmentation and subsequent embolization to the central venous system occurs in only 1% of cannulations, complications related to indwelling catheter emboli occur in up to 49% of such cases. Catheter fragments may be carried through the central venous system into the right heart and lodge in the pulmonary artery or one of its branches. Thus, catheter emboli should be extracted whenever clinically feasible. Fractures likely result from compression of the catheter between the clavicle and the first rib. Catheter fatigue and manufacturing flaws are infrequently responsible. PICC lines are being used with increased frequency for long-term venous access. These 2 to 5 French (F) diameter catheters are introduced via an antecubital vein and directed to the central venous system. The catheters are quite thin and flexible and may become looped, malpositioned, or displaced. PICC lines are not very radiopaque and at times can be quite difficult to perceive on chest radiography.

Clinical Findings

Most catheter emboli-related complications occur in the first year, and 65% occur in the first month post catheter placement. Such complications include infection (20%), thrombosis (16%), arrhythmias (16%), and endocardial or vascular perforation (10%). Virtually all catheter emboli in the right heart have associated complications and are responsible for 69% of all catheter emboli-related deaths. Catheter emboli in segmental pulmonary arteries are not associated with increased mortality.

Imaging Findings

- "Pinch off" sign: a kink or deformity of the catheter wall or lumen; suggestive of impending catheter fracture
- Change in catheter appearance, location, or length (**Figs. 109B** and **109C**)
- Visualization of catheter fragment on radiography or CT (**Figs. 109C** and **109D**)

Treatment

- Procedure of choice: percutaneous retrieval with a snare-loop
- Other techniques
  - Endoscopic forceps (e.g., superior vena cava and right atrial emboli)
  - Catheter grasping forceps (e.g., pulmonary vasculature)
  - Hooked-pigtail catheters and ureteric stone basket extractors
- Thoracotomy for catheter emboli that cannot otherwise be extracted
- Subacute bacterial endocarditis prophylaxis and low-dose warfarin to decrease the risk of potential thrombosis in patients with irretrievable catheter emboli

Prognosis

- Decreased risk of complications related to retained catheter emboli with time
- No statistically increased risk after 2 years

PEARLS_____

- Localization of embolized catheter fragments can be difficult and may require fluoroscopy or unenhanced CT.
- PICC line placements have no increased risk of pneumothorax, but are associated with a low risk of infection and thrombosis.

Suggested Readings

Aitken DR, Minton JP. The "pinch off sign": a warning of impending problems with permanent subclavian catheters. Am J Surg 1984;148:633–636

di Carlo I, Fisichella P, Russello D, Puleo S, Latteri F. Catheter fracture and cardiac migration: a rare complication of totally implantable venous devices. J Surg Oncol 2000;73:172–173

Egglin TKP, Dickey KW, Rosenblatt M, Pollak JS. Retrieval of intravascular foreign bodies: experience in 32 cases. AJR Am J Roentgenol 1995;164:1259–1264

Fisher KL, Leung AN. Radiographic appearance of central venous catheters. AJR Am J Roentgenol 1996;166:329–337

Roye GD, Breazeale EE, Byrnes JP, Rue LW. Management of catheter emboli. South Med J 1996;89:714–717

CASE 110 Malpositioned Pulmonary Artery Catheter

Clinical Presentation

A 62-year-old man who had undergone a remote coronary artery bypass was readmitted with chest pain and had a new pulmonary artery catheter placed.

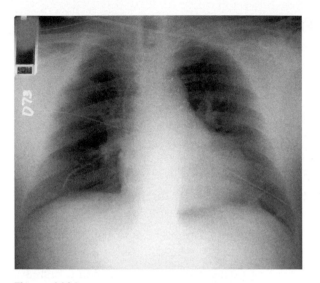

Figure 110A

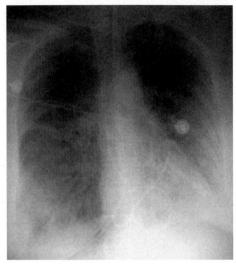

Figure 110B

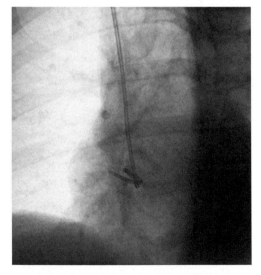

Figure 110C

Radiologic Findings

AP portable (**Fig. 110A**) chest radiograph demonstrates postoperative changes reflective of the previous bypass. The heart is enlarged without decompensation. The left subclavian–pulmonary artery catheter courses deep into the right interlobar pulmonary artery and should be retracted 9 cm. AP (**Fig. 110B**) chest radiograph of another patient in the intensive care unit with arrhythmias following placement of a pulmonary artery catheter shows catheter is looped on either side of the tricuspid valve. Fluoroscopic spot view (**Fig. 110C**) over the right heart after attempted catheter removal reveals the catheter is now knotted within the right atrium.

Diagnosis

Malpositioned pulmonary artery catheter

Differential Diagnosis

None

Discussion

Background

Pulmonary artery catheters are used to monitor the hemodynamic status of critically ill patients. Pressure tracings may help the clinician differentiate cardiogenic edema, noncardiogenic edema, and septicemia. Catheters may be introduced via an internal jugular, subclavian, or, less often, femoral venous approach, and are then "floated" distal to the pulmonic valve into the right or left main pulmonary artery. A balloon is located at the catheter tip, and when inflated (i.e., wedged), the resulting pulmonary artery wedge pressure (PAWP) serves as an indirect measurement of the left atrial and left-end diastolic volume.

Clinical Findings

When the balloon is deflated, the tip of the catheter optimally lies within 2 cm of the hilum. The complication rate of these catheters is 3 to 4.4%, but the complications can be serious and life threatening and include pneumothorax, hemothorax, pulmonary artery perforation and pseudoaneurysm formation, valvular damage, arrhythmias (e.g., ventricular ectopic beats, transient right bundle branch block), and knotting of the catheter. *Pulmonary artery perforation and pseudoaneurysm formation* (**Fig. 110D**) complicates approximately 0.06 to 0.2% of catheter placements and is caused by laceration of the vessel wall by an overinflated balloon, an eccentrically inflated balloon, or the catheter tip itself with subsequent bleeding into the lung parenchyma. Risk factors include female gender, pulmonary artery hypertension, systemic anticoagulation, long-term steroid therapy, induced hypothermia, age over 60 years, stiff catheters, repeated catheter manipulations, and distal catheter migration (**Figs. 110A** and **110D**). Patients may experience hemoptysis or hemothorax, and may exhibit new radiographic opacities in the region of the catheter tip (**Fig. 110E**). *Kinking* and *looping* are precursors of knotting (**Fig. 110B**). *Knotting* of a pulmonary artery catheter is a rare complication and occurs when an excessive length of catheter is inserted (**Figs. 110B** and **110C**). Predisposing factors include right ventricular dilatation, insertion of over 50 cm of catheter without achieving a wedge pressure, and introduction of an incompletely inflated balloon. The possibility of a knot must be considered whenever resistance is met on withdrawal. The catheter should never be forced, as forced removal may avulse the tricuspid valve, papillary muscle, and/or chordae tendineae.

Imaging Findings

RADIOGRAPHY

- Looped or kinked catheter in the cava, right heart, or rarely the pulmonary artery (**Fig. 110B**)
- Catheter embolization

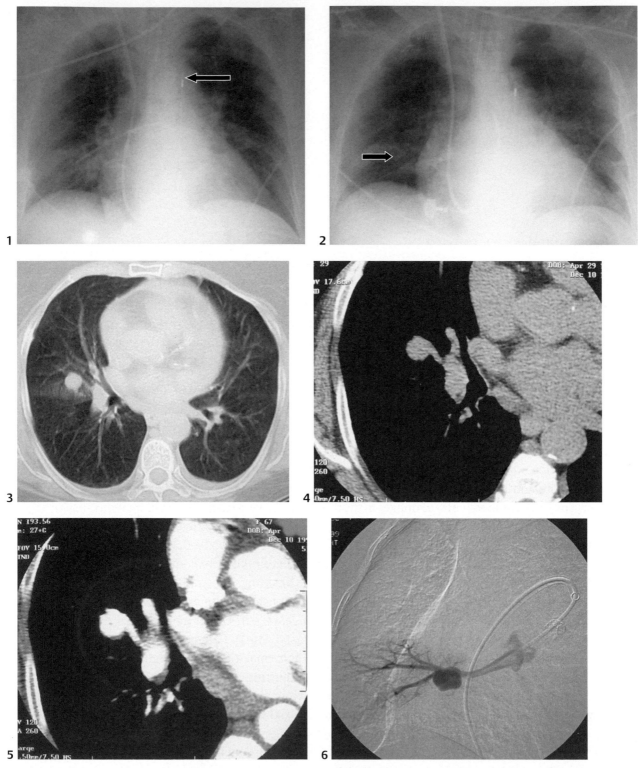

Figure 110D (1–6) AP chest radiograph **(1)** shows a right internal jugular–pulmonary artery catheter advanced deep into the right interlobar pulmonary artery. An ET tube and intraaortic balloon pump (arrow) is also present. Follow-up AP chest radiograph following retraction of the catheter **(2)** demonstrates a subtle nodular opacity (arrow) in the region of the preexisting catheter tip. Unenhanced chest CT **(3**, lung window, and **4**, mediastinal window) targeted to the right lung reveals a 1.5 cm right middle lobe nodule with surrounding ground glass. Notice the nodule's relationship to the adjacent vasculature. Contrast-enhanced chest CT **(5**, mediastinal window) targeted to the right lung shows intense enhancement of the nodule and its vascular etiology. Selective arteriogram **(6)** demonstrates a well-defined right middle lobe artery pseudoaneurysm, induced by a Swan-Ganz catheter. The pseudoaneurysm was subsequently embolized without ill sequelae.

- Pulmonary pseudoaneurysm: well-defined, persistent pulmonary nodule or mass adjacent to catheter tip (**Fig. 110D2**)
- Ground-glass opacity in the vicinity of the malpositioned catheter tip
- Pleural effusion may be present.

CT

- Visualization of looped, kinked, or malpositioned catheter
- Pulmonary artery pseudoaneurysm: enhancing mass that may be associated with thrombus or ground-glass opacity (**Figs. 110D3, 110D4,** and **110D5**)
- Ipsilateral effusion
- Use of coronal and sagittal reformations to aid in elucidating the vascular nature of the lesion

Treatment

- Pulmonary artery pseudoaneurysm
  - Affected lung placed in dependent position to protect the contralateral lung if bleeding ensues
  - Affected lung placed in nondependent position after placement of a double-lumen endotracheal (ET) tube; reduction of pulmonary artery pressure
  - Localization of source of bleeding (e.g., CT, pulmonary angiography)
  - Embolization of affected vessel
  - Occasionally direct repair of the vessel, temporary ligation of the involved artery, and/or resection of the affected lung segment
- Removal of knotted catheters
  - Pulling the catheter against an introducer sheath, reduction of size of the knot, followed by removal of the catheter and sheath
  - Guidewire insertion into catheter to untie knot
  - Use of Dotter basket to snare the catheter and remove it in two pieces
  - Venous cut-down
  - Open thoracotomy
  - Removal of a tightened knot behind an inflexible sheath; exercise caution, as procedure may be complicated by venous laceration and hemothorax

Prognosis

- Pulmonary artery catheter–induced pulmonary artery pseudoaneurysms; 45 to 65% mortality rate; survival dependent on clinical discovery and treatment before rupture of the pseudoaneurysm

PEARLS_____

- Contrast-enhanced chest CT is the imaging modality of choice for diagnosing pulmonary artery pseudoaneurysm. Pulmonary angiography may be considered as an alternative.
- The preferred technique to remove a knotted pulmonary artery catheter is to untie the knot.

Suggested Readings

Bhatti W, Sinha S, Rowlands P. Percutaneous untying of a knot in a retained Swan-Ganz catheter. Cardiovasc Intervent Radiol 2000;23:224–234

Castella M, Riambau V, Palacin J, Font C, Mulet J. True knot in a Swan-Ganz catheter on a central venous catheter: a simple trick for percutaneous removal. Intensive Care Med 1996;22: 830–831

Ferretti GR, Thony F, Link KM, et al. False aneurysm of the pulmonary artery induced by a Swan-Ganz catheter: clinical presentation and radiologic management. AJR Am J Roentgenol 1996; 167:941–945

Tan C, Bristow PJ, Segal P, Bell RJ. A technique to remove knotted pulmonary artery catheters. Anaesth Intensive Care 1997;25:160–162

CASE 111 Malpositioned Central Venous Catheter with Acute "Infusothorax"

Clinical Presentation

A 54-year-old woman had a central venous catheter placed for antibiotic therapy and now complains of right-sided chest discomfort and dyspnea.

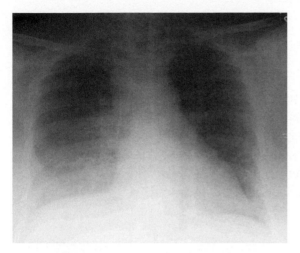

Figure 111A

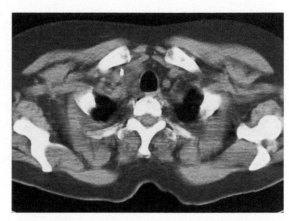

Figure 111B

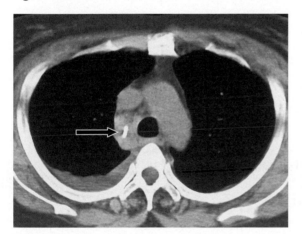

Figure 111C

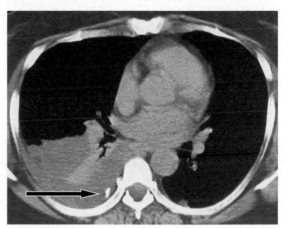

Figure 111D

(Figs. 111A, 111B, 111C, and 111D courtesy of Malcolm K. Sydnor, M.D., Medical College of Virginia Hospitals-Virginia Commonwealth University Health System; Richmond, Virginia.)

Radiologic Findings

AP (**Fig. 111A**) chest radiograph shows that the catheter that was introduced via right internal jugular approach has an anomalous course and position. Note the large right paratracheal hematoma and ground-glass opacity in the lower right thorax from a modest-sized ipsilateral pleural effusion. Unenhanced chest CT (**Figs. 111B** through **111D**) (mediastinal window) reveals initial intravascular purchase of the catheter within the right internal jugular vein (**Fig. 111B**). However, more caudally the catheter perforated the posterior wall of the brachiocephalic vein (not illustrated), coursing into the right paratracheal space and mediastinal pleural reflection (**Fig. 111C**). Note the extravascular catheter position (arrow), the right paratracheal hematoma, and the catheter course into the pleural space (**Fig. 111D**, arrow). Note the large ipsilateral pleural effusion.

Diagnosis

Malpositioned central venous catheter with complicating acute "infusothorax"

Differential Diagnosis

Traumatic hemothorax following central line placement

Discussion

Background

Central venous catheter–related complications may occur acutely (e.g., pneumothorax, hemothorax) or may be delayed (infection, fracture, and embolization). Similarly, traumatic perforation of the central vessel wall and intrapleural catheter malpositioning may occur acutely, at the time of catheterization, or may occur long after successful vascular cannulation. The delayed onset of a hydrothorax following central venous catheterization is more often related to lines introduced via a left-sided approach and the catheter tips juxtaposed against the superior vena cava wall.

Clinical Findings

Patients may develop dyspnea and tachycardia secondary to the hydrothorax. Patients may also complain of chest pain. There is typically poor or no blood return on aspiration from the suspect catheter. Biochemical analysis of the pleural effusion and comparison with the infusate is often diagnostic.

Imaging Findings

ACUTE CASES

- Anomalous course of central venous line (**Figs. 111A, 111C,** and **111D**)
- Pneumothorax
- Unilateral or bilateral pleural effusion temporally related to the central venous catheter placement (**Figs. 111A, 111C,** and **111D**)
- Ipsilateral paratracheal and/or mediastinal hematoma (**Figs. 111A** and **111C**)

DELAYED CASES

- Change in position of central venous catheter tip (i.e., curled or no longer parallels the vessel wall)
- Widened mediastinum
- Unexplained unilateral or bilateral pleural effusion

Treatment

- Stopping the infusion
- Supportive care with intravenous fluids, blood products, oxygen
- Removal of offending catheter
- Drainage of the pleural space; may rapidly improve the patient's respiratory status

Prognosis

- Life-threatening if not recognized

- Proper catheter placement within superior vena cava will avoid this complication.
- A subtle sign of catheter malposition is a slightly curled catheter tip.
- Delayed hydrothorax may occur long after successful catheter insertion and should be considered in patients with otherwise unexplained pleural or mediastinal effusions.
- Injection of a few milliliters of contrast media via the suspect catheter with immediate fluoroscopy or CT imaging may demonstrate leakage into the pleural space or mediastinum and may be useful in problematic cases.

Suggested Readings

Au FC, Badellino M. Significance of a curled central venous catheter tip. Chest 1988;93:890–891

Duntley P, Siever J, Korwes ML, Harpel K, Heffner JE. Vascular erosion by central venous catheters: clinical features and outcomes. Chest 1992;101:1633–1638

Flatley ME, Schapira RM. Hydropneumomediastinum and bilateral hydropneumothorax as delayed complications of central venous catheterization. Chest 1993;103:1914–1916

Krasna IH, Krause T. Life-threatening fluid extravasation of central venous catheters. J Pediatr Surg 1991;26:1346–1348

Tayama K, Inoue T, Yokoyama H, Yano T, Ichinose Y. Late development of hydrothorax induced by a central venous catheter: report of a case. Surg Today 1996;26:837–838

CASE 112 Malpositioned Intraparenchymal Chest Tube

Clinical Presentation

A 23-year-old woman was involved in a motor vehicle collision and suffered significant blunt thoracic trauma.

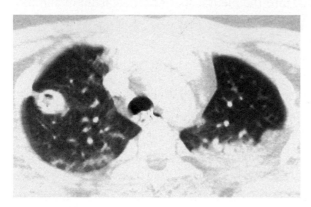

Figure 112A

Radiologic Findings

Contrast-enhanced chest CT (**Fig. 112A**, lung window) shows an intraparenchymal right-sided thoracostomy tube. Notice the debris within the chest tube lumen. Atelectatic changes are also present in the apical posterior segment left upper lobe.

Diagnosis

Malpositioned intraparenchymal chest tube

Differential Diagnosis

None

Discussion

Background

Malpositioning of thoracostomy tubes in extrathoracic, intraparenchymal (**Fig. 112A**), mediastinal, intrafissural (see Case 113), and subdiaphragmatic (**Fig. 112B**) locations occurs in 26 to 58% of placements under emergent conditions. Detection of such malpositioned tubes with a single-view radiograph is problematic, and malpositioning is often not appreciated. CT is more accurate in identifying malpositioned tubes and potential complications related to their anomalous course and position.

Clinical Findings

Most patients do not have any symptoms directly related to the intraparenchymal chest tube placement. The clinical clue may be a poorly functioning chest tube or a persistent air leak. The finding may be

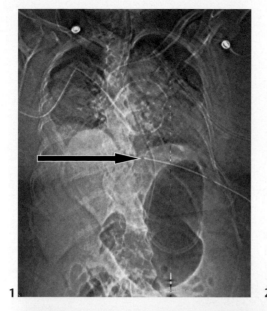

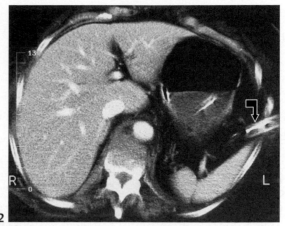

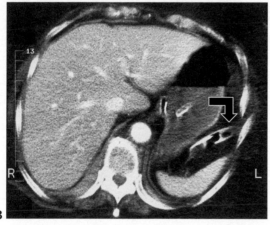

Figure 112B (1–3) Scout topogram **(1)** of a 72-year-old woman involved in a serious motor vehicle collision shows a kinked poorly functioning right chest tube and a subdiaphragmatic left chest tube (arrow). Contrast-enhanced chest CT (**2,3,** mediastinal window) demonstrates the left chest tube introduced below the diaphragm (arrow) as it courses between the stomach and spleen.

suggested on chest radiography or incidentally discovered on CT obtained for other reasons or in the evaluation of a persistent air leak or loculated pleural fluid collection. Intraparenchymal chest tube placement may be complicated by pulmonary hematoma, laceration, infection, and bronchopleural fistula.

Imaging Findings

RADIOGRAPHY

- Difficult recognition of tube malposition
- Ground-glass opacity or consolidation about the chest tube
- Persistent pneumothorax or pleural fluid collection

CT

- Often confused with intrafissural placement (**Fig. 112A;** see Case 113)
- Lung parenchyma completely surrounding the chest tube (**Fig. 112A**)
- Parenchymal vascular markings abruptly terminating at the margin of the chest tube
- Ground-glass opacities or consolidation representing intraparenchymal hemorrhage often parallel to malpositioned chest tube

Treatment

- Removal of the malpositioned tube

Prognosis

- Good if recognized and treated early

PEARL_____

- Intraparenchymal, mediastinal, subdiaphragmatic, and extrathoracic thoracostomy tubes must be removed.

Suggested Readings

Baldt MM, Bankier AA, Germann PS, Poschl GP, Skrbensky GT, Herold CJ. Complications after emergency tube thoracostomy: assessment with CT. Radiology 1995;195:539–543

Swensen SJ, Peters SG, LeRoy AJ, Gay PC, Sykes MW, Trastek VF. Subspecialty clinics: critical-care medicine. Radiology in the intensive-care unit. Mayo Clin Proc 1991;66:396–410

CASE 113 Malpositioned Intrafissural Chest Tube

Clinical Presentation

A 53-year-old woman involved in a motor vehicle collision 5 days earlier
has a persistent hemothorax that is not responding to chest tube drainage.

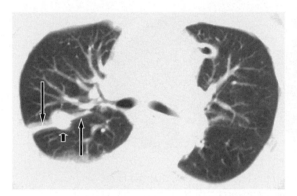

Figure 113A

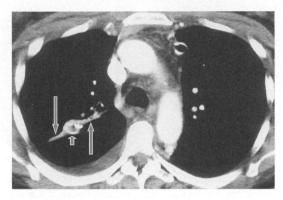

Figure 113B

Radiologic Findings

Contrast-enhanced chest CT (**Figs. 113A** and **113B** lung and mediastinal window) shows the right
chest tube (short arrow) lodged within the major fissure (long arrows). There is a small amount of
fluid localized within the fissure and a larger, more dependent hemothorax. The left chest tube is
well positioned.

Diagnosis

Malpositioned intrafissural chest tube

Differential Diagnosis

None

Discussion

Background

Thoracostomy tubes are used to evacuate air or fluid from the pleural space. Since air rises to the
nondependent aspect of the pleural cavity, simple pneumothoraces are best evacuated with tubes
directed anteriorly and superiorly. Because fluid gravitates to the most dependent portion of the
pleural space, uncomplicated effusions are best evacuated with tubes directed posteriorly and inferiorly. Thoracostomy tube failure may result from blockage of the tube by clot or debris, adhesions,
multiloculation, and incorrect positioning of the tube in the extrapleural soft tissues or interlobar
fissures.

435

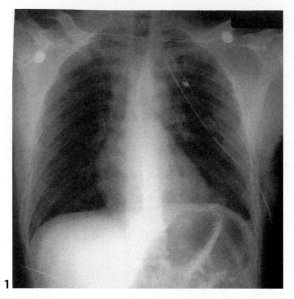
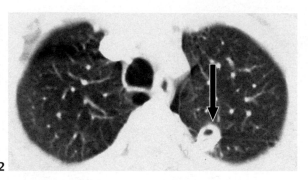

Figure 113C (1) Frontal chest radiograph of a 37-year-old man who was stabbed in the left chest shows that the chest tube follows the expected course and position of the oblique fissure. There is no residual pneumothorax. A small amount of subcutaneous air is present. **(2)** Contrast-enhanced chest CT (lung window) of the same patient shows the chest tube within the oblique fissure (arrow) and a small residual posterior medial pneumothorax.

Clinical Findings

Intrafissural chest tubes have no specific associated complications, although such tube placements may fail to completely evacuate the pleural space. There has been some controversy in the past; however, there is likely no increased incidence of empyema related to the intrafissural chest tube placement alone.

Imaging Findings

RADIOGRAPHY

- Difficult recognition on a single-view chest radiograph
- Chest tube paralleling the expected course and position of the interlobar fissure (**Fig. 113C1**)
- Persistent pleural fluid collection, pneumothorax, or air leak

CT

- Easier diagnosis; best appreciated on lung windows (**Figs. 113A** and **113D**)
- Chest tube within the interlobar fissure (**Figs. 113A** and **113C2**)
- Persistent pleural fluid collection, pneumothorax, or air leak (**Figs. 113A, 113B,** and **113C2**)

Treatment

- None for functioning tubes
- Removal and replacement of nonfunctioning tubes

Prognosis

- Good for functioning tubes
- Empyema secondary to inadequate drainage of an infected pleural space

Suggested Readings

Baldt MM, Bankier AA, Germann PS, Poschl GP, Skrbensky GT, Herold CJ. Complications after emergency tube thoracostomy: assessment with CT. Radiology 1995;195:539–543

Curtin JJ, Goodman LR, Quebbeman EJ, Haasler GB. Thoracostomy tubes after acute chest injury: relationship between location in a pleural fissure and function. AJR Am J Roentgenol 1994;163: 1339–1342

Swensen SJ, Peters SG, LeRoy AJ, Gay PC, Sykes MW, Trastek VF. Subspecialty clinics: critical-care medicine. Radiology in the intensive-care unit. Mayo Clin Proc 1991;66:396–410

CASE 114 Twiddler Syndrome

Clinical Presentation

A 48-year-old man with periods of bradycardia and asynchronous pacemaker activity without capture

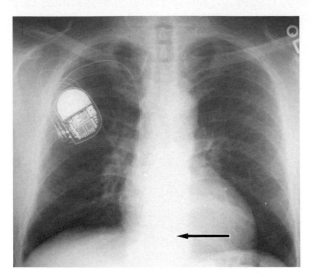

Figure 114A

Radiologic Findings

PA chest radiograph (**Fig. 114A**) demonstrates failure of the distal pacer lead (arrow) to cross the tricuspid valve plane (midthoracic spine) or course into the right ventricular chamber. Note the redundant loops of wire about the generator.

Diagnosis

Pacer lead twisting due to pulse generator rotation: twiddler syndrome

Differential Diagnosis

None

Discussion

Background

Twiddler syndrome is a rare complication of pacemaker and automatic internal cardioverter defibrillator (AICD) implantation. The reported incidence ranges between 0.14 and 1.1%. It results from the intentional or spontaneous rotation of the pacemaker. This causes traction on the electrodes, which may then dislodge or fracture, resulting in pacemaker malfunction.

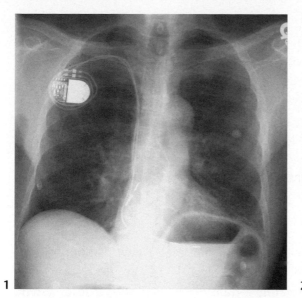 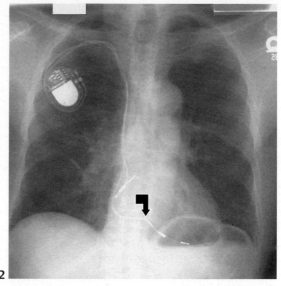

Figure 114B (1,2) PA chest radiograph **(1)** of a 68-year-old man with heart disease demonstrates a dual chamber cardiac pacemaker. Notice the generator orientation and the positioning of the right atrial and right ventricular leads. PA chest radiograph **(2)** obtained 1 year later when the pacer capture was inconsistent shows that the generator has rotated approximately 60 degrees clockwise, and there has been some retraction of the right ventricular lead with superior buckling (arrow). (Courtesy of Harold L. Floyd, M.D., Medical College of Virginia Hospitals-Virginia Commonwealth University Health System, Richmond, Virginia.)

Clinical Findings

Twiddler syndrome occurs more often in obese patients and elderly women (i.e., 60–85 years of age). Improper anchoring of the device, a large subcutaneous pocket, and loose subcutaneous tissue facilitate generator rotation. Localized discomfort may predispose the patient to unintentional manipulation of the device. If the patient is pacer dependent, the device malfunction may be associated with weakness, confusion, and syncope.

Imaging Findings

- Easily recognized on serial chest radiography by a change in the position of the generator (**Fig. 114B**) or by the presence of coiled, displaced, dislodged, or fractured electrodes
- Fracture of the pacing lead close to its connection with the generator
- Multiple redundant loops or coils in the subclavian region (**Fig. 114A**)
- Intracardiac twisting of a pacing lead

Treatment

- Surgical correction or pocket revision
- No pacemaker malfunction: opening of generator case and lead uncoiling
- Dysfunction caused by lead displacement: uncoiling and reimplantation of lead
- Fractured lead: replacement

Prognosis

- Good when recognized and corrected

Prevention

- Firm fixation of the generator and leads in the chest wall
- Smaller as opposed to larger subcutaneous implantation pockets
- Implanting the generator under the pectoralis major muscle
- Immobilizing the generator in the pocket with Dacron

PEARL_____

- The diagnosis should be considered in any patient with pacemaker or AICD malfunction.

Suggested Readings

Bayliss CE, Beanlands DS, Baird RJ. The pacemaker-twiddler's syndrome: a new complication of implantable transvenous pacemakers. Can Med Assoc J 1968;99:371–373

de Buitleir M, Canver C. Twiddler's syndrome complicating a transvenous defibrillator lead system. Chest 1996;109:1391–1394

Picone A, Boahene K. Defibrillator twiddler's syndrome: a rare cause of implantable cardioverter-defibrillator failure. Heart 1996;76:455–456

CASE 115 Malpositioned Intraaortic Balloon Pump

Clinical Presentation

A 59-year-old man who suffered an acute myocardial infarction

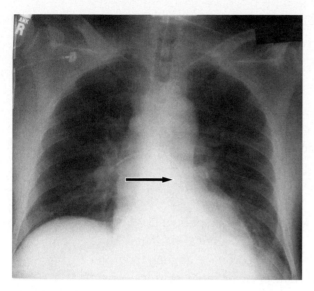

Figure 115A

Radiologic Findings

AP chest radiograph (**Fig. 115A**) reveals a low-lying intraaortic balloon pump (arrow). The endotracheal (ET) tube terminates 8.5 cm above the carina and should be advanced 3.0 cm. The tip of the femoral-pulmonary artery catheter overlies the right interlobar pulmonary artery. Note mild cardiomegaly and widening of the vascular pedicle, but no evidence of cardiac decompensation.

Diagnosis

Malpositioned intraaortic balloon pump

Differential Diagnosis

None

Discussion

Background

The intraaortic counterpulsation balloon pump (IABP) and catheter is the most commonly used mechanical assist device. Its primary purpose is to increase myocardial oxygen supply while reducing its demand. Its secondary purposes include improving cardiac output; improving ejection fraction; increasing coronary perfusion pressure and systemic perfusion; and reducing heart rate, pulmonary capillary wedge pressure, and systemic vascular resistance. Early indications for use include cardiac

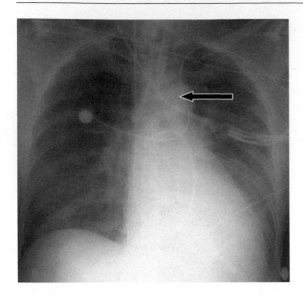

Figure 115B AP chest radiograph demonstrates an appropriately positioned IABP device (arrow) and pulmonary artery catheter. The heart is enlarged, and there is mild interstitial edema.

surgery, left ventricular failure, unstable angina, and failure to come off cardiopulmonary bypass. Prophylactic applications include stabilizing both cardiac and noncardiac surgical patients. More recent applications have included supporting cardiac patients during coronary angiography and percutaneous transluminal angioplasty, drug-induced cardiac failure, myocardial contusion, and septic shock, and as a bridge to heart transplant.

Clinical Findings

The 8.5 to 9.5 French (F) catheter is introduced percutaneously via the femoral or axillary artery or directly into the descending thoracic aorta at thoracotomy. It is advanced retrograde just distal to the left subclavian artery. A 26 to 28 mm inflatable balloon is mounted on the vascular catheter. Helium gas is pumped from the bedside console to the balloon. The balloon inflates with the onset of diastole and deflates during isometric contraction or early systole and is phasically pulsed in counterpulsation to the patient's cardiac cycle. Total or regional blood flow is improved during balloon inflation, as is collateral coronary artery circulation. Vascular complications associated with the use of the IABP are common and are most often related to femoral or iliac artery injury. The most common vascular complication is limb ischemia (14–45%). Iatrogenic injury of the thoracic aorta is less common but often fatal. Patients with extensive atherosclerotic disease are at increased risk. If the catheter is advanced too distal (e.g., aortic root), it may obstruct blood flow to the aortic arch and great vessels. The latter may be associated with acute cerebral vascular accident. If the catheter is not advanced far enough, the counterpulsation is less effective, and renal insufficiency may occur when the balloon occludes the renal arteries. Relative contraindications to the use of this device include severe aortic valvular insufficiency, known aortic dissection, and severe peripheral vascular disease.

Imaging Findings

- Catheter tip visible as an opaque 3 × 4 mm rectangle (**Figs. 115A** and **115B**)
- Optimal tip position in the proximal descending thoracic aorta, just below the left subclavian artery and the superior contour of the transverse aorta (**Fig. 115B**)
- Foreshortening or ring-like appearance of opaque rectangular catheter tip when catheter advances into aortic arch
- Loss of definition of the descending thoracic aorta in cases complicated by dissection

Treatment

- Prompt correction of catheters positioned too high or too low
- Surgical repair or covered endovascular stent placement in cases of vascular perforation

Prognosis

- Early mortality rate for perioperative cardiac failure requiring an intraaortic balloon pump as high as 52%
- Independent predictors of early death: preoperative serum creatinine level, left ventricular ejection fraction, perioperative myocardial infarction, timing of balloon pump insertion, and indication for operation
- Relatively good long-term prognosis for hospital survivors

Suggested Reading

Arafa OE, Pedersen TH, Svennevig JL, Fosse E, Geiran OR. Vascular complications of the intra-aortic balloon pump in patients undergoing open-heart operations: 15-year experience. Ann Thorac Surg 1999;67:645–651

Baskett RJ, Ghali WA, Maitland A, Hirsch GM. The intra-aortic balloon pump in cardiac surgery. Ann Thorac Surg 2002;74:1276–1287

Bautista-Hernandez V, Moya J, Martinell J, Polo ML, Fraile J. Successful stent-grafting for perforation of the thoracic aorta by an intra-aortic balloon pump. Ann Thorac Surg 2002;73:956–958

Cochran RP, Starkey TD, Panos AL, Kunzelman KS. Ambulatory intra-aortic balloon pump use as bridge to heart transplant. Ann Thorac Surg 2002;74:746–752

CASE 116 Left Ventricular Assist Device

Clinical Presentation

A 56-year-old man with ischemic heart disease and left ventricular failure who had recent cardiac surgery

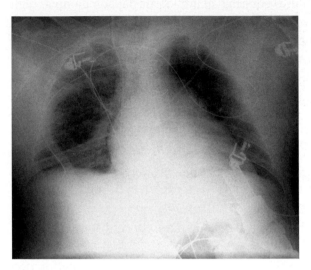

Figure 116A

Radiologic Findings

AP chest radiograph (**Fig. 116A**) demonstrates median sternotomy wires, numerous life support tubes and lines in appropriate position, and a left ventricular assist device in the left upper quadrant. The heart is enlarged, and there is mild interstitial edema.

Diagnosis

Left ventricular assist device; expected postsurgical changes and life support devices

Differential Diagnosis

None

Discussion

Background

Cardiac assist devices have become increasingly important in the management of patients with end-stage heart failure. Most current devices provide temporary left ventricular support for patients with cardiogenic shock from postcardiotomy syndrome, acute myocardial infarction complicated by cardiogenic shock, ischemic or idiopathic cardiomyopathy, and for those awaiting transplantation. Patients may need left ventricular, right ventricular, or biventricular support. Most patients receiving left ventricular assist devices (LVADs) have significant hemodynamic deterioration, loss of blood pressure, waning of cardiac output, and typically survive for only 24 to 48 hours.

444

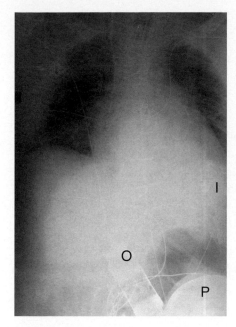

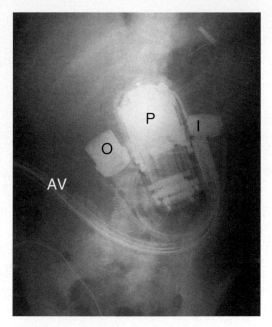

Figure 116B AP chest radiograph demonstrates an implanted LVAD in the left upper quadrant. The inflow tube (I), pump (P), and outflow tube (O) can be identified.

Figure 116C AP view of the abdomen demonstrates the components of an LVAD implanted in the abdomen. Notice the pump (P), external air vent tubing (AV), the inflow tube (I), and the outflow (O) tube.

Clinical Findings

The LVAD enhances the pumping efficiency of the left ventricle. The surgically implanted device requires a median sternotomy. A section of the left ventricular wall is removed, and the mouth of an *inflow tube* is sutured into the ventricular apex (**Fig. 116B**). The tube then descends through the diaphragm into the peritoneal cavity. Blood flows through the tube via a one-way valve into the implanted blood pump. The *pump* resides in the abdominal cavity, is connected to an external air vent (**Fig. 116C**), and is electronically controlled by two percutaneous lines. From the pump, blood passes through another one-way valve into an *outflow tube* that empties into the ascending aorta (**Fig. 116B**). Thus, the left ventricle is effectively bypassed. The aortic valve is surgically sealed to prevent backflow of blood into the ventricle from the aorta. *Biventricular assistance* can be accomplished with an *inflow tube* sutured into the pulmonary artery, a second implanted abdominal *pump,* and an *outflow tube* sutured into the right atrium. Complications include bleeding, asynchronous timing between the heart and the LVAD, infection, and cerebral vascular accidents.

Imaging Findings

- Postoperative changes reflective of the median sternotomy (**Figs. 116A** and **116B**)
- Appropriate life support tubes and lines (**Figs. 116A** and **116B**)
- Visualization of three major LVAD components (e.g., inflow tube, outflow tube, and pump) (**Figs. 116B** and **116C**)

Treatment

- Cardiogenic shock
- Cardiomyopathy
- High-risk cardiac patients as a bridge to transplantation

Prognosis

- Average length of implantation is 45 days.
- May allow patients to survive up to 4 years while awaiting transplantation

Suggested Reading

Cascade PN, Meaney JF, Jamadar DA. Methods of cardiopulmonary support: a review for radiologists. Radiographics 1997;17:1141–1155

Park SJ, Nguyen DQ, Bank AJ, Ormaza S, Bolman RM. Left ventricular assist device bridge therapy for acute myocardial infarction. Ann Thorac Surg 2000;69:1146–1151

Schmid C, Welp H, Klotz S, et al. Left ventricular assist stand-by for high-risk cardiac surgery. Thorac Cardiovasc Surg 2002;50:342–346

Stiller B, Lange PE, Hetzer R. Left ventricular assist device. N Engl J Med 2002;346:1023–1025

Williams M, Oz M, Mancini D. Cardiac assist devices for end-stage heart failure. Heart Dis 2001;3: 109–115

SECTION IX

Diffuse Lung Disease

CASE 117 Acute Interstitial Pneumonia (AIP)

Clinical Presentation

A 64-year-old woman with recurrent episodes of pulmonary consolidation

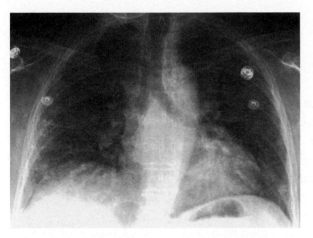

Figure 117A

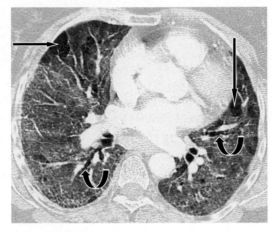

Figure 117B

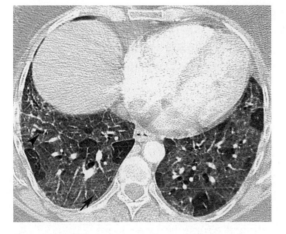

Figure 117C

Radiologic Findings

PA chest radiograph (**Fig. 117A**) demonstrates reduced lung volumes and diffuse, bilateral airspace and reticular opacities. Unenhanced HRCT (lung window) (**Figs. 117B** and **117C**) demonstrates diffuse bilateral ground-glass opacities with focal lobular areas of sparing (long arrows). Notice the interlobular septal thickening (short arrows) and the subtle areas of bronchial dilatation and traction bronchiectasis consistent with early fibrosis (curved arrows).

Diagnosis

Acute interstitial pneumonia (AIP)

Differential Diagnosis

- Permeability edema
- Diffuse pneumonia
- Pulmonary hemorrhage
- Acute hypersensitivity pneumonitis

Discussion

Background

The idiopathic interstitial pneumonias (IIPs) are the most common group of diffuse parenchymal lung diseases. The diffuse lung diseases were recently reclassified by a multidisciplinary panel of experts in a collaborative effort by the American Thoracic Society (ATS), the European Respiratory Society (ERS), and the American College of Chest Physicians (ACCP). The new classification includes seven distinct clinicopathologic entities: (1) idiopathic pulmonary fibrosis (IPF) or cryptogenic fibrosing alveolitis (CFA), (2) nonspecific interstitial pneumonia (NSIP), (3) cryptogenic organizing pneumonia (COP), (4) acute interstitial pneumonia (AIP), (5) lymphocytic interstitial pneumonia (LIP), (6) respiratory bronchiolitis–interstitial lung disease (RB-ILD), and (7) desquamative interstitial pneumonia (DIP).

Acute interstitial pneumonia (AIP) is an uncommon and rapidly progressive form of lung injury and represents an idiopathic form of acute respiratory distress syndrome (ARDS) and diffuse alveolar damage (DAD). Previously called Hamman-Rich syndrome, it was originally thought to represent rapidly progressive usual interstitial pneumonia (UIP) but is now recognized as a distinct clinicopathologic entity and is much less common than UIP.

Etiology

The etiology of AIP is unknown.

Clinical Findings

Affected patients are typically younger than those with UIP, and their clinical course is more acute. They present with a recent history of cough, fever, and dyspnea and progress rapidly to severe dyspnea, hypoxemia, and respiratory failure. Patients are often misdiagnosed as having severe community-acquired pneumonia but fail to respond to broad-spectrum antibiotic therapy.

The diagnosis of AIP requires negative bacterial, viral, and fungal cultures. In addition, other causes of ARDS must be excluded. Integration of biopsy results with the clinical, laboratory, and microbiologic findings allows the formulation of a final diagnosis.

Pathology

EXUDATIVE PHASE

- Hyaline membranes in alveoli, sparse cellular infiltrates in the interstitium

PROLIFERATIVE PHASE

- Proliferation of type 2 pneumocytes

FIBROTIC PHASE

- Loose, organizing fibrosis within the alveoli

Imaging Findings

RADIOGRAPHY

- Progressive diffuse bilateral parenchymal consolidation (similar to ARDS) (**Fig. 117A**)

CT/HRCT

- Scattered or diffuse ground-glass opacities (**Figs. 117B** and **117C**)
- Diffuse airspace consolidations
- Bilateral, symmetric, and basilar distribution
- Anteroposterior lung attenuation gradient may be evident.
- Architectural distortion, traction bronchiectasis (**Figs. 117B** and **117C**), and honeycombing in later stages
- Uncommonly lymphadenopathy, pleural effusion, and septal thickening

Treatment

- Supportive
- Corticosteroids may benefit some patients.

Prognosis

- Mortality 60 to 90%
- May develop severe parenchymal fibrosis, without progression in postrecovery period (unlike UIP)
- Significant functional abnormalities in survivors

Suggested Readings

International Multidisciplinary Consensus. Classification of the idiopathic interstitial pneumonias. Am J Respir Crit Care Med 2002;165:277–304

Johkoh T, Müller NL, Taniguchi H, et al. Acute interstitial pneumonia: thin section CT findings in 36 patients. Radiology 1999;211(3):859-863

Primack SL, Hartman TE, Ikezoe JA, et al. Acute interstitial pneumonia: radiographic and CT findings in nine patients. Radiology 1993;188:817–820

Travis WD, Colby TV, Koss MN, Rosado-de-Christenson ML, Müller NL, King TE Jr. Diffuse parenchymal lung diseases. In: King DW, ed. Atlas of Nontumor Pathology: Non-Neoplastic Disorders of the Lower Respiratory Tract, first series, fascicle 2. Washington, DC: American Registry of Pathology; 2002:103–106

CASE 118 Nonspecific Interstitial Pneumonia (NSIP)

Clinical Presentation

A 50-year-old male cigarette smoker (33 pack-year) with dyspnea and a 1-year history of rheumatoid-inflammatory arthritis

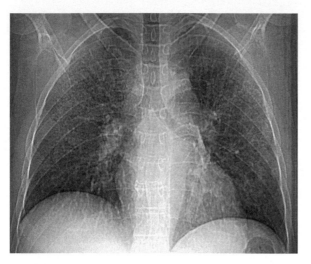

Figure 118A

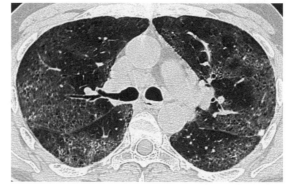

Figure 118B

Radiologic Findings

PA chest radiograph (**Fig. 118A**) demonstrates reduced lung volumes and diffuse bilateral reticular opacities. Unenhanced HRCT (lung window) (**Fig. 118B**) demonstrates bilateral patchy and juxtapleural ground-glass opacities, intralobular linear opacities, and fine honeycombing with a predominant peripheral and lower lung zone distribution.

Diagnosis

Nonspecific interstitial pneumonia (NSIP)

Differential Diagnosis

- Usual interstitial pneumonia (UIP)
- Desquamative interstitial pneumonia (DIP)
- Acute interstitial pneumonia (AIP)
- Respiratory bronchiolitis–interstitial lung disease (RB-ILD)
- Cryptogenic organizing pneumonia (COP)
- Hypersensitivity pneumonitis (HP)
- Connective tissue disease with associated fibrosis

Discussion

Background

Nonspecific interstitial pneumonia (NSIP) is one of the idiopathic interstitial pneumonias (IIPs) (see Case 117). Katzenstein first described NSIP in 1994. The term is used for cases of interstitial pneumonia in which diagnostic features of UIP, DIP, AIP, or cryptogenic organizing pneumonia (COP) are not present. It is associated with significantly longer survival than UIP.

Etiology

The etiology is unknown, but the pattern of NSIP is being recognized more frequently in patients with collagen vascular diseases and other systemic disorders.

Clinical Findings

Affected patients are typically middle-aged (median age: 45 years) men and women with a gradual onset of exertional dyspnea, cough, and fever. Pulmonary function tests reveal a restrictive pattern and reduced carbon monoxide diffusing capacity (DLCO). Many patients are current or former cigarette smokers.

Pathology

CELLULAR PATTERN

- Mild-to-moderate chronic inflammation of the alveolar interstitium
- Alveolar wall thickening
- No fibrosis

FIBROSING PATTERN

- Dense or loose interstitial fibrosis
- Alveolar wall thickening
- Relative preservation of lung architecture
- Temporally uniform histologic abnormalities

Imaging Findings

RADIOGRAPHY

- Variable and nonspecific
- Bilateral, patchy, or diffuse airspace and reticular opacities (**Fig. 118A**)

CT/HRCT

- Ground-glass attenuation, consolidation (**Fig. 118B**)
- Reticular opacities and honeycombing (**Fig. 118B**)
- Traction bronchiectasis
- Indistinguishable from UIP (32% cases), HP (20% cases), COP (14% cases), and others (12% cases)

Treatment

- Corticosteroids

Prognosis

- Improvement or recovery after corticosteroids in up to 75% of patients
- Five-year survival: 75%

PEARL_____

- NSIP is a diagnosis of exclusion: lacks features of UIP, DIP, COP, HP, or diffuse alveolar damage (DAD)

Suggested Readings

Katzenstein AL, Fiorelli RF. Nonspecific interstitial pneumonia/fibrosis: histologic features and clinical significance. Am J Surg Pathol 1994;18:136–147

Travis WD, Colby TV, Koss MN, Rosado-de-Christenson ML, Müller NL, King TE Jr. Diffuse parenchymal lung diseases. In: King DW, ed. Atlas of Nontumor Pathology: Non-Neoplastic Disorders of the Lower Respiratory Tract, first series, fascicle 2. Washington, DC: American Registry of Pathology; 2002:73–82

CASE 119 Pulmonary Alveolar Proteinosis

Clinical Presentation

A 28-year-old woman with dry cough and mild dyspnea

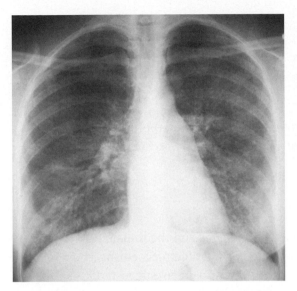

Figure 119A

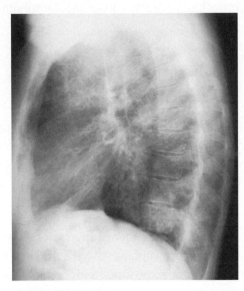

Figure 119B

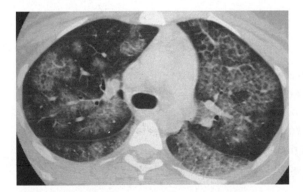

Figure 119C

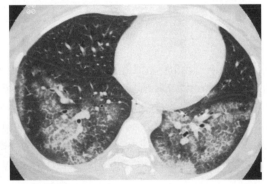

Figure 119D

(Figs. 119A, 119B, 119C, and 119D courtesy of H. Page McAdams, M.D., Duke University Medical Center, Durham, North Carolina)

Radiologic Findings

PA (**Fig. 119A**) and lateral (**Fig. 119B**) chest radiographs demonstrate bilateral symmetric airspace and reticular opacities without volume loss, lymphadenopathy, or pleural effusion. Unenhanced HRCT (lung window) (**Figs. 119C** and **119D**) demonstrates bilateral patchy ground-glass opacities with superimposed smooth septal thickening.

Diagnosis

Pulmonary alveolar proteinosis

455

Differential Diagnosis

- Pneumonia (infectious, eosinophilic, lipoid, organizing)
- Diffuse alveolar damage
- Edema (cardiogenic, noncardiogenic)
- Hemorrhage
- Multifocal neoplasia (bronchioloalveolar carcinoma, lymphoma)

Discussion

Background

Pulmonary alveolar proteinosis (also known as alveolar lipoproteinosis and alveolar phospholipoproteinosis) is characterized by the abnormal accumulation of lipid-rich granular eosinophilic material within the pulmonary alveoli.

Etiology

The etiology is unknown. The overproduction of surfactant by type 2 pneumocytes and the impaired clearance of surfactant by alveolar macrophages have both been postulated as possible mechanisms. An association with environmental exposures and cigarette smoking has also been suggested. Alveolar proteinosis may occur as an isolated condition or may be associated with immune deficiency, infection, and/or malignancy.

Clinical Findings

Affected patients are typically adults (although all age groups are affected) who present with an insidious onset of mild symptoms. Men are more commonly affected than women, with a male-to-female ratio of 2:1. Dry cough, dyspnea on exertion, chest pain, hemoptysis, and expectoration of gelatinous material are reported, and some patients develop respiratory failure. Constitutional symptoms of fatigue, weight loss, and low-grade fever may be present, as well as clubbing and cyanosis. Associated nocardial and mycobacterial infections may occur. Approximately one third of patients are asymptomatic.

Pathology

GROSS

- Heavy, congested lungs; cut sections may leak yellowish fluid
- Nodular consolidations of varying sizes

MICROSCOPIC

- Patchy or diffuse accumulation of eosinophilic periodic acid-Schiff (PAS)–positive proteinaceous material within alveolar spaces with well-demarcated "empty" spaces, cholesterol clefts, and globular foci of eosinophilic material
- Mild interstitial thickening
- No fibrosis
- Superimposed infection diagnosed by microscopic identification of specific bacteria

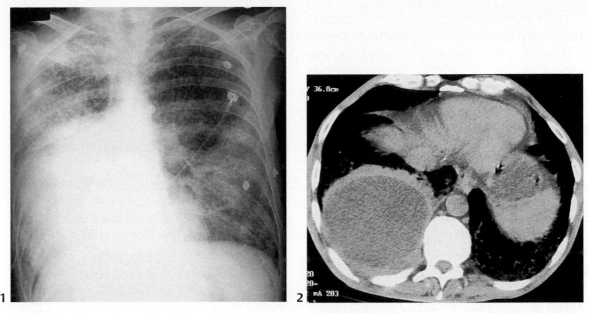

Figure 119E (1,2) PA chest radiograph **(1)** of a patient with alveolar proteinosis, fever, and leukocytosis demonstrates diffuse airspace and reticular opacities and a right lower lobe mass. Unenhanced chest CT (mediastinal window) **(2)** demonstrates a large spherical right lower lobe low-attenuation mass that represented a nocardia abscess.

Imaging Findings

RADIOGRAPHY

- Bilateral symmetrical patchy and diffuse airspace consolidations or ground-glass opacities; may manifest with nodular or reticular opacities (**Figs. 119A, 119B,** and **119E1**)
- Lower lobe predominance
- Normal lung volumes (**Figs. 119A** and **119B**)
- Rarely focal masses (**Fig. 119E**), lymphadenopathy, or pleural effusions

CT/HRCT

- Diffuse patchy bilateral ground-glass opacities with superimposed smooth thickening of interlobular septa ("crazy paving") (**Figs. 119C** and **119D**)
- Ground-glass opacities, airspace nodules, and confluent consolidations (**Figs. 119C** and **119D**)
- Distinct geographic demarcation between affected and normal lung parenchyma (**Figs. 119C** and **119D**)

Treatment

- Bilateral sequential whole-lung lavage under general anesthesia
- Repeated lobar lung lavage via bronchoscopy

Prognosis

- Generally favorable
- Spontaneous remission reported
- Repeated lavage procedures required in some cases

PITFALL

- The "crazy paving" pattern (described on HRCT) is not pathognomonic of alveolar proteinosis and has also been reported in neoplastic, infectious, idiopathic, inhalational, and hemorrhagic conditions.

Suggested Readings

Cheng SL, Chang HT, Lau HP, Lee LN, Yang PC. Pulmonary proteinosis: treatment by bronchofiberscopic lobar lavage. Chest 2002;122:1480–1485

Travis WD, Colby TV, Koss MN, Rosado-de-Christenson ML, Müller NL, King TE Jr. Idiopathic interstitial pneumonia and other diffuse parenchymal lung diseases. In: King DW, ed. Atlas of Nontumor Pathology: Non-Neoplastic Disorders of the Lower Respiratory Tract, fascicle 2, series 1. Washington, DC: American Registry of Pathology and Armed Forces Institute of Pathology, 2001:49–231

Webb WR, Müller NL, Naidich DP. Diseases characterized primarily by parenchymal opacification. In: Webb WR, Müller NL, Naidich DP, eds. High-Resolution CT of the Lung, 3rd ed. Philadelphia: Lippincott Williams and Wilkins, 2001:355–420

CASE 120 Eosinophilic Pneumonia

Clinical Presentation

An adult woman with a 3-year history of recurrent cough, bronchospasm, and peripheral eosinophilia

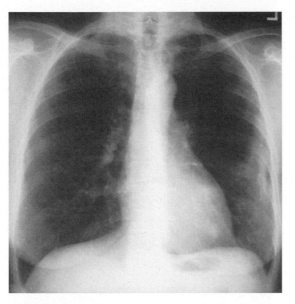

Figure 120A

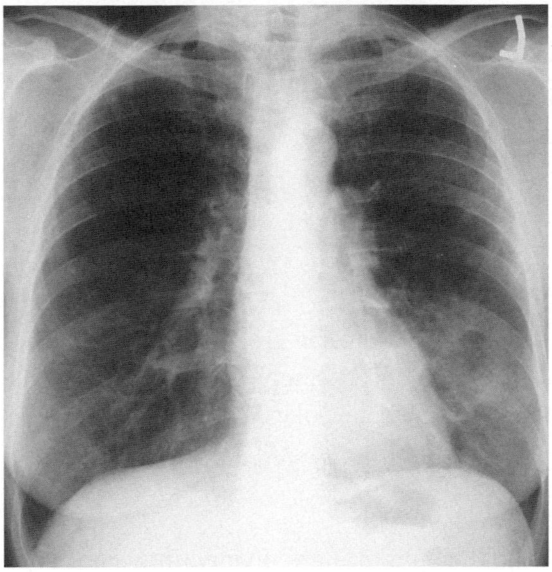

Figure 120B

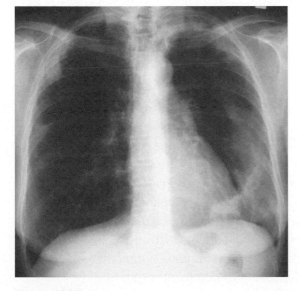

Figure 120C

Radiologic Findings

PA chest radiograph (**Fig. 120A**) demonstrates a peripheral consolidation in the left mid-to-lower lung. PA chest radiograph obtained 1 year later (**Fig. 120B**) demonstrates a subtle change in the morphology of the consolidation. PA chest radiograph obtained the following year (**Fig. 120C**) demonstrates progression of the left lung base consolidation and new bilateral peripheral upper lobe consolidations.

Diagnosis

Chronic eosinophilic pneumonia

Differential Diagnosis

- Infection (tuberculosis, other bacteria)
- Cryptogenic organizing pneumonia (COP)
- Pulmonary alveolar proteinosis
- Pulmonary hemorrhage
- Bronchioloalveolar carcinoma
- Pulmonary lymphoma

Discussion

Background

Eosinophilic lung diseases are a diverse group of disorders characterized by pulmonary consolidation associated with peripheral blood eosinophilia, tissue eosinophilia confirmed by lung biopsy, and/or increased eosinophils in bronchoalveolar lavage (BAL) fluid.

Etiology

Idiopathic eosinophilic pneumonias are divided into simple (Loeffler syndrome), acute, and chronic types. Idiopathic eosinophilic pneumonia may occur as a self-limited disorder or as a chronic process of greater than 1 month in duration; the latter is referred to as chronic eosinophilic pneumonia. Secondary eosinophilic pneumonia is reported in association with several conditions, including drug toxicity, parasitic or fungal infection, and vasculitis (Churg-Strauss syndrome).

Clinical Findings

Patients with Loeffler syndrome (LS) or simple eosinophilic pneumonia have minimal or absent pulmonary symptoms, and their pulmonary disease resolves spontaneously within 1 month. Acute eosinophilic pneumonia (AEP) is characterized by a rapid onset of fever, myalgias, pleuritic pain, and hypoxemia often progressing to respiratory failure and requiring mechanical ventilation. Chronic eosinophilic pneumonia (CEP) has an insidious onset of symptoms with cough, fever, dyspnea, weight loss, and asthma. The duration of symptoms is typically 3 months or longer. It affects adults in the fifth decade of life and women more commonly than men (2:1). Eosinophilic pneumonia may manifest as an allergic reaction to fungal antigens (usually *Aspergillus*) in patients with asthma, peripheral eosinophilia, and central bronchiectasis. It may also manifest with constitutional symptoms, fever, and respiratory complaints in patients with parasitic infestations. Mild to fulminant respiratory symptoms associated with eosinophilic pneumonia may develop in patients undergoing therapy with drugs such as methotrexate, nitrofurantoin, salicylates, sulfonamides, and many others. Patients with eosinophilic pneumonia respond promptly to corticosteroid therapy, a factor that helps confirm the diagnosis.

Pathology

GROSS

- Coalescent consolidations with a peripheral distribution

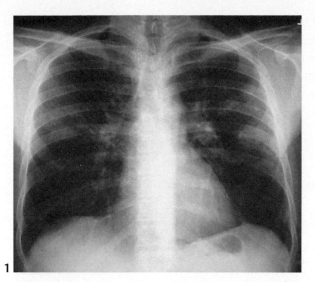
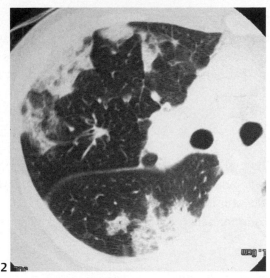

Figure 120D (1,2) PA chest radiograph **(1)** of a 32-year-old man who presented with cough, weight loss, and peripheral eosinophilia demonstrates patchy bilateral consolidations. Unenhanced HRCT (lung window) **(2)** targeted to the right lung demonstrates the peripheral distribution of the consolidations. The patient responded rapidly to corticosteroid therapy.

MICROSCOPIC

- Eosinophilic infiltration of the pulmonary alveoli and interstitium
- Absence of necrosis or fibrosis

Imaging Findings

RADIOGRAPHY

- LS: nonsegmental, multifocal migratory parenchymal consolidations that may exhibit a peripheral distribution, rarely single or multiple pulmonary nodules
- AEP: bilateral reticular opacities and pleural effusions with rapid progression to diffuse airspace disease
- CEP: bilateral nonsegmental airspace consolidations with a subpleural distribution in up to 60% of cases and a predilection for the upper and middle lung zones (**Figs. 120A, 120B, 120C,** and **120D1**); rarely nodules and pleural effusions
- Eosinophilic pneumonia secondary to drug reaction: consolidation, reticular and nodular opacities, lymphadenopathy, and pleural effusion
- Eosinophilic pneumonia secondary to parasitic infestation: fine diffuse reticular and nodular opacities with a lower lung zone predilection

CT/HRCT

- Peripheral distribution of airspace disease (which may not be evident on radiography) (**Fig. 120D2**)
- Patchy peripheral ground-glass opacities and consolidations with a middle and upper lung zone predilection in LS and CEP (**Fig. 120D2**)
- Band-like peripheral linear opacities in CEP, particularly with chronic or treated disease
- Ground-glass opacity (may be diffuse) with superimposed smooth septal thickening in AEP
- Nodular opacities in LS and AEP
- Pleural effusion in AEP and drug-induced eosinophilic pneumonia
- Lymphadenopathy in drug-induced eosinophilic pneumonia and rarely in CEP

Treatment

- Corticosteroids: prompt relief of symptoms and resolution of radiologic abnormalities
- Treatment of underlying conditions in cases of secondary eosinophilic pneumonia: antibiotics for patients with parasitic disease; steroids and drug withdrawal for those with drug-induced disease

Prognosis

- Generally favorable
- Spontaneous disease resolution or cure following first course of steroids in patients with LS and AEP and in many patients with CEP
- Common recurrences in CEP; may result in steroid dependence

Suggested Readings

Johkoh T, Müller NL, Akira N, et al. Eosinophilic lung diseases: diagnostic accuracy of thin-section CT in 111 patients. Radiology 2000;216:773–780

Kim Y, Lee KS, Choi D-C, Primack SL, Im J-G. The spectrum of eosinophilic lung disease: radiologic findings. J Comput Assist Tomogr 1997;21:920–930

Travis WD, Colby TV, Koss MN, Rosado-de-Christenson ML, Müller NL, King TE Jr. Idiopathic interstitial pneumonia and other diffuse parenchymal lung diseases. In: King DW, ed. Atlas of Nontumor Pathology: Non-Neoplastic Disorders of the Lower Respiratory Tract, fascicle 2, series 1. Washington, DC: American Registry of Pathology and Armed Forces Institute of Pathology, 2001: 49–231

CASE 121 Desquamative Interstitial Pneumonia (DIP)

Clinical Presentation

A 38-year-old woman, cigarette smoker, with increasing dyspnea for several months

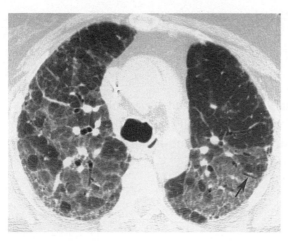

Figure 121A

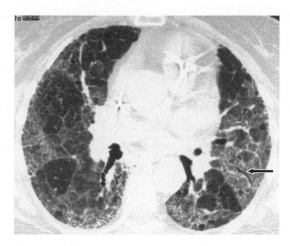

Figure 121B

(Figs. 121A and 121B courtesy of Diane C. Strollo, M.D., University of Pittsburgh Medical Center, Pittsburgh, Pennsylvania.)

Radiologic Findings

Unenhanced HRCT (lung window) (**Figs. 121A** and **121B**) demonstrates extensive bilateral areas of ground-glass attenuation, irregular juxtapleural linear opacities consistent with mild fibrosis, and traction bronchiectasis (arrow).

Diagnosis

Desquamative interstitial pneumonia (DIP)

Differential Diagnosis

- Chronic hypersensitivity pneumonitis
- Pulmonary drug toxicity
- Pulmonary hemorrhage
- Eosinophilic pneumonia

Discussion

Background

Desquamative interstitial pneumonia (DIP) is an idiopathic interstitial pneumonia (see Case 117) that occurs almost exclusively in current or former smokers and is characterized histologically by diffuse, marked intraalveolar accumulation of macrophages and minimal interstitial fibrosis. The term *desquamative* is a misnomer based on the previous but erroneous concept that the intraalveolar cells represented desquamated pneumocytes. Some authors have suggested that a more technically correct terminology for DIP would be alveolar macrophage pneumonia. The incidence of DIP is much lower than that of usual interstitial pneumonia (UIP). The diagnosis of DIP requires open or thoracoscopic lung biopsy.

Etiology

The etiology of DIP is unknown, but the majority of affected patients are current or former cigarette smokers.

Clinical Findings

Patients are typically younger, present with more acute pulmonary symptoms, and have milder pulmonary function abnormalities than those with UIP. Patients with DIP typically present with cough and dyspnea. Pulmonary function tests typically reveal a restrictive pattern and hypoxemia.

Pathology

- Diffuse, marked intraalveolar macrophage accumulation
- Mild thickening of the alveolar walls
- Mild interstitial thickening
- Very little fibrosis
- Little remodeling and/or architectural distortion

Imaging Findings

RADIOGRAPHY

- Normal chest radiograph in 3 to 22% of patients
- Bilateral, symmetric ground-glass opacification
- Bibasilar, irregular linear opacities
- Lower lung zone predominance
- Preserved lung volumes
- Nodules and honeycombing (10%)

CT/HRCT

- Bilateral lower lobe ground-glass opacities (**Figs. 121B** and **121C2**)
- Peripheral irregular linear opacities and architectural distortion (**Fig. 121C**)
- Honeycomb lung, traction bronchiectasis (33%) (**Figs. 121A** and **121C2**)
- Occasionally small cysts (**Fig. 121C**)

Treatment

- Cessation of smoking
- Corticosteroids

Prognosis

- Five- and 10-year survival of 95.2% and 69.6%, respectively (better than other interstitial pneumonias)

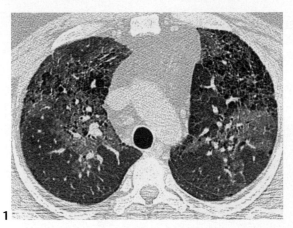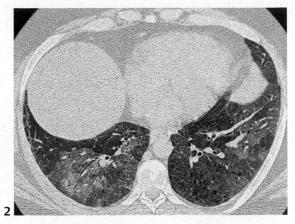

Figure 121C (1,2) Unenhanced HRCT (lung window) of a 29-year-old man with a 14-year history of cigarette smoking and increasing dyspnea for 1 year demonstrates extensive bilateral ground-glass opacities and irregular juxtapleural linear opacities consistent with mild fibrosis. Small cystic areas are demonstrated bilaterally, an uncommon but recognized imaging feature of DIP. The combination of ground-glass opacity and small cysts is suggestive of DIP. (Courtesy of Diane C. Strollo, M.D., University of Pittsburgh Medical Center, Pittsburgh, Pennsylvania.)

- Five-year survival of 100% reported in the absence of honeycombing
- Progression to end-stage fibrosis in some patients.

PEARL_____

- Findings of proximal acinar emphysema may also be present, as most patients with desquamative interstitial pneumonia are current or former cigarette smokers.

Suggested Readings

Hartman TE, Primack SL, Kang EY, et al. Disease progression in usual interstitial pneumonia compared with desquamative interstitial pneumonia: assessment with serial CT. Chest 1996;110:378–382

McAdams HP, Rosado-de-Christenson ML, Wehunt WD, Fishback NF. The alphabet soup revisited: the chronic interstitial pneumonias in the 1990s. Radiographics 1996;16:1009–1033

Travis WD, Colby TV, Koss MN, Rosado-de-Christenson ML, Müller NL, King TE Jr. Diffuse parenchymal lung diseases. In: King DW, ed. Atlas of Nontumor Pathology: Non-Neoplastic Disorders of the Lower Respiratory Tract, first series, fascicle 2. Washington, DC: American Registry of Pathology; 2002:109–115

CASE 122 Lymphocytic Interstitial Pneumonia (LIP)

Clinical Presentation

A 31-year-old woman with cough, dyspnea, and weight loss

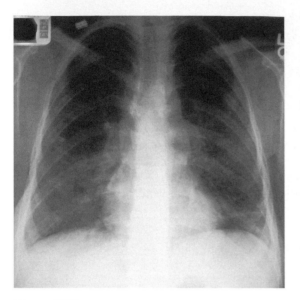

Figure 122A

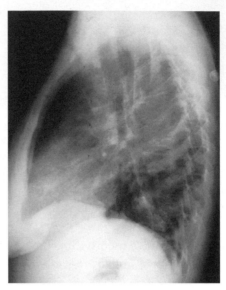

Figure 122B

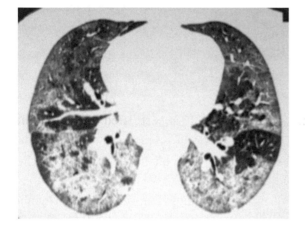

Figure 122C

Radiologic Findings

PA (**Fig. 122A**) and lateral (**Fig. 122B**) chest radiographs show diffuse, bilateral, perihilar, and lower lobe ground-glass opacities, incidental calcified upper lobe granulomas, and right paratracheal lymph nodes. Discoid atelectasis is present at the left base. Unenhanced chest CT (lung window) (**Fig. 122C**) reveals bilateral, patchy ground-glass opacities and consolidation that are more extensive in the lower lobes.

Diagnosis

Lymphocytic interstitial pneumonia (LIP)

Differential Diagnosis

- Immunocompetent patients
  - Nonspecific interstitial pneumonia (NSIP)
  - Hypersensitivity pneumonitis (HP)
  - Various drug reactions
  - Sarcoidosis
  - Low-grade B cell lymphoma; mucosa-associated lymphoid tissue (MALT)
  - Lymphangitic carcinomatosis
- Patients with HIV-AIDS
  - *Pneumocystis jiroveci* pneumonia
  - *Mycobacterium avium-intracellulare* complex infection
  - Fungal pneumonia

Discussion

Background

The incidence of LIP is unknown. It comprises several disorders associated with dysproteinemia, autoimmunity (e.g., connective tissue diseases, multicentric Castleman disease), and viral infections (e.g., human immunodeficiency virus). In a small subset of patients, LIP may occur as an idiopathic, nonneoplastic, inflammatory process.

Etiology

The etiology and pathogenesis are varied. An immunologic basis for LIP is postulated because of the association of LIP with other immunologic disorders (e.g., AIDS and Sjögren syndrome). Some cases likely represent a form of hypersensitivity pneumonitis, whereas other cases may be caused by viral infection (e.g., HIV, Epstein-Barr).

Clinical Findings

LIP is most often seen in HIV-positive children, and is considered an AIDS-defining diagnosis in children less than 13 years of age. Less than 1% of HIV-infected adults develop LIP. Adults who are not infected with HIV and develop LIP often have underlying autoimmune disease, most commonly Sjögren syndrome. Approximately 1% of adults with Sjögren syndrome have LIP, whereas up to 25% of adults with LIP have Sjögren syndrome. Whether idiopathic or related to an underlying systemic disease, most adults with LIP are women in the fourth to seventh decades of life, who present with cough and/or dyspnea (50–80%), and 60% of patients have dysproteinemia and hypergammaglobulinemia. B-cell lymphoma may develop in patients with LIP, especially those with Sjögren syndrome; 5% of patients with LIP develop disseminated malignant lymphoma.

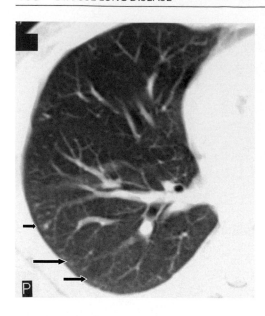

Figure 122D Unenhanced chest CT (lung window) targeted to the right lower lobe of a young man with LIP and multicentric Castleman disease demonstrates subtle ill-defined centrilobular nodules in the lower lobe (arrows).

Pathology

GROSS

- Pink-tan or tan-gray diffusely firm lungs
- Advanced disease: lung contraction and cobblestone appearance of the pleural surface

MICROSCOPIC

- Diffuse interstitial infiltrate of mononuclear cells with lymphocyte predominance
- Occasionally plasma cells predominate.

Imaging Findings

RADIOGRAPHY

- Preserved lung volume (**Figs. 122A** and **122B**)
- Nonspecific bilateral reticular-nodular and ground-glass opacities with or without consolidation (**Figs. 122A** and **122B**)
- Lower lung zone predilection (**Figs. 122A** and **122B**)
- Nodular pattern and lymphadenopathy more common in patients with AIDS
- Rare pleural effusions

HRCT

- Diffuse, bilateral, patchy areas of ground-glass opacity (**Fig. 122C**) and/or poorly defined centrilobular nodules (**Fig. 122D**)
- Small juxtapleural nodules (86%) (**Fig. 122D**)
- Peribronchovascular bundle thickening (86%)
- Mild interlobular septal thickening (82%)
- Cystic airspaces (68%)

Treatment

- Immunocompetent patients: corticosteroids with variable response
- Immunocompromised patients with AIDS and progressive symptoms: highly active antiretroviral therapy (HAART)

Prognosis

- Variable clinical course; spontaneous remissions reported
- Death within 5 years in one third to one half of affected immunocompetent adult patients from infectious complications secondary to immunosuppressive drug therapy, respiratory insufficiency, or malignant lymphoma
- Most immunocompromised patients with AIDS and LIP have mild disease that may spontaneously resolve.
- Rarely, LIP may evolve into lymphoma.

PEARLS_____

- Cystic airspaces are seen more commonly in LIP (82%) than in lymphoma (2%).
- Airspace consolidation is seen more commonly in lymphoma (66%) than in LIP (18%).
- Nodules measuring 10 to 30 mm are seen more commonly in lymphoma (41%) than in LIP (6%).
- Pleural effusions are seen more commonly in lymphoma.

Suggested Readings

Honda O, Johkoh T, Ichikado K, et al. Differential diagnosis of lymphocytic interstitial pneumonia and malignant lymphoma on high-resolution CT. AJR Am J Roentgenol 1999;173:71–74

Johkoh T, Müller NL, Pickford HA, et al. Lymphocytic interstitial pneumonia: thin-section CT findings in 22 patients. Radiology 1999;212:567–572

Travis WD, Colby TV, Koss MN, Rosado-de-Christenson ML, Müller NL, King TE Jr. Reactive lymphoid lesions. In: King DW, ed. Atlas of Nontumor Pathology: Non-Neoplastic Disorders of the Lower Respiratory Tract, first series, fascicle 2. Washington, DC: American Registry of Pathology; 2002: 266–276

Webb WR, Müller NL, Naidich DP. Disease characterized primarily by nodular or reticulonodular opacities. In: High-Resolution CT of the Lung, 3rd ed. Philadelphia: Lippincott Williams & Wilkins, 2001:276–277

CASE 123 Cryptogenic Organizing Pneumonia (COP)

Clinical Presentation

A 56-year-old woman treated for presumed community-acquired pneumonia for the past 2 months without improvement complains of dyspnea, a persistent nonproductive cough, and a recent 8-pound weight loss.

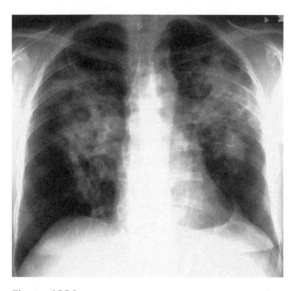

Figure 123A

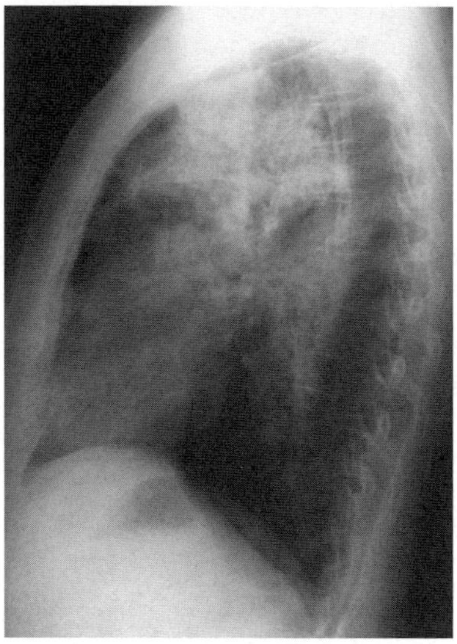

Figure 123B

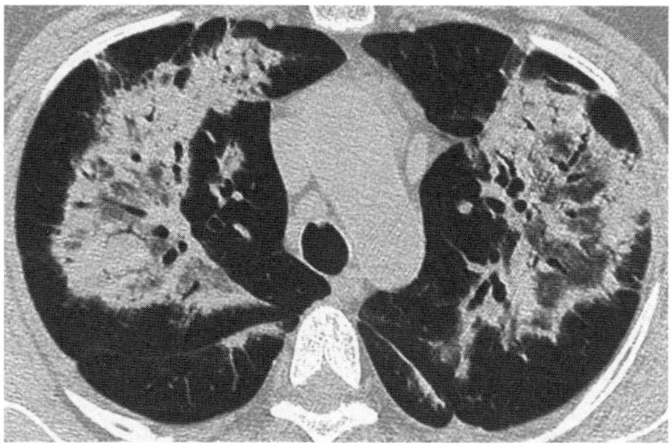

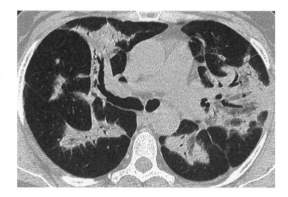

Figure 123C

Figure 123D

Radiologic Findings

PA (**Fig. 123A**) and lateral (**Fig. 123B**) chest radiographs demonstrate bilateral perihilar and upper lobe nonsegmental consolidations. Unenhanced HRCT (lung window) (**Figs. 123C** and **Fig. 123D**) reveals patchy bilateral airspace consolidations and ground-glass opacities with a peribronchial distribution. Bronchial wall thickening and bronchial dilatation are seen in the areas of parenchymal opacification.

Diagnosis

Cryptogenic organizing pneumonia (COP) (idiopathic bronchiolitis obliterans with organizing pneumonia)

Differential Diagnosis

- Acute interstitial pneumonia (AIP)
- Nonspecific interstitial pneumonia (NSIP)
- Diffuse alveolar damage (DAD)
- Chronic eosinophilic pneumonia (CEP)
- Desquamative interstitial pneumonia (DIP)/alveolar macrophage pneumonia (AMP)

Discussion

Background

Cryptogenic organizing pneumonia (COP) is a form of chronic interstitial lung disease. Because the clinical, functional, radiologic, and HRCT features of COP are primarily the result of an organizing pneumonia, the American Thoracic Society/European Respiratory Multidisciplinary Consensus Classification Committee proposed cryptogenic organizing pneumonia (COP) as an alternative designation to that of bronchiolitis obliterans with organizing pneumonia (BOOP) in idiopathic cases. The exact incidence and prevalence of COP are unknown. The diagnosis of COP is usually made on open lung biopsy.

Etiology

Most cases of COP are idiopathic. Numerous conditions may be associated with COP-like reactions, including, but not limited to, collagen vascular diseases, infection (e.g., HIV, *Pneumocystis jiroveci*, *Mycoplasma pneumoniae*), hypersensitivity pneumonitis, vasculitides (e.g., Wegener granulomatosis), intravenous drug abuse (e.g., cocaine), drug reactions, toxic fume inhalation, and lung and chest wall irradiation.

Clinical Findings

Patients affected with COP typically present in the fifth to sixth decades of life with symptoms of a community-acquired pneumonia. Most patients have had symptoms for less than 2 months, and many patients have had symptoms for only 1 to 2 weeks. A persistent nonproductive cough and dyspnea are common. A flu-like illness may herald the onset of COP. Weight loss of under 10 pounds is common. Inspiratory crackles may be heard, but wheezing is rare. Pulmonary function studies often show a restrictive pattern. Diffusing capacity for carbon monoxide (DLCO) is reduced. Hypoxemia is usually present. Fifty percent of patients with COP have leukocytosis. An elevated erythrocyte sedimentation rate (ESR) and positive C-reactive protein are common.

Pathology

GROSS

- Patchy, ill-defined nodular consolidations without scarring or honeycombing

MICROSCOPIC

- Granulation tissue polyps in the lumina of bronchioles and alveolar ducts
- Patchy areas of organizing pneumonia consisting of mononuclear cells and foamy macrophages
- Preservation of lung architecture

Imaging Findings

RADIOGRAPHY

- Nonspecific abnormalities
- Patchy, nonsegmental, unilateral, or bilateral airspace consolidations (**Figs. 123A** and **123B**)
- Small nodular opacities with or without airspace consolidations
- Less commonly irregular reticular opacities

HRCT

- Patchy unilateral/bilateral airspace consolidation (80%) (**Figs. 123C** and **123D**)
- Ground-glass opacity (60%) or crazy paving
- Juxtapleural or peribronchial distribution (63%) (**Figs. 123C** and **123D**)
- Bronchial wall thickening and dilatation in areas of airspace disease (**Figs. 123C** and **123D**)
- Centrilobular nodules ranging 1 to 10 mm diameter (50%)
- Large nodules or masses (8 mm–5 cm diameter) with irregular margins (88%); air bronchograms (45%); pleural tails (38%); spiculated margins (35%)
- Small pleural effusions (30–35%) or pleural thickening
- Irregular linear opacities (14%); honeycombing uncommon
- Disease often more severe in lower lung zones

Treatment

- Complete recovery and radiographic normalization in two thirds of patients treated with corticosteroids
- Persistent disease: one third of patients
- Cytotoxic drugs (e.g., cyclophosphamide, azathioprine) for corticosteroid failures: limited success

Prognosis

- Dramatic clinical response with improvement in days or weeks
- Relapses common 2 to 3 months after steroid withdrawal
- Worse prognosis in patients with primarily interstitial opacities

PEARLS

- Idiopathic pulmonary fibrosis (IPF) and COP/BOOP can appear clinically and functionally similar. The duration of symptoms and response to steroids in patients with COP aid in differentiation.
- The presence of consolidation and the paucity of reticular opacities differentiate COP from usual interstitial pneumonia (UIP) on imaging.

Suggested Readings

Arakawa H, Kurihara Y, Niimi H, Nakajima Y, Johkoh T, Nakamaura H. Bronchiolitis obliterans with organizing pneumonia versus chronic eosinophilic pneumonia: high-resolution CT findings in 81 patients. AJR Am J Roentgenol 2001;176:1053–1058

Lynch DA. High-resolution CT of idiopathic interstitial pneumonias. Radiol Clin North Am 2001;39: 1153–1170

Oikonomou A, Hansell DM. Organizing pneumonia: the many morphological faces. Eur Radiol 2002;12:1486–1496

Travis WD, Colby TV, Koss MN, Rosado-de-Christenson ML, Müller NL, King TE Jr. Reactive lymphoid lesions. In: King DW, ed. Atlas of Nontumor Pathology: Non-Neoplastic Disorders of the Lower Respiratory Tract, first series, fascicle 2. Washington, DC: American Registry of Pathology; 2002: 82–89

Webb WR, Müller NL, Naidich DP. Disease characterized primarily by nodular or reticulonodular opacities. In: High-Resolution CT of the Lung, 3rd ed. Philadelphia: Lippincott Williams & Wilkins, 2001:373–378

CASE 124 Diffuse Alveolar Hemorrhage

Clinical Presentation

A 22-year-old man with recent sore throat, chills, and fever, subsequently developed hematuria, dysuria, cough, dyspnea, hemoptysis, and respiratory failure.

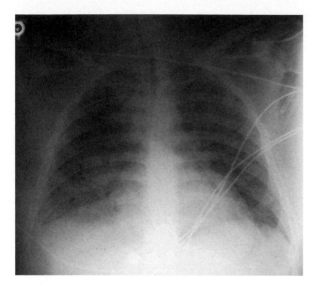

Figure 124A

Radiologic Findings

AP (**Fig. 124A**) chest radiograph reveals diffuse bilateral ground-glass opacities and right middle and lower lobe consolidation. Life support tubes and lines are appropriately positioned.

Diagnosis

Diffuse alveolar hemorrhage; Goodpasture syndrome

Differential Diagnosis

- Idiopathic pulmonary hemorrhage
- Other diffuse pulmonary hemorrhage syndromes
  - Wegener granulomatosis
  - Henoch-Schönlein purpura
  - Microscopic polyangiitis pauci-immune glomerulonephritis
  - Systemic lupus erythematosus
- Drugs
  - Drug-induced coagulopathy
  - Penicillamine
  - Nitrofurantoin

- Amiodarone
- Crack cocaine
- Environmental exposure
  - Paraquat
  - Pesticides
  - Leather conditioners
  - Isocyanates
- Bone marrow and heart-lung transplantation
- Dieulafoy disease (e.g., endobronchial vascular malformation)

Discussion

Background

Diffuse alveolar hemorrhage (DAH) is characterized by extensive intraalveolar hemorrhage. DAH may be acute, chronic, recurrent, idiopathic, or associated with a variety of systemic disorders.

Etiology

Goodpasture syndrome is an anti-basement membrane antibody disease (ABMABD) that affects the lung alone in 10% patients (e.g., DAH), the kidneys alone in 20 to 40% patients (e.g., glomerulonephritis), and both organ systems in 60 to 80% patients.

Clinical Findings

Most patients with DAH experience acute dyspnea, which may progress to respiratory failure, and hemoptysis. However, hemoptysis may be absent even with severe intraalveolar hemorrhage. Uveitis, fever, arthralgias, arthritis, and dermatologic leukocytoclastic vasculitis may be clues to the diagnosis. Elevated erythrocyte sedimentation rate, elevated white blood count, falling hematocrit levels, and impaired renal function may be seen. Elevated serum antineutrophil cytoplasmic antibody (ANCA) to myeloperoxidase may also be seen, depending on the underlying systemic disease. Hypoxemia is invariably present, often severe, and affected patients may require ventilatory support. Most patients with Goodpasture syndrome are young Caucasian men presenting with recent viral illness, cough, fever, respiratory alkalosis, hemoptysis (80–90%), and renal disease (e.g., azotemia, hematuria, proteinuria, granular casts). Alternatively, Goodpasture syndrome may occur in elderly women with kidney disease. The mean age at presentation is 35 years, and men are affected two to nine times as often as women. Over 90% of patients have antiglomerular basement membrane antibodies. Recurrent episodes of pulmonary hemorrhage may be associated with the development of interstitial fibrosis and eventual respiratory failure.

Pathology

GROSS

- Acute hemorrhage: dark red/purple lungs with blood in the airways
- Chronic hemorrhage: brown/firm lungs with or without fibrosis

MICROSCOPIC

- Intraalveolar red blood cells and hemosiderin-laden macrophages; coarse granular hemosiderin deposits; erythrophagocytosis; neutrophilic capillaritis

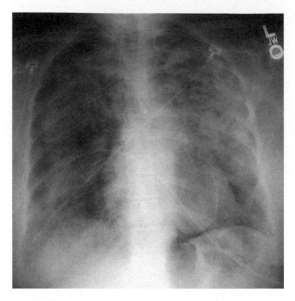

Figure 124B AP chest radiograph of a 57-year-old woman with Wegener granulomatosis and hemoptysis reveals diffuse bilateral airspace consolidations due to diffuse pulmonary hemorrhage.

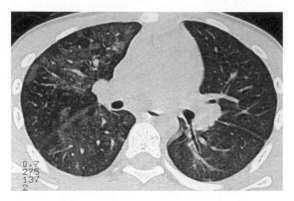

Figure 124C Unenhanced HRCT (lung window) of a 12-year-old boy with idiopathic pulmonary hemorrhage who presents with cough, dyspnea, fatigue, iron-deficiency anemia, and repeated bouts of hemoptysis demonstrates patchy ground-glass opacities in the right upper and lower lobes.

Imaging Findings

RADIOGRAPHY

- Patchy or diffuse bilateral ground-glass opacities or frank consolidation (**Figs. 124A** and **124B**)
- Widespread or perihilar/basilar opacities gradually resolve over 2 to 3 weeks after cessation of hemorrhage.
- Following acute hemorrhage, replacement of airspace opacities by interstitial opacities or septal thickening

CT/HRCT

- Patchy or diffuse ground-glass opacity or consolidation (**Fig. 124C**)
- Ill-defined centrilobular nodules
- Interlobular septal thickening develops over several days.
- Crazy-paving pattern

Treatment

- Directed toward underlying systemic disease
- Intravenous corticosteroids: acute fulminant disease
- Immunosuppressive therapy (e.g., cyclophosphamide, azathioprine)
- ABMABD: plasmapheresis to remove circulating antibodies and immunosuppressive agents
- Renal transplantation for patients who develop end-stage renal disease

Prognosis

- Fulminant clinical course
- Pulmonary fibrosis resulting from repeated hemorrhage

- Long-term survival in over 50% of patients with Goodpasture syndrome; dialysis dependence common
- Mean survival of 3 to 5 years in patients with idiopathic pulmonary hemorrhage
  - Death from massive pulmonary hemorrhage (25%)
  - Persistent active disease with repeated hemoptysis, complicating pulmonary fibrosis, and cor pulmonale (25%)
  - Persistent anemia and dyspnea (25%)
  - Recovery without recurrence (25%)

Suggested Readings

Ball JA, Young KR Jr. Pulmonary manifestations of Goodpasture's syndrome: antiglomerular basement membrane disease and related disorders. Clin Chest Med 1998;19:777–791

Travis WD, Colby TV, Koss MN, Rosado-de-Christenson ML, Müller NL, King TE Jr. Reactive lymphoid lesions. In: King DW, ed. Atlas of Nontumor Pathology: Non-Neoplastic Disorders of the Lower Respiratory Tract, first series, fascicle 2. Washington, DC: American Registry of Pathology, 2002: 176–186

Webb WR, Müller NL, Naidich DP. Disease characterized primarily by parenchymal opacification. In: High-Resolution CT of the Lung, 3rd ed. Philadelphia: Lippincott Williams & Wilkins, 2001:408

CASE 125 Alveolar Microlithiasis

Clinical Presentation

A 57-year-old woman with exercise intolerance and progressive dyspnea

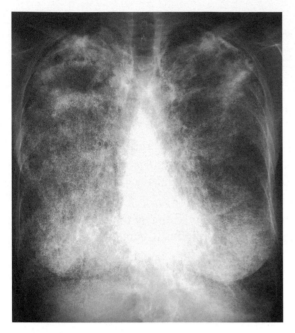

Figure 125A

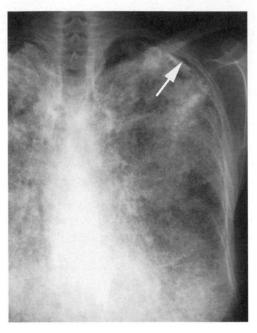

Figure 125B

Radiologic Findings

PA chest radiograph (**Fig. 125A**) and coned-down radiograph of the left lung (**Fig. 125B**) demonstrate dense diffuse bilateral micronodular parenchymal opacities with confluence and calcification in the lung apices. Note the "black pleura line" (arrow) adjacent to the apical calcification.

Diagnosis

Alveolar microlithiasis

Differential Diagnosis

- Metastatic calcification
- Pulmonary ossification
- Postinfectious or granulomatous calcification
- Amyloidosis

Discussion

Background

Alveolar microlithiasis is a rare disorder characterized by accumulation of calcium phosphate calcospherites within the alveolar spaces.

478

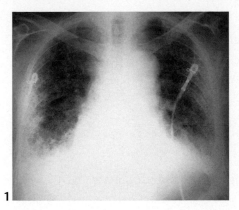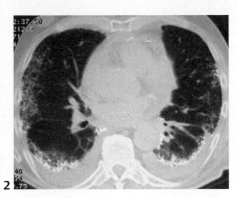

Figure 125C (1,2) AP chest radiograph **(1)** of a man with alveolar microlithiasis who presented with dyspnea demonstrates bilateral dense peripheral micronodular parenchymal opacities. Unenhanced chest CT (lung window) **(2)** demonstrates bilateral pleural effusions and the peripheral distribution of the calcified micronodules. (Courtesy of H. Page McAdams, M.D., Duke University Medical Center, Durham, North Carolina)

Etiology

The etiology is unknown.

Clinical Findings

Affected patients are typically adults although the disease has also been reported in children. Patients with alveolar microlithiasis may be asymptomatic or may present with cough, chest pain, and/or dyspnea. Some patients expectorate microliths. Alveolar microlithiasis may progress to interstitial fibrosis with resultant respiratory insufficiency and respiratory failure. Many cases have been reported in Europe, and a familial association is recognized.

Pathology

GROSS

- Individual calcospherites within airspaces on cut lung sections
- Hardened gritty appearance of affected lung

MICROSCOPIC

- Calcospherites: lamellar rounded calcific stones within individual alveoli
- Range from 0.01 to 0.3 mm in diameter
- Normal pulmonary interstitium or extensive interstitial fibrosis

Imaging Findings

RADIOGRAPHY

- Numerous well-defined micronodules measuring approximately 1 mm diffusely distributed throughout the lungs, so-called sandstorm appearance (may be superimposed on interstitial opacities), densest at the lung bases (**Fig. 125C1**)
- Overpenetrated radiography for visualization of individual microliths in cases of profuse lung involvement (**Fig. 125B**)
- "Lucent" mediastinum and "black pleura line" with profuse adjacent microlithiasis (**Fig. 125B**)
- Findings of pulmonary fibrosis and pulmonary hypertension

CT

- Widespread calcific nodules with peripheral, basilar, and posterior distribution and along bronchovascular bundles (**Fig. 125C2**)
- Ground-glass and micronodular opacities in early involvement
- Paraseptal emphysema, small juxtapleural cysts (some suggest the latter as the etiology of the "black pleura line")
- Reticular opacities, interstitial thickening

SCINTIGRAPHY

- Intense pulmonary uptake of technetium 99m (Tc-99m)-methylene diphosphonate (MDP)

Treatment

- No treatment for asymptomatic patients
- Lung transplantation for patients with respiratory insufficiency

Prognosis

- Generally favorable
- Successful lung transplantation reported

Suggested Readings

Cluzel P, Grenier P, Bernadac P, Laurent F, Picard JD. Pulmonary alveolar microlithiasis: CT findings. J Comput Assist Tomogr 1991;15:938–942

Mittal BR, Gupta D, Jindal SK. Radioisotope bone scanning in pulmonary alveolar microlithiasis. Clin Nucl Med 2000;25:474–475

Travis WD, Colby TV, Koss MN, Rosado-de-Christenson ML, Müller NL, King TE Jr. Idiopathic interstitial pneumonia and other diffuse parenchymal lung diseases. In: King WD, ed. Atlas of Nontumor Pathology: Non-Neoplastic Disorders of the Lower Respiratory Tract, first series, fascicle 2. Washington, DC: American Registry of Pathology and Armed Forces Institute of Pathology, 2001:49–231

CASE 126 Exogenous Lipoid Pneumonia

Clinical Presentation

A 52-year-old woman with a chronic, nonproductive cough

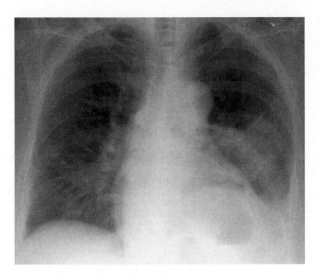

Figure 126A

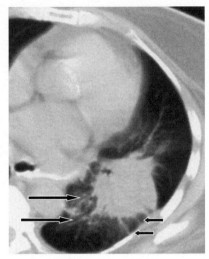

Figure 126B

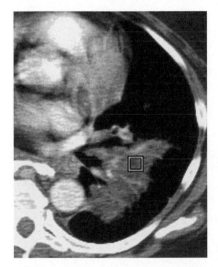

Figure 126C

Radiologic Findings

PA chest (**Fig. 126A**) radiograph shows an ill-defined left lower lobe consolidation and elevation of the ipsilateral diaphragm. Coned-down contrast-enhanced chest CT (lung window) (**Fig. 126B**) reveals a corresponding mass-like consolidation and surrounding ground-glass opacities with interlobular septal thickening (short arrows) and fibrosis (long arrows). Contrast-enhanced chest CT (mediastinal window) (**Fig. 126C**) shows low-attenuation areas in the consolidation. The region of interest demonstrated attenuation coefficients ranging between −11 and −72 Hounsfield units (HU).

Diagnosis

Exogenous lipoid pneumonia

Differential Diagnosis

- Infection
- Primary lung cancer
- Lymphoma

Discussion

Background

Exogenous lipoid pneumonia is an uncommon cause of parenchymal opacification secondary to the chronic aspiration or inhalation of animal, vegetable, or petroleum-based oils or fats.

Etiology

Mineral oil is responsible in most cases of exogenous lipoid pneumonia. Infants with feeding difficulties may aspirate oil when it is used as a lubricant. Elderly patients with constipation may aspirate oil ingested as a laxative. Other potential sources of exogenous lipoid pneumonia include oil-based nose drops, camphor and eucalyptus oil–based cough suppressants and nasal decongestants, lip gloss, and petroleum jelly applied to the face and nose for various reasons. Aspiration of animal oils may be associated with the ingestion of milk or milk products, and cod liver and shark liver oil. Most vegetable oil aspirations occur while eating or with regurgitation of gastric contents. Pure vegetable oil aspiration is uncommon. The pathogenesis of mineral and vegetable oil–related fibrosis is uncertain. The release of lysosomal enzymes by lipid-laden macrophages may be responsible for pulmonary fibrosis in some cases. Animal fats are hydrolyzed by lung lipases into fatty acids that may cause acute hemorrhagic pneumonitis.

Clinical Findings

Most patients with mineral oil aspiration are asymptomatic. Some patients complain of nonproductive cough and chest pain. The signs and symptoms associated with animal and vegetable oil aspiration are similar to those seen with acute bronchopneumonia (see Section 5).

Pathology

ASPIRATED MINERAL OIL

- Intraalveolar infiltrate of macrophages and mild inflammatory reaction
- Fine vacuolation within macrophages resulting from emulsified and phagocytosed oil
- Coalescence of small oil droplets into large, round oil droplets located within multinucleated giant cells

ASPIRATED ANIMAL AND VEGETABLE OIL

- Acute bronchopneumonia with edema, intraalveolar hemorrhage, and a mixed polymorphonuclear and mononuclear infiltrate
- Finely vacuolated macrophages
- Giant cell and granuloma formation

Imaging Findings

RADIOGRAPHY

- Relatively homogeneous airspace consolidation in one or more segments (**Fig. 126A**)
- Consolidation of variable size; may be several centimeters in diameter, and may exhibit poorly defined or sharply defined margins (**Fig. 126A**)
- Chronic cases: reticular opacities
- Multiple mass-like opacities; rare
- Cavitation in cases of secondary anaerobic infection

CT/HRCT

- Lower lobe predominance (**Figs. 126B** and **126C**)
- Patchy unilateral or bilateral airspace consolidation (**Figs. 126B** and **126C**)
- Consolidation with internal low or fat attenuation (i.e., attenuation less than the chest wall musculature but greater than the subcutaneous fat) (**Fig. 126C**)
- Ground-glass opacities with "crazy paving" pattern
- Centrilobular nodules
- Chronic cases: juxtapleural pulmonary fibrosis, architectural distortion, and honeycombing
- Foci of calcification rare

MR

- High signal intensity on both T1- and T2-weighted images (i.e., lipid content)
- Chemical-shift/in-phase/out-of-phase imaging useful to make a specific diagnosis

Treatment

- Discontinuation of offending agent
- Protection of airway to prevent aspiration

Prognosis

- Increased risk of infection with nontuberculous mycobacteria (e.g., *Mycobacterium fortuitum*, *Mycobacterium chelonae*) and of devolving primary lung cancer
- Chronic aspiration potentially complicated by restrictive lung disease and cor pulmonale
- Clinical course and outcome of animal and vegetable oil aspiration: similar to that seen with aspiration of gastric secretions

PEARLS_____

- Exogenous lipoid pneumonia predominantly affects the lower lobes; the posterior segments of upper lobes, superior segments of lower lobes, and middle lobes are affected less often.
- Lipoid pneumonia may be a cause of false-positive F-18-fluorodeoxyglucose (FDG) uptake on positron emission tomography (PET) imaging.

Suggested Readings

Fraser RS, Müller NL, Coleman N, Paré PD. Aspiration of solid foreign material and lipids. In: Fraser RS, Müller NL, Coleman N, Paré PD, eds. Fraser and Paré's Diagnosis of Diseases of the Chest, 4th ed. Philadelphia: Saunders, 1999: 2500–2507

Gaerte SC, Meyer CA, Winer-Muram HT, Tarver RD, Conces DJ Jr. Fat-containing lesions of the chest. RadioGraphics 2002; 22(Special No.): S61–78

Gimenez A, Franquet T, Prats R, Estrada P, Villalba J, Bague S. Unusual primary lung tumors: a radiologic-pathologic overview. Radiographics 2002;22:601–619

Tahon F, Berthezene Y, Hominal S, et al. Exogenous lipoid pneumonia with unusual CT pattern and FDG positron emission tomography scan findings. Eur Radiol 2002;12(suppl 4):S171–S173

Webb WR, Müller NL, Naidich DP. Disease characterized primarily by parenchymal opacification. In: High-Resolution CT of the Lung, 3rd ed. Philadelphia: Lippincott Williams & Wilkins, 2001: 393–396

CASE 127 Sarcoidosis

Clinical Presentation

A 52-year-old woman with dyspnea and uveitis

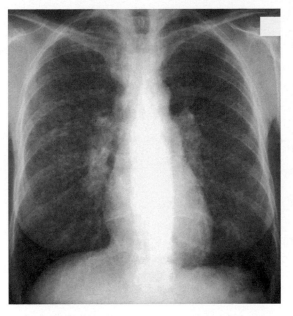

Figure 127A

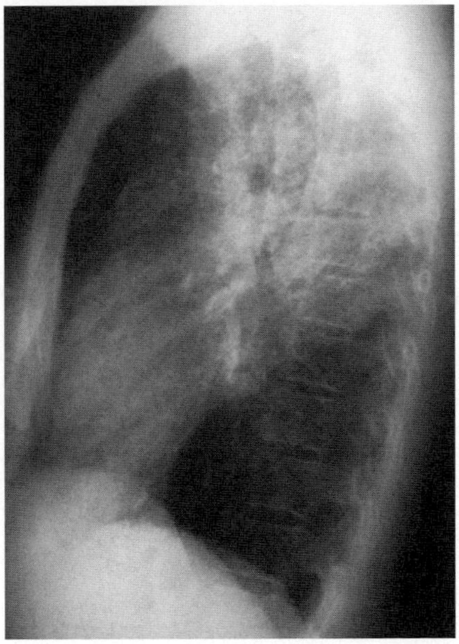

Figure 127B

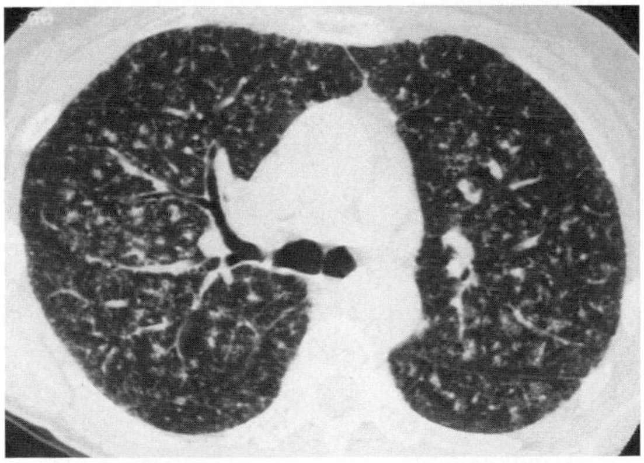

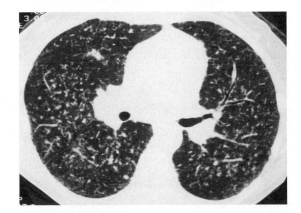

Figure 127C

Figure 127D

(From Miller BH, Rosado de Christenson ML, McAdams HP, Fishback NF. Thoracic sarcoidosis: radiologic-pathologic correlation. RadioGraphics 1995;15:421–437, with permission.)

Radiologic Findings

PA (**Fig. 127A**) and lateral (**Fig. 127B**) chest radiographs demonstrate profuse bilateral small pulmonary nodules most numerous in the upper and middle lung zones in association with symmetric bilateral hilar lymphadenopathy. Unenhanced HRCT (lung window) (**Figs. 127C** and **127D**) demonstrates multifocal micronodules along perilymphatic areas, the juxtapleural regions, the interlobular septa, and the bronchovascular bundles.

485

Diagnosis

Sarcoidosis

Differential Diagnosis

- Lymphangitic carcinomatosis
- Silicosis
- Lymphoproliferative disorder

Discussion

Background

Sarcoidosis is a systemic granulomatous disease that typically affects the lung and the lymphatic system.

Etiology

The etiology of sarcoidosis remains unknown. An abnormal immune response to an unidentified antigen is postulated. There may be a genetic predisposition, as familial cases have been reported.

Clinical Findings

Most affected patients with sarcoidosis are under the age of 40 years, with a peak of incidence between 20 and 29 years. The annual incidence of sarcoidosis in the United States is 35.5 per 100,000 persons for African Americans and 10.9 per 100,000 for Caucasians. Löfgren syndrome is an acute form of sarcoidosis characterized by fever, polyarthralgias, erythema nodosum, and bilateral hilar lymphadenopathy. Heerfordt syndrome is the association of fever, parotid enlargement, facial palsy, and anterior uveitis. Lupus pernio is a chronic form of sarcoidosis typified by indurated plaques and raised discoloration of the central face and ears. Dry cough, dyspnea, and chest pain occur in up to one half of patients with sarcoidosis, constitutional symptoms occur in one third, palpable lymphadenopathy occurs in one third, and skin lesions occur in one fourth. Some affected individuals with sarcoidosis are asymptomatic and are diagnosed incidentally on radiographs obtained for other reasons. Approximately 20% of patients develop pulmonary fibrosis with pulmonary insufficiency and pulmonary hypertension.

Pathology

GROSS

- Multiple small nodules along pleura, bronchi, vessels, and interlobular septa
- Multifocal lung nodules or large masses
- End-stage disease: fibrosis, architectural distortion, and cystic changes

MICROSCOPIC

- Well-formed noncaseating epithelioid granulomas along a perilymphatic distribution (juxta-pleural, interlobular septal, bronchovascular) and in lymph nodes
- Progression to fibrosis: 20% of cases
- Diagnosis of exclusion; requires correlation with clinical and radiologic findings and exclusion of sarcoid-like reactions and infectious granulomas

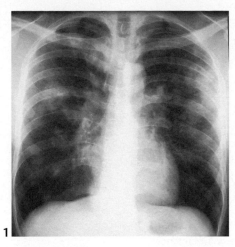
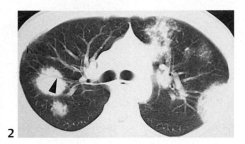

Figure 127E (1,2) PA chest radiograph **(1)** of a young woman with sarcoidosis who presented with cough demonstrates bilateral ill-defined nodular parenchymal opacities and bilateral hilar and subcarinal lymphadenopathy. Unenhanced chest CT (lung window) **(2)** demonstrates multifocal bilateral nodules and masses with a juxtapleural and peribronchial distribution and air bronchograms (arrow).

Imaging Findings

RADIOGRAPHY

- Radiographic staging
  - Stage 0: no visible intrathoracic abnormality
  - Stage 1: hilar or mediastinal lymphadenopathy
  - Stage 2: lymphadenopathy associated with parenchymal abnormalities (**Figs. 127A, 127B,** and **127E1**)
  - Stage 3: parenchymal abnormalities, no visible lymphadenopathy
  - Stage 4: upper lobe fibrosis, volume loss, hilar retraction, cystic change (**Fig. 127F1**)
- Intrathoracic lymphadenopathy
  - Eighty percent of patients at presentation, typically symmetric (**Figs. 127A, 127B,** and **127E1**)
  - Classic triad of right paratracheal and bilateral hilar lymphadenopathy, so-called 1-2-3 sign (also known as Garland triad) (**Fig. 127A**)
  - Intrathoracic lymphadenopathy
    - Bilateral hilar with or without mediastinal lymphadenopathy (95%) (**Figs. 127A** and **127E1**)
    - Aortopulmonary window lymphadenopathy (76%)
    - Common involvement of 4R, 5, 7, 10R, 11R, 11L American Thoracic Society (ATS) nodal stations
- Pulmonary involvement
  - Bilateral, symmetric small nodular and reticular opacities with a predilection for the upper and middle lung zones (**Figs. 127A** and **127B**)
  - Nodular (so-called alveolar) sarcoidosis: multifocal nodules or masses with or without air bronchograms (**Fig. 127E1**)
  - Rarely focal opacity, pleural effusion, pneumothorax, atelectasis, cavitation
  - Fibrosis with upper lobe volume loss, hilar retraction, and cystic change; may be complicated by mycetoma (**Fig. 127F1**)

CT/HRCT

- Bilateral discrete or irregular nodules along perilymphatic regions: juxtapleural, interlobular septa, bronchi, and vessels (**Figs. 127C** and **127D**)
- Ground-glass opacities, large nodules, and masses with perilymphatic distribution (**Fig. 127E2**)

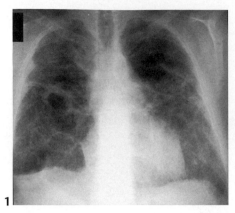
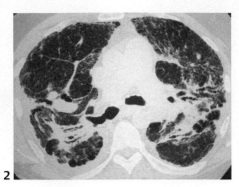

Figure 127F (1,2) PA chest radiograph **(1)** of a 49-year-old man with end-stage sarcoidosis demonstrates bilateral diffuse coarse central linear opacities and volume loss. Unenhanced HRCT (lung window) **(2)** demonstrates architectural distortion, perihilar conglomerate masses with posterior hilar retraction, traction bronchiectasis, and peripheral honeycomb lung. Note the residual micronodular opacities in the juxtapleural and septal regions.

- Pulmonary fibrosis: central and upper lobe distribution, architectural distortion, traction bronchiectasis, and large cystic spaces (**Fig. 127F2**)
  - Conglomerate central masses with superior/posterior hilar displacement
  - Peripheral honeycomb lung, bullae, and cystic spaces; may be complicated by saprophytic mycetoma

SCINTIGRAPHY

- Gallium-67 imaging; high sensitivity for active disease, low specificity
- Gallium-67 uptake patterns suggestive of sarcoidosis:
  - "Lambda" distribution: homogeneous uptake in perihilar infrahilar, and paratracheal lymph nodes
  - "Panda" distribution: bilateral symmetrical lacrimal gland and parotid gland uptake

Treatment

- Indicated in cardiac, ocular, central nervous system, and splenic involvement
- Corticosteroids; symptom relief, resolution of radiologic abnormalities, improved function
- Cytotoxic agents, chlorambucil, cyclophosphamide, and antimalarials
- Response to therapy typical; does not prevent recurrence

Prognosis

- Favorable prognosis in most patients, typical in:
  - Acute presentation
  - Löfgren syndrome
  - Erythema nodosum
- Poor prognosis typical in:
  - Insidious onset
  - Lupus pernio
  - Extrathoracic organ involvement
  - Pulmonary fibrosis
  - Non-Caucasian patient

- Mortality of approximately 10%
  - Pulmonary fibrosis
  - Cor pulmonale
  - Cardiac/central nervous system involvement, renal failure, pulmonary hemorrhage from mycetoma

Suggested Readings

Chiles C. Imaging features of thoracic sarcoidosis. Semin Roentgenol 2002;37:82–93

Patil SN, Levin DL. Distribution of thoracic lymphadenopathy in sarcoidosis using computed tomography. J Thorac Imaging 1999;14:114–117

Statement on sarcoidosis. Joint statement of the American Thoracic Society (ATS), the European Respiratory Society (ERS), and the World Association of Sarcoidosis and Other Granulomatous Disorders (WASOG), adopted by the ATS Board of Directors and by the ERS Executive Committee, February 1999. Am J Respir Crit Care Med 1999;160:736–755

Travis WD, Colby TV, Koss MN, Rosado-de-Christenson ML, Müller NL, King TE Jr. Idiopathic interstitial pneumonia and other diffuse parenchymal lung diseases. In: King DW, ed. Atlas of Nontumor Pathology: Non-Neoplastic Disorders of the Lower Respiratory Tract, first series, fascicle 2. Washington, DC: American Registry of Pathology and Armed Forces Institute of Pathology, 2001:49–231

Webb WR, Müller NL, Naidich DP. Diseases characterized primarily by parenchymal opacification. In: Webb WR, Müller NL, Naidich DP, eds. High-resolution CT of the Lung, 3rd ed. Philadelphia: Lippincott Williams & Wilkins, 2001;259–353

CASE 128 Hypersensitivity Pneumonitis

Clinical Presentation

A 36-year woman with cough and dyspnea

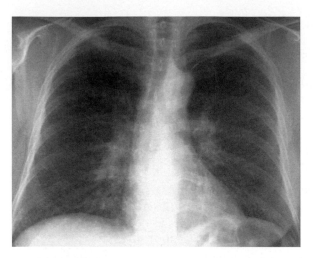

Figure 128A

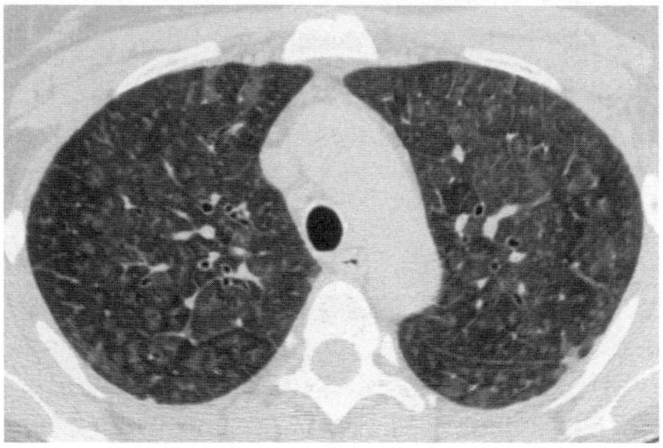

Figure 128B

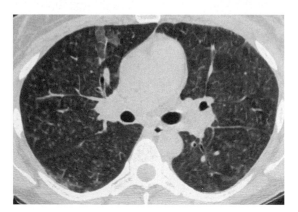

Figure 128C

Radiologic Findings

PA chest radiograph (**Fig. 128A**) demonstrates faint bilateral ground-glass opacities in the mid-to-lower lung zones. Unenhanced HRCT (lung window) (**Figs. 128B** and **128C**) demonstrates patchy ground-glass opacities and multiple centrilobular ground-glass nodular opacities.

Diagnosis

Hypersensitivity pneumonitis, subacute

Differential Diagnosis

- Respiratory bronchiolitis–interstitial lung disease (RB-ILD) (cigarette smokers)

490

- *Pneumocystis jiroveci* pneumonia (formerly *Pneumocystis carinii* pneumonia) (immune-compromised patients)
- Desquamative interstitial pneumonia (DIP)

Discussion

Background

Hypersensitivity pneumonitis (HP) (synonym: extrinsic allergic alveolitis) is an immunologic reaction to inhaled organic antigens that produces a diffuse interstitial granulomatous lung disease that varies in its intensity, clinical presentation, and natural history.

Etiology

There are a variety of known antigens including various bacteria, fungi, amoebae, animal proteins, and some chemicals. Most exposures are occupational in nature; others are related to hobbies or environmental exposures. Two of the most common forms of HP are farmer's lung and bird fancier's lung. Farmer's lung results from exposure to a bacterium in "moldy" hay; bird fancier's lung is caused by chronic exposure to proteins from bird feathers, serum, or excrement. Other forms of HP result from organisms growing in stagnant water (e.g., swimming pools, hot tubs, central heating units).

Clinical Findings

The clinical presentation may reflect an acute, subacute, or chronic form of HP. Pulmonary function tests typically show a restrictive pattern. Patients with acute HP typically have an acute onset of fever, chills, malaise, cough, and dyspnea usually following heavy exposures. Subacute HP has a more insidious clinical onset, with cough and breathlessness developing over days or weeks. Patients with chronic HP complain of progressive dyspnea.

Pathology

ACUTE

- Intraalveolar inflammatory exudate and edema

SUBACUTE

- Chronic bronchiolitis with peribronchiolar interstitial inflammation
- Scattered centrilobular inflammatory nodules with lymphocyte predominance

CHRONIC

- Interstitial fibrosis

Imaging Findings

RADIOGRAPHY

- Acute
  - Normal chest radiograph
  - Diffuse pulmonary opacities (may mimic pulmonary edema)
  - Mid-to-lower zone predominance of abnormalities
- Subacute
  - Diffuse ground glass opacity (**Fig. 128A**)
  - Small, poorly defined nodular opacities

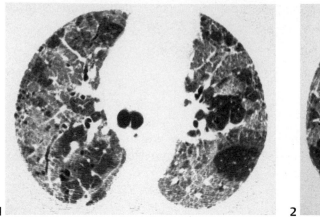 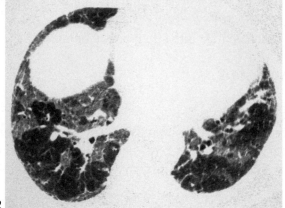

Figure 128D (1,2) Unenhanced HRCT (lung window) of a patient with chronic HP demonstrates patchy ground-glass opacities, reticular opacities, and traction bronchiectasis most pronounced in the mid-to-upper lung zones.

- Chronic
  - Coarse, irregular linear opacities
  - Honeycombing, reduced lung volumes
  - Mid-to-upper zone predominant but may mimic idiopathic pulmonary fibrosis (IPF)

CT/HRCT

- Acute and subacute
  - Poorly defined centrilobular opacities (**Figs. 128B** and **128C**)
  - Ground-glass opacities (**Figs. 128B** and **128C**)
  - Diffuse involvement (**Figs. 128B** and **128C**)
- Chronic
  - Fibrosis (mid-to-lower zone predominant) (**Fig. 128D**)
  - Reticular opacities: patchy, central, occasionally peripheral (**Fig. 128D**)
  - Areas of mosaic attenuation (**Fig. 128D**)

Treatment

- Cessation of exposure to offending antigen

Prognosis

- Resolution of symptoms and imaging abnormalities with discontinued exposure to antigen
- Pulmonary fibrosis with continued antigenic exposure

Suggested Readings

Adler BD, Padley SPG, Müller NL, Remy-Jardin M, Remy J. Chronic hypersensitivity pneumonitis: high resolution CT and radiographic features in 16 patients. Radiology 1992;185:91–95

Gurney JW. Hypersensitivity pneumonitis. Radiol Clin North Am 1992;30:1219–1230

Hansel DM, Wells AU, Padley SPG, Müller NL. Hypersensitivity pneumonitis: correlation of individual CT patterns with functional abnormalities. Radiology 1996;199:123–128

McAdams HP, Erasmus J. Chest case of the day: Williams-Campbell syndrome hypersensitivity pneumonitis. AJR Am J Roentgenol 1995;165:189–190

CASE 129 Usual Interstitial Pneumonia (UIP)

Clinical Presentation

A 68-year-old man with increasing dyspnea and fatigue

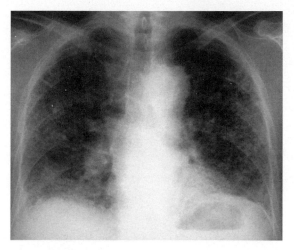

Figure 129A

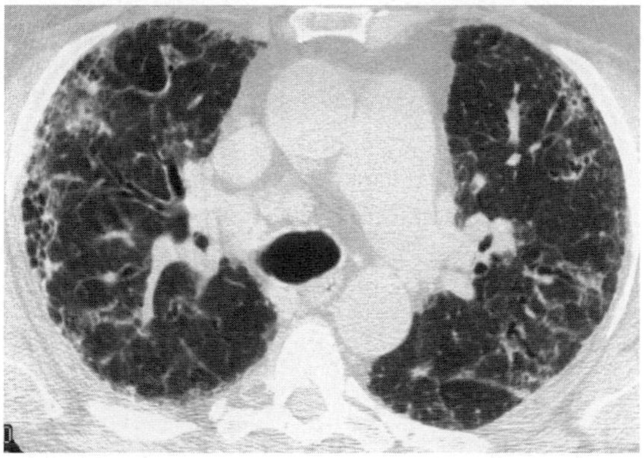

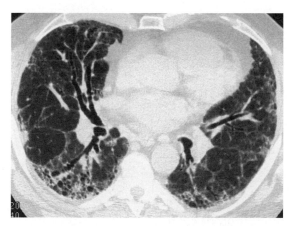

Figure 129C

Figure 129B

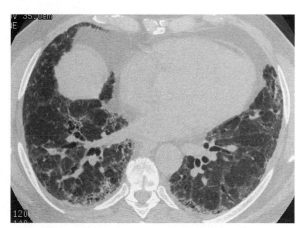

Figure 129D

Radiologic Findings

PA chest radiograph (**Fig. 129A**) demonstrates bilateral peripheral reticular opacities that are most severe in the lower lung zones and lung bases. Unenhanced HRCT (lung window) (**Figs. 129B, 129C, and 129D**) demonstrates irregular interlobular septal thickening, intralobular reticular opacities, traction bronchiectasis, and areas of fine honeycombing. The findings predominantly involve the juxtapleural aspects of the lower lung zones.

Diagnosis

Usual interstitial pneumonia (UIP); (idiopathic pulmonary fibrosis) (IPF)

493

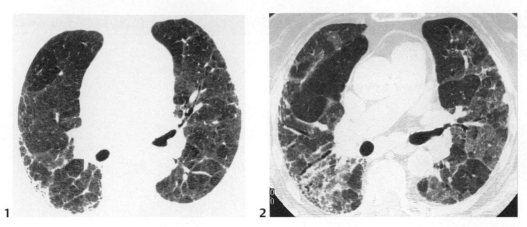

Figure 129E (1,2) Unenhanced HRCT (lung window) of a 78-year-old woman with UIP **(1)** demonstrates peripheral irregular opacities, ground-glass opacities, and architectural distortion. Follow-up HRCT 2 years later **(2)** demonstrates progressive involvement with increased traction bronchiectasis and ground-glass opacities.

Differential Diagnosis

- Collagen vascular disease with IPF
- Recurrent aspiration
- Pulmonary drug toxicity
- Asbestosis
- Chronic hypersensitivity pneumonitis

Discussion

Background

Usual interstitial pneumonia (UIP) is the most common of the idiopathic interstitial pneumonias (IIPs) (see Case 117). It is a histologic pattern of chronic fibrosing interstitial pneumonia that may be idiopathic (idiopathic pulmonary fibrosis, IPF) or may be a manifestation of connective tissue disease (e.g., rheumatoid arthritis, scleroderma), pulmonary drug toxicity, or asbestosis. Similarly, the HRCT findings of UIP are nonspecific and may be seen in the above entities. HRCT is accurate in the diagnosis of UIP. In one study, 47% of observers rendered a high confidence diagnosis of UIP based on clinical findings alone, 79% with the addition of radiographic data, and 88% with the addition of HRCT. While HRCT is more sensitive than chest radiography, a normal HRCT does not exclude UIP.

Etiology

The etiology of UIP is unknown. Viral, genetic, and immunologic factors have been implicated.

Clinical Findings

The idiopathic form of UIP (IPF) affects patients in the fifth to seventh decades of life, males more commonly than females. Affected patients present with progressive insidious dyspnea, cough, and fatigue. Pulmonary function tests show restrictive defects and decreased diffusing capacity for carbon monoxide (DLCO). Correlation of radiographic findings with clinical manifestations is often poor. Twenty to 30% of patients with UIP have collagen vascular disease, usually scleroderma or rheumatoid arthritis.

Pathology

GROSS

- Reduced lung volumes
- Cobblestone visceral pleural surface (retracting scars along the interlobular septa)

MICROSCOPIC

- Patchy interstitial fibrosis
- Fibroblastic foci
- Juxtapleural distribution
- Temporally heterogeneous histologic abnormalities

Imaging Findings

RADIOGRAPHY

- Early
  - Normal in 2 to 8% of pathologically proven cases
  - Irregular linear and reticular opacities
  - Ground-glass opacities
  - Peripheral and lower lung zone predominances
- Advanced
  - Coarse reticular or reticular and nodular opacities
  - Peripheral and lower lung zone predominance (**Fig. 129A**)
- End-stage fibrosis
  - Honeycomb cysts
  - Decreased lung volumes
  - Pleural effusions uncommon

CT/HRCT

- Irregular linear opacities (peripheral and subpleural) (**Fig. 129B**)
- Ground-glass opacities (may represent fibrosis or active alveolitis) (**Figs. 129B** and **129C**)
- Traction bronchiectasis and honeycombing in advanced disease (**Figs. 129B, 129C,** and **129D**)
- Predominance of basal and juxtapleural abnormalities (**Figs. 129B** and **129D**)
- Common mild mediastinal lymph node enlargement

Treatment

- Corticosteroids/cytotoxic drugs, with limited benefit
- Lung transplantation in selected patients

Prognosis

- Poor
- Respiratory failure from disease progression, edema, and superimposed infection
- High mortality; median survival after diagnosis of 3 to 6 years

- Irregular linear opacities, honeycomb cysts, and traction bronchiectasis indicate fibrosis and predict a poor therapeutic response.
- The extent and type of abnormality seen on HRCT correlates better with symptoms and physiologic indices than do radiographic findings.
- Combined with clinical and radiographic findings, HRCT can render a high confidence diagnosis of UIP, obviating open lung biopsy in most cases.

Suggested Readings

Katzenstein AL, Myers JL. Idiopathic pulmonary fibrosis: clinical relevance of pathologic classification. Am J Respir Crit Care Med 1998;157:1301–1315

McAdams HP, Rosado-de-Christenson ML, Wehunt WD, Fishback NF. The alphabet soup revisited: the chronic interstitial pneumonias in the 1990s. Radiographics 1996;16:1009–1033

Müller NL, Colby TV. Idiopathic interstitial pneumonias: high resolution CT and histologic findings. Radiographics 1997;17:1016–1022

Travis WD, Colby TV, Koss MN, Rosado-de-Christenson ML, Müller NL, King TE Jr. Diffuse parenchymal lung diseases. In: King DW, ed. Atlas of Nontumor Pathology: Non-Neoplastic Disorders of the Lower Respiratory Tract, first series, fascicle 2. Washington, DC: American Registry of Pathology; 2002:59–73

CASE 130 Respiratory Bronchiolitis–Interstitial Lung Disease (RB–ILD)

Clinical Presentation

A 33-year-old man with a long history of heavy tobacco abuse complains of worsening cough and increasing dyspnea.

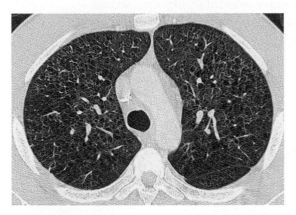

Figure 130A

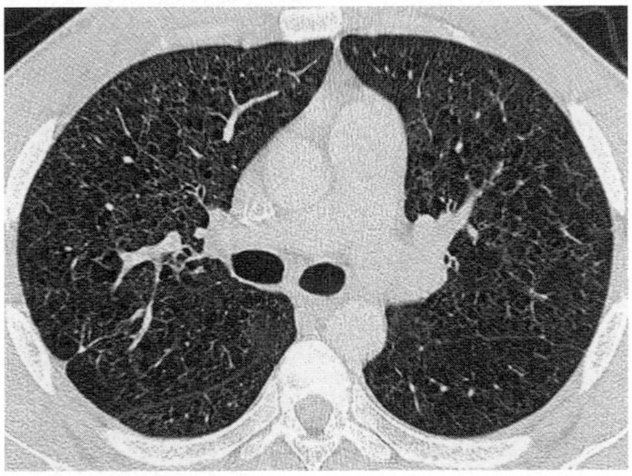

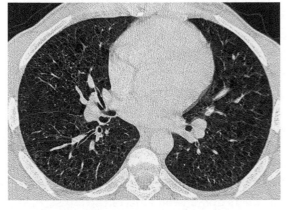

Figure 130C

Figure 130B

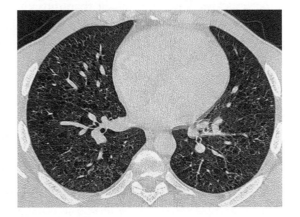

Figure 130D

Radiologic Findings

Unenhanced HRCT (lung window) (**Figs. 130A, 130B, 130C,** and **130D**) reveals diffuse proximal acinar emphysematous changes, fine diffuse centrilobular nodules, and bronchial wall thickening.

Diagnosis

Respiratory bronchiolitis–interstitial lung disease (RB-ILD)

Differential Diagnosis

- Desquamative interstitial pneumonia (DIP)
- Hypersensitivity pneumonitis (HP)

- Asbestosis
- Langerhans' cell histiocytosis (LCH)

Discussion

Background

Respiratory bronchiolitis–interstitial lung disease (RB-ILD) is a mild form of interstitial lung disease that occurs almost exclusively in heavy cigarette smokers. Because both RB-ILD and desquamative interstitial pneumonia (DIP) are related to tobacco abuse, many authorities believe both diseases are part of the spectrum of smoking-induced diffuse parenchymal lung disease, and that RB-ILD may be an early manifestation of DIP. The incidence and prevalence are unknown, and there is no sex predilection.

Etiology

The cause and pathogenesis are unknown, but the disease is strongly related to heavy tobacco abuse.

Clinical Findings

The mean age of patients at presentation is 36 years. Signs and symptoms include cough, dyspnea, and bibasilar, end-inspiratory crackles. Rales are coarser than those heard in other interstitial lung diseases and may be heard throughout inspiration and sometimes into early expiration. Pulmonary function studies may be normal. Alternatively, these studies may reveal an increased residual volume or a mixed obstructive-restrictive pattern. Mild hypoxemia at rest and exercise has also been reported.

Pathology

- Numerous finely pigmented macrophages in the respiratory bronchiole lumina and surrounding alveolar spaces
- Chronic inflammation and fibrosis in the bronchiole walls
- Fine brown cytoplasmic pigment and black particles in macrophages
- Goblet cell metaplasia and cuboidal cell hyperplasia along alveolar ducts and alveoli adjacent to the bronchioles

Imaging Findings

RADIOGRAPHY

- Normal in 20 to 30% patients
- Poorly defined ground-glass opacities or fine reticular or reticulonodular opacities and small peripheral ring shadows
- Bronchial wall thickening

HRCT

- Central bronchial wall thickening (90%); proximal to subsegmental bronchi (**Fig. 130**)
- Peripheral bronchial wall thickening (86%); distal to subsegmental bronchi
- Patchy ground-glass opacities (67–82%)
- Centrilobular nodules (86%) and tree-in-bud opacities (**Fig. 130**)
- Upper lobe predominant proximal acinar emphysema (57%) (**Fig. 130**)
- Patchy areas of hypoattenuation (38%) with lower lobe predominance
- Air trapping

Treatment

- Cessation of smoking
- Corticosteroids

Prognosis

- Favorable clinical course and excellent prognosis in most compliant patients
- Deterioration in some patients despite therapy

PEARL

- The diagnosis of RB-ILD requires a history of tobacco abuse, appropriate clinical signs and symptoms, and a lung biopsy that reveals RB-ILD and excludes other diffuse interstitial lung diseases.

Suggested Readings

Park JS, Brown KK, Tuder RM, Hale VA, King TE Jr, Lynch DA. Respiratory bronchiolitis-associated interstitial lung disease: radiologic features with clinical and pathologic correlation. J Comput Assist Tomogr 2002;26:13–20

Travis WD, Colby TV, Koss MN, Rosado-de-Christenson ML, Müller NL, King TE Jr. Reactive lymphoid lesions. In: King DW, ed. Atlas of Nontumor Pathology: Non-Neoplastic Disorders of the Lower Respiratory Tract, first series, fascicle 2. Washington, DC: American Registry of Pathology; 2002: 106–109

Webb WR, Müller NL, Naidich DP. Disease characterized primarily by parenchymal opacification. In: High-Resolution CT of the Lung, 3rd ed. Philadelphia: Lippincott Williams & Wilkins, 2001:382–384

CASE 131 Kaposi's Sarcoma

Clinical Presentation

A 36-year-old man with acquired immune deficiency syndrome (AIDS) and a CD4 count of 70 cells/μL presents with chest pain and dyspnea.

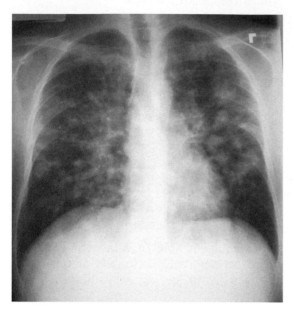

Figure 131A

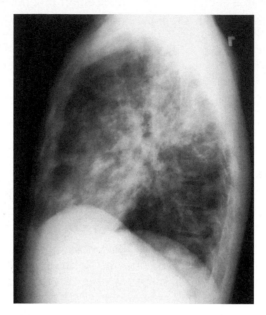

Figure 131B

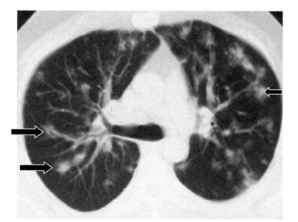

Figure 131C

Radiologic Findings

PA (**Fig. 131A**) and lateral (**Fig. 131B**) chest radiographs demonstrate bilateral, symmetric, poorly defined nodular opacities measuring up to 3 cm in diameter with a predominantly perihilar distribution. The bronchovascular bundles appear thickened. Contrast-enhanced chest CT (lung window) (**Fig. 131C**) from another patient with a similar history reveals ill-defined and irregular or "flame-shaped" nodular opacities in a predominantly perihilar and peribronchovascular bundle distribution.

500

Diagnosis

Kaposi's sarcoma

Differential Diagnosis

- Lymphoma
- Metastatic disease
- *Pneumocystis jiroveci* pneumonia
- *Mycobacterium tuberculosis* infection; nontuberculous mycobacterial infection
- Other bacterial and fungal pulmonary infections

Discussion

Background

Kaposi's sarcoma (KS) is a multicentric malignant neoplasm that originates from vascular and lymphatic endothelial cells. It occurs in 15 to 20% of human immunodeficiency virus (HIV)–infected male homosexuals, and in 1 to 3% of other HIV-infected individuals. The incidence of KS as an AIDS-defining illness has been decreasing over the last several years. Antiretroviral therapy may be at least partially responsible for this decline. Cutaneous or visceral KS usually precedes pulmonary involvement.

Etiology

There seems to be an association between infection with human herpes virus 8 DNA and the development of KS. The HIV regulatory protein (transactivator target, TAT), important for viral replication, is also likely responsible for the proliferation of KS cells.

Clinical Findings

Most patients with pulmonary KS are symptomatic and typically complain of dyspnea and cough. Blood-streaked sputum in a patient with cutaneous KS suggests endobronchial involvement. Endobronchial lesions may also be associated with focal wheezing on auscultation. Concomitant opportunistic infections (e.g., *Pneumocystis jiroveci* pneumonia) are not uncommon. KS lesions have a unique appearance on bronchoscopy. The lesions appear as irregularly shaped, flat, or slightly raised violaceous or bright-red plaques, located at the bifurcations of segmental and large subsegmental bronchi.

Pathology

GROSS

- Red or purplish lesions in the bronchovascular interstitium or pleura
- Ill-defined regions of parenchymal consolidation
- Purplish, irregularly shaped, flat or slightly raised plaques along the airway mucosa; typically located at bifurcations of segmental and large subsegmental bronchi

MICROSCOPIC

- Variable numbers of small, slit-like vascular spaces containing hemosiderin-laden macrophages and red blood cells insinuated between atypical spindle cells

Imaging Findings

RADIOGRAPHY

- Bilateral, symmetric, poorly defined nodular or linear opacities in a predominant perihilar distribution (**Figs. 131A** and **131B**)
- Nodules ranging between 0.5 and 3.0 cm in diameter, with a tendency to coalesce (**Figs. 131A** and **131B**)
- Bronchovascular bundle thickening may progress to perihilar consolidation.
- Interlobular septal thickening (e.g., Kerley B lines)
- Pleural effusions (30–70%); exudative and serous or serosanguineous
- Hilar and/or mediastinal lymphadenopathy (5–15%)

HRCT

- Ill-defined, irregular, "flame-shaped" or spiculated nodules in a predominantly perihilar and peribronchovascular distribution (85%) (**Fig. 131C**)
- Bronchial wall thickening (81%)
- Interlobular septal thickening (38%)
- Areas of ground-glass attenuation (23%) or parenchymal consolidation (35%)
- Pleural effusions (35%)
- Hilar and/or mediastinal lymphadenopathy (15–50%)

MR

- Parenchymal lesions; increased signal intensity on T1-weighted images and decreased signal intensity on T2-weighted images
- Marked increase in signal intensity on T1-weighted images after gadolinium administration

Treatment

- Regression after highly active antiretroviral therapy (HAART)
- Combination chemotherapy
- Paclitaxel

Prognosis

- Poor, with a median survival of 2 to 10 months
- Poor prognostic indicators
  - Pleural effusion
  - Severe breathlessness
  - CD4 counts < 100 cells/μL
  - Absence of cutaneous lesions
  - Previous opportunistic infection
  - Low white blood count or hemoglobin

PEARLS

- Irregular nodules greater than 1.0 cm in diameter in a peribronchovascular distribution strongly suggest this diagnosis.
- Focal and/or multifocal ground-glass opacities or consolidations are often secondary to concomitant infection with *Pneumocystis jiroveci* pneumonia.

Suggested Readings

Cannon MJ, Dollard SC, Black JB, et al. Risk factors for Kaposi's sarcoma in men seropositive for both human herpesvirus 8 and human immunodeficiency virus. AIDS 2003;17:215–222

Fraser RS, Müller NL, Coleman N, Paré PD. Pulmonary manifestations of human immunodeficiency virus infection. In: Fraser RS, Müller NL, Coleman N, Paré PD, eds. Fraser and Paré's Diagnosis of Diseases of the Chest, 4th ed. Philadelphia: Saunders, 1999:1676–1681

Kobayashi M, Takaori-Kondo A, Shindo K, Mizutani C, Ishikawa T, Uchiyama T. Successful treatment with paclitaxel of advanced AIDS-associated Kaposi's sarcoma. Intern Med 2002;41:1209–1212

Clinical Presentation

A 41-year-old man with metastatic adenocarcinoma from an unknown primary site with increasing dyspnea and cough

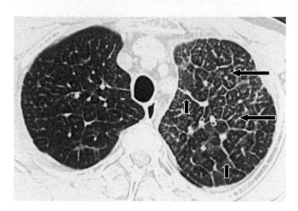

Figure 132A

Radiologic Findings

Unenhanced HRCT (lung window) (**Fig. 132A**) demonstrates asymmetric left upper lobe interlobular septal thickening with a thickened peribronchovascular interstitium (short arrows), pronounced polygonal arcades (long arrows), and preservation of the normal lung architecture.

Diagnosis

Lymphangitic carcinomatosis; adenocarcinoma

Differential Diagnosis

- Pulmonary edema
- Sarcoidosis
- Coal-workers' pneumoconiosis
- Lymphocytic interstitial pneumonia (LIP)
- Idiopathic pulmonary fibrosis (IPF)
- Pulmonary lymphoma

Discussion

Background

Pulmonary lymphangitic carcinomatosis (PLC) refers to the proliferation and spread of tumor in the pulmonary lymphatics. Virtually any metastatic neoplasm can demonstrate lymphangitic spread. The most common primary neoplasms associated with PLC are adenocarcinomas that originate in the lung, breast, stomach, pancreas, and prostate. PLC also occurs in patients with carcinomas of the thyroid and cervix and with metastatic adenocarcinoma from an unknown primary site.

Etiology

PLC typically results from the hematogenous spread of neoplasm to the lung with subsequent interstitial and lymphatic invasion. Direct lymphatic spread of tumor from mediastinal and hilar lymph nodes may also occur.

Clinical Findings

The most common clinical manifestation is dyspnea. Although initially insidious, it progresses rapidly and may result in severe respiratory distress in a few weeks. Some affected patients may also complain of cough.

Pathology

GROSS

- Slight to severe thickening of the interlobular septa and peribronchovascular connective tissue
- Common pleural involvement

MICROSCOPIC

- Neoplastic cells in clusters within lymphatic spaces and the interlobular and peribronchovascular interstitium
- Tumor emboli in adjacent small arteries and arterioles

Imaging Findings

RADIOGRAPHY

- Normal (i.e., 30–50% patients with pathologically proven PLC)
- Coarse bronchovascular markings with predominant perihilar and basal distribution (i.e., simulates pulmonary edema)
- Bilateral, unilateral, single lobe involvement
- Septal lines (i.e., Kerley B lines) usually present
- Coarse reticulonodular opacities
- Hilar and/or mediastinal lymphadenopathy (20–40%)
- Pleural effusion (30–50%)

HRCT

- Smooth or nodular peribronchovascular interstitial thickening (**Figs. 132A** and **132B**)
- Smooth or nodular interlobular septal and/or visceral pleural thickening (**Figs. 132A** and **132B**)
- Prominent centrilobular structures
- Characteristic septal thickening outlining distinct secondary pulmonary lobules (i.e., polygonal arcades) (**Fig. 132A**)
- Asymmetric diffuse, patchy, or unilateral involvement (50%) (**Fig. 132B**)
- Preservation of normal lung architecture (i.e., no architectural distortion or fibrosis)
- Hilar and/or mediastinal lymphadenopathy (40%)
- Pleural effusion (30%)

Treatment

- Supportive and directed toward the underlying malignancy

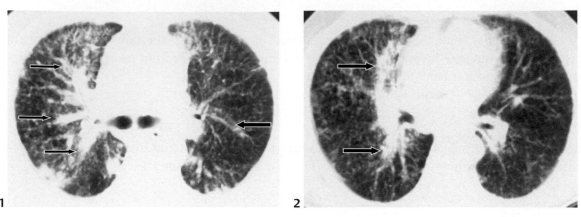

Figure 132B (1,2) Contrast-enhanced chest CT (lung window) at the carina **(1)** and through the middle and lower lobes **(2)** of a 54-year-old man with metastatic renal cell carcinoma demonstrates coarse, nodular peribronchovascular interstitial thickening (arrows), smooth as well as nodular interlobular septal thickening, and prominent centrilobular structures.

Prognosis

- Usually poor
- Death within 3 months in up to 50% of affected patients
- Survival for over 6 months in only 15% of affected patients

PEARL_____

- Preservation of lung architecture is an important CT finding used to differentiate PLC from other causes of diffuse interstitial lung disease. If there is architectural distortion or fibrosis, another diagnosis should be considered.

Suggested Readings

Fraser RS, Müller NL, Coleman N, Paré PD. Secondary neoplasms. In: Fraser RS, Müller NL, Coleman N, Paré PD, eds. Fraser and Paré's Diagnosis of Diseases of the Chest, 4th ed. Philadelphia: Saunders, 1999:1390–1397

Honda O, Johkoh T, Ichikado K, et al. Comparison of high resolution CT findings of sarcoidosis, lymphoma, and lymphangitic carcinoma: is there any difference of the involved interstitium: J Comput Assist Tomogr 1999;23:374–379

Webb WR, Müller NL, Naidich DP. Disease characterized primarily by nodular or reticulonodular opacities. In: High-Resolution CT of the Lung, 3rd ed. Philadelphia: Lippincott Williams & Wilkins, 2001:260–267

CASE 133 Pulmonary Langerhans' Cell Histiocytosis

Clinical Presentation

A 38-year-old female cigarette smoker with cough

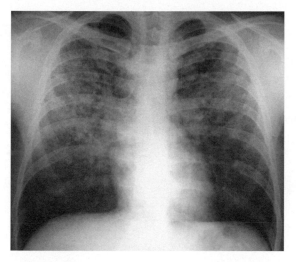

Figure 133A

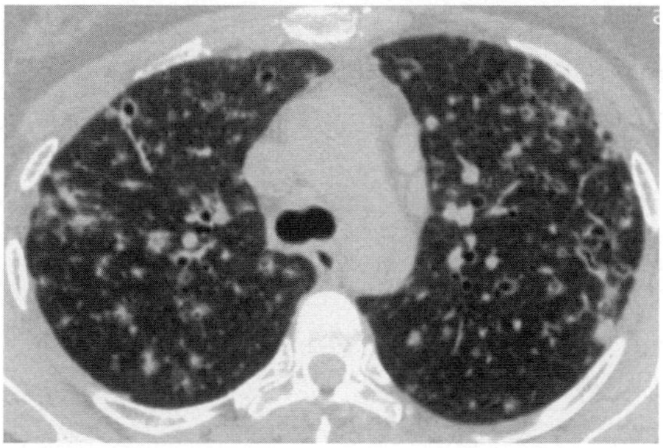

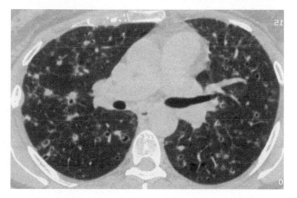

Figure 133C

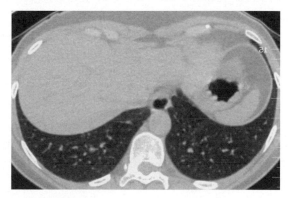

Figure 133B

Figure 133D

Radiologic Findings

PA (**Fig. 133A**) chest radiograph demonstrates bilateral reticular and nodular opacities predominantly involving the mid- and upper lung zones with relative sparing of the lung bases. Unenhanced HRCT (lung window) (**Figs. 133B, 133C,** and **133D**) demonstrates multiple irregular nodules and small cysts that vary in their configuration and are less profuse at the lung bases.

Diagnosis

Pulmonary Langerhans' cell histiocytosis

Differential Diagnosis

- Infection (*Mycobacterium tuberculosis, M. avium* complex, histoplasmosis)
- Sarcoidosis

- Silicosis
- Metastases
- Septic emboli

Discussion

Background

Langerhans' cell histiocytosis (LCH) (synonyms: pulmonary histiocytosis X, eosinophilic granuloma of lung) is a chronic, progressive interstitial lung disease that is strongly associated with cigarette smoking. It may involve the lungs in isolation or in combination with other organ systems (bone, pituitary gland, mucous membranes and skin, lymph nodes, and liver).

Etiology

While most affected patients are cigarette smokers, the specific etiology of LCH has not been established.

Clinical Findings

The majority of affected patients are young or middle-aged cigarette smokers; there is no sex predilection. Patients may be asymptomatic (25%) or present with dyspnea (40–87%), cough (56–70%), chest pain (10–20%), fatigue (30%), weight loss (20–30%), and fever (15%). Pneumothorax is a common complication in 25% of patients. Bone lesions occur in 4 to 13% of patients with PLCH; 20% involve the ribs and may be seen on chest radiography.

Pathology

- Peribronchiolar nodular proliferations of Langerhans' cells forming stellate nodules
- Cavitation of nodular proliferations
- Cyst formation
- Fibrosis in advanced cases

Imaging Findings

RADIOGRAPHY

- Diffuse, symmetric reticular or nodular opacities and cysts (**Fig. 133A**)
- Middle and upper lung zone predominance (**Fig. 133A**)
- Characteristic sparing of lung bases, especially near or adjacent to the costophrenic sulci (**Fig. 133A**)
- Secondary spontaneous pneumothorax (25% of affected patients)

CT/HRCT

- Nodules and cysts with normal intervening lung parenchyma (**Figs. 133B** and **133C**)
- Poorly defined centrilobular (1–15 mm) nodules
- Solid or cavitating nodules (**Figs. 133B** and **133C**)
- Progression from nodules to cysts
- Cyst of variable size, often with bizarre shapes (**Fig. 133E**)
- Thin, thick, or irregular cyst walls

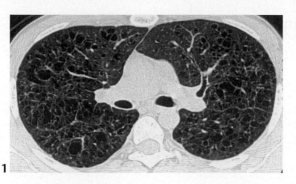 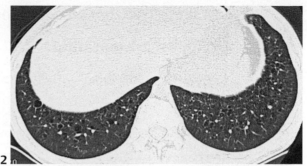

Figure 133E (1,2) Unenhanced HRCT (lung window) **(1)** of a 58-year-old physician with a long history of cigarette smoking and increasing dyspnea and cough demonstrates extensive bilateral cysts that vary in their size and configuration. There is relative sparing of the lung bases and costophrenic sulci **(2)**.

Treatment

- Cessation of smoking
- Corticosteroids of little value

Prognosis

- Spontaneous remission
- Regression with cessation of smoking.
- Progression to end-stage fibrotic lung disease

PEARL_____

- Cysts may be the only HRCT imaging feature of LCH in some cases (**Figs. 133E1** and **133E2**), but in most cases small nodules are also present. The combination of nodules and cysts is virtually diagnostic of LCH.

Suggested Readings

Abbott GF, Rosado-de-Christenson ML, Franks TJ, Frazier AA. Galvin JR. Pulmonary Langerhans' cell histiocystosis. Radiographics 2004;24:821–841

Brauner MW, Grenier P, Tijani K, Battesti JP, Veleye D. Pulmonary Langerhans' cell histiocytosis: evolution of lesions on CT scans. Radiology 1997;204:497–502

Travis WD, Colby TV, Koss MN, Rosado-de-Christenson ML, Müller NL, King TE Jr. Diffuse parenchymal lung diseases. In: King DW, ed. Atlas of Nontumor Pathology: Non-Neoplastic Disorders of the Lower Respiratory Tract, first series, fascicle 2. Washington, DC: American Registry of Pathology; 2002: 136–144

Vassallo R, Ryu JH, Colby TV, Hartman T, Limper AH. Pulmonary Langerhans' cell histiocytosis. N Engl J Med 2000;342:1969–1978

CASE 134 Lymphangioleiomyomatosis

Clinical Presentation

A 34-year-old woman with dyspnea

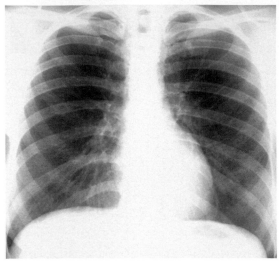

Figure 134A

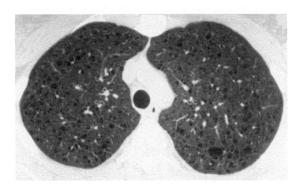

Figure 134B

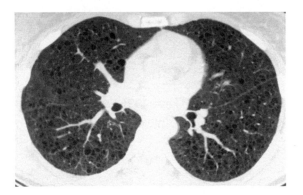

Figure 134C

Radiologic Findings

PA (**Fig. 134A**) chest radiograph demonstrates increased lung volumes without radiographic evidence of interstitial lung disease. Unenhanced HRCT (lung window) (**Figs. 134B** and **134C**) demonstrates small bilateral thin-walled cysts diffusely involving both lungs.

Diagnosis

Lymphangioleiomyomatosis (LAM)

Differential Diagnosis

- Pulmonary Langerhans' cell histiocytosis
- *Pneumocystis jiroveci* pneumonia (severe)
- Emphysema

510

Discussion

Background

Lymphangioleiomyomatosis (LAM) is a rare disease that affects young women of childbearing age and is characterized by abnormal proliferation of smooth muscle cells (LAM cells) along lymphatics in the chest and abdomen and also along vessels and bronchi in the lung. Lymphatic involvement can lead to chylous pleural effusions or ascites.

Etiology

The etiology of LAM is unknown.

Clinical Findings

LAM occurs almost exclusively in women of childbearing age with a mean age of 34 years. Patients may present with chronic dyspnea (59%), cough (39%), or less commonly with chest pain, hemoptysis and wheezing. Acute onset of chest pain and dyspnea may occur in association with spontaneous pneumothorax, a complication that occurs in 39%–53% of patients with LAM at presentation and in up to 81% during the course of the disease. The lungs are often hyperinflated. Pulmonary function tests (PFTs) reveal an obstructive or a mixed pattern. Approximately 2.3% of patients with tuberous sclerosis complex-associated LAM (TSC-LAM) have identical clinical, radiologic, and pathologic findings. Renal angiomyolipomas occur in 8%–57% of patients with spontaneous LAM and are found in 40%–80% of patients with TSC-associated LAM.

Pathology

GROSS

- Thin-walled cysts (0.5 to 0.2 cm) diffusely involving both lungs
- Enlarged lungs

MICROSCOPIC

- Abnormal proliferation of smooth muscle cells (LAM cells) in the pulmonary interstitium, lymphatics, and thoracic and retroperitoneal lymph nodes
- Cystic spaces (with LAM cells around the periphery of the spaces)

Imaging Findings

RADIOGRAPHY

- Normal chest radiograph in 20% of patients
- Diffuse bilateral reticular opacities (80%)
- Cystic airspaces, hyperinflation, pneumothorax (30–40%)
- Pleural effusion (10–20%) may be chylous
- Hyperinflation (**Fig. 134A**)

CT/HRCT

- Thin-walled cysts (0.2 to 2.0 cm) (**Figs. 134B, 134C,** and **134D**)
- Diffuse bilateral distribution throughout both lungs (upper and lower lungs equally affected)
- Pneumothorax
- Pleural effusion (may be chylous)

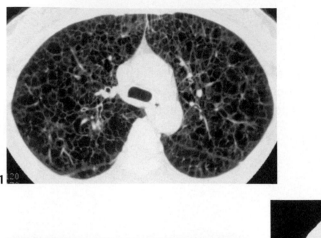

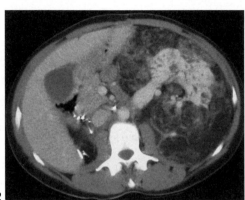

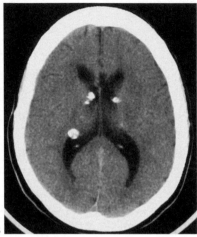

Figure 134D (1–3) Unenhanced HRCT (lung window) **(1)** of a woman with tuberous sclerosis demonstrates diffuse bilateral thin-walled cysts. Contrast-enhanced abdominal CT (soft tissue window) **(2)** demonstrates a large angiomyolipoma that virtually replaces the left kidney. Contrast-enhanced brain CT **(3)** reveals multiple calcified subependymal nodules representing tubers or hamartomas. This constellation of findings is characteristic of pulmonary involvement in patients with tuberous sclerosis (0.1–2.3%), which is indistinguishable from lymphangioleiomyomatosis physiologically, radiologically, and histologically.

Treatment

- Hormonal manipulation may improve or stabilize disease
- Lung transplantation

Prognosis

- Variable; frequent disease progression
- Median survival from time of diagnosis: 8 to 10 years
- Recurrence reported in transplanted lungs.

PEARLS AND PITFALLS

- Cysts of LAM are usually more regular in size and shape than the cysts of pulmonary Langerhans' cell histiocytosis.
- LAM typically involves both lungs diffusely; Langerhans' cell histiocytosis characteristically spares the lung bases.

- Nodules are not a characteristic feature of LAM but are common in pulmonary Langerhans' cell histiocytosis
- Pleural effusions are common in LAM but are uncommon in pulmonary Langerhans' cell histiocytosis.
- Emphysema can be distinguished from LAM by the polygonal shape of the affected pulmonary lobule in emphysema and by the presence of a central "dot" representing the core lobular artery in the emphysematous lobule.
- Areas of low attenuation in centrilobular emphysema have no perceptible walls; cysts of LAM have thin, perceptible walls.

Suggested Readings

Abbott GF, Rosado-de-Christenson ML, Frazier AA, Franks TJ et al. Lymphangioleiomyomatosis: Radiologic-Pathologic Correlation. Radiographics 2005;25:803–828

Lenoir S, Grenier P, Brauner MW, et al. Pulmonary lymphangiomyomatosis and tuberous sclerosis: comparison of radiographic and thin-section CT findings. Radiology 1990;175:329–334

Lynch DA, Brown KK, Lee JS, Hale VAE. Imaging of diffuse infiltrative lung disease. In: Lynch DA, Newell JD Jr, Lee JS, eds. Imaging of Diffuse Lung Disease. Hamilton, Ontario: Decker; 2000:114–115

Müller NL, Chiles C, Kulnig P. Pulmonary lymphangiomyomatosis: correlation of CT with radiographic and functional findings. Radiology 1990;175:335–339

Travis WD, Colby TV, Koss MN, Rosado-de-Christenson ML, Müller NL, King TE Jr. Diffuse parenchymal lung diseases. In: King DW, ed. Atlas of Nontumor Pathology: Non-Neoplastic Disorders of the Lower Respiratory Tract, first series, fascicle 2. Washington, DC: American Registry of Pathology; 2002: 47–160

SECTION X

Occupational Lung Disease

CASE 135 Silicosis

Clinical Presentation

An 80-year-old man with increasing dyspnea

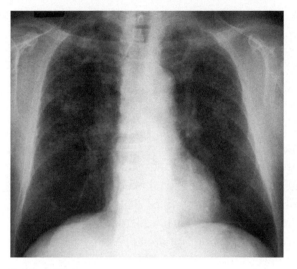

Figure 135A

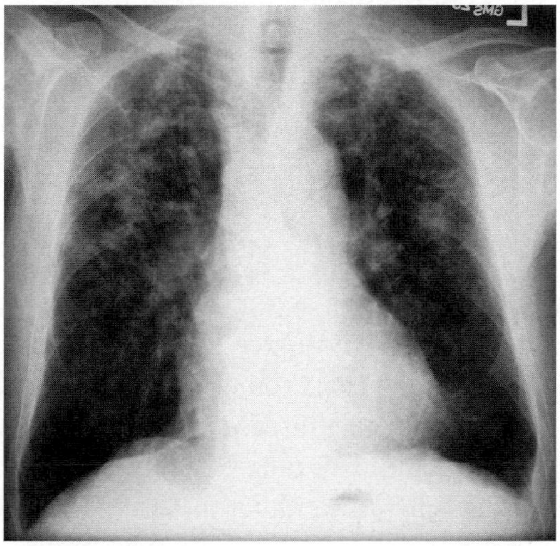

Figure 135B

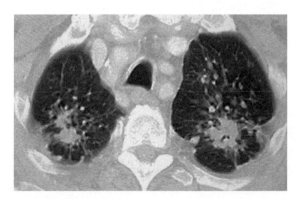

Figure 135C

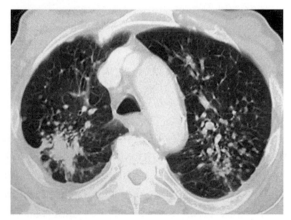

Figure 135D

Radiologic Findings

PA chest radiograph (**Fig. 135A**) demonstrates small bilateral, well-defined nodules (measuring approximately 1–6 mm) and coalescent nodular opacities (measuring more than 1 cm) predominantly involving the upper and mid-lung zones. PA chest radiograph obtained 8 years later (**Fig. 135B**) demonstrates an increase in the size and extent of the coalescent opacities on a background of small well-defined nodules and bilateral upper lobe parenchymal distortion. Contrast-enhanced chest CT (lung window) (**Figs. 135C** and **135D**) demonstrates bilateral upper lobe spiculated masses with associated adjacent pleural thickening and retraction, small well-defined nodules, and larger irregular opacities in the posterior aspects of both upper lobes.

517

Diagnosis

Silicosis, complicated

Differential Diagnosis

- Coal worker's pneumoconiosis (CWP)
- Sarcoidosis
- *Mycobacterium tuberculosis* infection

Discussion

Background

The term *pneumoconiosis* refers to the accumulation of dust in the lungs and the tissue reaction to its presence. The most frequently encountered inorganic dusts are silica, asbestos, coal, iron, and beryllium, and accumulation occurs most commonly through inhalation during occupational exposure. Silicosis is a chronic occupational lung disease that is characterized by pulmonary nodules that may coalesce to form lung masses and may progress to pulmonary fibrosis in patients with a history of inhalation of crystalline-free silica. Criteria for the diagnosis of silicosis are (1) appropriate exposure history, (2) radiologic findings consistent with silicosis, and (3) absence of other disease to explain the radiologic findings. *Simple silicosis* refers to cases in which small silicotic nodules (measuring less than 1 cm) are present and larger, conglomerate opacities are not demonstrated. Simple silicosis occurs in 10 to 20% of exposed workers. *Complicated silicosis* refers to the progression of disease with larger nodules that coalesce to form conglomerate masses (measuring more than 1 cm) in a process called progressive massive fibrosis (PMF). Complicated silicosis occurs in 1 to 2% of exposed workers.

Etiology

The most important factors in the development of silicosis are the intensity and duration of exposure to silica. The most abundant source of crystalline silica is quartz, and exposure is most common in the rock mining, quarrying, stone cutting, sandblasting, and ceramics industries. Pathogenetic factors include the size, shape, and concentration of dust particles, duration of exposure, and individual patient susceptibility. Relatively low levels of exposure result in classic chronic silicosis. Silica particles are ingested by alveolar macrophages; when the macrophages eventually break down, enzymes and other products are released, and the silica particles become available for re-ingestion by other macrophages. This repeating cycle explains the progression of silicosis, despite cessation of exposure to silica dust.

A rare, generalized form of alveolar proteinosis (silicoproteinosis; synonym: acute silicosis) may occur in individuals who experience a massive exposure to silica dust in enclosed spaces (e.g., sandblasters). In those individuals, the normal clearing mechanisms are overwhelmed, and silica particles are taken up by type II pneumocytes. Silicoproteinosis is a rapidly progressive condition that may result in death from respiratory failure within 1 to 2 years.

Clinical Findings

Patients with simple silicosis are typically asymptomatic. In cases of complicated silicosis, dyspnea usually occurs and typically develops following a latency period of 10 to 20 years. Individuals with silicoproteinosis (acute silicosis) may develop symptoms within a few weeks or months of exposure. Patients with silicosis have an increased susceptibility to infection with *Mycobacterium tuberculosis*, atypical mycobacteria, and fungi. The development of fever or weight loss in a patient with silicosis is suggestive of concomitant infection, especially by *M. tuberculosis*.

Pathology

SIMPLE SILICOSIS GROSS

- Discrete round, slate-gray fibrous nodules, measuring 3 to 6 mm in diameter, well demarcated on cut section; surrounded by a cuff of pigmentation when on the pleural surface
- Silicotic nodules composed of dense lamellar collagen; may demonstrate calcification, hyalinization, central degeneration
- Hilar lymph nodes typically involved by silicotic nodules with secondary calcification

MICROSCOPIC

- Background of dust-filled macrophages
- Nodules in a lymphangitic (i.e., along bronchovascular bundles, interlobular septa, and juxta-pleural regions) and random distribution
- Micronodules coalesce to form discrete rounded nodules of classic silicosis
- Weakly birefringent with polarized light

Progressive Massive Fibrosis

GROSS

- Individual and coalescent (conglomerate) masses (measuring more than 1 cm) associated with adjacent emphysema
- Predominant upper lobe and perihilar distribution
- Cavitation of conglomerate masses (suggestive of infection with tuberculosis)
- Pleural thickening

MICROSCOPIC

- Conglomerates of silicotic nodules
- Fibrosis
- Dust-ladden macrophages

Silicoproteinosis

GROSS

- Resembles pulmonary alveolar proteinosis
- Irregular zones of consolidation

MICROSCOPIC

- Granular, eosinophilic lipoproteinaceous material fills airspaces
- Poorly formed silicotic nodules and granulomas
- Mild interstitial inflammation and collagenization
- Weakly birefringent silica particles with polarized light

Silicotuberculosis

GROSS

- Silicotic nodules with central necrosis

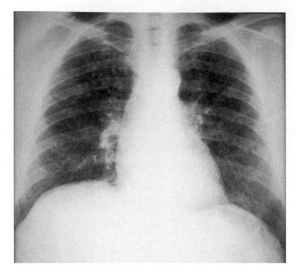

Figure 135E PA chest radiograph of a 72-year-old man with simple silicosis demonstrates diffuse bilateral small pulmonary nodules with a predominant upper lung zone distribution.

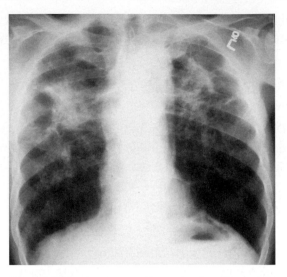

Figure 135F PA chest radiograph of a 67-year-old man with complicated coal worker's pneumoconiosis (CWP) demonstrates irregular spiculated conglomerate masses in the upper lung zones with peripheral emphysema and subtle nodularity.

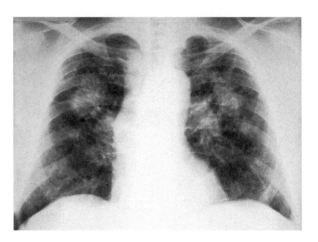

Figure 135G PA chest radiograph of a 62-year-old man with complicated silicosis demonstrates bilateral conglomerate masses predominantly involving the upper lung zones.

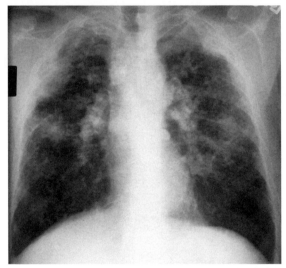

Figure 135H PA chest radiograph of a 58-year-old man with complicated silicosis demonstrates multiple bilateral pulmonary nodules, conglomerate masses, and bilateral hilar lymphadenopathy with peripheral ("eggshell") calcification.

MICROSCOPIC

- Histiocytic and epithelioid granualomatous reaction

Imaging Findings

RADIOGRAPHY

- Small, well-circumscribed nodules, typically measuring 2 to 5 mm (**Figs. 135A** and **135E**)
- Large opacities (measuring more than 1 cm) typically in middle portion or periphery of the upper lobes; eventual hilar migration with resultant emphysematous lung between mass and pleura (**Figs. 135B, 135F, 135G, 135H,** and **135I**)

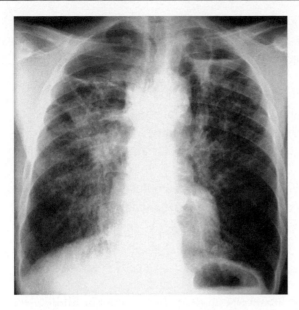

Figure 135I PA chest radiograph of a 64-year-old man with complicated silicosis and active tuberculosis (silicotuberculosis) demonstrates multiple small nodules predominantly involving the upper and middle lung zones with conglomerate opacities and biapical bullae. Note the bilateral hilar and mediastinal lymphadenopathy with peripheral calcification ("eggshell") in aorticopulmonary window lymph nodes. An air-fluid level in the left apical bulla prompted further evaluation, resulting in the diagnosis of silicotuberculosis.

- Predominant upper and posterior lung zone involvement (**Figs. 135A, 135B, 135E, 135F, 135G, 135H,** and **135I**)
- Frequent hilar and mediastinal lymphadenopathy; often calcified (peripheral "eggshell" calcification in 5%) (**Figs. 135H** and **135I**)
- Cavitation of PMF, apical pleural thickening, or rapidly changing radiographic abnormalities suggestive of *M. tuberculosis* infection (**Fig. 135I**)

CT/HRCT

- Small (2–5 mm) ill-defined or well-defined (centrilobular and juxtapleural) nodules (**Figs. 135C** and **135D**)
- Reticular opacities (**Figs. 135C** and **135D**)
- Diffuse distribution with upper lobe and posterior predominance (**Figs. 135C** and **135D**)
- Conglomerate irregular masses with central areas of cavitation (**Figs. 135C** and **135D**)
- Focal centrilobular emphysema
- Irregular or cicatricial emphysema
- Lymph node enlargement or calcification (calcification may be "eggshell," i.e., peripheral)

Treatment

- Cessation of exposure

Prognosis

- Good for patients with simple silicosis
- Significantly increased mortality rates in patients with advanced, complicated silicosis
- Recent decrease (1.5 deaths per million population in 1990 to 1.17 in 1999) in mortality rates reported by Centers for Disease Control and Prevention

PEARLS_____

- The 1980 International Labor Organization (ILO) International Classification of Radiographs of the Pneumoconioses is a system used worldwide to record the radiographic findings related to the inhalation of dusts. A set of 22 standard radiographs that demonstrate increasing profusion of round and irregular opacities are compared with the radiograph being evaluated, and a standardized scoring system is used. Several European countries are now employing a CT scoring system similar to the ILO system.

- Pulmonary tuberculosis is a serious complication of silicosis and should be suspected when nodular opacities increase in size rapidly or cavitate, if apical pleural thickening develops, or when there is a relatively rapid change in other radiographic abnormalities (**Fig. 135I**).

- Silicoproteinosis (acute silicosis) manifests as bilateral diffuse or perihilar airspace consolidation or ground-glass opacities.

- The radiographic and CT features of silicosis and coal worker's pneumoconiosis (CWP) are nearly identical. The prevalence of CWP has decreased since 1970, when federal mandates were established to reduce coal dust levels.

Suggested Reading

Fraser RS, Müller NL, Colman N, Paré PD. Inhalation of inorganic dust. In: Fraser RS, Müller NL, Colman N, Paré PD, eds. Fraser and Paré's Diagnosis of Diseases of the Chest, 4th ed. Philadelphia: Saunders, 1999:2386–2484

International Labor Organization. Guidelines for the Use of ILO International Classification of Radiographs of Pneumoconioses (Occupational Safety and Health Series, No. 22 (rev)). Geneva: ILO, 1980.

Kim JS, Lynch DA. Imaging of nonmalignant occupational lung disease. J Thorac Imaging 2002;17: 238–260

Laga AC, Allen T, Cagle PT. Silicosis. In: Cagle PT, ed. Color Atlas and Text of Pulmonary Pathology. Philadelphia: Lippincott Williams & Wilkins, 2005:397–399

National Institute for Occupational Safety and Health (NIOSH). Silicosis and related exposures. In: The Work-Related Lung Disease Surveillance Report, 2002. Washington, DC: U.S. Department of Health and Human Services (Centers for Disease Control and Prevention), 2003

Rosenman KD, Reilly MJ, Kalinowski DJ, Watt FC. Occupational and environmental lung disease: silicosis in the 1990s. Chest 1997;111:779–786

CASE 136 Asbestosis

Clinical Presentation

A 65-year-old man with cough and dyspnea who recently retired after a 30-year career in the boat-building industry

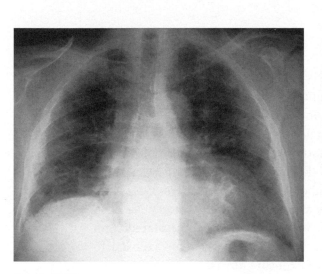

Figure 136A

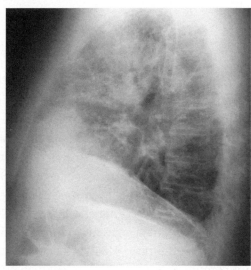

Figure 136B

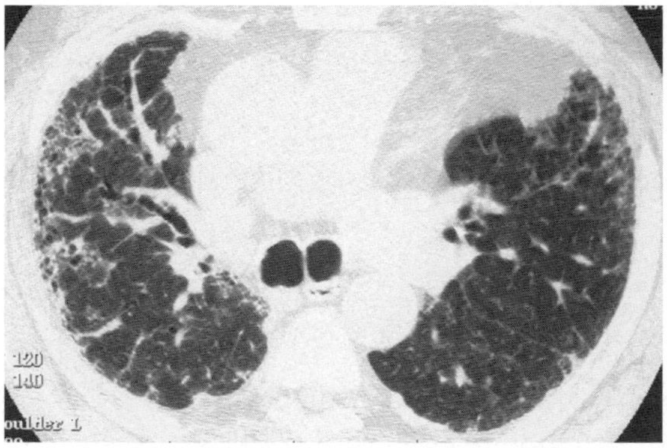

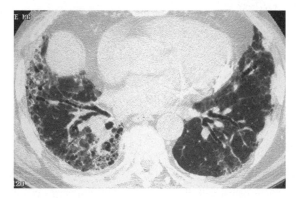

Figure 136C

Figure 136D

Radiologic Findings

PA (**Fig. 136A**) and lateral (**Fig. 136B**) chest radiographs demonstrate low lung volumes and bilateral reticular opacities that predominantly involve the peripheral lower lung zones. Calcified pleural plaques are demonstrated on the mid- and inferior pleural surfaces and along both diaphragms. Unenhanced HRCT (lung window) (**Figs. 136C** and **136D**) demonstrates extensive peripheral lower lobe architectural distortion, cystic changes, central traction bronchiectasis consistent with fibrosis, and pleural plaques.

Diagnosis

Asbestosis, asbestos-related pleural plaques

523

Differential Diagnosis

- Idiopathic pulmonary fibrosis (IPF)
- Connective tissue lung disease with associated fibrosis (scleroderma, rheumatoid arthritis)
- Drug toxicity
- Postirradiation pneumonitis

Discussion

Background

The inhalation of asbestos fibers is associated with a variety of pleural and parenchymal lung diseases. Pleural sequelae of asbestos exposure include noncalcified pleural plaques, calcified pleural plaques, diffuse pleural thickening, pleural effusion, and malignant mesothelioma. Parenchymal sequelae of asbestos exposure include rounded atelectasis, asbestosis, and an increased incidence of primary lung cancer. Asbestos fibers are a naturally occurring family of fibrous silicates that have been widely used in industry because of their heat-resistant properties. They are usually categorized as chrysotile (serpentine) or amphibole (needle-like) fibers. Chrysotile fibers are more easily cleared from the lung and less strongly associated with carcinogenesis than the amphibole fibers. Asbestos fibers may be found within alveoli and have been isolated from the pleura, omentum, and mesentery. Most urban-dwelling individuals have been exposed to asbestos as a frequent component of ambient air. High levels of exposure are associated with some occupations including asbestos mining and working with asbestos cement, insulation, friction products, and floor tiles.

Etiology

Asbestosis occurs almost exclusively in individuals exposed to high concentrations of asbestos mineral fibers, often occurring over the course of many years.

Clinical Findings

Patients affected with asbestosis complain of cough and dyspnea. Pulmonary function tests demonstrate restrictive lung disease, and patients become hypoxic with exercise. Auscultation reveals basal crackles or rales. Asbestos bodies may be encountered in bronchoalveolar lavage specimens, which indicates asbestos exposure but is not diagnostic of asbestosis.

Lung cancer occurs in a significantly larger number of asbestos-exposed individuals than in the general population. The risk of lung cancer increases with the severity of exposure to asbestos and with the presence of asbestosis. Primary lung cancer occurs 50 to 100 times more frequently in asbestos-exposed individuals who smoke than in the nonsmoking, nonexposed population. Asbestos-related lung cancers occur most frequently in the lower lobes, corresponding to the distribution of asbestosis.

Pathology

GROSS

- Juxtapleural fibrosis, predominantly involving the lower lobes and lung bases
- Mild parenchymal coarsening to honeycomb lung
- Parietal pleural thickening or pleural plaques

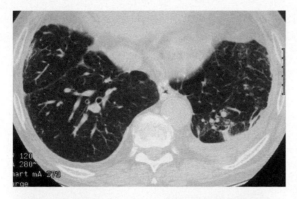

Figure 136E Unenhanced HRCT (lung window) of a 72-year-old man with asbestosis shows thickening of interlobular septa, nonseptal linear opacities including parenchymal bands, and juxtapleural lines and pleural thickening.

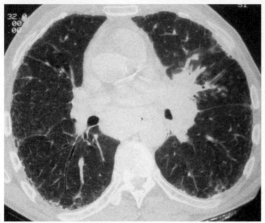
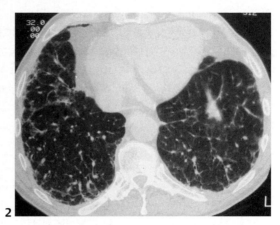

Figure 136F (1,2) Unenhanced HRCT (lung window) of a 66-year-old man with asbestosis demonstrates a left hilar mass (adenocarcinoma) **(1)** and findings of fibrosis characteristic of asbestosis (irregular interlobular septal thickening, intralobular interstitial thickening, parenchymal bands, and juxtapleural nonseptal linear opacities) **(1,2).** Note left pleural plaques **(1).**

MICROSCOPIC

- Asbestos bodies
- Fibrosis of respiratory bronchioles (early cases)
- Fibrosis of terminal bronchioles, alveolar ducts, and alveolar septa
- Complete obliteration of normal lung architecture (advanced cases)

Imaging Findings

RADIOGRAPHY

- Normal chest radiograph in 26% of proven cases
- Fine-to-medium reticular opacities predominantly involving the peripheral aspects of the lower lobes (**Figs. 136A** and **136B**)
- Pleural plaques (**Figs. 136A** and **136B**)
- Coarse reticulation and honeycomb lung (advanced cases)

CT/HRCT

- Juxtapleural dot-like opacities
- Juxtapleural nonseptal linear opacities (**Figs. 136E** and **136F**)
- Parenchymal bands (**Figs. 136C, 136D, 136E,** and **136F**)
- Findings of fibrosis: irregular interlobular septal thickening, intralobular interstitial thickening, irregular interfaces, traction bronchiectasis, and bronchiolectasis (**Figs. 136C** and **136D**)

- Predominance of findings in posterior and lateral basal segments of lower lobes
- Honeycomb lung (advanced disease) (**Figs. 136C, 136D, 136E,** and **136F**)
- Parietal pleural thickening or plaques (**Figs. 136C, 136D, 136E,** and **136F**)
- Earliest abnormalities posterior and basal (may require prone HRCT imaging to differentiate from physiologic atelectasis)

Treatment

- None

Prognosis

- Slow progression; may occur in the absence of further exposure
- Increasing dyspnea with advancing imaging abnormalities
- Recent increase in asbestosis-related deaths (annual age-adjusted death rate of 0.54 per million population in 1968 to 6.88 per million in 2000) reported by Centers for Disease Control and Prevention

PEARLS_____

- The pathologic diagnosis of asbestosis requires the demonstration of asbestos bodies in association with interstitial fibrosis with or without associated visceral pleural fibrosis.
- The imaging features of asbestosis may be indistinguishable from those of idiopathic pulmonary fibrosis and other diseases that manifest with a usual interstitial pneumonia (UIP) pattern on HRCT.
- The presence of parietal pleural thickening in association with interstitial fibrosis that is peripheral and predominant in the lower lung zones is highly suggestive of asbestosis.
- Prone HRCT is most sensitive for detecting early findings of asbestosis and distinguishes these from atelectasis in the dependent lung zones.

Suggested Reading

Akira M, Yamamoto S, Yokoyama K, et al. Asbestosis: high-resolution CT-pathologic correlation. Radiology 1990;176:389–394

Fraser RS, Müller NL, Colman N, Paré PD. Inhalation of inorganic dust. In: Fraser RS, Müller NL, Colman N, Paré PD, eds. Fraser and Paré's Diagnosis of Diseases of the Chest, 4th ed. Philadelphia: Saunders, 1999:2386–2484

Kim JS, Lynch DA. Imaging of nonmalignant occupational lung disease. J Thorac Imaging 2002;17: 238–260

National Institute for Occupational Safety and Health (NIOSH). Asbestosis and related exposures. In: The Work-Related Lung Disease Surveillance Report, 2002. Washington, DC: U.S. Department of Health and Human Services (Centers for Disease Control and Prevention), 2003

Webb WR, Müller NL, Naidich DP. Diseases characterized primarily linear and reticular opacities. In: Webb WR, Müller NL, Naidich DP, eds. High-Resolution CT of the Lung, 3rd ed. Philadelphia: Lippincott Williams & Wilkins, 2001:236–244

CASE 137 Farmer's Lung

Clinical Presentation

A 37-year-old man with acute dyspnea

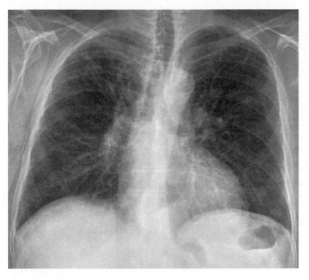

Figure 137A

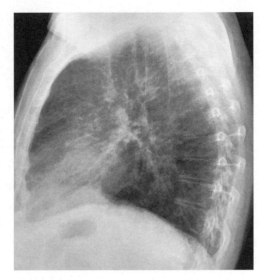

Figure 137B

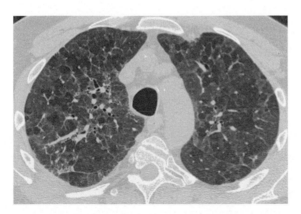

Figure 137C

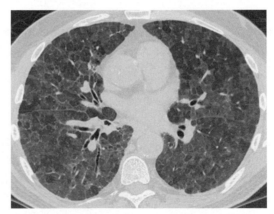

Figure 137D

(Figs. 137A, 137B, 137C, and 137D courtesy of Jud W. Gurney, M.D., University of Nebraska Hospital, Omaha, Nebraska.)

Radiologic Findings

PA (**Fig. 137A**) and lateral (**Fig. 137B**) chest radiographs demonstrate diffuse bilateral reticular opacities. Unenhanced HRCT (lung window) (**Figs. 137C** and **137D**) demonstrates patchy bilateral diffuse ground-glass opacities and a pattern of variable attenuation (i.e., mosaic perfusion) (**Fig. 137D**).

Diagnosis

Farmer's lung; hypersensitivity pneumonitis

527

Differential Diagnosis

- *Pneumocystis jiroveci* (formerly *Pneumocystis carinii*) pneumonia
- Desquamative interstitial pneumonia (DIP)
- Pulmonary drug toxicity
- Alveolar proteinosis

Discussion

Background

Farmer's lung is an occupational lung disease caused by exposure to moldy hay and inhalation of the associated antigen. Farmer's lung was one of the first recognized forms of hypersensitivity pneumonitis, a group of diseases characterized by an abnormal immunologic reaction to specific antigens in a variety of organic dusts. A long list of other forms of hypersensitivity pneumonitis now exists, including bird-fancier's lung, mushroom worker's lung, and detergent worker's lung. A striking similarity in the clinical, pathologic, and imaging features of these entities suggests a common pathogenesis (see Case 128). Hypersensitivity pneumonitis may develop acutely or may occur as a subacute or chronic disease, dependent on the duration of exposure and individual patient susceptibilities.

Etiology

Farmer's lung is caused by hypersensitivity to inhaled microorganisms (thermophilic actinomycetes) that grow in moldy hay. Affected patients are typically farmers who are exposed during the seasonal use of hay for feeding cattle.

Clinical Findings

Patients with farmer's lung are typically 40- to 50-year-old men who present with acute dyspnea after working with stored hay used for cattle feeding. Most cases occur during the winter or early spring (January to March). Affected patients typically present with fever, chills, cough, and dyspnea. Criteria for establishing the diagnosis of farmer's lung and other forms of hypersensitivity pneumonitis include (1) exposure to an organic dust of sufficiently fine particle size to allow deep penetration into the lung; (2) dyspnea often associated with cough, fever, and malaise occurring within hours after exposure to the offending antigen; (3) auscultatory crackles over both lung bases; (4) imaging evidence of diffuse ground-glass opacities or ill-defined small nodules; (5) reduced vital capacity on pulmonary function tests; (6) serum precipitins against the suspected antigen; (7) increased T lymphocytes and increased levels of immunoglobulins on bronchoalveolar lavage; (8) bronchiolitis and interstitial pneumonitis demonstrated on lung biopsy, with occasional granuloma formation; and (9) resolution of symptoms after cessation of exposure to the relevant antigen.

Pathology

- Acute: acute bronchiolitis (i.e., neutrophilic infiltrate in alveoli and respiratory bronchioles)
- Subacute: lymphocytic interstitial pneumonia, granulomas, organizing pneumonia, and fibrosis
- Chronic: bronchiolocentric cellular interstitial pneumonia, noncaseating granulomas, and intra-luminal budding fibrosis or organizing pneumonia

Imaging Features

RADIOGRAPHY

- Ground-glass opacities or ill-defined consolidations
- Interstitial linear/nodular opacities (**Figs. 137A** and **137B**)

CT/HRCT

- Subacute
  - Patchy or diffuse ground-glass opacity (**Figs. 137C** and **137D**)
  - Small centrilobular nodular opacities
  - Mosaic perfusion or a pattern of variable attenuation (i.e., lobular areas of decreased attenuation) (**Figs. 137C** and **137D**)
  - Air trapping on expiratory scans
- Chronic
  - Fibrosis without zonal predominance
  - Ground-glass opacities or centrilobular nodules
  - Patchy distribution

Treatment

- Cessation of exposure

Prognosis

- Good if prompt cessation of exposure; resolution of radiographic abnormalities within 10 days to 3 months
- Poor with repeated or continued exposure and progression to interstitial fibrosis

PEARL_____

- The extent of ground-glass opacities seen in patients with hypersensitivity pneumonitis does not always correlate with the results of pulmonary function studies, which may show restriction or obstruction.

Suggested Reading

Adler BD, Padley SPG, Müller NL, Remy-Jardin M, Remy J. Chronic hypersensitivity pneumonitis: high-resolution CT and radiographic features in 16 patients. Radiology 1992;185:91–95

Cormier Y, Brown M, Worthy S, Racine G, Müller NL. High-resolution computed tomographic characteristics in acute farmer's lung and in its follow-up. Eur Respir J 2000;16:56–60

Glazer CS, Rose CS, Lynch DA. Clinical and radiologic manifestations of hypersensitivity pneumonitis. J Thorac Imaging 2002;17:261–272

Hansel DM, Wells AU, Padley SPG, Müller NL. Hypersensitivity pneumonitis: correlation of individual CT patterns with functional abnormalities. Radiology 1996;199:123–128

CASE 138 Hard Metal Pneumoconiosis

Clinical Presentation

A 43-year-old man with cough and dyspnea

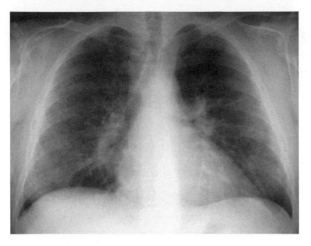

Figure 138A

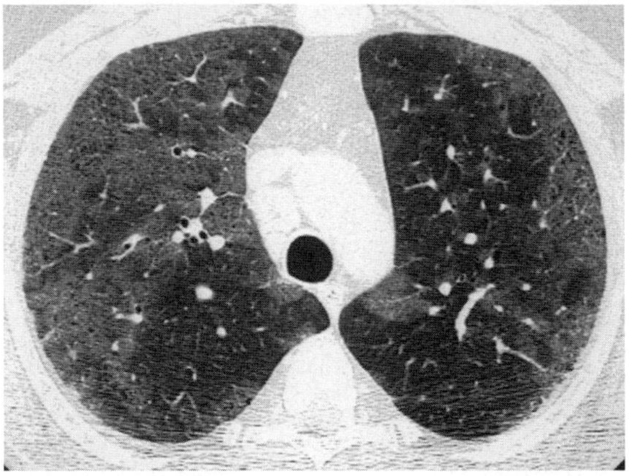

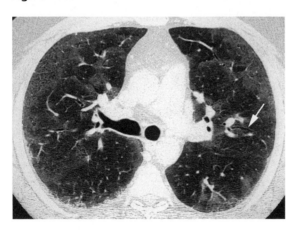

Figure 138C

Figure 138B

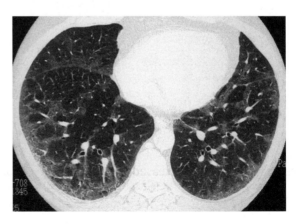

Figure 138D

Radiologic Findings

PA chest radiograph (**Fig. 138A**) demonstrates fine peripheral reticular opacities. Unenhanced HRCT (lung window) (**Figs. 138B, 138C,** and **138D**) demonstrates peripheral areas of ground-glass opacity involving the upper, middle, and lower lung zones with fine, peripheral honeycombing. An area of traction bronchiectasis is demonstrated in the left mid-lung (arrow) (**Fig. 138C**).

Diagnosis

Hard metal pneumoconiosis (cobalt-related)

Differential Diagnosis

- Desquamative interstitial pneumonia (DIP)
- Interstitial lung disease of other etiology
- Immunoglobulin (IgE)–mediated asthma
- Hypersensitivity pneumonitis

Discussion

Background

In the 1960s, Liebow originally classified giant cell interstitial pneumonia (GIP) as one of the idiopathic interstitial pneumonias. Today, it is recognized as an uncommon interstitial lung disease caused by exposure to hard metal. Hard metal pneumoconiosis is related to exposure to metals used primarily to grind, drill, cut, and polish other metals. Occupational exposure may occur during those activities or during hard metal manufacture. Occupations associated with exposure to hard metal include diamond polishing, saw and drill grinding, oil well drilling, and armor plating.

Etiology

Hard metal pneumoconiosis (synonym: giant cell interstitial pneumonia) is caused by exposure to hard metal, an alloy that consists primarily of tungsten, carbon, and cobalt. Animal studies suggest that cobalt is the constituent of hard metal that causes pulmonary disease. Diamond polishers are exposed to high levels of cobalt alone and develop interstitial lung disease identical to that which occurs in hard metal workers.

Clinical Features

Affected patients present with cough, dyspnea, wheezing, and allergic-type asthma and have a suggestive occupational exposure. Pulmonary function tests reveal both restrictive and obstructive lung disease, often with decreased diffusing capacity for carbon monoxide (DLCO). The diagnosis is usually confirmed by work history and analysis of lung tissue for metals by energy-dispersive x-ray analysis or other techniques.

Pathology

- Interstitial pneumonia with interstitial fibrosis
- Filling of alveolar spaces with macrophages and multinucleated giant cells
- Parenchymal distortion and honeycombing in advanced cases
- May resemble usual interstitial pneumonia (UIP)
- Common lymphoid reaction including germinal centers.

Imaging Features

RADIOGRAPHY

- Normal chest radiographs in some cases
- Diffuse reticular and nodular opacities (**Fig. 138A**)

- Lymphadenopathy
- Upper and middle zone predominant distribution; may resemble sarcoidosis
- Small cystic spaces representing honeycombing in advanced cases

CT/HRCT

- Variable appearance: may resemble nonspecific interstitial pneumonia (NSIP), UIP, or sarcoidosis
- Bilateral ground-glass opacities (**Figs. 138B, 138C,** and **138D**)
- Traction bronchiectasis (**Fig. 138C**)
- Peripheral cystic spaces (**Figs. 138B, 138C,** and **138D**)
- Findings of fibrosis or usual interstitial pneumonia
- Spontaneous pneumothorax

Treatment

- Removal of patient from offending workplace exposure
- Corticosteroids
- Cytotoxic therapy with cyclophosphamide or azathioprine for patients not responding to corticosteroids

Prognosis

- Recurrences in patients returning to the workplace
- Progressive symptoms leading to respiratory failure, which may be fatal
- Lung transplantation as last resort; recurrence reported in allograft has been reported

Suggested Reading

Akira M. Uncommon pneumoconioses: CT and pathologic findings. Radiology 1995;197:403–409

Fraser RS, Müller NL, Colman N, Paré PD. Inhalation of inorganic dust (pneumoconiosis). In: Fraser RS, Müller NL, Colman N, Paré PD, eds. Fraser and Paré's Diagnosis of Diseases of the Chest, 4th ed. Philadelphia: Saunders, 1999;2386–2484

Gotway MB, Golden JA, Warnock M, et al. Hard metal interstitial lung disease: high-resolution computed tomography appearance. J Thorac Imaging 2002;17:314–318

Kim KI, Kim CW, Lee MK, et al. Imaging of occupational lung disease. Radiographics 2001;21:1371–1391

SECTION XI

Adult Cardiovascular Disease

CASE 139 Pulmonary Thromboembolism with Infarction

Clinical Presentation

A 70-year-old woman admitted to the intensive care unit for possible myocardial infarction became acutely hypoxic and dyspneic on the second day following admission.

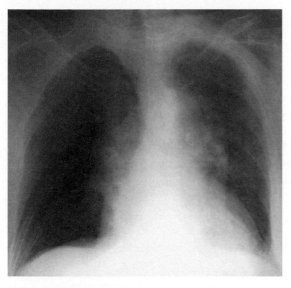

Figure 139A

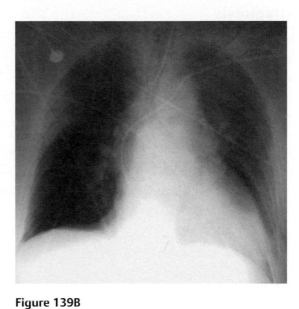

Figure 139B

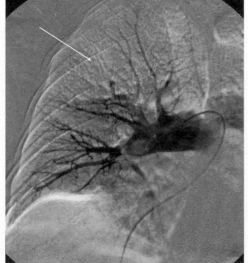

Figure 139C

Radiologic Findings

Admission AP chest radiograph (**Fig. 139A**) shows an enlarged cardiomediastinal silhouette and a relatively hyperlucent and oligemic right hemithorax. AP chest radiograph 2 days later (**Fig. 139B**) reveals a new peripheral wedge-shaped opacity in the axillary portion of the right upper lobe without intrinsic air bronchograms. An endotracheal tube and pulmonary catheter have been placed. Digital subtraction angiogram (**Fig. 139C**) demonstrates right upper lobe oligemia, a large clot in the proximal

535

upper lobe pulmonary artery, and scattered smaller emboli in the right middle and lower lobe arteries. Note the peripheral wedge-shaped area of nonperfusion or oligemia (arrow) (i.e., Westermark sign), which corresponds to the wedge-shaped opacity on the chest radiograph (**Fig. 139B**).

Diagnosis

Pulmonary thromboembolism with infarction (i.e., Hampton hump)

Differential Diagnosis

- Pulmonary thromboembolism with hemorrhage
- Acute lobar pneumonia

Discussion

Background

The precise incidence of deep venous thrombosis and acute pulmonary thromboembolism is unknown. Risk factors include immobilization, recent abdominal and pelvic surgery, trauma, HIV-AIDS, heart failure, hypercoagulable states, and oral contraceptives. Acute pulmonary thromboembolism is responsible for 2 to 7% of acute care hospital deaths.

Etiology

Ninety percent of pulmonary emboli originate from lower extremity deep veins.

Clinical Findings

Most episodes of pulmonary thromboembolism are asymptomatic and produce no appreciable radiographic changes. Ten to fifteen percent of symptomatic patients with angiographically proven emboli have normal chest radiographs. Signs and symptoms include acute dyspnea and pleuritic chest pain, anxiety, cough, tachycardia, tachypnea, hypoxia, abnormally high A-a gradient, and right ventricular strain on electrocardiogram (ECG).

Pathology

GROSS

- Large or medium-sized pulmonary artery involved; frequently in the right lung and lower lobes
- Deep reddish purple firm material containing some fibrin strands or lines of Zahn (alternating platelet and red cell layers)
- May be quite adherent to vessel wall if organization has begun
- Smaller strands of thrombus may extend into smaller vessels
- Lung parenchyma distal to embolus normal or demonstrates minimal atelectasis, intraalveolar hemorrhage, and/or edema
- Infarcts usually situated along the juxtapleural lung
- Infarcted lung manifests with coagulative necrosis (early) and peripheral granulation tissue (several days); reactive epithelial changes persist at infarct margin
- Long-standing infarcts; dense peripheral fibrosis, increase in pleural vascularity, fibrosis, and retraction

MICROSCOPIC

- Mixture of red blood cells, platelets, and fibrin
- Growth of capillaries, smooth muscle cells, and fibroblasts grow into the embolus from the pulmonary vessel wall over a few days
- Endothelialization of embolus surface
- Recanalization

Imaging Findings

RADIOGRAPHY

- Thromboembolism without infarction
  - Peripheral oligemia (Westermark sign) (**Fig. 139A**)
  - Enlargement of a major pulmonary artery (Fleischner sign)
  - Abrupt tapering of the occluded vessel (knuckle sign)
  - Volume loss and diaphragmatic elevation
  - Cardiac enlargement.
- Thromboembolism with hemorrhage or infarction
  - Any of the above signs, as well as parenchymal consolidation (i.e., Hampton hump) (**Fig. 139B**)
  - Ill-defined parenchymal opacities or homogeneous peripheral wedge-shaped opacity in early infarcts (**Fig. 139B**)
    - Base contiguous with visceral pleura
    - Apex points toward the ipsilateral hilum
    - Most infarcts in costophrenic sulcus of the right lower lobe involving one or two segments
- Opacities ranging from 3 to 5 cm in diameter; may develop as soon as 10 hours following the vascular occlusion
- Rarely air bronchograms and cavitation

Pulmonary Angiography

- Direct signs: intraluminal filling defects or abrupt vascular cut-offs (**Fig. 139C**)
- Indirect (nonspecific) signs: diminished capillary staining or delayed opacification

Prevention

- Prophylaxis with compression stockings, low-dose or low molecular weight heparin, and early mobilization

Treatment

- Anticoagulation
- Thrombolysis or thrombectomy in selected patients
- Inferior vena cava filters in patients with contraindications to anticoagulation therapy

Prognosis

- Recurrent emboli in one third of patients
- Mortality rates in untreated pulmonary emboli range from 18 to 38%.

PEARLS

- Most episodes of pulmonary thromboembolism do not result in radiographic abnormalities. Therefore, chest radiography has a limited role in establishing the diagnosis. The major value of chest radiography is in excluding other disease processes that can mimic pulmonary thromboembolism (e.g., pneumonia, pneumothorax, lobar collapse).
- The absence of air bronchograms combined with a peripheral region of homogeneous consolidation strongly suggests the diagnosis.
- Emboli associated with parenchymal hemorrhage and edema usually resolve in 4 to 7 days. Those associated with infarction may take as long as 5 weeks to resolve.

Suggested Readings

Fedullo PF, Rubin LJ, Kerr KM, Auger WR, Channick RN. The natural history of acute and chronic thromoboembolic disease: the search for missing link. Eur Respir J 2000;15:440–448

Fraser RS, Müller NL, Colman N, Paré PD. Thrombosis and thromboembolism. In: Fraser RS, Müller NL, Colman N, Paré PD, eds. Fraser and Pare's Diagnosis of Diseases of the Chest, 4th ed. Philadelphia: Saunders, 1999:1786–1799

CASE 140 Pulmonary Thromboembolic Disease: CT

Clinical Presentation

A 42-year-old woman with acquired immunodeficiency syndrome (AIDS) who presents with acute onset of right-sided pleuritic chest pain

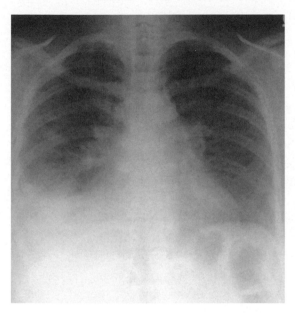

Figure 140A

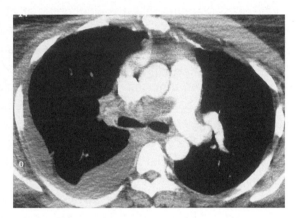

Figure 140B

Radiologic Findings

PA chest radiograph (**Fig. 140A**) shows a right pleural effusion. Contrast-enhanced chest CT (mediastinal window) (**Fig. 140B**) reveals a large filling defect occluding the right main pulmonary artery, right upper lobe artery origin, and the proximal right interlobar artery. A right pleural effusion is also seen.

Diagnosis

Acute pulmonary thromboembolic disease

Differential Diagnosis

None

Discussion

Background

Pulmonary thromboembolism (PTE) results from the transport of venous thrombi to the pulmonary arterial circuit. Thrombi may lodge in the main, lobar, segmental, or subsegmental pulmonary arteries. Pulmonary emboli are often multiple and have a predilection for the lower lobes. Fifteen percent of acute pulmonary thromboemboli are complicated by pulmonary infarction. The coexistence of HIV-AIDS–related illnesses (e.g., malignancies, opportunistic infections, drug therapy) may predispose to thromboembolic disease.

Etiology

Most emboli arise from clots in the deep venous system of the lower extremities. Other potential sites include the inferior vena cava, the pelvic veins, the right heart, and the upper extremities.

Clinical Findings

The physical examination of patients with PTE is often nonspecific. A significant number of patients will have normal vital signs. Patients that are diaphoretic at presentation are more likely to have significant emboli. Although patients may be febrile, the temperature is rarely more than 102° Fahrenheit. Tachypnea is frequent, but the respiratory rate is less than 20 in 30% of affected patients. The heart rate is normal in 70% of patients. An examination of the lower extremities is rarely helpful. PTE cannot be excluded based on a normal lower extremity exam. Calf swelling, tenderness, and asymmetry cannot distinguish between patients with PTE and those without thromboembolic disease. The presence of a palpable cord should increase the suspicion of PTE. Homan sign (i.e., pain in the posterior calf with forced dorsiflexion of the foot) is not accurate. The ECG is primarily used to exclude an acute myocardial infarction or possible pericarditis. The ECG changes of PTE are not specific but may reflect signs of right ventricular strain including the new onset of right bundle branch block, right axis deviation, shift in the transition zone to V5, and variations of the S1-Q3-T3 pattern. The arterial blood gas may be normal or near-normal in a significant percentage of patients. Twenty-five percent of patients with PTE have a room air partial pressure of oxygen (PO_2) greater than 80 mm Hg. Some patients may even have a PO_2 greater than 100 mm Hg on room air. Although a high PO_2 makes the diagnosis of PTE less likely, it does not exclude the diagnosis. Since the physical examination and laboratory data are unreliable in establishing the diagnosis of PTE, imaging studies play a crucial role in the evaluation of suspected disease.

Pathology

- Large emboli more frequent in the right lung and lower lobes
- Infarcts usually situated along the juxtapleural surface in the lung periphery
- Extensive hemorrhage in acute infarcts

Imaging Findings, Radiography

- See Case 139

CT

- Soft tissue attenuation thrombus within contrast-opacified vessel (**Figs. 140B, 140C,** and **140D**)
- Filling defect forming an acute angle with the vessel wall; most reliable sign
- Partial or complete filling defects
- Small, unilateral pleural effusions in 35 to 55% of patients with PTE disease (**Figs. 140B, 140C,** and **140D**); most common with infarction or hemorrhage

POTENTIAL CT PITFALLS

- Confusion of filling defects with hilar and infrahilar lymph nodes
- Poor vessel opacification and motion artifact mimicking or obscuring filling defects

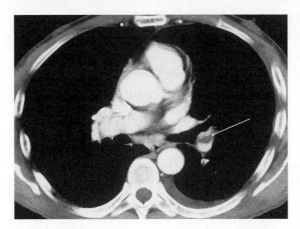

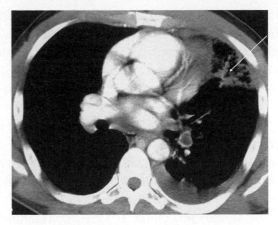

Figure 140C Contrast-enhanced chest CT (mediastinal window) of a 58-year-old man with a clinical suspicion of pulmonary *M. tuberculosis* infection shows a filling defect in the left interlobar pulmonary artery (arrow) produced by acute thromboembolism. A small left pleural effusion is also present.

Figure 140D Contrast-enhanced chest CT (mediastinal window) of a 32-year-old man with AIDS and hypoxia reveals an acute pulmonary embolus in the left interlobar pulmonary artery and lingular artery origin with a complicating lingular infarction (arrow) and left pleural effusion.

- Increased noise (i.e., quantum mottle) in obese patients
- Obscuration of vessels by adjacent parenchymal consolidation

Prevention

- Prophylaxis with compression stockings
- Low-dose or low molecular weight heparin
- Early mobilization

Treatment

- Anticoagulation
- Thrombolysis or thrombectomy in selected patients
- Inferior vena cava filters in patients with contraindications to anticoagulation therapy

Prognosis

- Recurrent emboli in one third of patients
- Mortality rates in untreated pulmonary embolus ranging from 18 to 38%

PEARLS_____

- Helical CT is a highly sensitive and specific imaging modality for diagnosing acute emboli in the main, lobar, and segmental arteries. Evaluation of subsegmental branches remains problematic but continues to improve with the newer multidetector scanners.
- CT is indicated for patients with symptoms suggestive of acute PTE disease and an intermediate-probability ventilation-perfusion (VQ) lung scan, low probability or normal VQ lung scan and a high clinical suspicion, severe chronic obstructive pulmonary disease, and in patients with extensive parenchymal lung disease on chest radiography.
- Acute and chronic pulmonary thromboemboli may manifest with filling defects that form a smooth or obtuse angle with the vessel wall, or complete cut-offs of vascular opacification.

- Clinically unsuspected acute pulmonary thromboembolism may be found on 0.4 to 0.6% of outpatient and 2 to 5% of inpatient CT studies.
- Other potential advantages of CT in the evaluation of patients with suspected PTE disease are its ability to detect other thoracic diseases that may mimic embolic disease (e.g., aortic dissection) and complications of embolic disease (e.g., effusion, infarction, cor pulmonale).

Suggested Readings

Blachere H, Latrabe V, Montaudon M, et al. Pulmonary embolism revealed on helical CT angiography: comparison with ventilation-perfusion radionuclide lung scanning. AJR Am J Roentgenol 2000;174: 1041–1047

Fraser RS, Müller NL, Colman N, Paré PD. Thrombosis and thromboembolism. In: Fraser RS, Müller NL, Colman N, Paré PD, eds. Fraser and Paré's Diagnosis of Diseases of the Chest, 4th ed. Philadelphia: Saunders, 1999:1808–1811

Garg K. CT of pulmonary thromboembolic disease. Radiol Clin North Am 2002;40:111–122

Saif MW, Bona R, Greenberg B. AIDS and thrombosis: retrospective study of 131 HIV-infected patients. AIDS Patient Care STDS 2001;15:311–320

Travis WD, Colby TV, Koss MN, Rosado-de-Christenson ML, Müller NL, King TE. Pulmonary hypertension and other vascular disorders. In: King DW, ed. Atlas of Nontumor Pathology: Non-Neoplastic Disorders of the Lower Respiratory Tract. First series, fascicle 2. Washington, DC: American Registry of Pathology; 2002;782–787

CASE 141 Chronic Pulmonary Thromboembolic Disease

Clinical Presentation

A 54-year-old man with chronic obstructive lung disease, a remote history of pulmonary thromboembolism, progressive dyspnea over the last 4 to 6 months

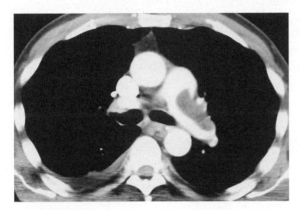

Figure 141A

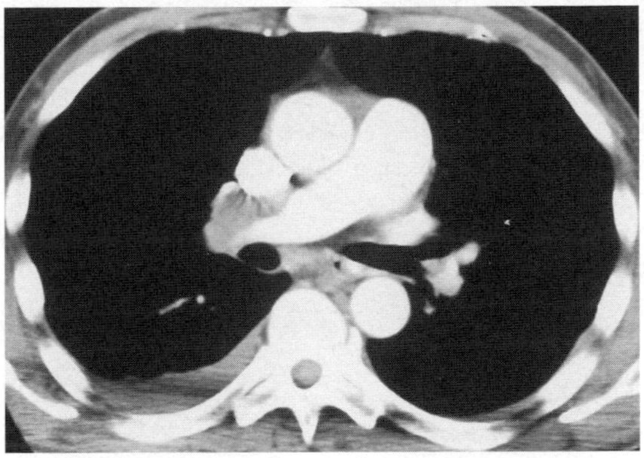

Figure 141B

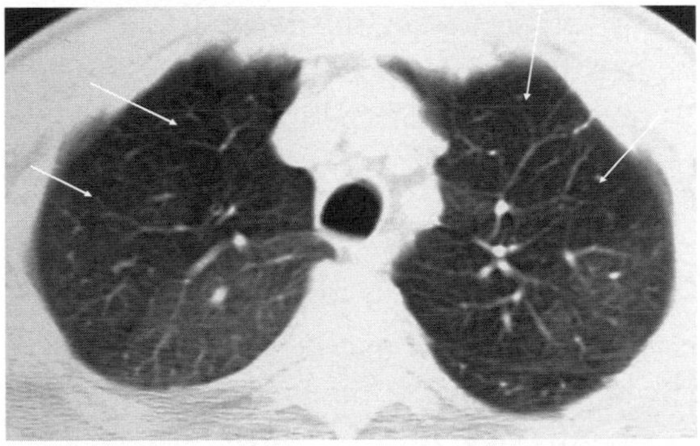

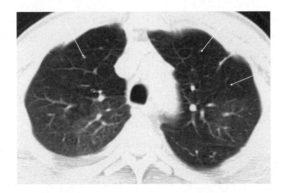

Figure 141C

Figure 141D

Radiologic Findings

Contrast-enhanced chest CT (mediastinal window) (**Figs. 141A** and **141B**) shows large soft tissue attenuation filling defects eccentrically located in the main pulmonary artery, left lobar and distal right lobar, and pulmonary arteries. Note the abrupt termination of the interlobar arteries bilaterally and the small dependent right pleural effusion. Contrast-enhanced chest CT (lung window) (**Figs. 141C** and **141D**) reveals mosaic parenchymal attenuation. Note the subtle decrease in caliber and number of vessels in the low-attenuation areas (arrows) compared with the normal higher attenuation lung.

Diagnosis

Chronic pulmonary thromboembolic disease (CPTE)

543

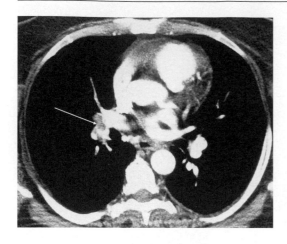

Figure 141E Contrast-enhanced chest CT (mediastinal window) of a 53-year-old woman with history of chronic PTE shows an eccentric soft tissue filling defect in the right middle and lower lobe artery origins. Enhancing tubular structure (arrow) within the intraluminal thrombus represents an area of recanalization.

Differential Diagnosis

None

Discussion

Background

The fate of pulmonary emboli depends on the status of the patient's fibrinolytic system, the degree of thrombus organization before its embolization, and the amount of new thrombus added in situ. Most emboli are degraded by one of three mechanisms: (1) lysis, (2) fragmentation and peripheral embolization, and (3) organization and recanalization.

Etiology

The majority of patients treated for acute PTE improve without sequelae. The remainder may develop chronic or recurrent emboli. Pulmonary emboli are considered chronic if at least two of the following features are present: (1) the clot is eccentrically located in the vessel wall (**Figs. 141A** and **141B**), (2) the intraluminal filling defect demonstrates recanalization (**Fig. 141E**), (3) the arterial diameter is reduced by at least 50%, (4) arterial webs or areas of stenosis are present, or (5) the stenosed artery is completely occluded.

Clinical Findings

Patients with CPTE usually do not present with signs or symptoms suggestive of acute PTE. These patients more frequently present with symptoms of pulmonary artery hypertension (e.g., progressive dyspnea on exertion and easy fatigability).

Pathology

GROSS

- Main pulmonary arteries and their branches contain fibrous webs and bands corresponding to organized thromboemboli, often with overlying recent thrombosis.
- Marked right ventricular hypertrophy is typical.

MICROSCOPIC

- Various stages of organized and recanalized thromboemboli in both the elastic and muscular arteries
- Patent pulmonary arteries develop medial hypertrophy, intimal thickening, and atherosclerotic plaques compatible with hypertensive changes.

Imaging Findings

CT (SENSITIVITY 78%; SPECIFICITY 100%)

- Eccentric (i.e., mural) thrombus contiguous with vessel wall (**Figs. 141A** and **141B**)
- Thrombi adherent to vessel wall (**Figs. 141A** and **141B**)
- Irregular margination (**Figs. 141A** and **141B**)
- Calcification; on occasion
- Intraluminal filling defect demonstrates vascular recanalization (**Fig. 141E**)
- Arterial webs or stenoses
- Marked reduction in arterial diameter
- Mosaic perfusion pattern (lung window) characterized by lobular or multilobular areas of variable lung attenuation; sharp margination between areas of low-attenuation lung with decreased vascularity and areas of normal attenuation and normal vessel size (**Figs. 141C** and **141D**)
- Airway abnormalities (e.g., cylindrical bronchiectasis).

PULMONARY ANGIOGRAPHY

- Eccentric (i.e., mural) thrombi contiguous with the vessel wall
- Multiple webs or stenoses
- Irregular vascular occlusions
- Varying pulmonary vessel calibers

MR ANGIOGRAPHY

- Features similar to those described for pulmonary angiography (see above)
- Affected segmental arteries of varying calibers

Treatment

- Thromboendarterectomy

Prognosis

- Surgical thromboendarterectomy; surgical mortality rate up to 10%
- In-hospital mortality from unrelieved pulmonary hypertension, intraoperative cardiac arrest, reperfusion pulmonary edema, and stroke

PEARLS_____

- Patients with CPTE often present with symptoms of progressive exertional dyspnea, right-sided heart failure, and cyanosis.
- Anticoagulants are not an effective treatment for CPTE; thromboendartectomy is the procedure of choice.

- The mosaic perfusion pattern may be secondary to vascular disease or small-medium airways disease. The latter often demonstrates air trapping on expiratory images, whereas the former usually does not.
- Chronic thromboembolic pulmonary hypertension (CTEPH) is the result of single or recurrent pulmonary thromboemboli that are thought to develop into organized pulmonary arterial obstructions by recurrent embolism and in situ thrombosis.
- Approximately 5% of patients with acute PTE ultimately develop CTEPH.

Suggested Readings

Fleischmann D, Scholten C, Klepetko W, Lang IM. Three-dimensional visualization of pulmonary thromboemboli in chronic thromboembolic hypertension with multiple detector-row spiral computed tomography. Circulation 2001;103:2993

Fraser RS, Müller NL, Colman N, Paré PD. Thrombosis and thromboembolism. In: Fraser RS, Müller NL, Colman N, Paré PD, eds. Fraser and Paré's Diagnosis of Diseases of the Chest, 4th ed. Philadelphia: Saunders, 1999:1811–1813

King MA, Ysrael M, Bergin CJ. Chronic thromboembolic pulmonary hypertension: CT findings. AJR Am J Roentgenol 1998;170:955–960

Remy-Jardin M, Remy J, Louvegny S, et al. Airway changes in chronic pulmonary embolism: CT findings in 33 patients. Radiology 1997;203:355–360

Roberts HC, Kauczor HU, Schweden F, Thelen M. Spiral CT of pulmonary hypertension and chronic thromboembolism. J Thorac Imaging 1997;12:118–127

CASE 142 Pulmonary Arterial Hypertension

Clinical Presentation

A 72-year-old woman with recent diagnosis of right breast carcinoma and an abnormal chest radiograph.

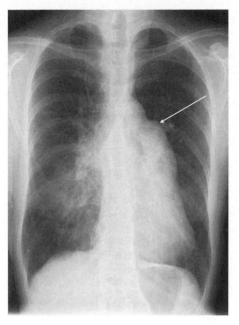

Figure 142A

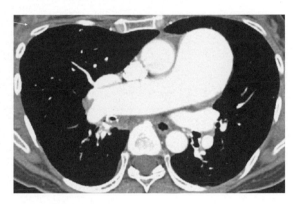

Figure 142B

Radiologic Findings

PA chest radiograph (**Fig. 142A**) shows marked enlargement of the central pulmonary arteries and rapid tapering of the peripheral upper lobe vessels. The enlarged main pulmonary artery creates a focal convexity (arrow) just below the aortic pulmonary window. Note the large size of the right interlobar artery adjacent to the bronchus intermedius. Contrast-enhanced chest CT (mediastinal window) (**Fig. 142B**) reveals massive enlargement of the main and right lobar pulmonary arteries compared with the diameter of the ascending aorta.

Diagnosis

Pulmonary arterial hypertension

Differential Diagnosis

- Primary or secondary pulmonary artery hypertension
- Pulmonic valvular disease

Table 142-1   Proposed Mechanisms and Causes of Pulmonary Arterial Hypertension

Precapillary Hypertension	Postcapillary Hypertension
Primary vascular disease	*Cardiac disease*
Left to right shunts	Left ventricular failure
Primary pulmonary hypertension	Mitral valve disease
Pulmonary artery stenosis or coarctation	Left atrial myxoma
Pulmonary thromboembolic disease	
HIV infection	
Immunologic abnormalities	
Vasculitis	
Pleuropulmonary disease	*Pulmonary venous disease*
Emphysema	Anomalous venous return
Cystic fibrosis	Veno-occlusive disease
Bronchiectasis	Sclerosing mediastinitis
Diffuse interstitial fibrosis	Constrictive pericarditis
Fibrothorax	
Chest wall deformities	
Alveolar hypoventilation	
Obesity/obstructive sleep apnea	
Neuromuscular disease	
High altitude	

Discussion

Background

Pulmonary arterial hypertension (PAH) is defined by a sustained systemic pulmonary artery pressure greater than 30 mm Hg or a mean pulmonary artery pressure greater than 20 mm Hg.

Etiology

PAH may develop secondary to one of three mechanisms: (1) increased pulmonary blood flow (e.g., intracardiac-extracardiac shunts), (2) decreased cross-sectional area of the pulmonary vasculature (e.g., chronic PTE disease), and (3) increased resistance to pulmonary venous drainage (e.g., mitral valvular disease). Alternatively, the etiology may be divided into precapillary causes (i.e., entities resulting in increased pulmonary blood flow or a decrease in cross-sectional area of the pulmonary vasculature) and postcapillary causes (i.e., entities that increase resistance to pulmonary venous drainage). Some of the causes of pulmonary artery hypertension based on these mechanisms are listed in **Table 142-1**. Most cases have an identifiable etiology and are referred to as secondary PAH (**Fig. 142C**). The remaining cases have no explanation and are classified as primary PAH.

Clinical Findings

Patients with primary PAH are usually women under the age of 40 who present with progressive dyspnea and fatigue; 10% of such patients may present with Raynaud's phenomenon. Familial and autosomal-dominant forms of primary PAH also exist. There is also an association between infection with the human immunodeficiency virus (HIV) and PAH. Only one third of these patients have had a prior AIDS-defining illness, and most have no concomitant pulmonary infection. In this patient population, the PAH is likely secondary to immunologic abnormalities.

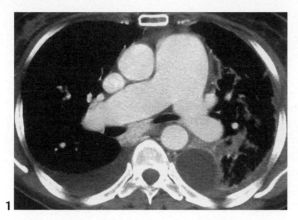 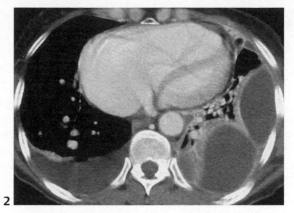

Figure 142C (1,2) Contrast-enhanced chest CT (mediastinal window) of a 39-year-old woman with untreated patent ductus arteriosus and resultant secondary PAH and Eisenmenger physiology who was admitted with empyema reveals marked enlargement of the main pulmonary artery and right heart. Compare the diameter of the pulmonary artery with that of the thoracic aorta. The interventricular septum is bowed as a result of the elevated right heart pressures. Note the multiloculated empyema.

Pathology

- Varies depending on underlying cause
- Dilatation of large elastic arteries (e.g., main pulmonary artery) with a diameter greater than that of the ascending aorta
- Thickening of the media of small muscular arteries and intimal fibrosis of elastic and large muscular arteries
- Cystic medial necrosis and pulmonary arterial atherosclerosis

Imaging Findings

RADIOGRAPHY

- Similar radiographic features regardless of etiology
- Enlargement of the central pulmonary arteries and rapid tapering of the vessels as they extend to the periphery (**Fig. 142A**)
- Pulmonary artery enlargement assessed on frontal radiographs by measurement of the right interlobar artery diameter tangential to the bronchus intermedius; upper limit of normal is 16 mm (men) and 15 mm (women)
- Intrapericardial location of left interlobar artery; inability to measure on frontal radiography; measurement on lateral radiography, identification of circular lucency created by the left upper lobe bronchus and measurement of diameter of the posterior margin of the vessel as it loops over the bronchus (i.e., hyparterial relationship); 18 mm is upper limit of normal
- Right ventricular enlargement; best appreciated on lateral chest radiography
- Rarely, calcifications in the main pulmonary artery or its hilar branches with severe chronic PAH; this most often occurs with Eisenmenger syndrome

CT/MR

- Main pulmonary artery enlargement measured at a right angle to the ascending aorta at the level where the main pulmonary artery bifurcates into the right and left main lobar branches (**Fig. 142D**)
- Main pulmonary artery diameter more than 29 mm has a sensitivity of 87%, specificity of 89%, and positive predictive value of 97% for PAH.
- Right ventricular hypertrophy; bowing of the interventricular septum (i.e., reversal of septal curvature) (**Fig. 142C2**)

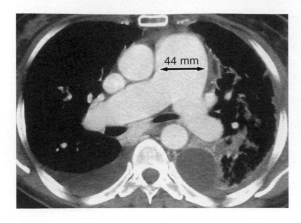

44 mm

Figure 142D Contrast-enhanced chest CT (mediastinal window) illustrates how to measure the diameter of the main pulmonary artery (double-headed arrow). The main pulmonary artery is markedly enlarged, measuring 44 mm. The normal diameter should be less than or equal to 29 mm. Compare the relative size of the main pulmonary artery to that of the ascending aorta.

- Pericardial thickening
- Mosaic perfusion (lung window)
- Interlobular septal thickening (i.e., linear septal opacities)
- Consolidation secondary to localized edema

Treatment

- Primarily supportive medical therapy, supplemental oxygen
- Transplantation

Prognosis

- Rapid deterioration in most patients
- One-year survival rate of 50% in patients with HIV infection

PEARLS_____

- The most striking radiologic feature of PAH is the disparity in size between the central and peripheral pulmonary arteries. However, the degree of vascular pruning does not correlate well with the severity of pulmonary hypertension.
- Significant PAH may exist even when chest radiograph is normal.
- Scrutiny of the imaging studies for concomitant cardiac, parenchymal, and pleural disease may provide insight into the underlying etiology.
- Echosonography is the most accurate noninvasive method of evaluating PAH.

Suggested Readings

Conte JV, Borja MJ, Patel CB, Yang SC, Jhaveri RM, Orens JB. Lung transplantation for primary and secondary pulmonary hypertension. Ann Thorac Surg 2001;72:1673–1680

Fraser RS, Müller NL, Colman N, Paré PD. Pulmonary hypertension. In: Fraser RS, Müller NL, Colman N, Paré PD, eds. Fraser and Paré's Diagnosis of Diseases of the Chest, 4th ed. Philadelphia: Saunders, 1999:1879–1891, 1914

Kruger S, Haage P, Hoffman R, et al. Diagnosis of pulmonary artery hypertension and pulmonary embolism with magnetic resonance angiography. Chest 2001;120:1556–1561

CASE 143 Cardiogenic Pulmonary Edema: Left Ventricular Failure

Clinical Presentation

A 52-year-old woman with recurrent episodes of left ventricular decompensation admitted with chest pain and a myocardial infarction

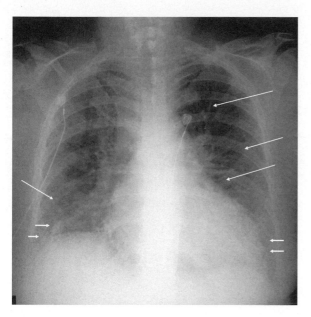

Figure 143A

Radiologic Findings

AP chest radiograph (**Fig. 143A**) reveals cardiomegaly with a left ventricular configuration. The peripheral vasculature is indistinct. Kerley A lines (long arrows) radiate from the central hilar region. Kerley B lines (short arrows) are present along the periphery of the chest wall and pleura. Both costophrenic sulci are ill defined.

Diagnosis

Cardiogenic pulmonary edema; left ventricular failure

Differential Diagnosis

- Hydrostatic edema of other etiologies
- Fulminant pneumonia
- Acute exacerbation of chronic obstructive pulmonary disease (COPD)
- Acute hemorrhage

551

Table 143-1   Causes of Pulmonary Edema

Hydrostatic Edema	Increased Permeability Edema
Cardiogenic	Aspiration of gastric contents
Left ventricular failure	Multiple trauma
Mitral valve disease	Prolonged hypotension
Left atrial myxoma	Multiple blood transfusions
Left atrial thrombus	Systemic sepsis
Decreased oncotic pressure	Drug overdose
Fluid overload	Near-drowning
Renal failure	Pancreatitis
Cirrhosis	Burns
Neurogenic	Fat emboli
Head trauma	Disseminated intravascular coagulation
Increased intracranial pressure	
Seizure	

Discussion

Background

Hydrostatic edema results from an increase in pulmonary microvascular pressure or a decrease in plasma oncotic pressure.

Etiology

The most common cause of interstitial and airspace edema is cardiogenic resulting from left heart failure (**Table 143-1**). An increase in pulmonary venous pressure may be secondary to transmitted back-pressure from the left ventricle as seen with systemic hypertension, cardiomyopathy, myocardial infarction, and aortic valvular disease or secondary to left atrial outflow obstruction as occurs with mitral stenosis (**Fig. 143B**), atrial myxoma or thrombus, and cor triatriatum. Transudation of fluid into the interstitium is the first stage of hydrostatic edema and invariably precedes airspace edema.

Clinical Findings

Acute presentations may be characterized by dyspnea, tachypnea, respiratory distress, use of accessory muscles for respiration, tachycardia, cyanosis, diaphoresis, elevated blood pressure, and in severe cases frothy blood-tinged sputum and frank hemoptysis. Patients may also demonstrate peripheral edema, hepatosplenomegaly, expiratory wheezes and crackles, and an S3 gallop. More insidious onset is characterized by dyspnea on exertion, orthopnea, and paroxysmal nocturnal dyspnea.

Pathology

- Transudation of fluid into perivascular interstitial tissue and interlobular septa
- Pleural thickening or effusion
- Patchy or confluent bilateral consolidations secondary to alveolar flooding and airspace edema

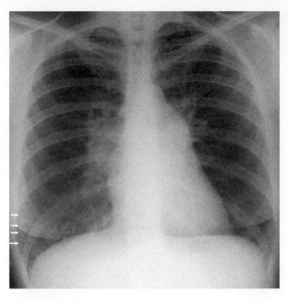

Figure 143B AP chest radiograph of a 39-year-old woman with rheumatic heart disease, mitral stenosis and interstitial pulmonary edema shows marked enlargement of the left atrial appendage and right interlobar pulmonary artery. Kerley B lines (arrows) are present in both lung bases.

Table 143-2 Radiologic Features of Hydrostatic Versus Increased Permeability Edema

Radiologic Feature	Hydrostatic Edema	Increased Permeability Edema
Increased cardiothoracic ratio	(+)	(−)
Vascular redistribution	(+) cardiogenic (−) volume overload (−) renal failure	(−)
Widened vascular pedicle	(+)	(−)
Kerley lines	(+)	(−)
Peribronchial cuffing	(+)	(−)
Perihilar haze	(+)	(−)
Airspace opacities and consolidation	Diffuse and perihilar or central and perihilar	Patchy and peripheral
Pleural effusions	(+)	(−)

(+) Feature present, (−) Feature absent

Imaging Findings (Table 143-2)

Principal radiologic patterns are interstitial edema and airspace edema:

- First manifestation: redistribution of blood flow; an increase in size of upper zone vessels compared with lower zone vessels and/or an increase in the end-on diameter of the upper lobe arteries and their adjacent bronchi (normally 1:1)
- Increasing vascular pedicle width (> 70 mm; supine AP chest radiographs); measured by drawing a line parallel to the origin of the left subclavian artery off the transverse aorta and a second horizontal line extending from the right lateral border of the superior vena cava as it crosses the right main bronchus. The horizontal measurement between these two lines is the vascular pedicle width (**Fig. 143C**).
- Indistinct vascular markings, peribronchial wall thickening (i.e., > 1 mm) (**Fig. 143D**), and Kerley A and B lines (**Figs. 143A** and **143B**) as the pulmonary venous pressure increases and fluid accumulates in the perivascular interstitial tissue and interlobular septa
- Perihilar or lower lung zone "haze" as fluid accumulates in the parenchymal interstitial tissues and alveolar walls; usually precedes airspace edema.

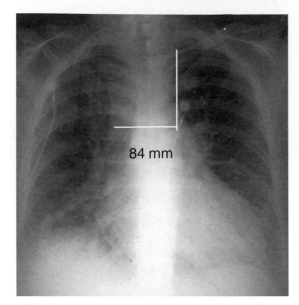

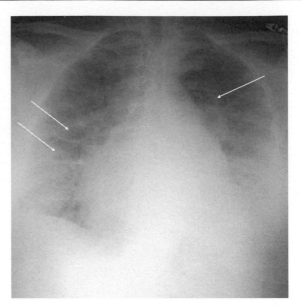

Figure 143C AP chest radiograph illustrates how to measure the vascular pedicle width. The pedicle is measured by drawing two lines. The first line parallels the origin of the left subclavian artery from the transverse aorta. The second line extends from the right lateral border of the superior vena cava as it crosses the right main bronchus. The width of these two lines is 84 mm in this patient with hydrostatic edema. The normal width on a portable supine chest radiograph is less than or equal to 70 mm.

Figure 143D AP chest radiograph of a 52-year-old woman status post–remote mitral valve replacement complicated by collagenous degradation of the porcine valve and pulmonary edema shows an increased cardio-thoracic ratio and widened vascular pedicle. The peripheral vasculature is indistinct; there is peribronchial cuffing and a perihilar haze. Curvilinear Kerley A lines (long arrows) and bilateral pleural effusions are present.

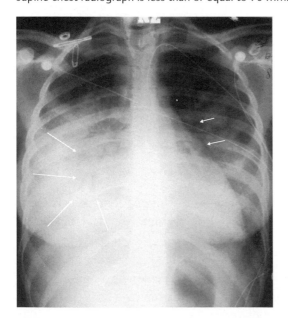

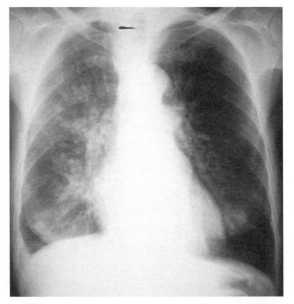

Figure 143E AP chest radiograph of a 57-year-old woman with progressive dyspnea secondary to mitral insufficiency and resultant airspace edema reveals cardiomegaly and slight fullness of the left atrial appendage. The peripheral vasculature is indistinct. There are marked bronchial cuffing (short arrows) and perihilar consolidation with air bronchograms (long arrows).

Figure 143F AP chest radiograph of a 60-year-old woman with emphysema, heart failure, and gravitational pulmonary edema who breathes easier when lying on her right side reveals hyperinflated lungs, indistinct, congested right perihilar vasculature, bronchial cuffing, septal lines, and an ipsilateral pleural effusion.

Table 143-3 Unusual Patterns of Pulmonary Edema

Ipsilateral unilateral pulmonary edema	Contralateral unilateral pulmonary edema	Right upper lobe edema
Systemic-to-pulmonary shunts (e.g., congenital heart defects)	Acute pulmonary thromboembolism	Mitral regurgitation
Bronchial obstruction (e.g., drowned lobe)	Localized emphysema	Underlying parenchymal disease spared this lobe
Prolonged decubitus positioning	Pleural disease	
Unilateral aspiration	Swyer-James syndrome	
Pulmonary contusion	Extrinsic pulmonary artery obstruction (e.g., mass, nodes, thoracic aorta aneurysm)	
Rapid thoracentesis of pleural air or fluid	Lobectomy	
Unilateral thoracic sympathectomy	Unilateral thoracic sympathectomy	

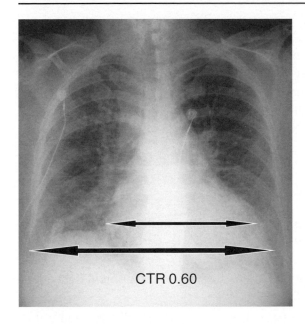

CTR 0.60

Figure 143G AP chest radiograph illustrates how to measure the cardiothoracic ratio (CTR). The cardiac size is first determined by measuring the width of the cardiac silhouette at its widest point (short double-headed arrow). The thoracic cage is then measured at its widest point from the inner margin of the right ribs to the inner margin of the left ribs (long double-headed arrow). The ratio of these two values defines the CTR, which is 0.60 in this patient with hydrostatic edema.

- Bilateral, patchy or confluent, symmetric, perihilar, and lower lung areas of consolidation; airspace edema with air bronchograms in 30% of patients (**Fig. 143E**)
- Edema typically bilateral and symmetric; asymmetric or unilateral (**Fig. 143F**) patterns of edema may be seen (**Table 143-3**)
- Increase in cardiothoracic ratio > 0.55 (**Fig. 143G**)

Treatment

- Reduction of cardiac workload
- Improvement of cardiac performance (e.g., positive inotropic agents, correction of arrhythmias, underlying valvular defects)
- Control excess salt and water (e.g., dietary sodium restriction, diuretics)

Prognosis

- Dependent on underlying cause

PEARLS_____

- Supine radiographic signs helpful in differentiating hydrostatic edema from increased permeability edema include an increased cardiothoracic ratio (> 0.55) coupled with a vascular pedicle width > 70 mm, interstitial edema, and pleural effusions. The first two radiographic signs are the most sensitive and specific.
- Vascular pedicle width is not affected by the phase of respiration. However, patient rotation will affect the vascular pedicle width. It is reduced with right anterior oblique rotation and increased with left anterior oblique rotation.
- Radiographic features of pulmonary venous hypertension and their physiologic relationship to pulmonary venous wedge pressure can be remembered by applying the "rule of 6's" (add 5 mm Hg at each stage in cases of chronic heart failure):
  - 6–< 12 mm Hg: normal pulmonary venous wedge pressure
  - > 12–< 18 mm Hg: vascular redistribution (e.g., cephalization)
  - > 18–< 24 mm Hg: indistinct vascular markings, peribronchial cuffing, Kerley lines, and pleural effusions
  - > 24–30 mm Hg: airspace edema
- Acute volume overload can simulate cardiogenic edema radiographically.
- The radiographic signs of pulmonary edema may resolve rapidly with appropriate therapy but may lag 12 to 24 hours behind clinical improvement in some cases.
- Unilateral or asymmetric patterns of edema may be difficult to differentiate from pneumonia. A change in the pattern of edema following diuresis or with an alteration in the patient's positioning may aid in differentiation.

Suggested Readings

Fraser RS, Müller NL, Colman N, Paré PD. Pulmonary edema. In: Fraser RS, Müller NL, Colman N, Paré PD, eds. Fraser and Paré's Diagnosis of Diseases of the Chest, 4th ed. Philadelphia: Saunders, 1999:1956–1976

Gluecker T, Capasso P, Schnyder P, et al. Clinical and radiologic features of pulmonary edema. Radiographics 1999;19:1507–1531

Ketai LH, Godwin JD. A new view of pulmonary edema and acute respiratory distress syndrome. J Thorac Imaging 1998;13:147–171

CASE 144 Noncardiogenic Pulmonary Edema

Clinical Presentation

A 62-year-old woman with dialysis-dependent chronic renal disease and new onset of dyspnea

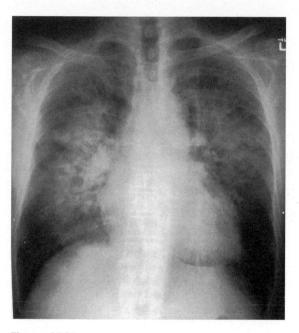

Figure 144A

Radiologic Findings

PA chest radiograph (**Fig. 144A**) reveals an abnormal cardiothoracic ratio and hyperinflated lungs. There is airspace edema involving the perihilar portion of both lungs with sparing of the lung periphery.

Diagnosis

Noncardiogenic edema of renal disease

Differential Diagnosis

- Hydrostatic edema of other etiologies
- Pulmonary hemorrhage
- Aspiration pneumonia
- Multilobar pneumonia

Discussion

Background

Hydrostatic edema may be associated with both acute and chronic renal disease (see Case 143, **Table 143-1**).

Etiology

The edema develops from a combination of left ventricular failure, decreased protein oncotic pressure, increased intravascular volume, and capillary leak. Uremic patients may develop edema secondary to chronic high-output failure, hypervolemia, coronary artery disease, and left ventricular hypertrophy. Acute hydrostatic edema is not an infrequent manifestation of renal disease secondary to bilateral renal artery stenosis.

Clinical Findings

Basal rales are the traditional hallmark of early pulmonary edema. Patients may also exhibit tachypnea and signs of peripheral edema including anasarca.

Pathology

- Transudation of fluid into perivascular interstitial tissue and interlobular septa
- Pleural thickening or effusion
- Patchy or confluent bilateral consolidations secondary to alveolar flooding and airspace edema

Imaging Findings (see Case 143, Table 143-2)

- Enlarged cardiothoracic ratio (e.g., cardiomegaly, pericardial effusion)
- Increasing or widened vascular pedicle (> 70 mm) on serial radiographs
- Kerley lines and peribronchial cuffing
- Central perihilar airspace opacification; "bat wing" or "butterfly" pattern of airspace edema when the outer 2 to 3 cm of lung parenchyma is spared (**Fig. 144A**)
- Pleural effusions

Treatment

- Renal failure:
  - Supportive
  - Control excess salt and water (e.g., dietary sodium restriction, diuretics, dialysis)
  - Transplantation
- Volume overload:
  - Supportive
  - Diuretics
  - Colloids in select cases

Prognosis

- Left ventricular hypertrophy; risk factor for death in patients dependent on chronic dialysis

PEARLS

- Hydrostatic edema resulting from a decrease in oncotic pressure is most often seen following the infusion of large volumes of intravenous fluid in postoperative, trauma, and elderly patients. Concomitant temporary high-output left ventricular failure likely also plays a role.
- Hydrostatic edema may also occur in the setting of acute liver failure, chronic liver failure, and cirrhosis, and following liver transplantation.

Suggested Readings

Fraser RS, Müller NL, Colman N, Paré PD. Pulmonary edema. In: Fraser RS, Müller NL, Colman N, Paré PD, eds. Fraser and Paré's Diagnosis of Diseases of the Chest, 4th ed. Philadelphia: Saunders, 1999:1956–1976

Gluecker T, Capasso P, Schnyder P, et al. Clinical and radiologic features of pulmonary edema. Radiographics 1999;19:1507–1531

Ketai LH, Godwin JD. A new view of pulmonary edema and acute respiratory distress syndrome. J Thorac Imaging 1998;13:147–171

CASE 145 Increased Permeability Edema

Clinical Presentation

A 33-year-old man with pancreatitis, hypoxia, increasing ventilation requirements, and normal pulmonary venous wedge pressures

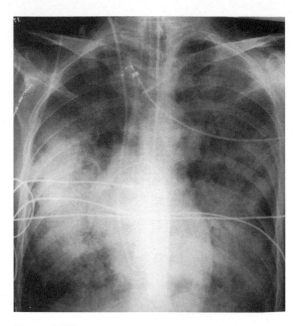

Figure 145A

Radiologic Findings

AP chest radiograph (**Fig. 145A**) shows bilateral, patchy, relatively peripheral, parenchymal opacities with asymmetric coalescence in the right mid-lung. The heart size is normal, as is the vascular pedicle width. There is no interstitial edema or pleural effusion. Multiple life support tubes and lines are well positioned.

Diagnosis

Increased permeability edema; acute respiratory distress syndrome

Differential Diagnosis

- Pulmonary hemorrhage
- Aspiration
- Hospital-acquired pneumonia

Discussion

Background

Increased permeability edema is best exemplified by acute respiratory distress syndrome (ARDS). Common risk factors for ARDS include shock, sepsis, near-drowning, multiple trauma, smoke or noxious gas inhalation, aspiration of gastric contents, pancreatitis, and disseminated intravascular coagulation (see Case 143, **Table 143-1**).

Etiology

Increased permeability edema (i.e., normal-pressure edema) results from an increase in microvascular permeability and the accumulation of proteinaceous fluid in the extravascular space.

Clinical Findings

Affected patients may exhibit severe arterial desaturation resistant to high concentrations of oxygen, stiff or noncompliant lungs, and difficulty in ventilation. They may also have normal pulmonary venous wedge pressures and radiographic evidence of diffuse airspace disease.

Pathology

GROSS

- Exudative (acute) phase (first week after onset of respiratory failure)
  - Large and heavy lung (2–3 times normal weight)
  - Lung congestion and edema
  - External lung surface distends overlying pleura
  - Cut lung surface: noncrepitant; dark red to blue
- Proliferative (organizing) phase (end of first week after onset of respiratory failure)
  - Lung surface: noncrepitant, rubbery, firm; patchy red-brown or yellow-gray
  - Cut lung surface: pale, spongy; fine cysts; airspaces measure 1 to 2 mm with thick walls; irregular dense scarring
  - Pleural surface: coarse, cobblestone appearance

MICROSCOPIC

- Exudative (acute) phase (first week after onset of respiratory failure)
  - Light microscopy
    - Alveolar capillary congestion
    - Interstitial and alveolar edema
    - Intraalveolar hemorrhage
    - Hyaline membranes (histologic hallmark)
  - Electron microscopy
    - Type 1 pneumocyte injury: necrosis; sloughed alveolar surface
    - Endothelial cell injury
    - Edema and exudation of plasma proteins into alveolar interstitium and spaces
    - Denuded basement membrane

- Type 2 pneumocyte necrosis
- Intercellular junction widening and swelling
- Increase in number of pinocytotic vesicles
- Proliferative (organizing) phase (end of first week after onset of respiratory failure)
  - Light microscopy
    - Organization of interstitial and alveolar space exudate organizes
    - Extensive type 2 pneumocyte and fibroblast proliferation
  - Electron microscopy
    - Type 2 pneumocytes express surfactant
    - Squamous metaplasia
    - Considerable cytologic atypia
    - Interstitial fibroblast and myofibroblast proliferation
    - Exudate transforms into granulation tissue
    - Alveolar duct fibrosis
- Fibrotic (chronic) phase (survivors 3–4 weeks on mechanical ventilation)
  - Light microscopy
    - Extensive remodeling by dense fibrous tissue
    - Haphazard arrangement of alveolar spaces and bronchioles
    - Honeycomb changes
    - Juxtapleural necrosis
  - Electron microscopy
    - Basement membrane disruption
    - Thick collagen deposition along alveolar walls
    - Progressive alveolar duct and interstitial fibrosis

Imaging Findings (see Case 143, Table 143-1)

RADIOGRAPHY

- First 12 to 24 hours (following onset of respiratory failure)
  - Decrease in lung volume; otherwise normal (unless precipitated by a pulmonary process such as aspiration or pneumonia)
- 24 hours (following onset of respiratory failure)
  - Patchy airspace consolidation becomes rapidly confluent and diffuse (**Fig. 145A**).
  - Consolidation most severe in peripheral lung
  - Frequent air bronchograms
  - Uncommon septal lines and pleural effusions (**Fig. 145A**)
- Normal heart size and vascular pedicle width (**Fig. 145A**)
  - 5 to 7 days (following onset of respiratory failure)
    - Consolidation replaced by less dense, ground-glass opacification
    - Thin-walled cystic airspaces or lucencies (i.e., manifestation of barotrauma)
  - 2 to 3 weeks (following onset of respiratory failure)
    - Reticular opacities (i.e., reflecting fibrosis)

CT

- Consolidation more heterogeneous and patchy than radiography suggests
- Consolidation favors dependent lung zones.
- Bronchiole dilatation in areas of abnormal lung (i.e., reflecting fibrosis)
- Small unilateral or bilateral pleural effusions (50%)
- Manifestations of barotrauma (e.g., pulmonary interstitial air, pneumomediastinum, pneumothorax, pneumatoceles, subcutaneous air)

Treatment

- Primarily supportive, including use of mechanical ventilation and supplemental oxygen
- No drugs are effective in combating ARDS; steroids, inhaled nitric oxide, and prone ventilation beneficial in some patients
- Correction of underlying predisposing medical problem (e.g., pancreatitis)

Prognosis

- Mortality rate exceeds 40%; death is often secondary to sepsis and/or multiorgan failure.
- Survivors may recover normal lung function; some suffer permanent lung damage and pulmonary fibrosis.

PEARLS_____

- Characteristically, there is a delay of up to 12 hours from the clinical onset of respiratory failure to the appearance of chest radiographic abnormalities.
- Pleural effusion on chest radiography suggests concomitant hydrostatic edema, complicating pneumonia (e.g., hospital-acquired), pulmonary thromboembolism, or subdiaphragmatic disease.

Suggested Readings

Fraser RS, Müller NL, Colman N, Paré PD. Pulmonary edema. In: Fraser RS, Müller NL, Colman N, Paré PD, eds. Fraser and Paré's Diagnosis of Diseases of the Chest, 4th ed. Philadelphia: Saunders, 1999:1976–1999

Gluecker T, Capasso P, Schnyder P, et al. Clinical and radiologic features of pulmonary edema. Radiographics 1999;19:1507–1531

Ketai LH, Godwin JD. A new view of pulmonary edema and acute respiratory distress syndrome. J Thorac Imaging 1998;13:147–171

Nakos G, Tsangaris I, Kostanti E, et al. Effect of the prone position on patients with hydrostatic pulmonary edema compared with patients with acute respiratory distress syndrome and pulmonary fibrosis. Am J Respir Crit Care Med 2000;161:360–368

CASE 146 Reexpansion Pulmonary Edema

Clinical Presentation

A 53-year-old man with a tension pneumothorax

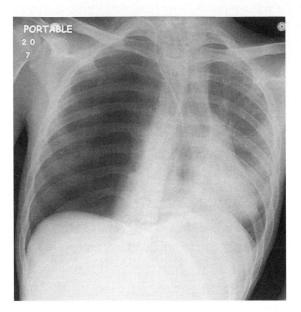

Figure 146A

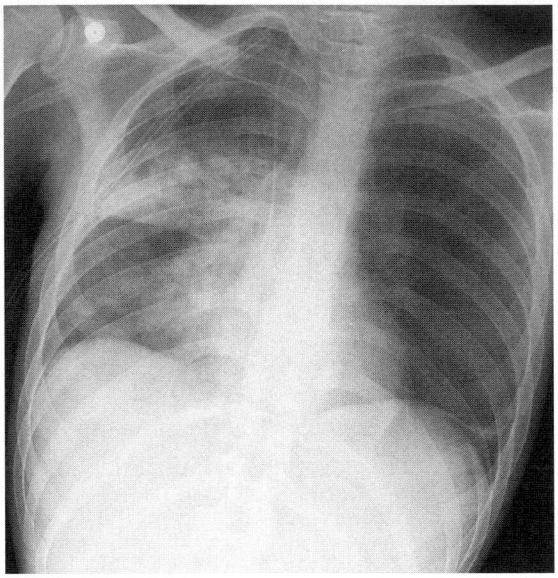

Figure 146B

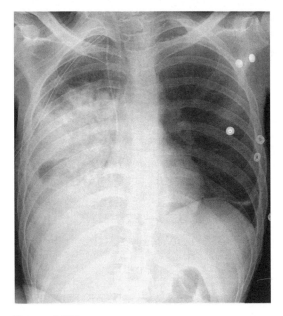

Figure 146C

Radiologic Findings

AP chest radiograph (**Fig. 146A**) reveals a right-sided tension pneumothorax, marked leftward mediastinal shift, and left lower lobe volume loss. AP chest radiograph 24 hours later (**Fig. 146B**), immediately following chest tube placement, shows relief of the pneumothorax. However, right perihilar, upper lobe, and lower lobe airspace consolidations are now present. AP chest radiograph 10 hours following the chest tube placement (**Fig. 146C**) shows progressive right airspace consolidation, ipsilateral lower lobe volume loss, and a right pleural effusion.

Diagnosis

Reexpansion pulmonary edema

Differential Diagnosis

None

Discussion

Background

Reexpansion pulmonary edema represents a form of unilateral pulmonary edema that occurs following the rapid evacuation of air or fluid from the ipsilateral pleural space. In most cases, the pneumothorax or hydrothorax is moderate or large in volume (i.e., occupying at least 50% of the affected hemithorax) and has been present for several days. However, reexpansion edema may develop after the evacuation of pneumothoraces present for only a few hours. Reexpansion pulmonary edema can be prevented by the slow withdrawal of pleural air or fluid.

Etiology

Reexpansion pulmonary edema is likely related to a sudden increase in negative intrapleural pressure transmitted to the interstitial space, an alteration in alveolar surface tension, and increased capillary permeability.

Clinical Findings

Reexpansion pulmonary edema may be preceded clinically by chest tightness and spasmodic coughing.

Pathology

- Reperfusion injury to the pulmonary endothelium due to local production of toxic oxygen free radicals

Imaging Findings

RADIOGRAPHY

- Airspace edema localized to ipsilateral lung; develops within 2 to 4 hours after lung reexpansion
- Consolidation usually affects entire reexpanded lung; only one lobe affected on occasion (**Figs. 146B** and **146C**)
- Consolidation resolves over 5 to 7 days
- Ipsilateral pleural effusion or pneumothorax

CT

- Patchy distribution of areas of consolidation
- Ground-glass opacities with interlobular septal lines (i.e., crazy paving) in affected lung
- Ipsilateral pleural effusion or pneumothorax

Prognosis

- Most often without clinical consequences
- Catastrophic circulatory collapse: mortality rates approaching 20%

Suggested Readings

Fraser RS, Müller NL, Colman N, Paré PD. Pulmonary edema. In: Fraser RS, Müller NL, Colman N, Paré PD, eds. Fraser and Paré's Diagnosis of Diseases of the Chest, 4th ed. Philadelphia: Saunders, 1999:2001–2002

Gascoigne A, Appleton A, Taylor R, Batchelor A, Cook S. Catastrophic circulatory collapse following re-expansion pulmonary oedema. Resuscitation 1996;31:265–269

Rozenman J, Yellin A, Simansky DA, Shiner RJ. Re-expansion pulmonary oedema following spontaneous pneumothorax. Respir Med 1996;90:235–238

Tremey B, Guglielminotti J, Belkacem A, Maury E, Offenstadt G. Acute respiratory failure after re-expansion pulmonary oedema localized to a lobe. Intensive Care Med 2001;27:325–326

CASE 147 Negative Pressure Pulmonary Edema

Clinical Presentation

A 49-year-old woman with a large thyroid goiter and dyspnea was intubated in preparation for a thyroidectomy and became acutely hypotensive. The procedure was aborted, and she was treated with intravenous fluids and subsequently extubated. The extubation was complicated by laryngospasm, necessitating reintubation.

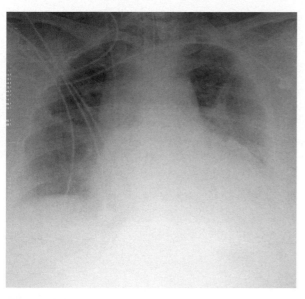

Figure 147A

Radiologic Findings

AP chest radiograph (**Fig. 147A**) shows rightward deviation of the tracheal air column secondary to the thyroid goiter, modest cardiomegaly, and hydrostatic pulmonary edema. Life support devices are appropriately positioned.

Diagnosis

Negative pressure pulmonary edema

Differential Diagnosis

Other causes of hydrostatic pulmonary edema

Discussion

Background

This form of pulmonary edema is associated with severe upper airway obstruction.

567

Etiology

Negative pressure pulmonary edema is often precipitated by laryngospasm, especially in patients having surgical procedures performed on or around the extrathoracic trachea. The edema usually develops following relief of the laryngospasm by reintubation. In such patients, the negative intrapleural pressure is markedly increased by the forceful inspiratory effort exerted against the obstructed extrathoracic airway. This results in an influx of fluid from the pulmonary capillaries into the lung and resultant pulmonary edema. Negative pressure edema may also develop following relief of the extrathoracic airway obstruction. A modified Valsalva maneuver is likely responsible in these patients. The high-negative intrapulmonary pressures generated during inspiration before relief of the obstruction are countered by an expiratory component. When the obstructing lesion is removed, this counterforce is no longer present, and pulmonary blood flow rapidly increases, resulting in pulmonary edema.

Clinical Findings

Cardiac dysfunction likely contributes to the pulmonary edema. Very negative intrathoracic pressures profoundly affect left heart function, generating pressures of -140 cm of water or greater. This is equivalent to adding an afterload of approximately 100 mm Hg to the left heart.

Imaging Findings

- Features associated with noncardiogenic hydrostatic pulmonary edema (see Case 143)
- Increase in cardiothoracic ratio (**Fig. 147A**)
- Vascular pedicle widening (**Fig. 147A**)
- Indistinct vascular markings (**Fig. 147A**)
- Perihilar haze (**Fig. 147A**)
- Pleural effusion (**Fig. 147A**)
- Thoracic inlet mass and/or subglottic stenosis

Treatment

- Prompt recognition
- Intravenous diuretics
- Oxygen therapy
- Low levels of peak end-expiratory pressure (PEEP) (5 cm H_2O) used in most cases

Prognosis

- Good with prompt recognition and treatment

PEARL_____

- Negative pressure pulmonary edema may complicate the induction of anesthesia, manipulation of endotracheal tubes, and various head and neck as well as oral maxillofacial surgical procedures.

Suggested Readings

DeVane GG. Acute postobstructive pulmonary edema. CRNA 1995;6:110–113

Dicpinigaitis PV, Mehta DC. Postobstructive pulmonary edema induced by endotracheal tube occlusion. Intensive Care Med 1995;21:1048–1050

Fraser RS, Müller NL, Colman N, Paré PD. Pulmonary edema. In: Fraser RS, Müller NL, Colman N, Paré PD, eds. Fraser and Paré's Diagnosis of Diseases of the Chest, 4th ed. Philadelphia: Saunders, 1999:2002–2003

Sharma ML, Beckett N, Gormley P. Negative pressure pulmonary edema following thyroidectomy. Can J Anaesth 2002;49:215

CASE 148 Left Aortic Nipple

Clinical Presentation

A 17-year-old man who is experiencing chest pain

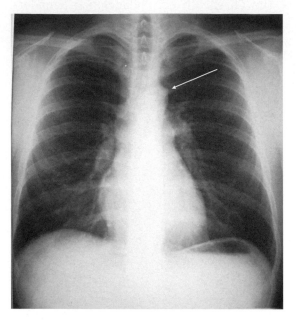

Figure 148A

Radiologic Findings

PA chest radiograph (**Fig. 148A**) demonstrates a small, localized protuberance off the transverse aorta (arrow).

Diagnosis

Normal chest radiograph; incidental aortic nipple

Differential Diagnosis

None

Discussion

Background

The left first intercostal space drains into the left supreme or highest intercostal vein. The left second through fourth intercostal spaces drain into a common vessel, the left superior intercostal vein. This vessel usually communicates with the accessory hemiazygos vein as it descends along the spine and arches around the transverse aorta to empty into the left brachiocephalic vein. As the left superior intercostal–accessory hemiazygos vein passes anteriorly from the spine and parallels the transverse aorta, it may be seen en face in approximately 10% of frontal chest radiographs.

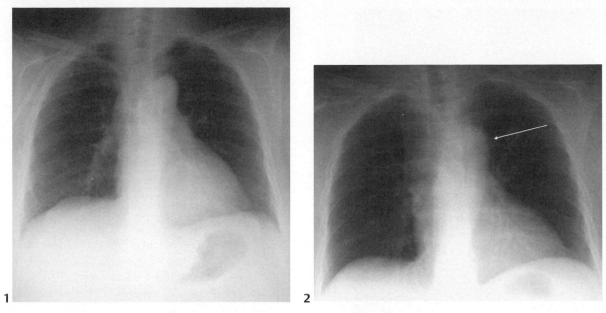

Figure 148B (1,2) Baseline PA chest radiograph **(1)** of a 42-year-old morbidly obese woman on chronic hemodialysis with a well-positioned right subclavian catheter. PA chest radiograph 2 months later **(2)** when she has right upper extremity swelling reveals interval removal of the hemodialysis catheter and formation of an acquired aortic nipple (arrow). Venography (not shown) demonstrated recruitment of collateral blood flow via the left superior intercostal vein due to right innominate–superior vena caval catheter-induced venous stenosis.

Etiology

The aortic nipple is formed by the left superior intercostal and accessory hemiazygos veins.

Clinical Findings

Like the vascular pedicle and the azygos vein, an increase in size of the left superior intercostal vein may serve as a marker of a given patient's intravascular volume. Gradual formation or enlargement of the aortic nipple over time may indicate recruitment of collateral blood flow via this venous system in patients with obstruction of the innominate vein and superior or inferior vena cava (**Fig. 148B**) by stricture-stenosis, thrombus or tumor, Budd-Chiari syndrome, portal hypertension, hypoplasia of the left innominate vein, congenital absence of the azygos vein, and azygos continuation of the inferior vena cava (**Fig. 148C**).

Imaging Findings

RADIOGRAPHY

- Variable-sized local protuberance in contour of superomedial or inferolateral aorta (**Figs. 148A, 148B2,** and **148C**)
- Commonly measures less than 5 mm in diameter on erect chest frontal radiographs (**Figs. 148A** and **148B2**)

Treatment

- None
- Endovascular stenting-angioplasty of affected vessel in patients with venous-related stricture-stenosis

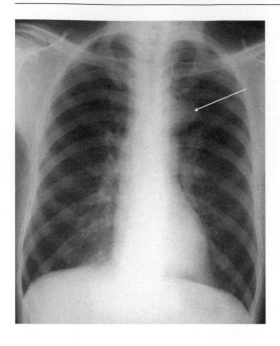

Figure 148C PA chest radiograph of a 38-year-old man with abdominal pain and congenital hemiazygos-azygos continuation of the inferior vena cava demonstrates a 4.0 cm oblong left-sided mediastinal mass just above the aortic arch (arrow) due to aneurysmal dilatation of the left superior intercostal vein.

Prognosis

- Good

Suggested Readings

Arslan G, Cubuk M, Ozkaynk C, Sindel T, Luleci E. Absence of the azygos vein. Clin Imaging 2000;24: 157–158

Fraser RS, Müller NL, Colman N, Paré PD. The mediastinum. In: Fraser RS, Müller NL, Colman N, Paré PD, eds. Fraser and Paré's Diagnosis of Diseases of the Chest, 4th ed. Philadelphia: Saunders, 1999:209–211

Medrea M, Meydam K, Schmitt WG. MRI visualization of the aortic nipple. Cardiovasc Intervent Radiol 1988;11(1):29–31

CASE 149 Aneurysm of the Thoracic Aorta

Clinical Presentation

A 66-year-old man with hypertension and coronary artery disease complaining of chest pain

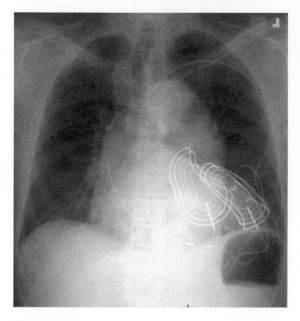

Figure 149A

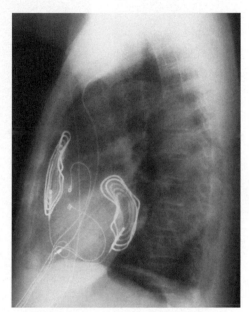

Figure 149B

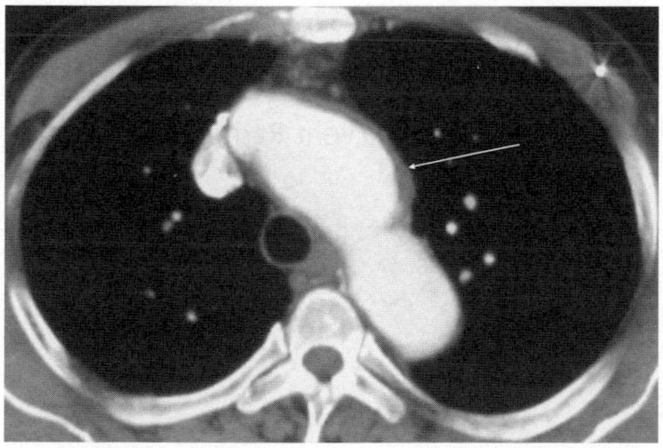

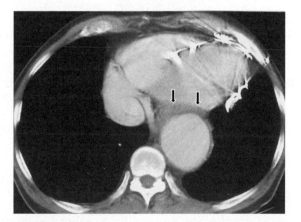

Figure 149C

Figure 149D

Radiologic Findings

PA (**Fig. 149A**) and lateral (**Fig. 149B**) chest radiographs demonstrate cardiomegaly, a single-lead ventricular pacer, and fusiform dilation of the thoracic aorta from the aortic knob to the hiatus. Contrast-enhanced chest CT (mediastinal window) (**Figs. 149C** and **149D**) reveals diffuse enlargement of the thoracic aorta and mural thrombus (arrows).

573

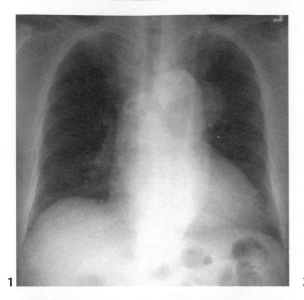

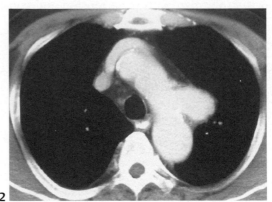

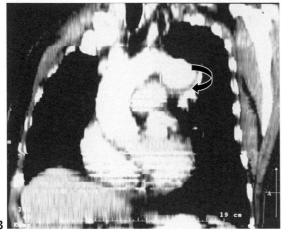

Figure 149E (1–3) PA chest radiograph **(1)** of a 63-year-old hypertensive man shows a 5 cm mass related to the transverse aorta. The thoracic aorta is ectatic and demonstrates mural calcifications. Contrast-enhanced axial (mediastinal window) **(2)** and multiplanar reconstruction MPR coronal (mediastinal window) **(3)** chest CT reveals a focal eccentric outpouching in the lateral wall of the transverse aorta from a saccular aneurysm of the thoracic aorta. Note the mural thrombus (curved arrow).

Diagnosis

Fusiform aneurysm of the thoracic aorta

Differential Diagnosis

Fusiform aneurysm of the thoracic aorta with complicating dissection

Discussion

Background

Dilatation of the thoracic aorta lumen greater than five times normal defines an aneurysm. A diameter greater than normal but less than 2 standard deviations above the mean defines ectasia. An ectatic aorta enlarges in both the transverse and longitudinal axes. Aneurysms may be classified by shape as fusiform or saccular. Fusiform aneurysms are characterized by cylindrical dilation. Such aneurysms may involve a short segment of the aorta or can affect its entire length. An aneurysm is present when the aortic diameter is greater than 5 cm. Saccular aneurysms are characterized by a focal outpouching in the aortic wall (**Fig. 149E**).

Etiology

Most descending thoracic aortic aneurysms are true aneurysms and result from atherosclerosis. Ascending aortic aneurysms are less common and may occur secondary to atherosclerosis, cystic medial degeneration, and, rarely, infection.

Clinical Findings

Atherosclerotic disease usually affects long segments of the aortic arch and descending thoracic aorta. Associated aneurysms are usually fusiform, and more often seen in elderly men with hypertension, coronary artery disease, hypercholesterolemia, and long-standing tobacco abuse. Thoracic aortic aneurysms are also found in association with abdominal aortic aneurysms. Patients with thoracic aorta aneurysms may be asymptomatic or may complain of substernal, back, or shoulder pain. Patients with larger aneurysms may complain of compressive symptoms (e.g., dyspnea, dysphagia, hoarseness) or may develop superior vena cava syndrome. Descending thoracic aortic aneurysms may be complicated by dissection, aortobronchopulmonary fistula, rupture, and death. Complications related to ascending aortic aneurysms include dissection, rupture, aortic insufficiency, tamponade, and death.

Pathology

- Aneurysms classified based on vessel wall integrity
- True aneurysms: intact aortic wall
- False (pseudoaneurysms): perforation into tunica intima and media surrounded by adjacent mediastinal tissues

Imaging Findings

RADIOGRAPHY

- Widened superior mediastinum or left paraaortic stripe (**Fig. 149A**)
- Mediastinal mass in continuity with or in close proximity to thoracic aorta (**Fig. 149E1**)
- Ascending aorta and proximal arch aneurysms project anteriorly and rightward.
- Distal arch and descending thoracic aorta aneurysms project posteriorly and leftward (**Fig. 149E1**).
- Curvilinear peripheral calcifications
- Extrinsic compression of the trachea, bronchi, or esophagus
- Complications related to rupture (e.g., hemothorax)

CT/MR

- CT procedure of choice to evaluate aorta arch and descending thoracic aorta
- MR preferred for evaluation of ascending aortic and sinotubular junction
- Aorta dilatation (**Figs. 149C** and **149D**)
- Intramural circumferential or crescent thrombus (**Figs. 149C, 149D, 149E2,** and **149E3**)
- Perianeurysmal hemorrhage and/or infection
- Evaluate size, extent, location, and type of aneurysm (**Figs. 149C, 149D, 149E2,** and **149E3**)
- Potential complications (e.g., dissection, rupture into mediastinum, pleura, or extrapleural space)

Treatment

- Aneurysms of ascending aorta or arch > 6 cm in diameter: surgical replacement of aorta with a synthetic conduit; and possibly aortic valve replacement in selected cases

- Aneurysms of descending thoracic aorta > 6 cm in diameter: surgical replacement of aorta or endovascular stenting

Prognosis

- Natural history untreated thoracic aortic aneurysms: growth and eventual rupture
- Untreated 50% 5-year and 75% 10-year mortality rate
- Open surgical repair is the gold standard; 5 to 20% operative morality rate
- Operative mortality rate exceeds 50% in patients requiring emergent surgery and/or those with significant comorbid factors.
- Percutaneous covered endovascular stents recently introduced as a surgical alternative; lower 30-day mortality rate.

PEARLS_____

- Normal thoracic aorta dimensions
  - Aortic root 37 ± 3 mm
  - Ascending aorta 24 ± 6 mm
  - Descending thoracic aorta 24 ± 3 mm
- Radiologic description of a thoracic aortic aneurysm should include location, proximal-most and distal-most extent, type of aneurysm, its mediastinal relationships, and associated complications.
- Thoracic aorta aneurysms should be assessed for resection if ≥ 6 cm in diameter.
- Thoracic or thoracoabdominal aortic aneurysms are more difficult to treat than abdominal aortic aneurysms.
- One of the greatest risks in elective surgery for descending thoracic aorta lesions (e.g., aneurysms, dissections, traumatic injuries) is spinal cord ischemia and paralysis from injury to the artery of Adamkiewicz. This artery usually arises from the thoracic aorta between the T8 and L1 levels. The reattachment of large intercostal or lumbar arteries during graft placement may reduce the incidence of paraplegia to 16% in extensive thoracic aortic vascular reconstructions and/or resections.

Suggested Readings

Fraser RS, Müller NL, Colman N, Paré PD. Masses situated predominantly in the middle-posterior mediastinal compartment. In: Fraser RS, Müller NL, Colman N, Paré PD, eds. Fraser and Paré's Diagnosis of Diseases of the Chest, 4th ed. Philadelphia: Saunders, 1999:2951–2955

Miller WT. Thoracic aortic aneurysms: plain film findings. Semin Roentgenol 2001;36:288–294

Milner R, Bavaria JE, Baum RA, et al. Thoracic aortic stents. Semin Roentgenol 2001;36:340–350

Nguyen BT. Computed tomography diagnosis of thoracic aortic aneurysms. Semin Roentgenol 2001;36:309–324

Roberts DA. Magnetic resonance imaging of thoracic aortic aneurysm and dissection. Semin Roentgenol 2001;36:295–308

CASE 150 Mycotic Aneurysm of the Thoracic Aorta

Clinical Presentation

A 52-year-old man admitted to the hospital 9 months ago and treated for bacterial endocarditis. Chest radiograph at that time (not illustrated) revealed hyperinflated lungs and a normal-appearing mediastinum and thoracic aorta. He now complains of nonspecific chest discomfort and has a low-grade fever.

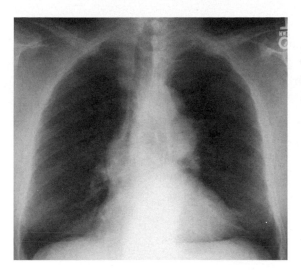

Figure 150A

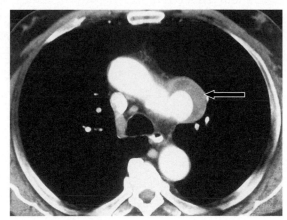

Figure 150B

Radiologic Findings

PA chest radiograph (**Fig. 150A**) shows a 4.5 cm left hilar mass following the contour of the descending thoracic aorta. Contrast-enhanced chest CT (mediastinal window) (**Fig. 150B**) shows a saccular outpouching off the lateral wall of the thoracic aorta that creates the apparent mass seen on chest radiography. Note the thick wall about the saccular aneurysm (arrow).

Diagnosis

Mycotic aneurysm of the thoracic aorta

Differential Diagnosis

Other causes of saccular aneurysms

Discussion

Background

Most mycotic aneurysms are saccular in morphology. Historically, various fungi and *Mycobacterium tuberculosis* were responsible for most cases of mycotic aneurysms. Today, most mycotic aneurysms

577

result from *Staphylococcus aureus* and *Streptococcus* species infections. Predisposing conditions include bacterial endocarditis, intravenous drug abuse, atherosclerosis, and immunosuppression (e.g., malignancy, alcoholism, chemotherapy, autoimmune disease).

Etiology

Mycotic aneurysms may form when organisms spread contiguously from infected lymph nodes or the spine to the thoracic aorta and destroy the internal elastic lamella and portions of the tunica media and adventitia.

Clinical Findings

Patients with mycotic aneurysms often present with insidious signs and symptoms that tend to be nonspecific. The early diagnosis requires a high clinical index of suspicion. Many patients are febrile, and blood cultures are often positive. Untreated mycotic aneurysms may be complicated by uncontrolled sepsis and rupture.

Pathology

- False aneurysms
- Periaortic inflammation
- Periaortic abscesses

Imaging Findings

RADIOGRAPHY

- Superior mediastinal widening
- Abnormal contour to transverse aorta or descending thoracic aorta (**Fig. 150A**)
- Mediastinal mass adjacent to thoracic aorta (**Fig. 150A**)
- Border of mass indistinguishable from thoracic aorta (**Fig. 150A**)
- Pleural effusion (hemothorax) in cases complicated by rupture
- Ground glass opacity and/or parenchymal consolidation (i.e., signs of pulmonary infection)

CT/MR

- Periaortic soft tissue mass or irregular enhancement of the aortic wall with a normal-size aorta in early cases
- Intimal calcifications displaced or disrupted; progressive infection
- Aortic lumen enlarges, forming a noncalcified saccular aneurysm (**Fig. 150B**).
- Enhancing aortic wall thickens due to inflammation (**Fig. 150B**).
- Rare: periaortic gas or lymph node enlargement

Treatment

- Intravenous antibiotics and possibly debridement of infected tissue
- Aneurysmectomy and placement of a synthetic interposition graft

Prognosis

- Untreated: mortality rates approach 70%

PEARL

- If unrecognized, the aortic lumen continues to enlarge until it ruptures.

Suggested Readings

Aliaga L, Cobo F, Miranda C, Lara J. Mycotic aneurysm of the aortic arch. Infection 2000;28:240–242

Koral K, Hall TR. Mycotic pseudoaneurysms of the aortic arch: an unusual complication of invasive pulmonary aspergillosis. Clin Imaging 2000;24:279–282

Semba CP, Sakai T, Slonim SM, et al. Mycotic aneurysms of the thoracic aorta: repair with use of endovascular stent-grafts. J Vasc Interv Radiol 1998;9:33–40

CASE 151 Acute Aortic Dissection (DeBakey Type I)

Clinical Presentation

A 60-year-old hypertensive man with pancreatitis and an abrupt onset of severe chest pain that penetrates from the sternum through to the spine.

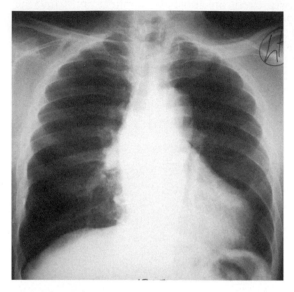

Figure 151A

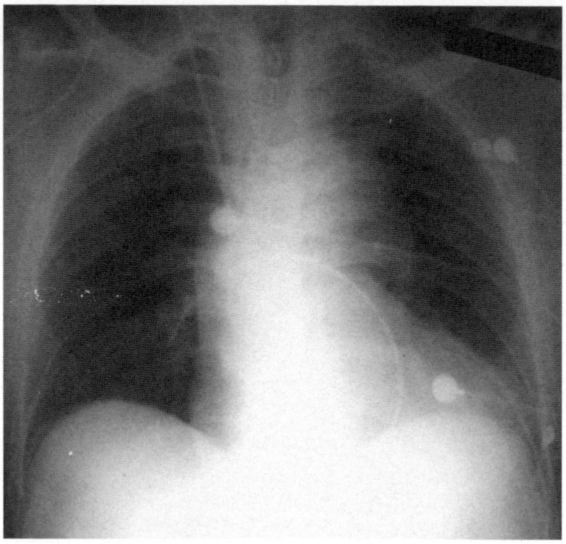

Figure 151B

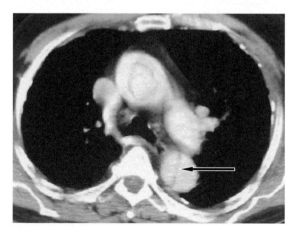

Figure 151C

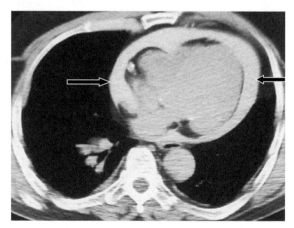

Figure 151D

Radiologic Findings

Admission AP chest radiograph (**Fig. 151A**) shows an elongated thoracic aorta and cardiomegaly. AP chest radiograph (**Fig. 151B**) obtained for evaluation of chest pain reveals a marked change in the mediastinal width and contour. Contrast-enhanced chest CT (mediastinal window) (**Fig. 151C**) shows an abnormal second lumen in the ascending aorta and opacification of both lumina in the ascending aorta. Notice the linear filling defect (i.e., intimal flap) in the descending aorta (arrow). Contrast-enhanced chest CT (mediastinal window) (**Fig. 151D**) obtained immediately following cardiac arrest and unsuccessful resuscitation reveals an intensely enhancing pericardial effusion (i.e., hemopericardium) (arrows).

580

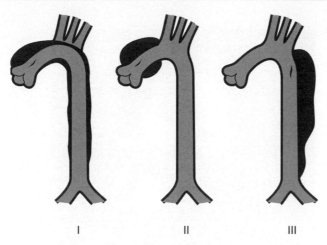

Figure 151E The three types of DeBakey dissections.

Diagnosis

Acute aortic dissection (DeBakey type I); complicating hemopericardium and tamponade

Differential Diagnosis

None

Discussion

Background

The incidence of aortic dissection (AD) is between 5 and 10/million population/year. AD occurs two to three times more often than rupture of an abdominal aortic aneurysm, and is two to three times more common in men. One half of aortic dissections in women under 40 years of age occur during pregnancy. There are two systems of classification. The DeBakey system (**Fig. 151E**) is based on the extent of the dissection, and the Stanford system characterizes aortic dissections by their proximal extent. DeBakey type I dissections (29–34%) involve the ascending aorta and extend around the arch and continue distally. DeBakey type II dissections (12–21%) involve the ascending aorta only (**Fig. 151F**). DeBakey type III dissections (> 50%) begin beyond the thoracic aorta branch vessels and continue down the descending aorta and may extend as far distally as the femoral arteries (**Fig. 151G**). Stanford type A dissections (70%) involve the ascending aorta, regardless of where the entry tear begins and how far distally the dissection extends. Stanford type B dissections (20–30%) begin after the arch vessels and are equivalent to DeBakey type III. An AD less than 2 weeks old is considered acute, whereas an AD more than 2 weeks old is considered chronic.

Etiology

Aortic dissection is a life-threatening condition that most often results from a tear in the tunica intima. High-pressure blood passes into the tunica media, creating a false channel for passage of blood separate from the true aortic lumen. There may be only one tear into the false lumen or multiple entry and distal reentry tears. Most dissections arise in the ascending aorta, above the sinotubular ridge, or in the descending aorta beyond the ligamentum arteriosum.

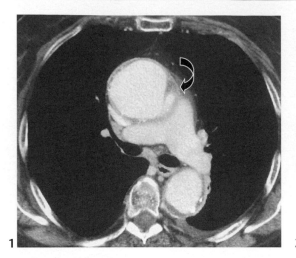
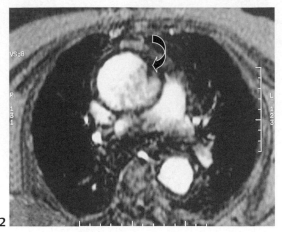

Figure 151F (1,2) Contrast-enhanced chest CT (mediastinal window) **(1)** of a 72-year-old hypertensive woman with an abrupt onset of chest pain reveals aneurysmal dilatation of the ascending aorta with a subtle intimal flap (curved arrow). Axial gradient-echo MR image **(2;** TR 12; TE 3.9**)** also shows the ascending aorta intimal flap (curved arrow) related to the contained DeBakey type II (Stanford type A) aortic dissection.

Clinical Findings

Aortic dissections occur most often in hypertensive patients and in patients with Marfan syndrome. Other risk factors for AD include congenital bicuspid aortic valve, aortic valvular stenosis, and coarctation of the aorta, pregnancy, Ehlers-Danlos syndrome, Turner syndrome, Behçet disease, aortitis, crack cocaine abuse, and cardiac surgery. Patients with AD are usually symptomatic, complaining of sudden, sharp, tearing intractable chest pain, often penetrating to the back or radiating to the neck or jaw. Deficits of major arterial pulses occur in two thirds of patients and are more common with type A dissection. Aortic insufficiency murmur is heard in two thirds of patients with proximal aortic dissections. Additional complications of AD include retrograde dissection (e.g., aortic insufficiency, coronary artery occlusion, rupture into the pericardial sac (**Fig. 151D**) or pleural space), occlusion of major branch vessels, limb and organ ischemia, rupture of the aorta, and saccular aneurysm formation.

Pathology

- Intimal tear
- Channel or cleavage plane in tunica media (i.e., false lumen)
- One or more tears in tunica media; entry and exit sites
- Vasa vasorum bleeding into tunica media (less common)
- Vasa vasorum rupture; thickening of aortic wall without rupture

Imaging Findings

RADIOGRAPHY

- Normal (25%)
- Widening of superior mediastinum and aorta; most common (**Fig. 151G1**)
- Double contour to aortic arch (**Fig. 151G1**)
- Central displacement of calcified plaque from outer aortic contour > 10 mm
- Disparity in size between ascending and descending aorta (**Fig. 151G1**)

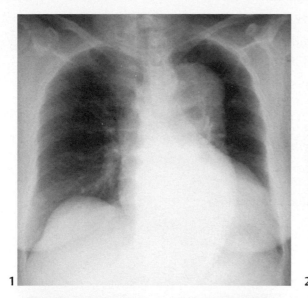

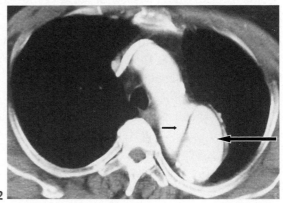

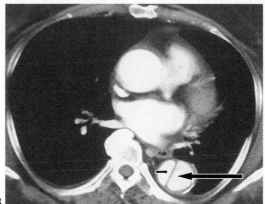

Figure 151G (1–3) AP chest radiograph **(1)** of a 63-year-old woman with uncontrolled hypertension and abrupt onset of chest pain shows fusiform enlargement of the thoracic aorta with a disparity in size between the ascending and descending aorta. The superior mediastinum is wide, and the trachea is displaced rightward. Contrast-enhanced chest CT (mediastinal window) at the aortic arch **(2)** and left atrium **(3)** reveals a DeBakey type III (Stanford type B) dissecting thoracic aortic aneurysm. Note the smaller true lumen (short arrows) and the larger false lumen (long arrows).

CT (SENSITIVITY 98%; SPECIFICITY 87–100%; ACCURACY 100%)

- Linear filling defect (i.e., intimal flap) and false lumen; characteristic finding (**Figs. 151C, 151G2, and 151G3**)
- Differential enhancement of true and false lumina
- Internally displaced intimal calcifications
- Left pleural or pericardial effusion in complicated dissection

MR (SENSITIVITY 98%; SPECIFICITY 98%)

- Comparable to contrast-enhanced CT
- Better for evaluation of aortic root and ascending aorta (**Fig. 151F2**)
- T1-weighted imaging (ECG gating); intimal flap and two lumina
- Gradient-echo MR or gadolinium-enhanced MR angiography (MRA); differentiates slow flow from thrombus

TRANSTHORACIC ECHOCARDIOGRAPHY (TTE)

- Type A dissection: sensitivity 60–85%, specificity 83%
- Type B dissection: sensitivity 50%, specificity 60–90%
- Assesses ascending aorta but cannot image aorta arch and descending aorta
- False-positives from reverberation echoes off calcified atheromatous plaque

TRANSESOPHAGEAL ECHOCARDIOGRAPHY (TEE) (SENSITIVITY 94%; SPECIFICITY 77%)

- Better than TTE for evaluating aortic arch and descending aorta
- False-positive from reverberation echoes created by calcified atheromatous plaque

AORTOGRAPHY (SENSITIVITY 80–90%; SPECIFICITY 75–94%)

- Intimal medial flap
- Failure of false lumen to opacify or compression of true lumen by false lumen
- "Double-barrel" aorta (i.e., opacification of two aortic lumina)
- Branch vessel occlusion or obstruction
- Aortic valvular regurgitation
- Abnormal catheter position outside the anticipated aortic course

Treatment

TYPE A

- Repair of ascending aorta and aortic arch in two stages
  - Bentall-DeBono procedure is the first stage.
    - Dissected aorta is removed and replaced with a composite graft of woven Dacron attached to a mechanical aortic valve.
    - Coronary arteries are reimplanted and sewn directly to the graft.
  - Second stage
    - Arch is replaced with a Dacron graft.
    - Branch vessels are replanted to graft itself.
- Alternative two-stage repair
  - Stage 1 involves inserting a tubular, dangling aortic graft prosthesis ("elephant trunk") into the distal aorta while replacing the ascending aorta and arch.
  - Distal elephant trunk used during the second stage 6 weeks later when replacing sections of the distal aorta via a left thoracotomy.
- Aortic valve undamaged; Dacron tube graft sewn directly onto aortic root

TYPE B

- Medical
  - Antihypertensive agents
  - Diet
  - Exercise
- Surgical replacement of diseased aorta with Dacron graft and replantation of branch vessels required when medical therapy fails (e.g., unrelenting pain, occlusion of major vessel, limb or visceral ischemia, leakage, or rupture)
- Stent-graft placement; promising surgical alternative in high-risk patients

Prognosis

TYPE A

- Untreated: rapidly fatal; death rate 1% per hour for the first 48 hours; 75% of untreated patients die within 2 weeks
- Long-term survival of treated patients: 60% at 5 years; 40% at 10 years
- Operative mortality rate < 10%

TYPE B

- Medical treatment: 80 to 90% 30 day survival
- Untreated type B dissections: 40% mortality rate
- Surgical repair may be complicated by paraplegia (see Case 149).

PEARLS_____

- Normal chest radiography does not exclude the diagnosis of aortic dissection.
- Change in size or appearance of the aorta on serial chest radiographs is the most helpful chest radiographic finding.
- Marfan syndrome is the leading cause of aortic dissection in persons under 40 years of age.
- The incidence of aortic dissection is nine times higher in patients with bicuspid aortic valve.
- False positive CT studies created by streak artifact, cardiac motion, pericardial recess
- False negative CT studies created by suboptimal contrast opacification; atheromatous disease
- Caution: Slow blood flow in the false lumen mimics thrombus on spin-echo MR sequences.

Suggested Readings

Fraser RS, Müller NL, Colman N, Paré PD. Masses situated predominantly in the middle-posterior mediastinal compartment. In: Fraser RS, Müller NL, Colman N, Paré PD, eds. Fraser and Paré's Diagnosis of Diseases of the Chest, 4th ed. Philadelphia: Saunders, 1999:2955–2957

Hsue PY, Salinas CL, Bolger AF, Benowitz NL, Waters DD. Acute aortic dissection related to crack cocaine. Circulation 2002;105:1592–1595

Mizuno T, Toyama M, Tabuchi N, Wu H, Sunamori M. Stented elephant trunk procedure combined with ascending aorta and arch replacement for acute type A aortic dissection. Eur J Cardiothorac Surg 2002;22:504–509

CASE 152 Type B Intramural Hematoma

Clinical Presentation

A 64-year-old hypertensive man who developed chest pain while straining during defecation

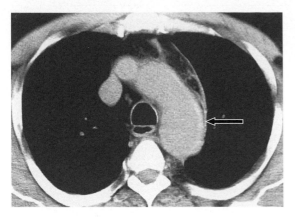

Figure 152A

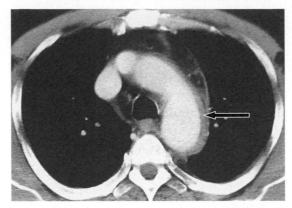

Figure 152B

Radiologic Findings

Unenhanced chest CT (mediastinal window) (**Fig. 152A**) shows a high attenuation crescent along the aortic arch (arrow). Contrast-enhanced chest CT (mediastinal window) at the same anatomic level (**Fig. 152B**) reveals the crescent of subintimal hemorrhage appears lower in attenuation than the opacified aortic lumen (arrow).

Diagnosis

Type B intramural hematoma

Differential Diagnosis

None

Discussion

Background

Intramural hematoma (IMH) represents an aortic dissection without an intimal tear. The ascending and descending thoracic aorta are equally affected. Less than 10% of cases of IMH involve the aortic arch. Those associated with atherosclerotic ulcers more often occur in the descending thoracic aorta. The classification of intramural hematoma follows the Stanford system for aortic dissection.

Etiology

Proposed mechanisms of IMH include weakening of the tunica intima with spontaneous rupture of the vasa vasorum leading to subintimal hemorrhage, fracture of an intimal plaque, and intramural extension of hemorrhage adjacent to a penetrating atherosclerotic ulcer.

Clinical Findings

Most patients with IMH are hypertensive and range between 55 and 65 years of age. However, patients with calcific pericarditis may also have associated constrictive pericarditis, in which case presenting symptoms are similar to those of aortic dissection, including chest pain (50–74%) and back pain (44–84%). Type A IMH progresses to dissection or rupture more often than type B lesions.

Pathology

- Rupture of vasa vasorum
- Subintimal hemorrhage
- Intimal plaque fracture
- Penetrating ulcer with intramural blood

Imaging Findings

CHEST RADIOGRAPHY

- Mediastinal widening ($>$ 80%)
- Left pleural effusion (33%)
- Pericardial effusion ($<$ 25%)

CT

- Crescent-shaped region of increased attenuation on unenhanced scans (reflecting acute subintimal hemorrhage) (**Fig. 152A**)
- Region of mural thickening is lower in attenuation than the opacified aortic lumen on contrast-enhanced scans (**Fig. 152B**)
- Increased attenuation of surrounding mediastinal fat; (edema or hemorrhage)
- Displaced intimal calcifications
- Left pleural effusion or hemothorax in complicated IMH

MR

- T1-weighted imaging: crescentic or circumferential mural thickening in aortic wall
  - Isointense to skeletal muscle (less than or equal to 1 week old)
  - Hyperintense to skeletal muscle (more than 1 week old)
- No change in signal intensity or cine gradient-echo images
- Intimal flap not visualized

Treatment

- Type A: emergent surgical intervention or endovascular stent-graft
- Type B: medical management

Prognosis

- 18% progress to dissection; 15% rupture
- 30-day mortality of untreated intramural hematoma: 36% (type A); 12% (type B)
- Surgical repair reduces mortality rate of type A intramural hematoma: 18%
- Medical management reduces mortality rate of type B intramural hematoma: 8%
- Type B intramural hematoma may resolve spontaneously.

PEARLS_____

- Intramural hematoma is a potential precursor of aortic dissection and is managed as such.
- Intramural hematoma can be difficult to distinguish from atherosclerotic plaque or thrombus. Plaque is typically absent in the ascending aorta. Intramural hematoma tends to be smooth, whereas plaque is often irregular.
- Useful CT signs for predicting progression to dissection and/or rupture include a thick intramural hematoma, compression of the true lumen, and/or pleural and pericardial effusion.
- Follow-up CT may reveal a decrease in intramural hematoma, development of a penetrating ulcer or fusiform aneurysm, or progression to true dissection.

Suggested Readings

Choi SH, Choi SJ, Kim JH, et al. Useful CT findings for predicting the progression of aortic intramural hematoma to overt aortic dissection. J Comput Assist Tomogr 2001;25:295–299

Coady MA, Rizzo JA, Elefteriades JA. Pathologic variants of thoracic aortic dissections: penetrating atherosclerotic ulcers and intramural hematomas. Cardiol Clin 1999;17:637–657

Kaji S, Akasaka T, Horibata Y, et al. Long-term prognosis of patients with type A aortic intramural hematoma. Circulation 2002;106:1248–1252

CASE 153 Mitral Stenosis

Clinical Presentation

A 35-year-old woman with dyspnea on exertion

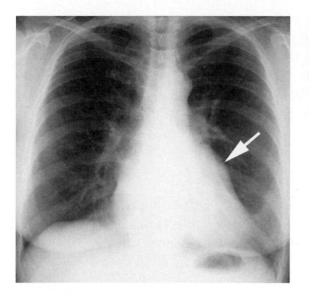

Figure 153A

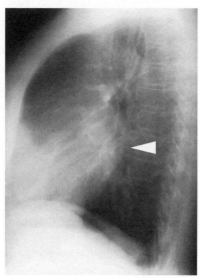

Figure 153B

(Figs. 153A and 153B courtesy of Diane C. Strollo, M.D., University of Pittsburgh Medical Center, Pittsburgh, Pennsylvania.)

Radiologic Findings

PA (**Fig. 153A**) and lateral (**Fig. 153B**) chest radiographs demonstrate mild cardiomegaly, an enlarged left atrial appendage (arrow) (**Fig. 153A**), moderate left atrial enlargement (arrowhead) (**Fig. 153B**), and normal pulmonary vascularity.

Diagnosis

Mitral stenosis

Differential Diagnosis

- Left atrial enlargement from another etiology
  - Myxoma
  - Left atrial thrombus

Discussion

Background

The mitral valve is characterized by its bicuspid morphology with anterior and posterior leaflets. The anterior mitral valve leaflet is in fibrous continuity with the posterior and left aortic valve leaflets. In normal hemodynamics, diastolic elevation of left atrial pressure forces the mitral valve open, and

589

systolic elevation of left ventricular pressure forces it closed. Mitral stenosis refers to valvular obstruction of antegrade blood flow within the left heart and is a lesion of pressure overload. Volume overload follows and results in left atrial enlargement. Rheumatic mitral stenosis almost always has a secondary component of mitral insufficiency.

Etiology

While mitral stenosis may be congenital, it more commonly results from rheumatic heart disease, a complication of rheumatic fever. Rheumatic fever is a systemic inflammatory disorder caused by group A beta-hemolytic *Streptococcus*. Approximately 30% of affected patients develop rheumatic heart disease. The mitral valve is most commonly affected (50%), followed by combined involvement of the mitral and aortic valves (20–50%). Tricuspid valve involvement may result in trivalvular disease. The pulmonic valve is rarely affected.

Clinical Findings

Rheumatic fever typically affects patients between the ages of 5 and 15 years. Only 50% of patients with rheumatic mitral stenosis are aware of a past episode of rheumatic fever. Affected patients remain asymptomatic for at least one decade but eventually develop dyspnea. With sustained volume overload, the left atrium enlarges and atrial fibrillation may ensue. Turbulent flow may result in the formation of a left atrial thrombus, particularly within the atrial appendage, and subsequent systemic embolization may occur. Untreated patients develop secondary pulmonary arterial hypertension leading to right ventricular hypertrophy, followed by right ventricular failure with systemic venous hypertension, peripheral edema, hepatic congestion, ascites, and fatigue. Pulmonary hemosiderosis is a late consequence of untreated mitral stenosis due to repeated episodes of hemorrhage that manifest with hemoptysis.

Pathology

- Rheumatic mitral stenosis
  - Endocardial vegetations with erosion at line of valve closure
  - Commissural fusion and fibrosis
  - Shortening and adhesions of chordae tendineae
  - Resultant funnel-shaped mitral valve with apex toward the left ventricle
- Congenital mitral stenosis
  - Hypoplastic left heart
  - Parachute mitral stenosis: insertion of all chordae tendineae into a single papillary muscle

Imaging Findings

RADIOGRAPHY

- Normal heart size in early disease
- Cardiomegaly secondary to right ventricular failure (late) (**Figs. 153A** and **153B**)
- Left atrial appendage enlargement (**Figs. 153A** and **153C**)
- Left atrial enlargement (**Figs. 153A, 153B,** and **153C**): double contour with the right atrium, elevated left main bronchus
- Findings of pulmonary venous hypertension (**Fig. 153C**), typically cephalization of blood flow
- Findings of pulmonary arterial hypertension
- Calcified mitral valve (rarely detected on radiography)

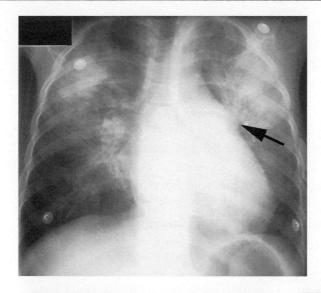

Figure 153C PA chest radiograph of a young man with mitral stenosis and atrial fibrillation demonstrates pulmonary edema with preferential involvement of the upper lobes. Note left atrial enlargement (arrow) and cardiomegaly. (Courtesy of Diane C. Strollo, M.D., University of Pittsburgh Medical Center, Pittsburgh, Pennsylvania.)

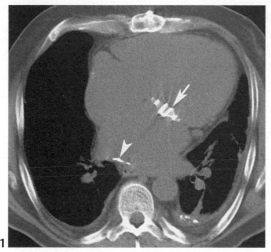
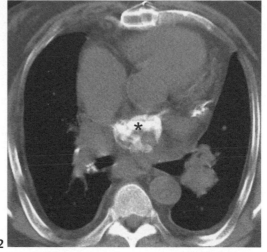

Figure 153D (1,2) Unenhanced chest CT (mediastinal window) demonstrates left atrial enlargement **(1)**, a prosthetic mitral valve **(1,** arrow), left atrial wall calcification **(1,** arrowhead), and densely calcified left atrial thrombus **(2,** *). (Courtesy of Helen T. Winer-Muram, M.D., Indiana University Medical Center, Indianapolis, Indiana.)

- Calcified left atrial wall; calcified left atrial thrombus
- Pulmonary infarction
- Pulmonary hemosiderosis: 2 to 5 mm densely calcified nodules in mid- and lower lung, more frequently on the right

CT

- Left atrial enlargement (**Fig. 153D1**)
- Mitral valve leaflet calcification
- Visualization of intraatrial thrombus (may be calcified) (**Fig. 153D2**) or left atrial wall calcification (**Fig. 153D1**)
- Right ventricular hypertrophy followed by right ventricular failure, right chamber enlargement, and systemic venous hypertension
- Assessment of cardiac function and valvular stenosis with or without insufficiency with helical and electron beam CT

ANGIOGRAPHY

- Left atrial enlargement with normal-to-small left ventricle
- Doming of mitral valve leaflets on left ventriculography
- Mitral stenosis with or without insufficiency on ventriculography

MR

- Spin-echo and double inversion recovery techniques: assessment of atrial volume, identification of atrial thrombus, visualization of right ventricular hypertrophy or enlargement
- Gradient-echo technique
  - High-velocity jet across stenotic mitral valve: diastolic signal void extending from leaflets into left ventricle
  - Assessment of mitral valve morphology and maximum leaflet separation
- Velocity-encoded cine MRI: mean pressure gradients, blood flow velocity

Treatment

- Mitral valvuloplasty
- Mitral valve commissurotomy
- Mitral valve replacement

Prognosis

- Fifteen to 20% 5-year survival in untreated patients with resting dyspnea

Suggested Readings

Del Negro AA. Physiology of mitral stenosis. In: Taveras JM, Ferrucci JT, eds. Radiology on CD-ROM: Diagnosis, Imaging, Intervention, vol. 2. Philadelphia: Lippincott Williams & Wilkins, 2000:chapter 65

Edwards BS, Edwards JE. Pathology of mitral stenosis. In: Taveras JM, Ferrucci JT, eds. Radiology on CD-ROM: Diagnosis, Imaging, Intervention, vol. 2. Philadelphia: Lippincott Williams & Wilkins, 2000:chapter 64.

Globits S, Higgins CB. Magnetic resonance imaging of valvular heart disease. In: Taveras JM, Ferrucci JT, eds. Radiology on CD-ROM: Diagnosis, Imaging, Intervention, vol. 2. Philadelphia: Lippincott Williams & Wilkins, 2000:chapter 28

Miller SW. Radiography and angiography of valvular heart disease. In: Taveras JM, Ferrucci JT, eds. Radiology on CD-ROM: Diagnosis, Imaging, Intervention, vol. 2. Philadelphia: Lippincott Williams & Wilkins, 2000:chapter 26

CASE 154 Aortic Stenosis

Clinical Presentation

An asymptomatic 55-year-old woman

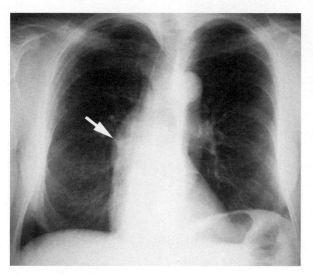

Figure 154A

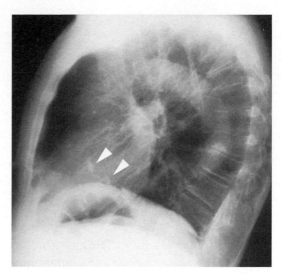

Figure 154B

(Figs. 154A and 154B courtesy of Diane C. Strollo, M.D., University of Pittsburgh Medical Center, Pittsburgh, Pennsylvania.)

Radiologic Findings

Posteroanterior (PA) (**Fig. 154A**) and lateral (**Fig. 154B**) chest radiographs demonstrate dilatation of the ascending aorta (arrow) (**Fig. 154A**) and dense calcification of the aortic valve (arrowheads) (**Fig. 154B**). The heart size and pulmonary vascularity are normal.

Diagnosis

Aortic stenosis, bicuspid aortic valve

Differential Diagnosis

Hypertension

Discussion

Background

The aortic valve has a tricuspid morphology with right, left, and posterior leaflets. In normal hemodynamics, systolic elevation of left ventricular pressure forces the valve open, and diastolic elevation of systemic pressure (relative to left ventricular pressure) forces it closed. Aortic stenosis refers to obstruction to antegrade blood flow between the left ventricle and the systemic circulation and may be valvular, supravalvular, or subvalvular (asymmetric septal hypertrophy). Aortic stenosis is a lesion

593

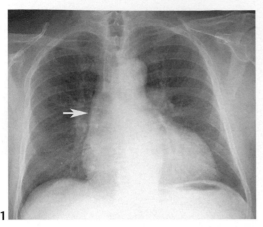 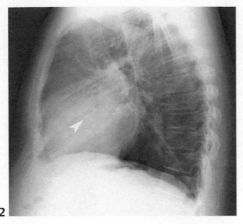

Figure 154C (1,2) PA **(1)** and lateral **(2)** chest radiographs of an elderly man with aortic stenosis and recurrent left ventricular failure demonstrate a left ventricular cardiac configuration, post-stenotic dilatation of the ascending aorta (arrow), aortic valve calcification (arrowhead), and cardiomegaly consistent with secondary aortic insufficiency. (Courtesy of Helen T. Winer-Muram, M.D., Indiana University Medical Center, Indianapolis, Indiana.)

of pressure overload. Aortic stenosis almost always exhibits a component of secondary aortic insufficiency as calcium deposits on the stenotic valve often interfere with normal closure.

Etiology

Congenital aortic stenosis may manifest with a unicuspid (patients under 15 years), bicuspid (patients between 15 and 65 years), or a tricuspid (patients over 65 years) aortic valve. More than 95% of patients with congenital aortic stenosis have unicuspid or bicuspid aortic valves. The latter occur in 1.5% of live births, and aortic stenosis is the most common complication. Acquired aortic stenosis may occur as a sequela of rheumatic heart disease or as a degenerative condition in patients over the age of 65 years.

Clinical Findings

Patients with aortic stenosis may be entirely asymptomatic and are diagnosed because of an ejection murmur or an abnormal chest radiograph. Asymptomatic patients are usually under the age of 20 years. Approximately 75% of patients with congenital and rheumatic aortic stenosis are males, whereas degenerative aortic stenosis affects males and females equally. Degenerative stenosis is associated with hypertension, smoking, and blood lipid abnormalities. Sustained pressure overload results in left ventricular hypertrophy, increased cardiac work (to generate higher than normal systolic pressures), and increased oxygen consumption (to supply an increased left ventricular mass), which may produce chest pain. Subsequent left ventricular failure results in dyspnea. Patients with moderate to severe aortic stenosis may not be able to increase their cardiac output in response to exercise-induced peripheral vasodilatation. These patients develop ventricular tachycardia, which may progress to ventricular fibrillation and result in presyncope, syncope, or sudden death.

Pathology

- Unicuspid valve: eccentric or central orifice
- Bicuspid valve: abnormal hemodynamics, cusp thickening, fibrosis, and calcification

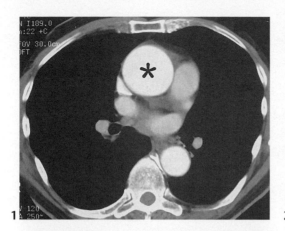
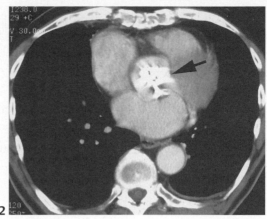
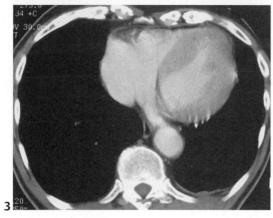

Figure 154D (1–3) Contrast-enhanced chest CT (mediastinal window) of an asymptomatic middle-aged man with aortic stenosis demonstrates post-stenotic dilatation of the ascending aorta (**1**, *), dense calcification of the stenotic aortic valve (**2**, arrow), and left ventricular hypertrophy **(3).** (Courtesy of Diane C. Strollo, M.D., University of Pittsburgh Medical Center, Pittsburgh, Pennsylvania.)

- Rheumatic aortic stenosis (tricuspid valve)
    - Thickened valve leaflets with fibrosis and calcification
    - Commissural fusion
    - Extension of disease from affected mitral valve (7 years after development of mitral stenosis)
- Degenerative stenosis: calcific deposits on aortic surface of otherwise normal valve leaflets with resultant poor mobility

Imaging Findings

RADIOGRAPHY

- Normal heart size; left ventricular configuration: spherical ventricular border, concave left mid-heart border, border-forming or dilated ascending aorta (**Figs. 154A** and **154B**)
- Dilatation of ascending aorta (**Figs. 154A** and **154C1**)
- Calcification of aortic valve leaflets (**Figs. 154B** and **154C2**)
- Cardiomegaly with left heart failure or associated aortic insufficiency (**Fig. 154C**)
- Infants with congenital aortic stenosis: cardiomegaly and pulmonary edema

CT

- Post-stenotic dilatation of ascending aorta (**Fig. 154D1**)
- Aortic valve calcification (**Fig. 154D2**)
- Left ventricular hypertrophy (**Fig. 154D3**)

MR

- Spin-echo or double inversion recovery techniques: left ventricular hypertrophy and post-stenotic aortic dilatation
- Gradient-echo technique:
  - Thick, dark aortic valve leaflets
  - Systolic turbulent flow and signal loss distal to aortic valve, signal void post-stenotic jet within signal-enhanced ascending aorta
  - Assessment of type of aortic stenosis (valvular, supravalvular, subvalvular) and valve morphology
- Velocity-encoded cine MR: quantification of aortic stenosis

ANGIOGRAPHY

- Domed thickened aortic valve during systole
- Eccentric contrast jet
- Evaluation of coronary arteries

Treatment

- Aortic valve replacement
- Coronary bypass for significant coronary artery stenosis

Prognosis

- Symptomatic untreated patients survive up to 5 years.
- 1 to 3% surgical mortality with aortic valve replacement

Suggested Readings

Del Negro AA. Physiology of severe aortic stenosis. In: Taveras JM, Ferrucci JT, eds. Radiology on CD-ROM: Diagnosis, Imaging, Intervention, vol. 2. Philadelphia: Lippincott Williams & Wilkins, 2000: chapter 25

Globits S, Higgins CB. Magnetic resonance imaging of valvular heart disease. In: Taveras JM, Ferrucci JT, eds. Radiology on CD-ROM: Diagnosis, Imaging, Intervention, vol. 2. Philadelphia: Lippincott Williams & Wilkins, 2000:chapter 28

Miller SW. Radiography and angiography of valvular heart disease. In: Taveras JM, Ferrucci JT, eds. Radiology on CD-ROM: Diagnosis, Imaging, Intervention, vol. 2. Philadelphia: Lippincott Williams & Wilkins, 2000:chapter 265

Roberts WC. Morphologic aspects of aortic valve stenosis. In: Taveras JM, Ferrucci JT, eds. Radiology on CD-ROM: Diagnosis, Imaging, Intervention, vol. 2. Philadelphia: Lippincott Williams & Wilkins, 2000:chapter 24

White R. Magnetic resonance imaging of aortic valve stenosis. In: Taveras JM, Ferrucci JT, eds. Radiology on CD-ROM: Diagnosis, Imaging, Intervention, vol. 2. Philadelphia: Lippincott Williams & Wilkins, 2000:chapter 27A

CASE 155 Calcified Left Ventricular Wall Aneurysm

Clinical Presentation

Preoperative chest radiograph of an asymptomatic 79-year-old man admitted for a total hip arthroplasty

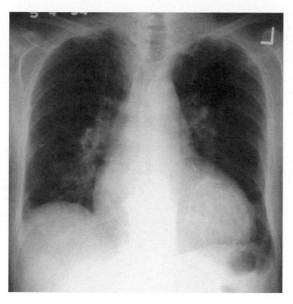

Figure 155A

Radiologic Findings

PA (**Fig. 155A**) chest radiograph demonstrates laminated rings of calcium outlining the anterior and apical walls of the left ventricle.

Diagnosis

Calcified left ventricular wall aneurysm

Differential Diagnosis

- Left ventricular pseudoaneurysm
- Pericardial calcification

Discussion

Background

Left ventricular aneurysms usually involve the anterior and apical myocardial walls. The inferior and inferior posterior myocardial walls are less often affected. Calcification of the anterolateral and apical regions usually does not occur until several years after infarction.

597

Etiology

Left ventricular aneurysms may develop as a sequela of transmural myocardial infarction and may be present within 48 hours of the infarction. These aneurysms are usually circumscribed, noncontractile, with a wide mouth and demonstrate localized dyskinesis on real-time imaging (e.g., echocardiography, ventriculography, cine MR).

Clinical Findings

Left ventricular aneurysms occur more frequently in women and in patients without previous angina. Most patients also have disease involving the left anterior descending coronary artery with severe stenosis or total occlusion.

Pathology

- True left ventricular aneurysm
  - Anterolateral and apical myocardial walls
- False left ventricular aneurysm
  - Posterolateral myocardial walls
  - Pericardial adhesions
  - Remote infarction: scarring, calcification
  - Thrombus along aneurysm wall

Imaging Findings

RADIOGRAPHY

- Localized bulge along left heart border
- Shelf-like or squared-off appearance to mid-lateral margin of left heart border
- Rim or laminated rings of calcification (e.g., remote infarction) (**Fig. 155A**)
- Left ventricular enlargement
- Hydrostatic edema; cardiac decompensation (see Case 143)

ECHOCARDIOGRAPHY/VENTRICULOGRAPHY/CINE MR

- Wide communication with the ventricular chamber
- Affected segment is akinetic or severely hypokinetic.

Treatment

- Resection
- Linear repair
- Dor's circular patch repair

Prognosis

- Systemic embolization of aneurysmal thrombus
- Rare; rupture (4%)

PEARL

- Myocardial calcifications lie > 2 mm below the external cardiac contour, are linear or laminated, and are limited to the left ventricle.

Suggested Readings

Brown SL, Gropler RJ, Harris KM. Distinguishing left ventricular aneurysm from pseudoaneurysm: a review of the literature. Chest 1997;111:1403–1409

Cohen AJ, Rubin O, Hauptman E, Harpaz D, Turkisher V, Schachner A. Ventricular aneurysm repair: a new approach. J Card Surg 2000;15:209–216

Ha JW, Cho SY, Lee JD, Kang MS. Left ventricular aneurysm after myocardial infarction. Clin Cardiol 1998;21:917

Nakajima O, Sano I, Akioka H. Images in cardiovascular medicine: marked calcified left ventricular aneurysm. Circulation 1997;95:1974

Tikiz H, Atak R, Balbay Y, Genc Y, Kutuk E. Left ventricular aneurysm formation after anterior myocardial infarction: clinical and angiographic determinants in 809 patents. Int J Cardiol 2002;82:7–14

CASE 156 Pericardial Calcifications: Remote Tuberculosis

Clinical Presentation

An asymptomatic 61-year-old woman with a remote history of tuberculosis

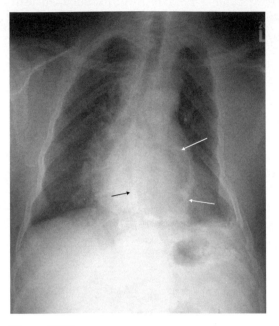

Figure 156A

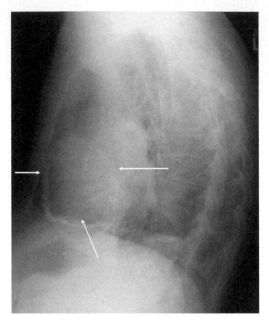

Figure 156B

Radiologic Findings

PA (**Fig. 156A**) and lateral (**Fig. 156B**) chest radiographs demonstrate thick, amorphous calcifications over most of the heart's surface (arrows) and along the atrioventricular groove. The left chest wall is deformed secondary to remote trauma. Amorphous pleural calcifications are also present in the posterior and lateral left hemithorax secondary to a remote traumatic hemothorax. Note the asymmetric left apical pleural fibrosis.

Diagnosis

Pericardial calcifications secondary to remote tuberculous pericarditis; calcific pleuritis secondary to remote trauma

Differential Diagnosis

- Pericardial calcifications secondary to other causes of remote pericarditis
- Myocardial calcifications

Discussion

Background

Calcium may deposit along the pericardial surface as a sequela of infectious or inflammatory process. Thin, linear "eggshell" calcifications are more often associated with viral and uremic pericarditis. Shaggy, thick, amorphous calcifications are more often associated with tuberculous pericarditis and were once considered pathognomonic. Calcium deposits tend to be most obvious in the atrioventricular groove, where fat usually occurs. The left atrium is not entirely covered by pericardium; thus calcium deposits are not usually located in this region.

Etiology

Thin, linear, or "eggshell" pericardial calcifications around the margin of the heart are most often seen in the setting of viral or uremic pericarditis. Historically, the more shaggy, amorphous calcific pericardial deposits have been associated with tuberculous pericarditis.

Clinical Findings

Calcific pericarditis is often asymptomatic and found incidentally on chest radiography obtained for other reasons. However, patients with calcific pericarditis may be associated with constrictive pericarditis, in which case patients may have dyspnea, ascites, hepatomegaly, peripheral edema, and heart failure. Patients with calcific pericarditis and constrictive pericarditis are typically more symptomatic than those without calcified pericarditis.

Pathology

ACUTE PERICARDITIS

- Pericardial inflammation
- Diffuse fibrin deposition
- Fibrinous material deposited on pericardial surface (i.e., "bread and butter" appearance)
- Increase in pericardial vascularity
- Large number of neutrophils

CHRONIC

- Pericardial inflammation, thickening, scarring
- Calcifications deposited along myocardial wall; thin, linear, amorphous
- Constrictive pericarditis

Imaging Findings

RADIOGRAPHY

- Diffuse, thin, eggshell calcifications
- Thick amorphous calcified masses (**Figs. 156A** and **156B**)
- Thicker and more irregular than myocardial calcifications (see Case 155, **Fig. 155A**)
- Calcifications not restricted to left ventricular surface; usually spare cardiac apex and left atrium
- Fifty percent of patients with constrictive pericarditis have visible calcifications

CT (CONSTRICTIVE PERICARDITIS)

- Pericardial thickening (i.e., 0.5–2.0 cm)
- Pericardial calcification
- Signs of systemic venous hypertension (e.g., dilated right and left atria, vena cava dilatation, hepatomegaly, pleural effusion, ascites)
- Small tubular right ventricle

MR

- Features similar to those seen on CT
- Pericardial effusion can mimic pericardial thickening on T1-weighted imaging.
- Less sensitive detection of pericardial calcification

Treatment

- Calcific pericarditis by itself does not require treatment.
- Constrictive pericarditis may necessitate pericardiectomy in selected patients.

Prognosis

- Untreated constrictive pericarditis is life threatening.

PEARLS

- Pericardial calcification can be an incidental finding and does not imply constrictive pericarditis in the absence of heart failure.
- Calcific pericarditis in a patient with high filling pressures is diagnostic of constrictive pericarditis.

Suggested Reading

MacGregor JH, Chen JT, Chiles C, Kier R, Godwin JD, Ravin CE. The radiographic distinction between pericardial and myocardial calcifications. AJR Am J Roentgenol 1987;148:675–677

CASE 157 Pericardial Effusion

Clinical Presentation

A 47-year-old man with uremia and new onset of shortness of breath

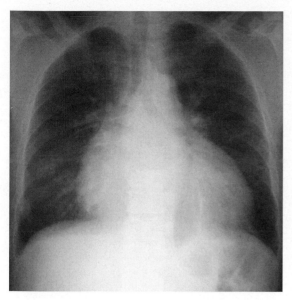

Figure 157A

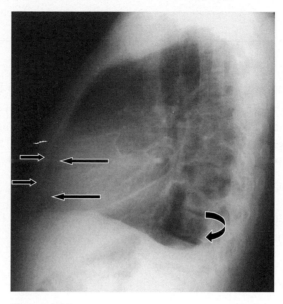

Figure 157B

Radiologic Findings

PA (**Fig. 157A**) and lateral (**Fig. 157B**) chest radiographs show globular enlargement of the cardio-mediastinal silhouette. Note the marked separation of the black retrosternal fat stripe (short arrows) from the black epicardial fat stripe (long arrows) by a thick white interface (i.e., "Oreo cookie" sign). Small bilateral pleural effusions are best appreciated on the lateral radiograph (curved arrows). There is no interstitial edema.

Diagnosis

Uremic pericardial effusion

Differential Diagnosis

- Pericardial effusion of other etiology
- Global cardiomegaly-cardiomyopathy

Discussion

Background

The pericardium consists of two layers. The visceral pericardium is attached to the surface of the heart and the proximal great vessels. The parietal pericardium forms the free wall of the pericardial sac. The sac itself normally contains 20 to 50 mL of fluid. The most common cause of pericardial effusion is myocardial infarction with left ventricular failure. Fifty percent of patients with chronic

Table 157-1   Causes of Pericardial Effusion

Serous	Hemorrhagic	Fibrinous	Chylous
Heart failure	Acute infarction	Infectious	Neoplastic
Hypoalbuminemia	Cardiac surgery	Uremia	Cardiothoracic surgery
Irradiation	Trauma	Rheumatoid arthritis	Superior vena cava
Myxedema	Coagulopathy	Systemic lupus erythematosus	obstruction
Drug reactions	Neoplasm	Hypersensitivity reaction	Congenital
		HIV	

renal failure develop uremic pericarditis. Coxsackie virus group B, *Staphylococcus*, and *Haemophilus influenzae* are common infectious agents associated with pericardial effusion. Today, tuberculous pericarditis is unusual except in the HIV-AIDS population, in which pericardial effusion of any etiology is a poor prognostic sign.

Etiology

An increased volume of pericardial fluid and alterations in the composition of the fluid may occur in the setting of numerous diseases (**Table 157-1**).

Clinical Findings

Tamponade occurs when the volume of fluid in the pericardial sac compromises blood return to the right heart, affecting cardiac output. It is usually caused by serous or bloody fluid. If fluid accumulates slowly, the pericardial sac can accommodate large volumes of fluid without hemodynamic consequences.

Imaging Findings

RADIOGRAPHY

- Normal until volume of fluid > 250 mL
- Symmetric enlargement of the cardiac silhouette (e.g., "water bottle" morphology) (**Fig. 157A**)
- Separation of retrosternal and epicardial fat stripe > 2 mm: (e.g., "Oreo cookie" sign) (**Fig. 157B**)
- Cardiomegaly with normal pulmonary vascularity (**Fig. 157A**)

CT

- Small effusions first collect dorsal to left ventricle and along left atrium
- Larger effusions collect ventral and lateral to right ventricle
- Largest effusions may envelop the myocardium ("halo" sign) (**Fig. 157C**)
- Loculations most often form along right anterolateral pericardium
- Pericardial thickening, nodularity, enhancement

MR

- Transudates: low signal intensity on T1-weighted imaging
- Exudates: higher signal intensity on T1-weighted imaging

Treatment

- Directed toward the underlying cause (see **Table 157-1**)
- Pericardiocentesis or pericardial window in select cases

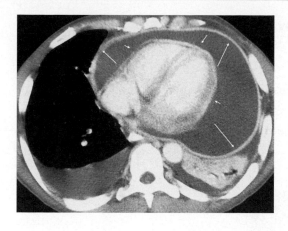

Figure 157C Contrast-enhanced chest CT (mediastinal window) of a 42-year-old man with HIV infection and dyspnea with a tuberculous pericardial effusion and tamponade shows a massive pericardial fluid collection enveloping the myocardium ("halo sign") and subtle effacement of the right atrium and right ventricle. Note the thickened and enhancing visceral (short arrows) and parietal (long arrows) pericardium.

Prognosis

- Depends on underlying cause (see **Table 157-1**)

PEARLS

- Echocardiography is the imaging modality of choice for detecting pericardial effusion, but it tends to underestimate the volume of pericardial fluid when compared to CT.
- Reliable distinction between benign and malignant pericardial effusion is not possible on the basis of Hounsfield units alone.

Suggested Readings

Barbaro G. Cardiovascular manifestations of HIV infection. Circulation 2002;106:1420–1425

Karia DH, Xing YQ, Kuvin JT, Nesser HJ, Pandian NG. Recent role of imaging in the diagnosis of pericardial disease. Curr Cardiol Rep 2002;4:33–40

Lawler LP, Horton KM, Corl FM, Fishman EK. Review: the pericardium—a computed tomography perspective. Crit Rev Diagn Imaging 2001;42:229–258

CASE 158 Postpericardiotomy Syndrome

Clinical Presentation

A 47-year-old man six weeks status post myocardial infarction and subsequent revascularization surgery and pacemaker placement complains of chest pain and a low-grade fever. Recent thoracentesis revealed a bloody exudate.

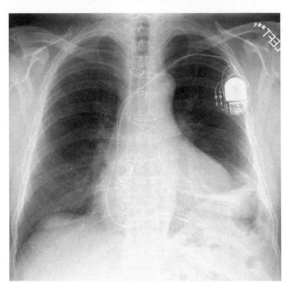

Figure 158A

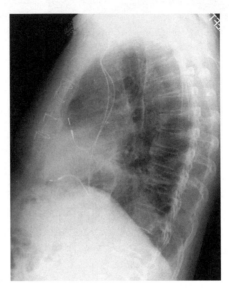

Figure 158B

Radiologic Findings

PA (**Fig. 158A**) and lateral (**Fig. 158B**) chest radiographs show an enlarged cardiomediastinal silhouette and a left pleural effusion.

Diagnosis

Postpericardiotomy syndrome (i.e., postmyocardial infarction or Dressler syndrome)

Differential Diagnosis

Recurrent ischemia

Discussion

Background

Postpericardiotomy syndrome occurs in approximately 3 to 4% of patients following myocardial infarction and a slightly higher percentage of patients following surgical procedures that violate the pericardium. It has also been reported following percutaneous balloon pericardiotomy, temporary and permanent transvenous pacing, and pulmonary infarction.

Etiology

The pathogenesis of postpericardiotomy syndrome is unknown, but likely represents an immunologic reaction.

Clinical Findings

The average onset of clinical symptoms in patients with postpericardiotomy syndrome is 20 days following injury, surgery, or instrumentation. However, the range is between 1 week and several months. More than 90% of affected patients complain of chest pain, and two thirds are febrile. Most have dyspnea, crackles, and a pericardial rub. A pleural rub and elevated white blood count are seen in nearly half of all patients. The pleural fluid is typically exudative and hemorrhagic with a pH > 7.40.

Pathology

- Low pleural fluid complement
- High pleural/serum antimyocardial antibody ratio

Imaging Findings

RADIOGRAPHY

- Abnormal (94%)
- Pleural effusion (83%) (**Figs. 158A** and **158B**)
- Parenchymal opacities (74%)
- Enlarged cardiomediastinal silhouette (49%) (**Fig. 158A**)

Treatment

- Nonsteroidal antiinflammatory drugs (NSAIDs); mainstay
- Pleural and/or pericardiocentesis in select cases

Prognosis

- Postpericardiotomy syndrome is often self limited
- May relapse as late as 2 years after the initial episode

Suggested Readings

Bajaj BP, Evans KE, Thomas P. Postpericardiotomy syndrome following temporary and permanent transvenous pacing. Postgrad Med J 1999;75:357–358

Dressler W. The post-myocardial infarction syndrome: a report on forty-four cases. AMA Arch Intern Med 1959;103:28–42

Fraser RS, Müller NL, Colman N, Paré PD. Pleural effusion. In: Fraser and Paré's Diagnosis of Diseases of the Chest, 4th ed. Philadelphia: Saunders, 1999:2766

Wang A, Harrison JK, Toptine JH, Bashore TM. Post-pericardiotomy syndrome after percutaneous balloon pericardiotomy. J Invasive Cardiol 1999;11:144–146

CASE 159 Sternal Dehiscence

Clinical Presentation

A 57-year-old man who is 10 days post cardiac revascularization complains of pain and the sensation of movement in his anterior chest wall, especially when coughing.

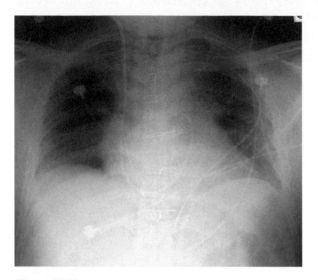

Figure 159A

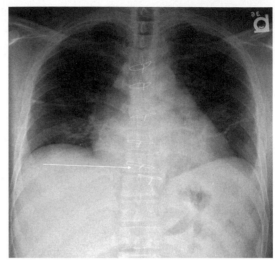

Figure 159B

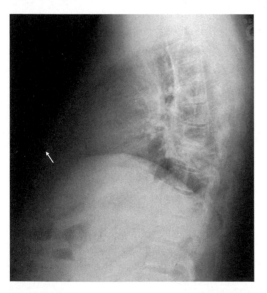

Figure 159C

(Figs. 159A, 159B, and 159C courtesy of Cynthia K. Brooks, M.D., Medical College of Virginia Hospitals, Virginia Commonwealth University Health System; Richmond, Virginia.)

Radiologic Findings

AP chest radiograph (**Fig. 159A**) obtained on the second postoperative day following cardiac revascularization shows an enlarged cardiomediastinal silhouette. Note the alignment of the median sternotomy wires. PA (**Fig. 159B**) and lateral (**Fig. 159C**) chest radiographs on the 10th postoperative day reveal displacement of the sixth sternotomy wire (long arrow) and a fracture in the fifth wire (short arrow).

Diagnosis

Sternal wound dehiscence without mediastinitis

Differential Diagnosis

Mediastinitis

Discussion

Background

Median sternotomy is the preferred surgical approach to expose the mediastinum, pericardium, heart, and great vessels. Surgical complications occur in 5% of patients and include wound dehiscence, mediastinitis, and sternal osteomyelitis.

Etiology

Deep sternal wound infections arise from hematogenous seeding of the wound or from direct extension of an adjacent infection. *Staphylococcus* species are responsible in most cases. Dehiscence usually develops within the first 7 to 10 days following surgery. Risk factors for sternal dehiscence include hypertension, tobacco abuse, insulin-dependent diabetes, obesity, intraaortic balloon pump, immunosuppression, prolonged mechanical ventilation, female gender, and harvest of both internal mammary arteries.

Clinical Findings

Signs and symptoms of sternal dehiscence include wound pain with or without drainage, sternal instability, palpable sternal clicking with deep breathing or coughing, fever, and leukocytosis.

Pathology

- Superficial and deep soft tissue inflammation/infection
- Abscess formation
- Draining sinus tracts
- Osteomyelitis

Imaging Findings

RADIOGRAPHY

- Sternal wire displacement (i.e., offset of one or more wires relative to others in vertical axis) (**Fig. 159B**)
- Sternal wire rotation (i.e., alteration in axis of a wire compared with its original orientation)
- Sternal wire disruption (i.e., fracture, unraveling) (**Fig. 159C**)
- Mediastinal widening; acute mediastinitis (see Section 12, Case 180)
- Mediastinal air-fluid levels; acute mediastinitis (see Section 12, Case 180)

CT

- Presternal complications: draining sinus tracts, abscesses
- Retrosternal complications: hematoma, abscess, draining sinus tracts, mediastinitis, pericardial effusion, empyema
- Limited value in evaluation of sternal osteomyelitis

Treatment

- Debridement of devitalized infected soft tissue and bone
- Culture-specific antibiotics
- Flap closure (e.g., muscle, musculocutaneous, omental flap transpositions)

Prognosis

- Mortality rate < 10% with appropriate early and aggressive treatment

PEARLS_____

- Small collections of parasternal air normally resorb within the first 7 postoperative days
- A shift in position of sternal wire(s) on sequential postoperative radiographs is best appreciated when the current radiograph is compared with the first postoperative exam.
- Parasternal soft tissue edema, localized hematoma, sternal nonunion, minimal pericardial thickening: normal postoperative findings for first 2 to 3 weeks
- Radiographic abnormalities may precede the clinical diagnosis of sternal dehiscence in more than two thirds of patients.
- The "midsternal stripe" is a normal 2 to 4 mm radiographic gap seen in 30 to 60% of postoperative chest radiographs and is of no clinical significance.
- First rib fractures are seen on 6% of chest radiographs following routine median sternotomy.

Suggested Readings

Boiselle PM, Mansilla AV. A closer look at the midsternal stripe sign. AJR Am J Roentgenol 2002;178: 945–948

Boiselle PM, Mansilla AV, Fisher MS, McLoud TC. Wandering wires: frequency of sternal wire abnormalities with sternal dehiscence. AJR Am J Roentgenol 1999;173:777–780

Boiselle PM, Mansilla AV, White CS, Fisher MS. Sternal dehiscence in patients with and without mediastinitis. J Thorac Imaging 2001;16:106–110

Fraser RS, Müller NL, Colman N, Paré PD. Complications of therapeutic, biopsy, and monitoring procedures. In: Fraser RS, Müller NL, Colman N, Paré PD, eds. Fraser and Paré's Diagnosis of Diseases of the Chest, 4th ed. Philadelphia: Saunders, 1999:2660–2661

CASE 160 Wegener Granulomatosis

Clinical Presentation

A 72-year-old woman with cough, sinusitis, and renal insufficiency

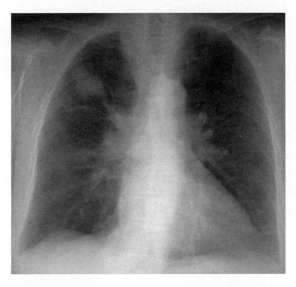

Figure 160A

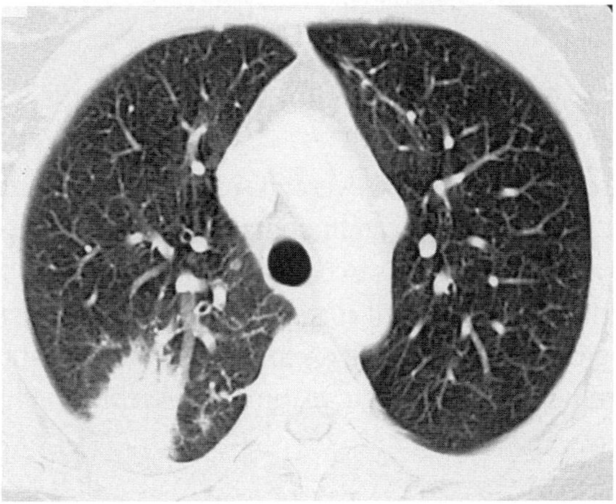

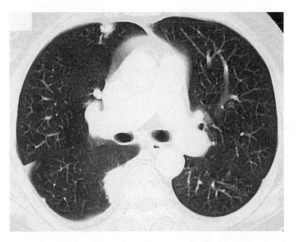

Figure 160C

Figure 160B

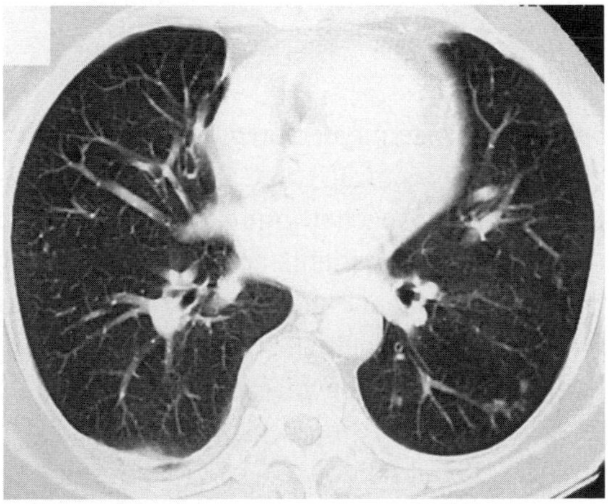

Figure 160D

Radiologic Findings

PA chest radiograph (**Fig. 160A**) demonstrates a right upper lobe mass-like consolidation with associated volume loss. Unenhanced chest CT (lung window) (**Figs. 160B, 160C,** and **160D**) demonstrates a peripheral wedge-shaped right upper lobe consolidation and multifocal peripheral juxtapleural and angiocentric pulmonary masses and nodules.

Diagnosis

Wegener granulomatosis

Differential Diagnosis

- Multifocal primary or secondary neoplasia
- Multifocal bacterial pneumonia
- Bland or septic emboli
- Pulmonary infarcts
- Pulmonary vasculitis (Churg-Strauss syndrome, necrotizing sarcoid granulomatosis)
- Cryptogenic organizing pneumonia (COP)

Discussion

Background

The pulmonary vasculitides include several disorders characterized by inflammation of the pulmonary blood vessel walls. While Wegener granulomatosis is the most common pulmonary vasculitis, Churg-Strauss syndrome and necrotizing sarcoid granulomatosis may also affect the lung. The diagnosis of pulmonary vasculitis requires careful correlation of clinical presentation and imaging findings with the underlying histologic findings and the exclusion of more common infectious granulomatous diseases, many of which often exhibit histologic features of vasculitis.

Etiology

The etiology of pulmonary vasculitis is unknown.

Clinical Findings

Wegener granulomatosis is a systemic necrotizing vasculitis that commonly affects the lung. Although many organs are affected, the clinical triad of febrile sinusitis, pulmonary disease, and glomerulonephritis characterizes classic Wegener granulomatosis. A limited form of Wegener granulomatosis affects primarily the lung. Affected patients are typically adults in the fourth and fifth decades of life, and men are slightly more commonly affected than women. Early symptoms usually relate to upper respiratory tract involvement and include rhinitis, sinusitis, and otitis. Approximately 60 to 80% of affected patients develop pulmonary involvement with cough, dyspnea, hemoptysis, chest pain, and fever. Wegener granulomatosis may produce tracheobronchial stenosis resulting in stridor, dyspnea, wheezing, and hemoptysis. Renal failure is a late manifestation of the disease. A cytoplasmic pattern of antineutrophil cytoplasmic autoantibody (c-ANCA or proteinase 3 ANCA) when confirmed by standard enzyme-lined immunosorbent assay (ELISA) has a diagnostic specificity of 99%.

Pathology

GROSS

- Multifocal gray-white, solid or cavitary pulmonary nodules or masses
- Coalescence of pulmonary nodules or masses into large areas of necrosis
- Pulmonary hemorrhage
- Airway involvement with resultant stenosis

MICROSCOPIC

- Vasculitis with granulomatous inflammation of medium-sized and small pulmonary arteries, veins, and capillaries
- Geographic necrosis

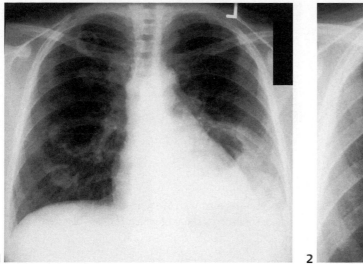
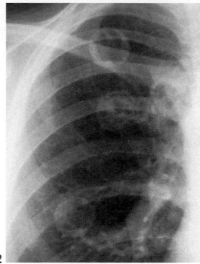

Figure 160E (1,2) PA **(1)** and coned-down PA **(2)** chest radiographs of a 20-year-old woman with Wegener's granulomatosis demonstrate a large cavitary left lower lobe mass and bilateral multifocal cavitary nodules with thin but irregular walls **(2).**

- Neutrophilic microabscesses
- Alveolar hemorrhage

Imaging Findings

RADIOGRAPHY

- Bilateral multifocal, well-defined pulmonary nodules or masses (**Figs. 160A** and **160E**)
- Cavitation (50%): typically thick, irregular walls; may evolve to thin-walled cysts (**Fig. 160E**)
- Multifocal consolidations (**Fig. 160A**)
- Bilateral diffuse airspace opacities from pulmonary hemorrhage
- Visualization of airway stenosis or secondary obstruction, atelectasis, or consolidation
- Rarely lymphadenopathy

CT/HRCT

- Multifocal irregular pulmonary nodules or masses (**Figs. 160C, 160D,** and **160F**)
- Cavitation: typically in nodules over 2 cm in diameter; thick irregular cavity walls (**Fig. 160F**)
- Angiocentric (feeding vessels entering the lesions) and juxtapleural distribution of nodules and/or masses (**Figs. 160D** and **160F**)
- Pleural-based wedge-shaped nodules or consolidations (**Figs. 160B** and **160C**)
- CT "halo sign": ground-glass attenuation surrounding pulmonary lesions
- Focal or diffuse airway stenosis or endoluminal nodules or masses with secondary consolidation or atelectasis
- Pleural effusion in less than 10% of cases

Treatment

- Combination therapy with cytotoxic drugs (cyclophosphamide, azathioprine) and corticosteroids
  - May be complicated by opportunistic infection
  - May relapse

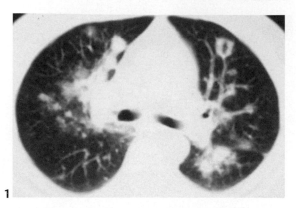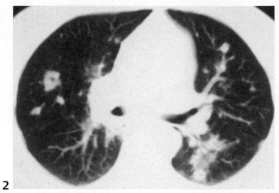

Figure 160F (1,2) Unenhanced chest CT (lung window) of a 45-year-old man with Wegener's granulomatosis demonstrates bilateral multifocal irregular nodules, masses, and consolidations, some of which exhibit cavitation and an angiocentric distribution (feeding vessels entering the lesions).

Prognosis

- Ninety to 95% 5-year survival in treated patients
- Poor prognosis in patients with pulmonary hemorrhage and/or renal failure

PEARLS_____

- Progression of imaging abnormalities or development of air-fluid levels within cavitary lesions in patients with Wegener granulomatosis who are undergoing therapy should suggest superimposed pulmonary infection.
- Churg-Strauss syndrome (allergic angiitis and granulomatosis) begins as a prodromal disease characterized by asthma, allergic rhinitis, and peripheral eosinophilia, and evolves to a systemic vasculitis. Cardiac involvement is more common than in Wegener granulomatosis, and sinus and renal disease are less severe. Affected patients are young adults with recurrent consolidations, airspace opacities, and/or pulmonary nodules, which may exhibit a peripheral distribution as seen in eosinophilic pneumonia.
- Necrotizing sarcoid granulomatosis is characterized by isolated pulmonary involvement and typically affects middle-aged women who present with cough, dyspnea, chest pain, and fever. Chest radiographs demonstrate multifocal bilateral pulmonary nodules or masses, which may cavitate and may be associated with hilar lymphadenopathy.

Suggested Readings

Frazier AA, Rosado de Christenson ML, Galvin JR, Fleming MV. Pulmonary angiitis and granulomatosis: radiologic-pathologic correlation. Radiographics 1998;18:687–710

Mayberry JP, Primack SL, Müller NL. Thoracic manifestations of systemic autoimmune diseases: radiographic and high-resolution CT findings. Radiographics 2000;20:1623–1635

Savage COS, Harper L, Adu D. Primary systemic vasculitis. Lancet 1997;349:553–558

Travis WD, Colby TV, Koss MN, Rosado-de-Christenson ML, Müller NL, King TE Jr. Pulmonary vasculitis. In: King WD, ed. Atlas of Nontumor Pathology: Non-Neoplastic Disorders of the Lower Respiratory Tract, fascicle 2, series 1. Washington, DC: American Registry of Pathology and Armed Forces Institute of Pathology, 2001:233–264

CASE 161 Acute Chest Syndrome of Sickle Cell Anemia

Clinical Presentation

A 19-year-old man with sickle cell anemia and recent cough, fever, and chest pain

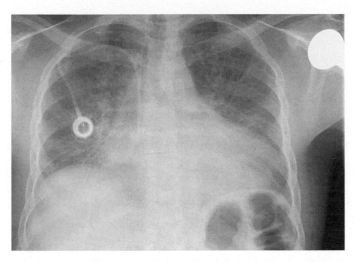

Figure 161A (Courtesy of Diane C. Strollo, M.D., University of Pittsburgh Medical Center, Pittsburgh, Pennsylvania.)

Radiologic Findings

PA chest radiograph (**Fig. 161A**) demonstrates moderate cardiomegaly, low lung volumes, and bilateral patchy perihilar consolidations. A central venous catheter is appropriately positioned. Note the left humeral head replacement for management of epiphyseal infarction and subsequent fracture.

Diagnosis

Acute chest syndrome

Differential Diagnosis

- Bacterial pneumonia
- Pulmonary infarction

Discussion

Background

Sickle cell anemia is a hemolytic anemia that results from the production of abnormal hemoglobin molecules that deform the red blood cells and impair their transit through vascular channels. Resultant vascular occlusion produces tissue ischemia and infarction. The acute chest syndrome is the second leading cause of hospitalization in patients with sickle cell anemia.

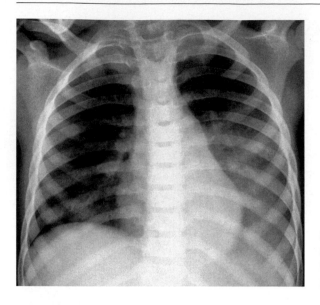

Figure 161B PA chest radiograph of a child with sickle cell disease and acute chest syndrome demonstrates a left lower lobe consolidation. (Courtesy of Gael J. Lonergan, M.D., Austin Radiological Association Austin, Texas.)

Etiology

The cause of acute chest syndrome is poorly understood. It may follow bacterial or viral pneumonia in up to 40% of cases. Because patients admitted for pain crisis may later develop the acute chest syndrome, osseous infarction with fat embolism has been proposed as a possible etiology. Pulmonary vascular occlusion is probably a component of acute chest syndrome and may be the initiating insult in some cases. Acute chest syndrome may follow general anesthesia in up to 10% of affected patients.

Clinical Findings

Acute chest syndrome occurs more frequently in children than in adults, and 50% of children with sickle cell anemia experience at least one episode during their lifetime. Patients present acutely with fever, chest pain, cough, and dyspnea and may progress to respiratory failure and death. The majority of patients (70%) are hypoxemic.

Pathology

GROSS

- Vascular congestion
- Pulmonary hemorrhage
- Pulmonary infarction

MICROSCOPIC

- Vascular occlusion and thrombosis
- Pulmonary infarction

Imaging Findings

RADIOGRAPHY

- Bilateral patchy consolidation with predilection for the middle and lower lobes (**Figs. 161A** and **161B**)
- Frequent pleural effusions
- Visualization of osseous findings of sickle cell anemia such as medullary humeral head infarcts (**Fig. 161A**) and H-shaped thoracic vertebrae

CT/HRCT

- Consolidation
- Areas of vascular attenuation attributed to hypoperfusion
- Late focal or diffuse pulmonary fibrosis

Treatment

- Hydration
- Transfusion
- Supplemental oxygen; mechanical ventilation and extracorporeal membrane oxygenation (ECMO) in severe cases
- Analgesia
- Antibiotic therapy for underlying or suspected infection

Prognosis

- Response to therapy and hospital discharge within 1 week is typical.
- Leading cause of death in patients with sickle cell anemia; mortality rate higher in adults (4.3%) than in children (1.8%)
- Death from chronic pulmonary disease (pulmonary fibrosis, pulmonary hypertension) secondary to repeated episodes

PEARLS_____

- Chest radiographs may initially be normal in patients with acute pain crises who later develop acute chest syndrome.
- Bacterial and/or viral pneumonia must be excluded in all patients with suspected acute chest syndrome.

Suggested Readings

Fraser RS, Müller NL, Colman N, Paré PD. Thrombosis and thromboembolism. In: Fraser RS, Müller NL, Colman N, Paré PD, eds. Fraser and Paré's Diagnosis of Diseases of the Chest, 4th ed. Philadelphia: Saunders, 1999:1773–1843

Lonergan GJ, Cline DB, Abbondanzo SL. Sickle cell anemia. Radiographics 2001;21:971–994

CASE 162 Hepatopulmonary Syndrome

Clinical Presentation

A 52-year-old woman with cirrhosis, portal hypertension, and distal esophageal and gastric varices with progressive dyspnea

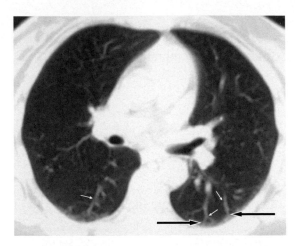

Figure 162A

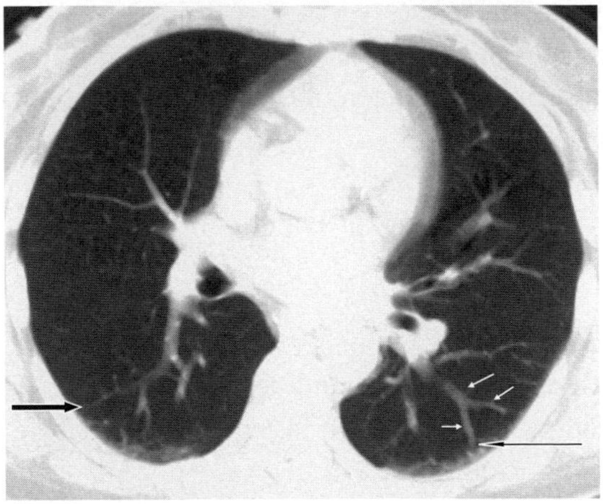

Figure 162B

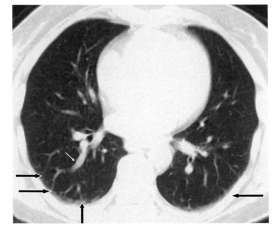

Figure 162C

Radiologic Findings

Contrast-enhanced chest CT (lung window) (**Figs. 162A, 162B,** and **162C**) shows dilated peripheral lower lobe pulmonary vessels (short arrows). An abnormally large number of terminal artery branches extend to the pleural surface (large arrows). There is some associated nodularity and ground-glass opacity.

Diagnosis

Hepatopulmonary syndrome (HPS)

Differential Diagnosis

None

Discussion

Background

The triad of hepatic dysfunction, intrapulmonary vascular dilatation, and hypoxemia characterizes the hepatopulmonary syndrome (HPS). The prevalence of HPS in patients with terminal liver disease ranges between 4 and 47%. There are two types based on arteriography. Type I is the most common pattern, observed in 85% of patients, in which the peripheral juxtapleural vessels have a spidery appearance. Type II is less common, observed in 15% of patients, and is characterized by small, discrete pulmonary arteriovenous fistulas.

Etiology

The pathogenesis of the intrapulmonary vascular dilatation in HPS is unknown. The hypoxemia likely develops as a result of impaired diffusion and perfusion in the dilated vessels.

Clinical Findings

Most patients with HPS have cirrhosis, complain of progressive dyspnea, and manifest hypoxemia. Patients may also complain of platypnea and have orthodeoxia. Pulmonary artery pressures are usually normal or reduced.

Pathology

- No intrinsic lung disease
- Variable degrees of pulmonary vascular dilatation
- Variable degrees of pulmonary capillary dilatation
- Impaired hypoxic pressor response

Imaging Findings

RADIOGRAPHY

- Normal; most common
- Bibasilar nodular or reticular opacities
- Enlarged central pulmonary arteries

ARTERIOGRAPHY

- Enlarged central pulmonary arteries
- Peripheral arteriolar dilatation
- "Spidery" appearance of lower lobe peripheral juxtapleural vessels (type I)
- Small, discrete lower lobe pulmonary arteriovenous fistulas (type II)

CT/HRCT

- Dilatation of the peripheral lower lobe pulmonary vessels (**Figs. 162A, 162B,** and **162C**)
- Increased number of visible terminal artery branches (**Figs. 162A, 162B,** and **162C**)

- Peripheral lower lobe vessels may extend to pleural surface (**Figs. 162A, 162B,** and **162C**).
- Increased lower lobe segmental arterial diameter when compared with the diameter of the adjacent bronchi
- Cirrhosis, hepatosplenomegaly, varices, ascites

Treatment

- Patients with PaO_2 < 55 mm Hg, or PaO_2 > 55 mm Hg accompanied by polycythemia, cor pulmonale, or cognitive impairment should receive 100% oxygen therapy.
  - If PaO_2 increases to > 150 mm Hg and hypoxia is corrected, ambulatory oxygen therapy is continued (i.e., type I disease).
  - If hypoxia is not corrected, or PaO_2 < 150 mm Hg after receiving 100% oxygen, the patient should be studied with pulmonary angiography for potential embolotherapy (i.e., type II disease).
- Liver transplantation

Prognosis

- Liver transplantation is the most effective therapy; syndrome is corrected in more than 80% of patients within 15 months of transplantation.
- Liver transplantation does not correct the diffusion abnormalities.

PEARL_____

- The association of spider nevi, digital clubbing, hypoxemia, and portal hypertension is highly suggestive of HPS.

Suggested Readings

Castro M, Krowka MJ. Hepatopulmonary syndrome: a pulmonary vascular complication of liver disease. Clin Chest Med 1996;17:35–48

Lee KN, Lee HJ, Shin WW, et al. Hypoxemia and liver cirrhosis (hepatopulmonary syndrome) in eight patients: comparison of the central and peripheral pulmonary vasculature. Radiology 1999;211: 549–553

McAdams HP, Erasmus J, Crockett R, et al. The hepatopulmonary syndrome: radiologic findings in ten patients. AJR Am J Roentgenol 1996;166:1379–1385

SECTION XII

Abnormalities and Diseases of the Mediastinum

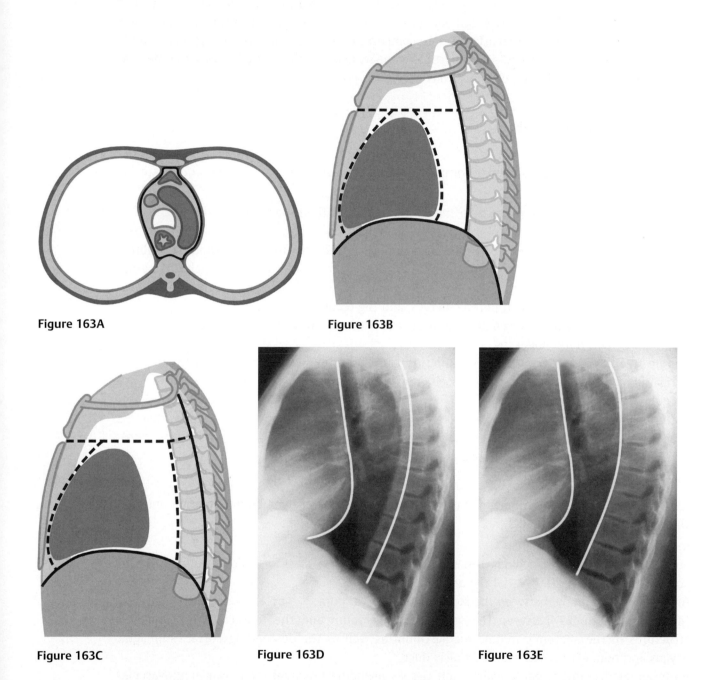

Figure 163A

Figure 163B

Figure 163C

Figure 163D

Figure 163E

The Mediastinum

Fig. 163A is an axial illustration of the mediastinum at the level of the aortic arch. A sagittal illustration (**Fig. 163B**) of the four anatomic mediastinal compartments is compared with a sagittal illustration (**Fig. 163C**) of the four surgical mediastinal compartments. A lateral chest radiograph (**Fig. 163D**) with superimposed lines illustrates the radiographic mediastinal compartments according to Felson. A lateral chest radiograph with superimposed lines (**Fig. 163E**) illustrates the radiographic mediastinal compartments according to Fraser, Müller, Colman, and Paré.

Discussion

Background

The mediastinum is the space between the lungs and pleural surfaces and is bound by the sternum anteriorly and the vertebral column posteriorly (**Fig. 163A**). It extends from the thoracic inlet to the diaphragm and contains the thymus, lymph nodes, heart, great vessels, trachea, esophagus, and other soft tissues. The division of the mediastinum into compartments is arbitrary, as no anatomic boundaries divide the space. The method of mediastinal compartmentalization varies among the medical disciplines, and several radiologic classifications have been proposed.

The Mediastinal Compartments

ANATOMIC DIVISION

Anatomists describe four mediastinal compartments: superior, anterior, middle, and posterior (**Fig. 163B**).

- Anterior, middle, and posterior compartments located below the superior mediastinum
- Exclusion of paravertebral areas
- Superior mediastinum—between the sternal manubrium and the first four thoracic vertebrae, from an oblique plane through the first rib superiorly to a horizontal plane through the sternal angle inferiorly; contains thymus, portions of the great vessels, portions of the trachea and esophagus, portions of the vagus and phrenic nerves, and the recurrent laryngeal nerve
- Anterior mediastinum—between the sternum and the pericardium; contains areolar tissue, lymphatics, and lymph nodes
- Middle mediastinum—between the anterior and posterior compartments; contains the pericardium, heart, origins of great vessels, tracheal bifurcation, lymph nodes, portions of the phrenic nerves, and azygos arch
- Posterior mediastinum—between the posterior aspect of the pericardium and the spine; contains descending aorta, a portion of the esophagus, thoracic duct, azygos and hemiazygos veins, portions of the vagus nerves, the splanchnic nerves, and lymph nodes

SURGICAL DIVISION

Surgeons describe four mediastinal compartments based on areas of operability: superior, anterior, middle, and posterior (**Fig. 163C**).

- Inclusion of paravertebral areas
- Superior mediastinum—includes the superior aspect of the anterior, middle, and posterior compartments above the level of the aortic arch
- Anterior mediastinum—between the sternum and pericardium
- Middle mediastinum—between the anterior mediastinum and the thoracic spine; includes structures in the anatomic middle mediastinum as well as the descending aorta, esophagus, azygos and hemiazygos veins, and thoracic duct
- Posterior mediastinum—paravertebral soft tissues including proximal intercostal neurovascular structures, lymph nodes, sympathetic chain and branches

RADIOGRAPHIC DIVISIONS

- Felson

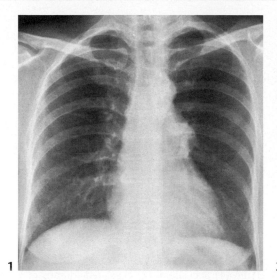

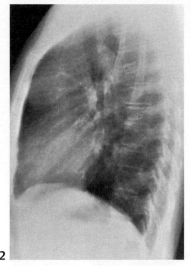

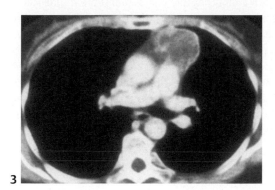

Figure 163F (1–3) PA **(1)** and lateral **(2)** chest radiographs of an asymptomatic 53-year-old woman with thymoma demonstrate a left anterior mediastinal mass. The mass projects over the retrosternal space on the lateral chest radiograph **(3)** and would be localized in the anterior mediastinum based on both the Felson and the Fraser et al classifications. Contrast-enhanced chest CT (mediastinal window) **(3)** demonstrates a heterogeneous well-defined prevascular mass occupying the left lobe of the thymus. Based on the patient's age, absence of symptoms, and absence of lymphadenopathy, thymoma would be the preferred diagnosis. (From Rosado-de-Christenson ML, Galobardes J, Moran CA. Thymoma: radiologic-pathologic correlation. Radiographics 1992;12:151–168, with permission.)

- Benjamin Felson divided the mediastinum based on the lateral chest radiograph (**Fig. 163D**). Because anterior mediastinal masses frequently projected over the heart on lateral radiography, the heart was included in the radiographic anterior mediastinal compartment (**Fig. 163F**). The paravertebral region (not anatomically in the mediastinum) was included within the posterior mediastinum.
  - Anterior mediastinum—structures anterior to a line drawn along the anterior tracheal wall and continued along the posterior heart border
  - Posterior mediastinum—structures posterior to a line connecting points on each thoracic vertebral body approximately 1 cm behind their anterior margins
  - Middle mediastinum—structures contained between the above-mentioned lines (**Fig. 163G**)
- Fraser, Müller, Colman, and Paré
  - This classification recognizes that the distinction between compartments is difficult to establish on radiography and that mediastinal masses may occupy more than one compartment. It combines the middle and posterior compartments and describes a separate paravertebral region. Masses are described as occurring predominantly in one of the compartments (**Fig. 163E**).

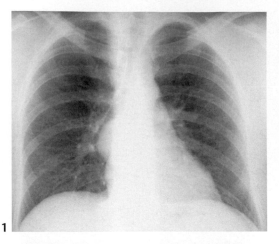
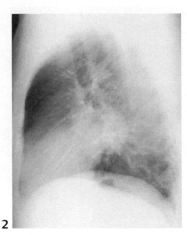

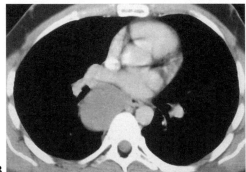

Figure 163G (1–3) PA **(1)** and lateral **(2)** chest radiographs of an asymptomatic 40-year-old man with a bronchogenic cyst demonstrate a spherical subcarinal mass. Based on the lateral chest radiograph **(2)**, the mass would be localized in the middle mediastinum based on the Felson classification and predominantly in the middle-posterior mediastinum based on the Fraser et al classification. Contrast-enhanced chest CT (mediastinal window) **(3)** demonstrates a homogeneous spherical subcarinal mass of soft tissue attenuation that does not exhibit contrast enhancement and produces mass effect on the left atrium. The mass is posterior to the heart and extends into the paravertebral region. Based on its location and morphology as well as the absence of contrast enhancement, a congenital cyst is the most likely diagnosis.

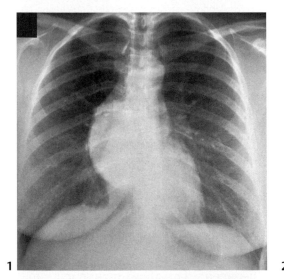
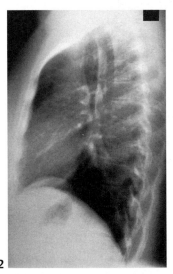

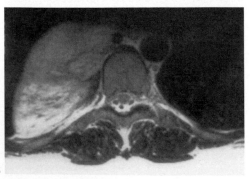

Figure 163H (1–3) PA **(1)** and lateral **(2)** chest radiographs of an asymptomatic young woman with a ganglioneuroma demonstrate an elongated right paravertebral mass. Based on its location on the lateral chest radiograph **(2)**, the lesion occupies both the middle and posterior mediastinal compartments based on the Felson classification and predominantly the paravertebral region based on the Fraser et al classification. Subtle expansion of the seventh posterior intercostal space **(1)** suggests a neurogenic neoplasm. Axial T1-weighted MR **(3)** demonstrates a heterogeneous mass of high signal intensity situated predominantly in the right paravertebral region.

- Anterior mediastinum—structures anterior to a line that extends along the anterior wall of the trachea and continues along the posterior heart border
- Middle-posterior mediastinum—structures located between the above-mentioned line and a line drawn along the anterior aspects of the thoracic vertebral bodies
- Paravertebral region—overlaps the vertebral bodies on the lateral chest radiograph (**Fig. 163H**)

Cross-Sectional Imaging

Cross-sectional imaging with CT and MR imaging allows visualization of the normal mediastinal structures and accurate localization of mediastinal abnormalities.

- Anterior mediastinum—between the chest wall anteriorly and the anterior tracheal wall and pericardium posteriorly
- Middle mediastinum—bound anteriorly by the pericardium and posteriorly by the posterior tracheal wall and pericardium
- Posterior mediastinum—bound anteriorly by the plane between the trachea and esophagus and the pericardium and posteriorly by the paraspinal regions

Radiographic localization of a mediastinal lesion within one of these compartments is the first step in the formulation of a differential diagnosis, which may be refined by incorporation of demographic and clinical information. Cross-sectional imaging allows analysis of a lesion's morphologic characteristics, its precise anatomic localization, and, in some cases, identification of the structure of origin. This permits further refinement of the differential diagnosis, and on occasion a specific diagnosis can be proposed.

Suggested Readings

Aquino SL, Duncan G, Taber KH, Sharma A, Hayman LA. Reconciliation of the anatomic, surgical, and radiographic classifications of the mediastinum. J Comput Assist Tomogr 2001;25:489–492

Felson B. Chest Roentgenology. Philadelphia: Saunders, 1973:380–420

Fraser RS, Müller NL, Colman N, Paré PD. Masses situated predominantly in the anterior compartment. In: Fraser RS, Müller NL, Colman N, Paré PD, eds. Fraser and Paré's Diagnosis of Diseases of the Chest, 4th ed. Philadelphia: Saunders, 1999:2875–2937

Rosado-de-Christenson ML, Galobardes J, Moran CA. Thymoma: radiologic-pathologic correlation. Radiographics 1992;12:151–168

Woodburne RT, Burkel WE. Essentials of Human Anatomy, 9th ed. New York: Oxford University Press, 1994:370–371

Clinical Presentation

An asymptomatic 68-year-old man

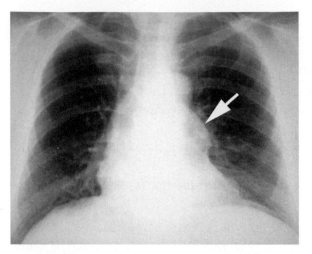

Figure 164A

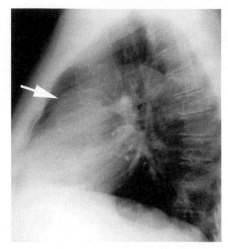

Figure 164B

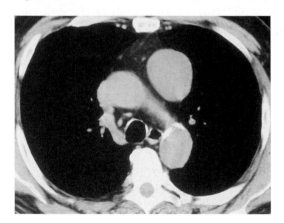

Figure 164C

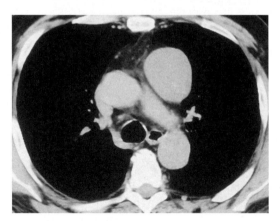

Figure 164D

Radiologic Findings

PA (**Fig. 164A**) and lateral (**Fig. 164B**) chest radiographs demonstrate a well-defined left anterior mediastinal mass (arrows). Contrast-enhanced chest CT (mediastinal window) (**Figs. 164C** and **164D**) demonstrates a well-circumscribed ovoid homogeneous soft tissue mass located in the left lobe of the thymus. A tissue plane separates the mass from the mediastinal great vessels.

Diagnosis

Thymoma, encapsulated

Differential Diagnosis

- Thymoma, invasive
- Thymic carcinoid, thymic carcinoma
- Lymphoma

Discussion

Background

Thymoma is an epithelial neoplasm of the thymus. It represents the most common primary neoplasm of the thymus and the most common primary neoplasm of the anterior mediastinum.

Etiology

The etiology of thymoma remains unknown. Thymoma is associated with systemic and autoimmune disorders (parathymic syndromes), such as myasthenia gravis, hypogammaglobulinemia, and pure red cell aplasia, as well as with a variety of nonthymic neoplasms.

Clinical Findings

Patients with thymoma are typically adult men and women who usually present after the age of 40 years, although all age groups are affected. While many patients with thymoma are asymptomatic, approximately one third present with chest pain, cough, dyspnea, or symptoms related to local invasion by the tumor (including superior vena cava syndrome). Approximately 15% of patients with myasthenia gravis have thymoma, and up to 50% of patients with thymoma develop myasthenia gravis. Approximately 10% of patients with thymoma have hypogammaglobulinemia, and approximately 5% have pure red cell aplasia.

Pathology

GROSS

- Spherical or ovoid, smooth, or lobular mass
- Surrounded by a fibrous capsule (*encapsulated* thymoma) in two thirds of cases
- Tumor growth through fibrous capsule (*invasive* thymoma) into adjacent fat, cardiovascular structures, pleura (tumor implants), lung, and/or abdomen
- Pale tan, pink-gray cut surface compartmentalized by fibrous trabeculae
- Frequent cystic areas; may be predominantly cystic with mural tumor nodules

MICROSCOPIC

- No histologic features of malignancy
- World Health Organization classification (1999) based on epithelial cell morphology and lymphocyte-to-epithelial cell ratios
  - Type A: spindle/oval epithelial cells with few or no lymphocytes
  - Type AB: features of type A thymoma with lymphocyte-rich areas
  - Type B1: resembles normal thymus with cortical and medullary areas

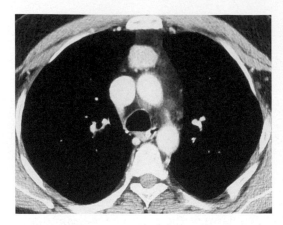

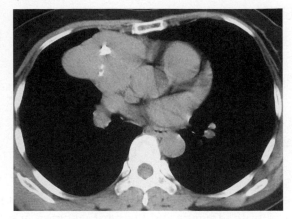

Figure 164E Contrast-enhanced chest CT (mediastinal window) of an elderly woman with myasthenia gravis demonstrates a small lobular thymic soft tissue mass, which represented an occult thymoma.

Figure 164F Unenhanced chest CT (mediastinal window) of an asymptomatic 48-year-old woman with an incidentally discovered thymoma demonstrates a large lobular right anterior mediastinal mass with multifocal central calcifications. Note that this encapsulated thymoma exhibits focal obliteration of adjacent tissue planes.

- Type B2: plump epithelial cells with a heavy lymphocyte population
- Type B3: round/polygonal epithelial cells with a minor lymphocyte component
- Microscopic documentation of capsular invasion defines invasive thymoma

Imaging Findings

RADIOGRAPHY

- Well-defined lobular unilateral anterior mediastinal mass; variable size (**Figs. 164A** and **164B**)
- Located anywhere from thoracic inlet to cardiophrenic angle
- Irregular borders against the lung, ipsilateral diaphragmatic elevation, and associated pleural-based nodules/masses suggest local invasion.
- Normal chest radiography in cases of occult thymoma (25% of thymomas)

CT

- Well-defined prevascular (typically unilateral) anterior mediastinal (in anatomic location of thymus) soft tissue mass
  - Homogeneous with uniform contrast enhancement (**Figs. 164C, 164D,** and **164E**)
  - Heterogeneous (**Figs. 164F, 164G,** and **164H1**)
    - Cystic change, hemorrhage, necrosis (**Figs. 164G** and **164H1**)
    - Predominantly cystic mass (mural nodules)
    - Calcification; peripheral capsular, or central (**Figs. 164F** and **164H1**)
  - Lobular (**Figs. 164E, 164F, 164G,** and **164H1**) or smooth contours (**Figs. 164C** and **164D**)
  - Exclusion of local invasion [adjacent fat, cardiovascular structures (**Fig. 164H1**), lung] or pleural implantation (**Fig. 164H2**), which may progress to circumferential pleural thickening

MR

- T1-weighted images: intermediate signal intensity similar to skeletal muscle
- T2-weighted images: increased signal intensity

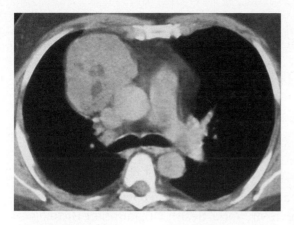

Figure 164G Contrast-enhanced chest CT (mediastinal window) of an asymptomatic 70-year-old man with an encapsulated thymoma demonstrates a large lobular right anterior mediastinal mass with central foci of low attenuation that corresponded to cystic changes.

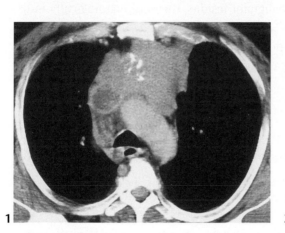
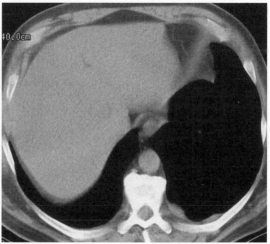

Figure 164H (1,2) Contrast-enhanced chest CT (mediastinal window) of a middle-aged man with invasive thymoma who presented with superior vena cava syndrome demonstrates a large anterior mediastinal mass with irregular contours, multifocal central calcifications, vascular invasion **(1)**, and multiple left pleural tumor implants **(2)**.

- Cystic areas with low signal intensity on T1- and high signal intensity on T2-weighted images
- Exclusion of local invasion

Staging (Masaoka system)

- Stage I: encapsulated thymoma without microscopic capsular invasion
- Stage II: macroscopic invasion into surrounding fat or mediastinal pleura, microscopic invasion into capsule
- Stage III: macroscopic invasion of neighboring organs
- Stage IVa: pleural or pericardial dissemination
- Stage IVb: lymphogenous or hematogenous metastases

Treatment

- Complete surgical excision
- Postoperative radiation for invasive thymoma to decrease likelihood of local recurrence
- Chemotherapy for tumor progression following surgery and for unresectable thymoma

Prognosis

- Encapsulated and minimally invasive (adjacent fat) thymoma: 95 to 100% 5-year survival; small percentage of local recurrences
- Invasive thymoma (pericardium, lung, cardiovascular structures): 50 to 60% 5-year survival, worse with pleural/pericardial tumor dissemination
- Reported recurrences 10 to 20 years after initially successful treatment

PEARLS

- The term *thymoma* is generally reserved for primary epithelial thymic neoplasms without overt atypia of the epithelial component. However, the 1999 World Health Organization Histological Typing of Tumors of the Thymus classifies thymic carcinomas as type C thymomas.
- Although invasive thymomas may be regarded as malignant lesions, they are histologically indistinguishable from encapsulated thymomas.
- Obliteration of adjacent tissue planes on cross-sectional imaging is not diagnostic of local invasion; identification of intact tissue planes does not exclude local invasion.

Suggested Readings

Okumura M, Ohta M, Tateyama H, et al. The World Health Organization histologic classification system reflects the oncologic behavior of thymoma: a clinical study of 273 patients. Cancer 2002; 94:624–632

Rosai J, Sobin LH. Histological Typing of Tumours of the Thymus: International Histological Classification of Tumours, 2nd ed. New York: Springer 1999

Shimosato Y, Mukai K. Tumors of the thymus and related lesions. In: Rosai J, ed. Atlas of Tumor Pathology: Tumors of the Mediastinum, fascicle 21, series 3. Washington, DC: American Registry of Pathology and Armed Forces Institute of Pathology, 1997:33–247

Strollo DC, Rosado-de-Christenson ML. Tumors of the thymus. J Thorac Imaging 1999;14:152–171

Thomas CR, Wright CD, Loehrer PJ Sr. Thymoma: state of the art. J Clin Oncol 1999;17:2280–2289

Tomiyama N, Müller NL, Ellis SJ, et al. Invasive and noninvasive thymoma: distinctive CT features. J Comput Assist Tomogr 2001;25:388–393

CASE 165 Thymic Malignancy: Carcinoid

Clinical Presentation

A 45-year-old man with Cushing syndrome

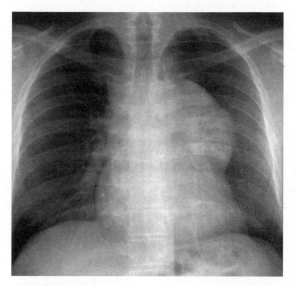

Figure 165A

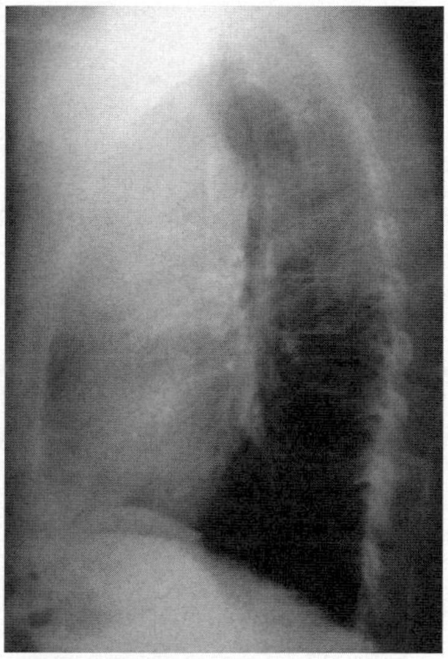

Figure 165B

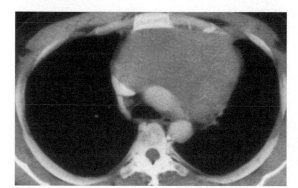

Figure 165C

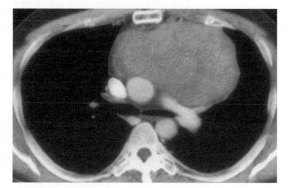

Figure 165D

Radiologic Findings

PA (**Fig. 165A**) and lateral (**Fig. 165B**) chest radiographs demonstrate a large, well-defined anterior mediastinal mass that extends predominantly to the left side. Note the mass effect on the trachea (**Fig. 165B**). Contrast-enhanced chest CT (mediastinal window) (**Figs. 165C** and **165D**) demonstrates a large lobular heterogeneous anterior mediastinal mass with marked mass effect on the great vessels and the airways.

Diagnosis

Thymic carcinoid

Differential Diagnosis

- Thymoma
- Lymphoma
- Seminoma
- Thymic carcinoma

Discussion

Background

Thymic carcinoid is a rare primary malignant neuroendocrine thymic neoplasm.

Etiology

The etiology of thymic carcinoid is unknown. It is histologically indistinguishable from bronchial carcinoid but exhibits a higher frequency of atypical histology and more aggressive behavior.

Clinical Findings

Thymic carcinoid affects men more commonly than women (3:1 male-to-female ratio) over a wide age range, with a mean age of 43 years. Most patients are symptomatic at presentation with cough, dyspnea, chest pain, and/or symptoms related to invasion of adjacent structures. Approximately 50% of thymic carcinoids are functionally active and may initially manifest with Cushing syndrome or in association with the syndrome of multiple endocrine neoplasia (MEN).

Pathology

GROSS

- Large anterior mediastinal mass; ranging in size from 6 to 20 cm
- Approximately 50% encapsulated; most are well circumscribed; local invasion in approximately 30%
- Gray-white on cut section with foci of hemorrhage or necrosis

MICROSCOPIC

- Tumor cells arranged in ribbons, solid sheets, or nests amid fibrous trabeculae
- Polygonal cells with eosinophilic cytoplasm, rounded nuclei, and stippled nuclear chromatin
- Most are atypical thymic carcinoids with numerous mitoses and areas of necrosis.

Imaging Findings

RADIOGRAPHY

- Large anterior mediastinal mass (indistinguishable from thymoma) (**Figs. 165A** and **165B**)
- Typically well-defined borders on radiography, even when locally invasive (**Figs. 165A** and **165B**)

CT

- Typically large homogeneous or heterogeneous anterior mediastinal mass (indistinguishable from thymoma) (**Figs. 165C** and **165D**)
- Lymphadenopathy
- Invasion of adjacent structures, pleural effusion/tumor implants, distant metastases

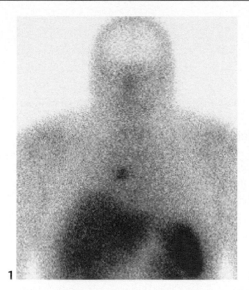 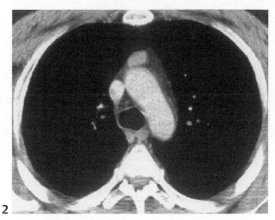

Figure 165E (1,2) Octreotide scintigraphy **(1)** of a middle-aged man who presented with Cushing syndrome demonstrates focal abnormal mediastinal uptake. Contrast-enhanced chest CT (mediastinal window) **(2)** demonstrates an ovoid soft tissue nodule in the right lobe of the thymus, that corresponds to the area of abnormal uptake and represented a radiographically occult thymic carcinoid.

SCINTIGRAPHY

- Evaluation of patients with clinical evidence of ectopic adrenocorticotropic hormone (ACTH) production
- Uptake of octreotide: In-111-diethylenetriamine pentaacetic acid (DTPA)-D-Phe[1] in occult thymic carcinoids (nonspecific finding; uptake in other primary and metastatic thymic neoplasms) (**Fig. 165E**)

Treatment

- Aggressive surgical excision
- Adjuvant radiation therapy and chemotherapy

Prognosis

- Frequent disease progression, recurrence, and metastases
- Poor prognosis; 31% 5-year survival
- Aggressive behavior and worse prognosis in patients with MEN syndrome or clinical Cushing syndrome

PEARLS

- Thymic carcinoid exhibits a high incidence of local recurrence. Follow-up cross-sectional imaging every 6 to 12 months is recommended.
- Thymic carcinoid may be radiologically indistinguishable from thymoma. The presence of a clinical hormone syndrome suggests the diagnosis; visualization of lymphadenopathy should suggest a thymic or anterior mediastinal malignancy (carcinoid, carcinoma, lymphoma).

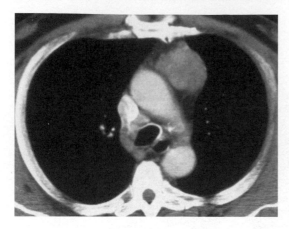

Figure 165F Contrast-enhanced chest CT (mediastinal window) of a 50-year-old man with chest pain and thymic carcinoma demonstrates a lobular left anterior mediastinal heterogeneous soft tissue mass with pretracheal lymphadenopathy but no imaging evidence of local invasion. While the lesion itself is indistinguishable from thymoma, the presence of lymphadenopathy should suggest the diagnosis of a thymic malignancy or lymphoma.

• Thymic carcinoma (World Health Organization type C thymoma) exhibits cytologic atypia and histologic features analogous to carcinomas of other organs and lacks immature lymphocytes characteristically found in thymomas. Radiologically, it manifests as a large anterior mediastinal mass with frequent central necrosis, calcification, local invasion, lymphadenopathy **(Fig. 165F)**, and distant metastases.

Suggested Readings

Jung K-J, Lee KS, Han J, Kim J, Kim TS, Kim EA. Malignant thymic epithelial tumors: CT-pathologic correlation. AJR Am J Roentgenol 2001;176:433–439

Rosado-de-Christenson ML, Abbott GF, Kirejczyk WM, Galvin JR, Travis WD. Thoracic carcinoids: radiologic-pathologic correlation. Radiographics 1999;19:707–736

Rosai J, Sobin LH. Histological Typing of Tumours of the Thymus: International Histological Classification of Tumours, 2nd ed. New York: Springer, 1999

Shimosato Y, Mukai K. Tumors of the thymus and related lesions. In: Rosai J, ed. Atlas of Tumor Pathology: Tumors of the Mediastinum, fascicle 21, series 3. Washington, DC: American Registry of Pathology and Armed Forces Institute of Pathology, 1997:33–247

Strollo DC, Rosado-de-Christenson ML. Tumors of the thymus. J Thorac Imaging 1999;14:152–171

CASE 166 Thymolipoma

Clinical Presentation

An asymptomatic 12-year-old boy

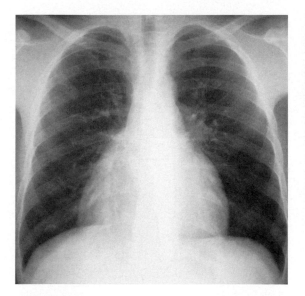

Figure 166A

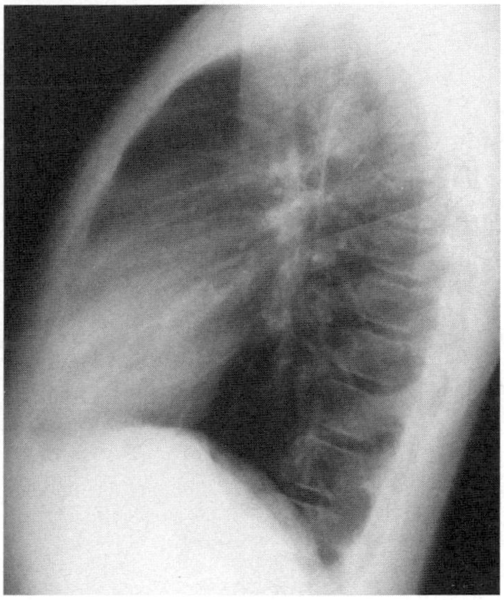

Figure 166B

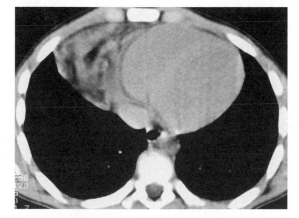

Figure 166C

Radiologic Findings

PA (**Fig. 166A**) and lateral (**Fig. 166B**) chest radiographs demonstrate a right anterior-inferior mediastinal mass, which conforms to the shape of the heart and mimics cardiomegaly. Note that the lesion is not visible on the lateral chest radiograph (**Fig. 166B**). Contrast-enhanced chest CT (mediastinal window) (**Fig. 166C**) demonstrates a well-defined right paracardiac mass composed of soft tissue elements intermixed with areas of fat attenuation. Note mild mass effect on the heart and an intact adjacent tissue plane formed by epicardial fat.

Diagnosis

Thymolipoma

637

Differential Diagnosis

- Morgagni hernia
- Lipoma/liposarcoma
- Mature teratoma

Discussion

Background

Thymolipomas are rare benign primary thymic neoplasms characterized by their soft consistency and preferential growth in the inferior aspect of the anterior mediastinum. These lesions may reach very large sizes in spite of minimal symptoms.

Etiology

The etiology of thymolipoma is unknown.

Pathology

GROSS

- Encapsulated lobular soft tissue thymic mass
- Yellow cut surface

MICROSCOPIC

- Mature adipose and thymic tissue in roughly equal proportions
- May exhibit adipose tissue predominance with minute foci of thymic tissue

Clinical Findings

Thymolipoma usually occurs in young adults in the third decade of life. Men and women are equally affected. Patients may be entirely asymptomatic. Symptomatic patients typically present with complaints related to mass effect by large lesions and may complain of cough, dyspnea, and/or chest pain.

Imaging Features

RADIOGRAPHY

- Well-defined unilateral or bilateral anterior inferior mediastinal mass (**Figs. 166A** and **166B**)
- Conforms to the shape of adjacent structures; may mimic cardiomegaly (**Figs. 166A** and **166B**) or diaphragmatic elevation
- Positional changes in shape due to soft consistency

CT

- Circumscribed anterior mediastinal mass with an anatomic connection to the thymus
- Admixture of linear, whorled, or rounded soft tissue elements and fat attenuation (**Fig. 166C**)
- Less commonly predominant fat attenuation with small internal soft tissue foci

MR

- T1-weighted images: high signal intensity areas intermixed with intermediate signal intensity foci (roughly isointense to muscle)
- Documentation of absence of local invasion

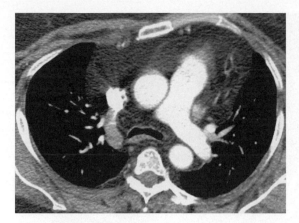

Figure 166D Contrast-enhanced chest CT (mediastinal window) of an obese 58-year-old woman with mediastinal lipomatosis demonstrates fat attenuation surrounding normal mediastinal structures without resultant mass effect. Note excess fat deposition in the paravertebral regions.

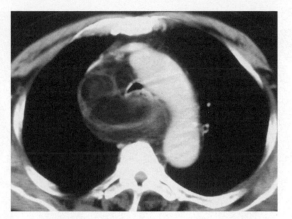

Figure 166E Contrast-enhanced chest CT (mediastinal window) of an asymptomatic man with a mediastinal lipoma demonstrates a middle mediastinal mass of predominant fat attenuation with internal soft tissue elements, which produces mass effect on the airway and the great vessels.

Treatment

- Surgical excision
- Observation of patients who are not surgical candidates

Prognosis

- Excellent
- No reports of malignant transformation

PEARLS

- The diagnosis of thymolipoma should be considered in any asymptomatic patient with an anterior inferior mediastinal mass that conforms to the shape of adjacent structures and produces little mass effect. The demonstration of fat and soft tissue elements within the lesion and an anatomic connection to the thymus strongly supports the diagnosis.
- The differential diagnosis of fat-containing soft tissue mediastinal masses includes:
    - Mediastinal lipomatosis—deposition of nonneoplastic unencapsulated mature adipose tissue particularly in the superior mediastinum, pleuropericardial angles, and paravertebral regions in association with obesity or endogenous/exogenous hypercortisolism; imaging studies demonstrate mediastinal enlargement produced by tissue of homogeneous fat attenuation/signal without mass effect (**Fig. 166D**).
    - Mediastinal lipoma—a rare mesenchymal mediastinal neoplasm composed of encapsulated adipose tissue, vascular structures, and fibrous septa, which typically affects asymptomatic adults (although large tumors may produce symptoms of compression); CT/MR demonstrate a noninvasive mass of predominant fat attenuation with small internal soft tissue foci (**Fig. 166E**).
    - Mediastinal liposarcoma—a rare mesenchymal malignant neoplasm of variable degrees of differentiation and histologic makeup that typically affects older individuals who present with dyspnea, chest pain, cough, or constitutional complaints; imaging features correlate with the histologic composition of the tumor and range from masses of predominant fat attenuation/

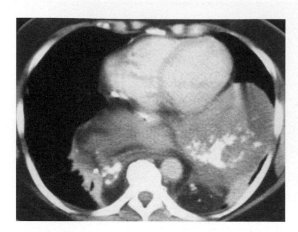

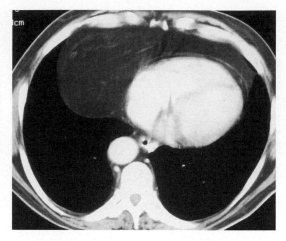

Figure 166F Contrast-enhanced chest CT (mediastinal window) of an elderly man with weight loss, dysphagia, and a mediastinal liposarcoma demonstrates a large middle-posterior (and paravertebral) mediastinal mass of predominant soft tissue attenuation with multifocal coarse calcifications and areas of fat attenuation. Note marked mass effect on the esophagus and heart and adjacent subsegmental atelectasis.

Figure 166G Contrast-enhanced chest CT (mediastinal window) of an asymptomatic 74-year-old woman with a Morgagni hernia demonstrates a right cardiophrenic angle mass of predominant fat attenuation with internal thin linear strands of soft tissue attenuation, which represented omental vessels.

signal to soft tissue masses with minimal or absent foci of fat attenuation/signal; soft tissue components are often dominant, and mass effect is typical (**Fig. 166F**).

- Morgagni hernia—a developmental abnormality characterized by a defect in the anteromedial diaphragm through which abdominal contents (including omental fat) may herniate (**Fig. 166G**). Affected patients are typically asymptomatic but may also present with nonspecific abdominal and thoracic complaints. Radiography typically demonstrates a right cardiophrenic angle mass. CT/MR demonstrate fat corresponding to omental herniation and may show bowel loops within the mass and discontinuity of the adjacent diaphragm.

Suggested Readings

Eisenstat R, Bruce D, Williams LE, Katz DS. Primary liposarcoma of the mediastinum with coexistent mediastinal lipomatosis. AJR Am J Roentgenol 2000;174:572–573

Fraser RS, Müller NL, Colman N, Paré PD. Anterior mediastinal masses. In: Fraser RS, Müller NL, Colman N, Paré PD, eds. Fraser and Paré's Diagnosis of Diseases of the Chest, 4th ed. Philadelphia: Saunders, 1999:2851–2937

Rosado-de-Christenson ML, Pugatch RD, Moran CA, Galobardes J. Thymolipoma: analysis of 27 cases. Radiology 1994;193:121–126

Shimosato Y, Mukai K. Tumors of the thymus and related lesions. In: Rosai J, ed. Atlas of Tumor Pathology: Tumors of the Mediastinum, fascicle 21, series 3. Washington, DC: American Registry of Pathology and Armed Forces Institute of Pathology, 1997:33–247

CASE 167 Thymic Hyperplasia

Clinical Presentation

A 35-year-old woman with Graves disease

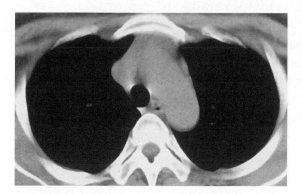

Figure 167A

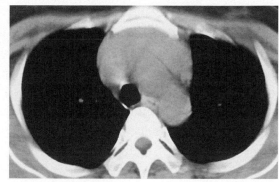

Figure 167B

Radiologic Findings

Unenhanced chest CT (mediastinal window) (**Fig. 167A**) demonstrates morphologically normal soft tissue in the anterior mediastinum consistent with thymic remnant. Unenhanced chest CT (mediastinal window) performed 1 year later (**Fig. 167B**) and after the diagnosis of Graves disease demonstrates an anterior mediastinal soft tissue mass, which exhibits convex lateral borders.

Diagnosis

Lymphoid (follicular) thymic hyperplasia

Differential Diagnosis

- Thymoma
- Lymphoma
- Seminoma (a diagnostic consideration in male patients)

Discussion

Background

Lymphoid thymic hyperplasia, also known as lymphofollicular or autoimmune thymitis and thymic lymphoid hyperplasia, refers to abnormal numbers of secondary lymphoid follicles with germinal centers within an otherwise normal thymus. Lymphoid hyperplasia may or may not result in thymic enlargement.

True thymic hyperplasia is an uncommon condition characterized by a global increase in the size and weight of the thymus (based on the expected thymic size for the individual's age), but with a normal microscopic appearance. The term *rebound thymic hyperplasia* is used specifically for hyperplasia that occurs following chemotherapy, steroid therapy, or recovery from a severe systemic stress or insult.

641

Etiology

The etiology of lymphoid hyperplasia is unknown, but it is typically found in association with myasthenia gravis. In fact, after exclusion of patients with thymoma, as many as 84% of the remaining patients with myasthenia gravis exhibit typical histologic features of lymphofollicular thymitis. Lymphoid hyperplasia is also associated with a series of autoimmune and systemic disorders including hyperthyroidism (Graves disease), acromegaly, systemic lupus erythematosus, scleroderma, rheumatoid arthritis, and cirrhosis.

True thymic hyperplasia may occur as a rebound phenomenon secondary to thymic atrophy caused by chemotherapy for malignancy (testicular carcinoma, breast carcinoma, lymphoma, and other malignancies). In these cases, thymic enlargement typically occurs between 2 weeks and 14 months following chemotherapy. It has been postulated that it is caused by chemotherapy-induced gonadal atrophy and a resultant increase in luteinizing hormone secretion. True thymic hyperplasia is also reported after treatment of hypercortisolism (Cushing syndrome) and following conditions of severe stress including sepsis and burns.

Pathology

GROSS

- Lymphoid hyperplasia
  - Typically normal thymus, but thymic enlargement reported
  - Normal gross thymic architecture
- True thymic hyperplasia
  - Increased thymic size and weight (exceeding upper limits of normal)

MICROSCOPIC

- Lymphoid hyperplasia
  - Increased number of secondary lymphoid follicles with germinal centers in an otherwise normal thymus
- True thymic hyperplasia
  - Histologically normal thymus

Clinical Findings

Patients with lymphoid hyperplasia typically have a normal or mildly enlarged thymus gland and usually have no symptoms related to the thymus. These patients are usually adults and may present with symptoms related to the associated condition (e.g., myasthenia gravis, Graves disease). Patients with true thymic hyperplasia are typically children, adolescents, and young adults and are usually asymptomatic, but may present with dyspnea and/or dysphagia.

Imaging Features

RADIOGRAPHY

- Normal chest radiographs (in lymphoid hyperplasia)
- Focal or diffuse anterior mediastinal widening (in true hyperplasia)
  - Most commonly appreciated in children
  - May or may not be visible in adults

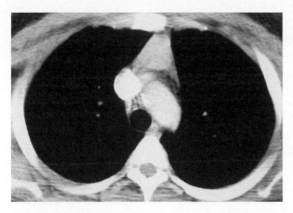

Figure 167C Contrast-enhanced chest CT (mediastinal window) of a 24-year-old woman with myasthenia gravis demonstrates prominent thymic soft tissue with normal morphology. Thymectomy revealed lymphoid hyperplasia.

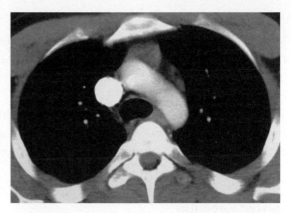

Figure 167D Contrast-enhanced chest CT (mediastinal window) in a young man status postsurgery and chemotherapy for testicular malignancy demonstrates a new soft tissue thymic nodule. Surgical excision revealed true thymic hyperplasia. (Courtesy of Diane C. Strollo, M.D., University of Pittsburgh Medical Center, Pittsburgh, Pennsylvania.)

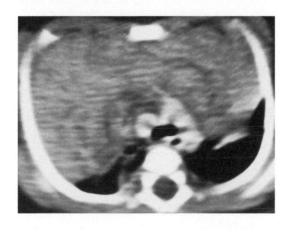

Figure 167E Contrast-enhanced chest CT (mediastinal window) of a 7-week-old girl with severe respiratory distress demonstrates massive thymic enlargement with resultant mass effect on the mediastinal vessels and the central airways. The resected thymus was histologically normal, and the diagnosis of true thymic hyperplasia was rendered.

CT

- Typically normal-appearing thymus (in lymphoid hyperplasia)
- Thymic enlargement based on measured thymic thickness (in true hyperplasia and occasionally in lymphoid hyperplasia) (**Figs. 167B, 167C, 167D,** and **167E**)

Treatment

- Recognition and observation in patients with appropriate history
- Thymectomy in selected patients with myasthenia gravis
- Excision in patients with symptomatic airway compression

Prognosis

- Relates to associated disease process in patients with lymphoid hyperplasia
- Excellent in true thymic hyperplasia, which may be a marker of improved survival in some patients with malignancy

PEARLS_____

- Thymic thickness refers to the short axis measurement of a thymic lobe; thymic width refers to the long axis measurement of a thymic lobe. The maximal normal thymic thickness in individuals under 20 years of age is 1.8 cm. The maximal normal thymic thickness in individuals over 20 years is 1.3 cm.
- Thymic hyperplasia represents a diagnostic dilemma in patients who have been treated for mediastinal lymphoma or other neoplasms, as residual or recurrent malignancy must be excluded. In these cases, biopsy is often recommended.

Suggested Readings

Budavari AI, Whitaker MD, Helmers RA. Thymic hyperplasia presenting as anterior mediastinal mass in 2 patients with Graves disease. Mayo Clin Proc 2002;77:495–499

Fraser RS, Müller NL, Colman N, Paré PD. Anterior mediastinal masses. In: Fraser RS, Müller NL, Colman N, Paré PD, eds. Fraser and Paré's Diagnosis of Diseases of the Chest, 4th ed. Philadelphia: Saunders, 1999:2851–2937

Hara M, McAdams HP, Vredenburgh JJ, Herndon JE, Patz EF Jr. Thymic hyperplasia after high-dose chemotherapy and autologous stem cell transplantation: incidence and significance in patients with breast cancer. AJR Am J Roentgenol 1999;173:1341–1344

Rosai J, Sobin LH. Histological Typing of Tumours of the Thymus: International Histological Classification of Tumours, 2nd ed. New York: Springer, 1999

Shimosato Y, Mukai K. Non-neoplastic conditions of the thymus. In: Rosai J, ed. Atlas of Tumor Pathology: Tumors of the Mediastinum, fascicle 21, series 3. Washington, DC: American Registry of Pathology and Armed Forces Institute of Pathology, 1997:23–31

CASE 168 Benign Germ Cell Neoplasms: Mature Teratoma

Clinical Presentation

A 74-year-old woman who presented with cough and chest pain

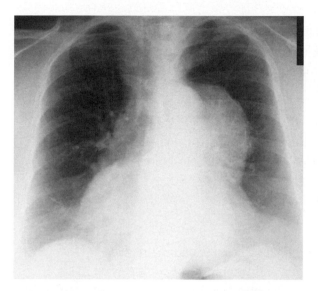

Figure 168A

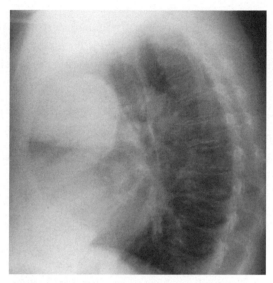

Figure 168B

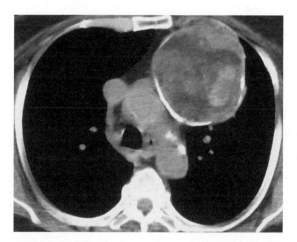

Figure 168C

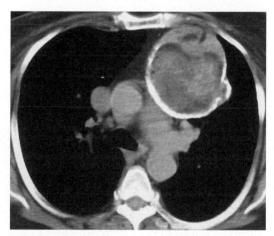

Figure 168D

Radiologic Findings

PA (**Fig. 168A**) and lateral (**Fig. 168B**) chest radiographs demonstrate a large left anterior mediastinal mass with a thin peripheral curvilinear calcification. Unenhanced chest CT (mediastinal window) (**Figs. 168C** and **168D**) demonstrates a heterogeneous spherical mass in the left lobe of the thymus. Note the peripheral curvilinear calcification and internal areas of soft tissue, fluid, and fat attenuation.

Diagnosis

Mature teratoma

Differential Diagnosis

None

Discussion

Background

Germ cell neoplasms typically occur in the gonad, but may also affect extragonadal sites, typically the anterior mediastinum (near or within the thymus). Mature teratoma is a benign neoplasm that accounts for approximately 70% of all primary mediastinal germ cell neoplasms.

Etiology

The etiology of germ cell neoplasms is poorly understood. It is theorized that extragonadal mature teratomas may arise from primitive germ cells that are "misplaced" along midline structures during their embryologic migration from the yolk sac to the gonad.

Clinical Findings

Patients with mature teratoma are typically children and young adults (usually under the age of 40 years). Patients may be asymptomatic or may present with signs and symptoms of compression of adjacent structures including chest pain, dyspnea, and cough, or because of symptoms related to tumor rupture.

Pathology

GROSS

- Encapsulated unilocular or multilocular cystic mass
- May contain well-differentiated structures (hair, teeth, bone)
- Cysts filled with brown lipid-rich fluid or grumous material

MICROSCOPIC

- Tissues derived from (often three) embryonic germ cell layers
  - Ectoderm: skin, dermal appendages
  - Mesoderm: bone, cartilage, adipose tissue
  - Endoderm: respiratory epithelium, gastrointestinal mucosa

Imaging Findings

RADIOGRAPHY

- Well-defined unilateral anterior mediastinal mass (**Figs. 168A** and **168B**)
- Calcification in 22% (**Figs. 168A** and **168B**)
- Mass effect with resultant consolidation and/or atelectasis
- Occasional pleural effusion (does not necessarily denote tumor rupture)

CT

- Well-defined heterogeneous anterior mediastinal mass (**Figs. 168C, 168D, 168E,** and **168F**)
- Multilocular cystic mass (85%); fluid attenuation (89%) (**Figs. 168C, 168D, 168E,** and **168F**)
- Fat attenuation (76%) (**Figs. 168C, 168D, 168E,** and **168F**); fat-fluid levels (11%)
- Calcification (53%) (**Figs. 168C, 168D,** and **168E**)

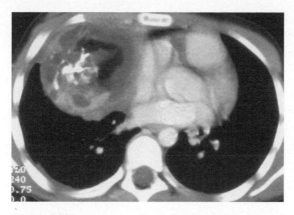

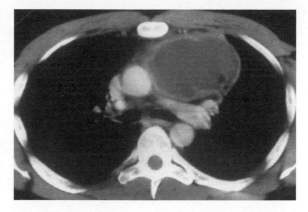

Figure 168E Contrast-enhanced chest CT (mediastinal window) of a 10-year-old girl with chest discomfort and a mediastinal mature teratoma demonstrates a spherical multilocular cystic anterior mediastinal mass with fluid, fat, soft tissue, and calcium attenuation. Note mass effect on the heart and the small ipsilateral pleural effusion.

Figure 168F Contrast-enhanced chest CT (mediastinal window) of a young man who presented with chest discomfort demonstrates a large left anterior mediastinal mature teratoma. The lesion is predominantly cystic, exhibits a thin soft tissue capsule, and contains a small focus of fat attenuation.

- Soft tissue elements (**Figs. 168C, 168D, 168E,** and **168F**)
  - Thin capsule and internal tissue septa
  - Rarely nodular soft tissue in capsule and septa
  - Increased conspicuity of soft tissue elements after intravenous contrast administration

MR

- Heterogeneous mediastinal mass
- High signal intensity content on T1-weighted images (corresponding to fat) and variable signal intensity on T2-weighted images; not diagnostic of fat, may be seen in hemorrhagic cysts
- Fat saturation MR imaging such as phase-shift gradient-echo imaging or proton-selective fat-saturation imaging for detection of fat and distinction from hemorrhage

Treatment

- Complete surgical excision

Prognosis

- Excellent in mature teratoma
- Excellent in immature teratoma of infancy and childhood
- Poor in immature teratoma of adulthood and in all teratomas with malignant elements

PEARLS

- Demonstration of fat attenuation within a well-circumscribed cystic mediastinal mass is virtually diagnostic of mature teratoma (**Fig. 168F**).
- While most mature teratomas exhibit fat, calcium, or both, approximately 15% do not. Thus, mature teratoma should be considered in the differential diagnosis of any multilocular cystic anterior mediastinal mass.
- Rupture of a mature teratoma may result in increased heterogeneity within the mass, adjacent consolidation and/or atelectasis, and a higher frequency of pleural and/or pericardial effusions.

- Immature teratoma consists of more than 10% of immature neuroectodermal and mesenchymal tissues. These neoplasms may be indistinguishable from mature teratoma on imaging studies or may manifest as predominantly solid masses. They often exhibit a highly aggressive behavior in affected adults.
- Malignant immature teratoma and teratoma with additional malignant components may represent malignant degeneration of a former immature or mature teratoma and may contain foci of carcinoma, sarcoma, or other malignant germ cell histologies. While these tumors may exhibit fat and/or calcium attenuation and may mimic mature teratoma on imaging studies, they often display a predominance of enhancing soft tissue elements, may show extensive areas of necrosis, and may exhibit indistinct margins, obliteration of tissue planes, or frank local invasion.

Suggested Readings

Choi S-J, Lee JS, Song KS, Lim T-H. Mediastinal teratoma: CT differentiation of ruptured and unruptured tumors. AJR Am J Roentgenol 1998;171:591–594

Jeung M-Y, Gasser B, Gangi A, et al. Imaging of cystic masses of the mediastinum. Radiographics 2002; 22:S79–S93

Moeller KH, Rosado-de-Christenson ML, Templeton PA. Mediastinal mature teratoma: imaging features. AJR Am J Roentgenol 1997;169:985–990

Shimosato Y, Mukai K. Tumors of the thymus and related lesions. In: Rosai J, ed. Atlas of Tumor Pathology: Tumors of the Mediastinum, fascicle 21, series 3. Washington, DC: American Registry of Pathology and Armed Forces Institute of Pathology, 1997:33–247

Strollo DC, Rosado-de-Christenson ML. Primary mediastinal malignant germ cell neoplasms: imaging features. Chest Surg Clin N Am 2002;12:645–658

Strollo DC, Rosado-de-Christenson ML. Tumors of the thymus. J Thorac Imaging 1999;14:152–171

CASE 169 Malignant Germ Cell Neoplasms

Clinical Presentation

A 35-year-old man with facial swelling and flushing

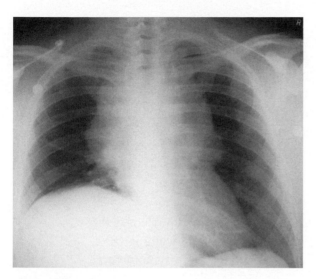

Figure 169A

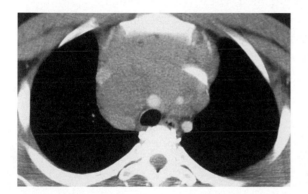

Figure 169B

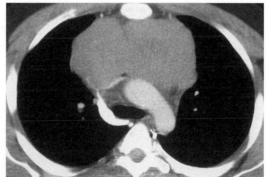

Figure 169C

Radiologic Findings

PA (**Fig. 169A**) chest radiograph demonstrates a large, lobular, well-defined anterior mediastinal mass that extends to both sides of the midline and is associated with elevation of the right hemidiaphragm. Contrast-enhanced chest CT (mediastinal window) (**Figs. 169B** and **169C**) demonstrates a bulky anterior mediastinal mass of homogeneous soft tissue attenuation and lobular borders. The mass encases the right brachiocephalic artery, the left common carotid artery, and the brachiocephalic veins (**Fig. 169B**) and invades the superior vena cava (**Fig. 169C**).

Diagnosis

Seminoma

Differential Diagnosis

- Lymphoma
- Thymoma, invasive

Discussion

Background

Seminoma is an uncommon neoplasm that represents approximately 40% of primary mediastinal malignant germ cell neoplasms of a single histology.

Nonseminomatous malignant germ cell neoplasms (GCNs) are aggressive neoplasms and include embryonal carcinoma, endodermal sinus (yolk sac) tumor, and choriocarcinoma. These lesions typically exhibit more than one germ cell histology and may contain foci of seminoma.

Clinical Findings

Seminoma affects men almost exclusively. These patients are usually in the third and fourth decades of life who typically present with symptoms related to mass effect or local invasion including chest pain, dyspnea, and superior vena cava syndrome. Up to 30% of affected patients are asymptomatic at presentation.

Nonseminomatous malignant GCNs affect almost exclusively young men. These patients usually present with symptoms of mediastinal compression and/or invasion, or with systemic complaints or symptoms related to metastatic disease. Patients may also present with precocious puberty or gynecomastia. Approximately 20% of patients have Klinefelter syndrome, may also develop a concurrent hematologic malignancy.

Pathology

GROSS

- Seminoma
  - Large, soft, well-circumscribed mass
  - Homogeneous cut surface
  - Uncommon central hemorrhage, necrosis, cystic change
- Nonseminomatous malignant GCN
  - Large, irregular often locally invasive mass
  - Heterogeneous cut surface with extensive hemorrhage and necrosis

MICROSCOPIC

- Seminoma
  - Sheets of large uniform polygonal cells
  - Distinct borders, clear or finely granular cytoplasm, central nuclei, infrequent mitoses
  - Loose stroma with dense lymphocytic infiltrate
- Nonseminomatous malignant GCN
  - Embryonal carcinoma: large cells disposed in sheets, tubules, and papillary structures with frequent mitoses
  - Endodermal sinus tumor: communicating spaces with epithelial lining
  - Choriocarcinoma: mononuclear cytotrophoblastic cells and giant multinucleated syncytiotrophoblastic cells with abundant hemorrhage

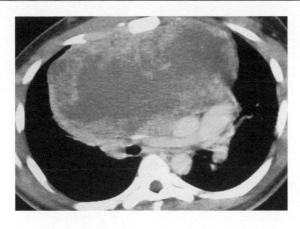

Figure 169D Contrast-enhanced chest CT (mediastinal window) of a 21-year-old man with chest pain, dyspnea, and a nonseminomatous malignant GCN demonstrates a bulky, heterogeneous anterior mediastinal mass with peripheral frond-like enhancing soft tissue, central irregular low attenuation, and marked mass effect on the adjacent structures.

Imaging Findings

RADIOGRAPHY

- Seminoma
  - Bulky, often well-defined anterior mediastinal mass (**Fig. 169A**)
  - Extends to both sides of midline (**Fig. 169A**)
  - Mass effect
- Nonseminomatous malignant GCN
  - Large, bulky anterior mediastinal mass
  - Extends to both sides of midline
  - Well- or ill-defined margins
  - Mass effect
  - Frequent associated pleural effusion

CT

- Seminoma
  - Large, homogeneous soft tissue mass (**Figs. 169B** and **169C**)
  - Rarely (8%) central necrosis or cystic change
  - Local invasion (**Fig. 169C**)
  - Lymphadenopathy
- Nonseminomatous malignant GCN
  - Large, locally invasive, heterogeneous soft tissue mass (**Fig. 169D**)
  - Contrast-enhanced studies: central low attenuation (corresponding to necrosis) and peripheral frond-like nodular enhancement (**Fig. 169D**)
  - Obliteration of adjacent tissue planes or frank local invasion (mediastinum, lung, chest wall) (**Fig. 169D**)
  - Pleural and/or pericardial effusion
  - Lymphadenopathy

Treatment

- Seminoma
  - Radiation therapy
  - Chemotherapy
- Nonseminomatous malignant GCN
  - Chemotherapy
  - Surgical excision of residual necrotic or viable tumor

Prognosis

- Seminoma
  - 60 to 80% 5-year survival
- Nonseminomatous malignant GCN
  - Poor; documented cases of long-term survival

PEARLS_____

- Evaluation of serologic markers (alpha-fetoprotein, β subunit of human chorionic gonadotropin) is useful in the diagnosis of mediastinal malignant GCN and may suggest the histologic types represented.
- The diagnosis of malignant mediastinal GCN often prompts testicular evaluation to exclude a primary malignancy. However, most testicular GCNs metastatic to the mediastinum exhibit intervening retroperitoneal lymph node metastases.

Suggested Readings

Shimosato Y, Mukai K. Tumors of the thymus and related lesions. In: Rosai J, ed. Atlas of Tumor Pathology: Tumors of the Mediastinum, fascicle 21, series 3. Washington, DC: American Registry of Pathology and Armed Forces Institute of Pathology, 1997:33–247

Strollo DC, Rosado-de-Christenson ML. Primary mediastinal malignant germ cell neoplasms: imaging features. Chest Surg Clin N Am 2002;12:645–658

Strollo DC, Rosado-de-Christenson ML. Tumors of the thymus. J Thorac Imaging 1999;14:152–171

CASE 170 Neoplastic Lymphadenopathy: Lymphoma

Clinical Presentation

A 38-year-old man with chest discomfort

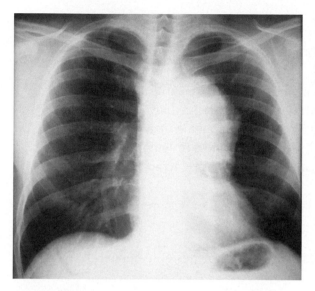

Figure 170A

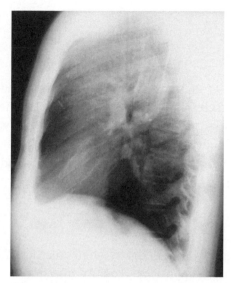

Figure 170B

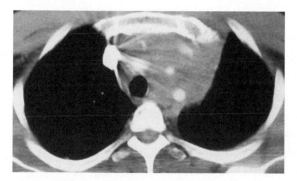

Figure 170C

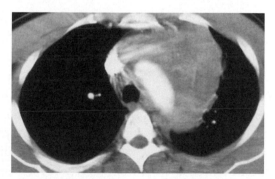

Figure 170D

Radiologic Findings

PA (**Fig. 170A**) and lateral (**Fig. 170B**) chest radiographs demonstrate a large lobular left anterior mediastinal mass. The mass exhibits linear and punctate calcifications seen best on the lateral radiograph (**Fig. 170B**). Contrast-enhanced chest CT (mediastinal window) (**Figs. 170C** and **170D**) demonstrates a large mediastinal soft tissue mass of irregular borders that occupies the anterior, middle, and posterior compartments, produces mass effect, and encases the mediastinal great vessels.

Diagnosis

Hodgkin lymphoma

Differential Diagnosis

- Non-Hodgkin lymphoma
- Metastatic mediastinal lymphadenopathy: lung cancer, extrathoracic malignancy
- Thymoma, invasive
- Thymic malignancy

Discussion

Background

Non-Hodgkin lymphoma is the most frequent lymphoma and accounts for up to 75% of all cases. Hodgkin lymphoma represents approximately 25% of lymphomas. However, mediastinal involvement from systemic lymphoma is much more common in patients with Hodgkin lymphoma than in those with non-Hodgkin lymphoma. The most common cell type of mediastinal Hodgkin lymphoma is nodular sclerosis. The most common mediastinal non-Hodgkin lymphomas are lymphoblastic lymphoma, and diffuse large B-cell lymphoma.

Etiology

The etiologies of Hodgkin and non-Hodgkin lymphomas are unknown. Some subtypes of lymphoma are associated with immunosuppression and HIV infection.

Clinical Findings

Hodgkin lymphoma affects men and women in a bimodal age distribution, with peak incidences in adolescence and young adulthood and a smaller incidence peak after the fifth decade of life. Many patients present because of palpable enlarged peripheral lymph nodes, typically in the neck. Chest pain and systemic complaints occur in approximately one third of affected individuals.

Non-Hodgkin lymphoma affects both sexes and all ages. Most patients have advanced systemic lymphoma at the time of presentation and are typically symptomatic because of constitutional complaints, palpable lymphadenopathy, and/or extranodal disease. Lymphoblastic lymphoma (precursor T-lymphoblastic lymphoma) typically affects boys (male children and adolescents). Diffuse large B-cell lymphoma [primary mediastinal (thymic) large B-cell lymphoma] typically affects young adults, with a slight female predominance. Both groups of patients often present with thoracic complaints related to compression and/or invasion of mediastinal structures.

Pathology

Lymphomas represent a diverse and heterogeneous group of neoplasms. Multiple pathologic classifications are currently in use. A comprehensive discussion of the pathologic classification of lymphoma is beyond the scope of this book. The terms listed below are generally derived from terminology shared by the Working Formulation, the Kiel classification, and the Revised European-American Lymphoma (REAL) classification.

GROSS

- Hodgkin lymphoma (nodular sclerosis)
  - Distinct tumor nodules separated by interconnecting white tissue bands
  - Thymic enlargement with or without cystic change

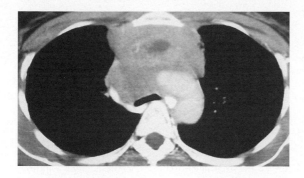

Figure 170E Contrast-enhanced chest CT (mediastinal window) of a young woman with Hodgkin lymphoma who presented with superior vena cava syndrome demonstrates a large heterogeneous prevascular soft tissue mass that obstructs the superior vena cava and produces mass effect on the airways and the mediastinal great vessels. The central area of low attenuation may represent necrosis or cystic change. Note marked enhancement of the azygos and hemiazygos veins.

- Multifocal enlarged lymph nodes
- Coalescent soft tissue mass with or without local invasion
- Non-Hodgkin lymphoma
  - Large infiltrative and locally invasive mediastinal mass; necrosis

MICROSCOPIC

- Hodgkin lymphoma (nodular sclerosis)
  - Cellular nodules surrounded by bands of interconnecting collagenous connective tissue
  - Polymorphic cells, lymphocytes, plasma cells, eosinophils
  - Diagnostic or lacunar Reed-Sternberg cells
- Non-Hodgkin lymphoma
  - Lymphoblastic lymphoma (precursor T-lymphoblastic lymphoma): lymphoblasts with round or convoluted nuclei and scant cytoplasm; infiltrative growth
  - Diffuse large B-cell lymphoma [primary mediastinal (thymic) large B-cell lymphoma]: large cells with vesicular nuclei, prominent nucleoli, basophilic cytoplasm, and numerous mitoses

Imaging Findings

RADIOGRAPHY

- Hodgkin lymphoma
  - Intrathoracic involvement in 75% of cases
  - Anterior mediastinal enlargement with "filling" of the retrosternal space on lateral chest radiography (**Figs. 170A** and **170B**)
  - Lobular contours, frequent growth to both sides of the midline, mass effect (**Fig. 170A**)
- Non-Hodgkin lymphoma
  - Intrathoracic involvement in less than half of cases
  - Anterior and middle mediastinal lymph node enlargement

CT

- Hodgkin lymphoma
  - Intrathoracic involvement in up to 85% of patients
  - Lymphadenopathy affecting contiguous prevascular, paratracheal, and other intrathoracic lymph nodes (**Figs. 170C, 170D,** and **170E**)
  - Nodal coalescence, homogeneous anterior mediastinal soft tissue mass (**Figs. 170C** and **170D**)
  - Heterogeneity; cystic change, necrosis (**Fig. 170E**)

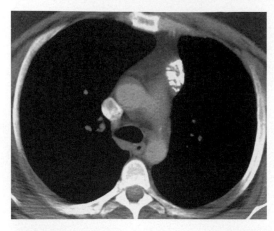

Figure 170F Contrast-enhanced chest CT (mediastinal window) of a 31-year-old woman 4 years following successful treatment of Hodgkin lymphoma demonstrates dense calcification in the left anterior mediastinum, in an area of prior involvement by lymphoma.

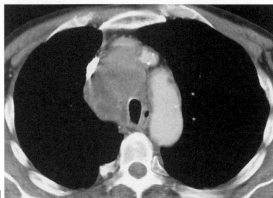

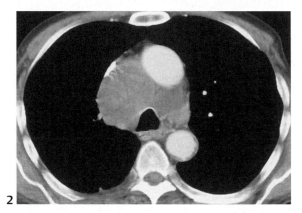

Figure 170G (1,2) Contrast-enhanced chest CT (mediastinal window) of a 71-year-old man with weight loss, superior vena cava syndrome, and non-Hodgkin lymphoma demonstrates pretracheal and aorticopulmonary window lymphadenopathy.

- Local invasion of cardiovascular structures, pleura, lung, and/or chest wall (**Fig. 170E**)
- Calcification rare; usually occurs 1 year after therapy, affects less than 1% of patients (**Fig. 170F**)
- Non-Hodgkin lymphoma
  - Findings indistinguishable from those of Hodgkin lymphoma (**Fig. 170G**)
  - Isolated involvement of mediastinal lymph nodes other than prevascular and paratracheal

MR

- Increased signal intensity on T2-weighted images in active disease
- Low signal intensity on T1- and T2-weighted images in residual fibrous tissue after successful therapy
- High signal on T2-weighted images in inflammatory and cystic tissue following therapy

Treatment

- Hodgkin lymphoma
  - Radiation therapy
  - Chemotherapy
  - Chemotherapy followed by radiation therapy in bulky (i.e., mediastinal mass width more than 33% of the maximum chest diameter or a 10 cm mass) mediastinal disease
- Non-Hodgkin lymphoma
  - Radiation therapy and/or chemotherapy
  - Palliative treatment for indolent lymphoma

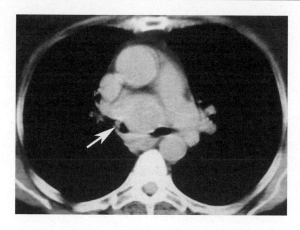

Figure 170H Unenhanced chest CT (mediastinal window) of a 64-year-old woman with hemoptysis and metastatic renal cell carcinoma demonstrates pretracheal and subcarinal lymphadenopathy. Note the small well-defined endoluminal nodule (arrow) in the right mainstem bronchus, which represents an endobronchial metastasis.

Prognosis

- Hodgkin lymphoma
  - Over 90% cure rates achieved in early-stage disease
  - Up to 60% cure rates in advanced disease; cure achievable in recurrent disease
- Non-Hodgkin lymphoma
  - Poor prognosis in aggressive non-Hodgkin lymphoma, but greater potential for cure than in indolent lymphoma

PEARLS_____

- Most patients with Hodgkin lymphoma present with palpable peripheral lymphadenopathy. In these cases, the diagnosis is established by lymph node biopsy prior to thoracic imaging. However, up to 10% of affected patients have primary mediastinal Hodgkin lymphoma without superficial lymph node involvement and present with a mediastinal mass.
- Mediastinal lymphoma with nodal coalescence may be indistinguishable from other malignant and locally invasive anterior mediastinal masses. Lymphoma must be considered in the differential diagnosis, particularly when there is imaging evidence of adjacent lymphadenopathy or involvement of multiple lymph node groups (**Figs. 170C, 170D, 170E,** and **170G**).
- Lymphoma is not a surgical lesion. If lymphoma is suspected, biopsy should be recommended for definitive diagnosis.
- Thoracic Hodgkin lymphoma may recur in the originally affected mediastinum, other mediastinal compartments, or in the lung.
- Mediastinal lymphoma may manifest with locally invasive disease and superior vena cava syndrome (**Figs. 170E** and **170G**).
- Advanced lung cancer with mediastinal metastases may manifest as a locally invasive dominant mediastinal mass, particularly in cases of small cell carcinoma (see Case 75).
- Extrapulmonary malignancies (particularly renal cell, testicular, and head and neck carcinomas) may metastasize to intrathoracic lymph nodes (without concomitant pulmonary metastases) and may manifest as dominant mediastinal abnormalities that mimic lymphoma and metastatic lung cancer (**Fig. 170H**).

Suggested Readings

Harris NL, Jaffe ES, Stein H, et al. A revised European-American classification of lymphoid neoplasms: a proposal from the international lymphoma study group. Blood 1994;84:1361–1392

Fraser RS, Müller NL, Colman N, Paré PD. Anterior mediastinal masses. In: Fraser RS, Müller NL, Colman N, Paré PD, eds. Fraser and Paré's Diagnosis of Diseases of the Chest, 4th ed. Philadelphia: Saunders, 1999:2875–2937

Fraser RS, Müller NL, Colman N, Paré PD. Lymphoproliferative disorders and leukemia. In: Fraser RS, Müller NL, Colman N, Paré PD, eds. Fraser and Paré's Diagnosis of Diseases of the Chest, 4th ed. Philadelphia: Saunders, 1999:1269–1330

Shimosato Y, Mukai K. Tumors of the thymus and related lesions. In: Rosai J, ed. Atlas of Tumor Pathology: Tumors of the Mediastinum, fascicle 21, series 3. Washington, DC: American Registry of Pathology and Armed Forces Institute of Pathology, 1997:33–247

Strollo DC, Rosado de Christenson ML. Tumors of the thymus. J Thorac Imaging 1999;14:152–171

CASE 171 Nonneoplastic Lymphadenopathy: Mediastinal Fibrosis

Clinical Presentation

A middle-aged man with superior vena cava syndrome

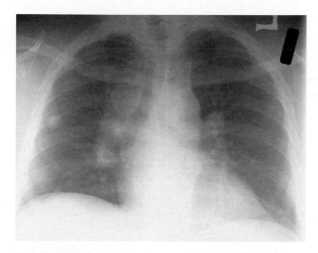

Figure 171A

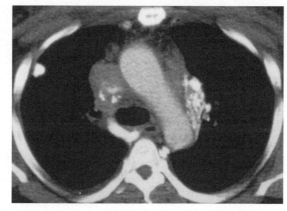

Figure 171B

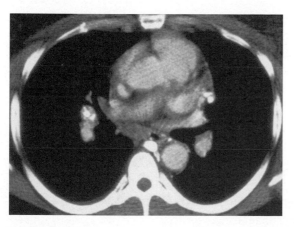

Figure 171C

(Figs. 171A, 171B, and 171C from Rossi SE, McAdams HP, Rosado-de-Christenson ML, Franks TJ, Galvin JR. Fibrosing mediastinitis. Radiographics 2001;21:737–757, with permission.)

Radiologic Findings

PA chest radiograph (**Fig. 171A**) demonstrates a well-defined lobular right paratracheal soft tissue mass, multifocal mediastinal calcifications, and a densely calcified right upper lobe solitary pulmonary nodule. Contrast-enhanced chest CT (mediastinal window) (**Figs. 171B** and **171C**) demonstrates a right paratracheal soft tissue mass with multifocal internal calcifications, which obliterates the lumen of the superior vena cava and prominent mediastinal collateral vessels (**Fig. 171B**). Note intense contrast enhancement of the azygos system, the calcified solitary pulmonary nodule (**Fig. 171B**), and the right hilar lymph node calcifications (**Fig. 171C**).

Diagnosis

Mediastinal fibrosis

Differential Diagnosis

- Lung cancer
- Lymphoma
- Metastatic mediastinal lymphadenopathy
- Other nonneoplastic lymphadenopathies: mycobacterial infection (see Cases 60 and 61), fungal disease (see Cases 62, 63, and 64), sarcoidosis (see Case 127), silicosis (see Case 135)

Discussion

Background

Mediastinal fibrosis represents the proliferation of dense fibrous tissue in the mediastinum with resultant focal or infiltrative masses, that may be locally invasive.

Etiology

Mediastinal fibrosis may be associated with granulomatous infection, typically with *Histoplasma capsulatum* (and rarely with other fungi and *Mycobacterium tuberculosis*). Mediastinal fibrosis also occurs as an idiopathic condition, which may be related to other fibroinflammatory disorders such as retroperitoneal fibrosis.

Clinical Findings

Mediastinal fibrosis typically affects young patients, but it is reported in all age groups. Patients present with signs and symptoms of obstruction of vital mediastinal structures, including the trachea, main bronchi, esophagus, systemic veins, and pulmonary arteries and veins. Symptoms include cough, dyspnea, recurrent infection, hemoptysis, chest pain, and dysphagia.

Pathology

GROSS

- Localized or infiltrative white dense mediastinal soft tissue mass

MICROSCOPIC

- Paucicellular fibrous tissue with infiltration and obliteration of normal adipose tissue
- Mononuclear cell infiltrates
- Diagnosis of exclusion; rule out granulomatous infection and malignant neoplasia

Imaging Findings

RADIOGRAPHY

- Nonspecific mediastinal widening often affecting the middle compartment (**Fig. 171A**)
- Associated pulmonary granulomas and/or mediastinal lymph node calcifications (**Fig. 171A**)

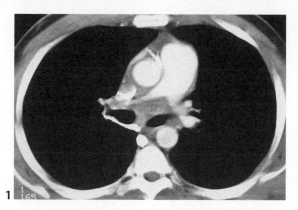 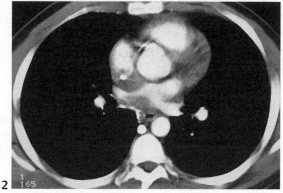

Figure 171D (1,2) Contrast-enhanced chest CT (mediastinal window) of a 30-year-old man with mediastinal fibrosis who presented with superior vena cava syndrome demonstrates soft tissue infiltration of the mediastinum that encases and partially obstructs the superior vena cava **(1)**, the right main pulmonary artery **(1)**, and the right superior pulmonary vein **(2)**.

CT

- Localized or diffuse, locally invasive soft tissue mass (**Figs. 171B, 171C,** and **171D**)
- May demonstrate calcification (**Figs. 171B, 171C,** and **171D**)
- Evaluation of location and extent of involvement; exclusion of vascular, airway, or esophageal involvement (**Figs. 171B** and **171D**)
- Indirect findings:
  - Enhanced vascular collaterals, enlargement of uninvolved vessels (**Figs. 171B** and **171C**)
  - Abnormal lung attenuation: wedge-shaped opacities representing infarcts, ground-glass opacities, thickening of interlobular septa, postobstructive pneumonia, and/or atelectasis related to arterial, venous, or bronchial obstruction

MR

- Heterogeneous infiltrative mass of intermediate signal intensity on T1-weighted images
- May demonstrate areas of high and very low signal intensity on both T1- and T2-weighted images
- Low signal intensity foci on T2-weighed images corresponding to calcification or fibrosis

Treatment

- Systemic antifungal agents with reported cases of disease stabilization
- Surgical excision of localized disease; may require vascular and/or airway reconstruction
- Laser therapy, balloon dilatation, and stenting of obstructed vessels and bronchi
- Venous bypass grafts for vena cava occlusion

Prognosis

- Mortality of up to 30%; recurrent infection, hemoptysis, cor pulmonale

PEARLS_____

- Locally invasive mediastinal soft tissue with associated calcification in a young patient from an area of endemic histoplasmosis (see Case 62) suggests the diagnosis of mediastinal fibrosis. In the absence of calcification, malignant neoplasia must be considered, and biopsy is indicated.

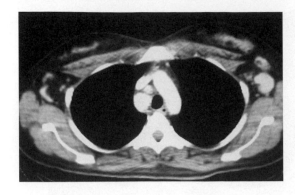

Figure 171E Contrast-enhanced chest CT (mediastinal window) of an asymptomatic 35-year-old man with localized Castleman disease demonstrates enlarged enhancing right paratracheal and left axillary lymph nodes.

- Castleman disease (angiofollicular or giant lymph node hyperplasia) is a form of lymphadenopathy that represents a diverse group of lymphoproliferative disorders classified as hyaline vascular (over 90%) and plasma cell variants, localized and disseminated forms. Localized Castleman disease typically affects the middle mediastinum and hila of women who may be asymptomatic or present with symptoms of compression or local invasion. Imaging may demonstrate a solitary well-defined mass (**Fig. 171E**) without associated lymphadenopathy, a dominant mass with associated lymphadenopathy, or multiple enlarged lymph nodes confined to one mediastinal compartment. Contrast enhancement is demonstrated in virtually all cases (**Fig. 171E**) and calcification in up to 10%.

Suggested Readings

Atasoy C, Fitoz S, Erguvan B, Akyar S. Tuberculous fibrosing mediastinitis: CT and MRI findings. J Thorac Imaging 2001;16:191–193

McAdams HP, Rosado de Christenson ML, Fishback NF, Templeton PA. Castleman disease of the thorax: radiologic features with clinical and histopathologic correlation. Radiology 1998;209:221–228

Rossi SE, McAdams HP, Rosado-de-Christenson ML, Franks TJ, Galvin JR. Fibrosing mediastinitis. Radiographics 2001;21:737–757

CASE 172 Congenital Cysts: Bronchogenic Cyst

Clinical Presentation

A 25-year-old woman with cough

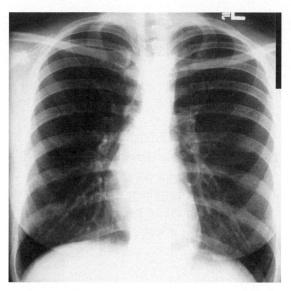

Figure 172A

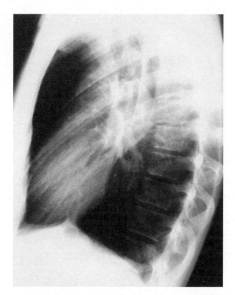

Figure 172B

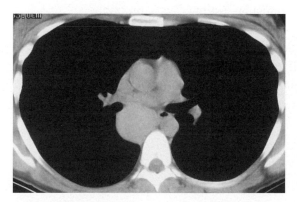

Figure 172C

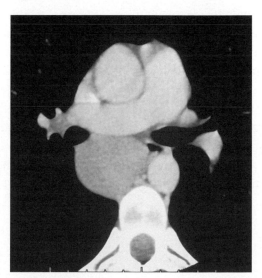

Figure 172D

Radiologic Findings

PA (**Fig. 172A**) and lateral (**Fig. 172B**) chest radiographs demonstrate a well-defined middle mediastinal (subcarinal) mass that projects to the right of the midline and produces mass effect on the bronchus intermedius. Unenhanced (**Fig. 172C**) and contrast-enhanced chest CT (**Fig. 172D**) (mediastinal window) demonstrate a spherical nonenhancing homogeneous subcarinal mass of soft tissue attenuation.

663

Diagnosis

Bronchogenic cyst

Differential Diagnosis

- Other foregut cysts; esophageal, gastroenteric
- Pericardial cyst
- Lymphadenopathy

Discussion

Background

Congenital cysts represent approximately 20% of mediastinal masses affecting adults. Bronchogenic cyst is the most common congenital mediastinal cyst and is typically located in the middle compartment near the carina, but may also affect other mediastinal compartments, the pericardium, diaphragm, pleura, and the lung. Other foregut-derived congenital cysts include esophageal and gastroenteric cysts, that occur in the wall of the esophagus and posterior mediastinum, respectively. Pericardial cysts are typically located in the cardiophrenic angle. Thymic cysts usually affect the anterior mediastinum and often represent acquired lesions.

Etiology

Bronchogenic cyst is thought to result from abnormal budding of the primitive foregut or the developing tracheobronchial tree. The original connection to the foregut is usually obliterated, resulting in a blind-ending, fluid-filled, thin-walled cyst. Esophageal cysts may also derive from the primitive foregut as a result of anomalous esophageal development. Pericardial cysts are thought to result from disordered formation of the primitive coelomic cavities. While unilocular thymic cysts probably represent congenital anomalies related to the fetal thymopharyngeal duct, multilocular thymic cysts are generally considered acquired lesions related to trauma (including thoracotomy), thymic neoplasia, and radiation therapy for lymphoma. Multilocular thymic cysts affect approximately 1% of children with HIV infection in association with the diffuse infiltrative lymphocytosis syndrome. They are also described in other immune-mediated disorders such as Sjögren syndrome, aplastic anemia, and myasthenia gravis.

Pathology

GROSS

- Bronchogenic cyst
  - Spherical, unilocular, thin-walled cyst; smooth external and/or trabeculated internal surfaces
  - Variable fluid content ranging from white and translucent to brown and hemorrhagic and from thin to gelatinous consistency
  - Frequent fibrous connection to adjacent foregut-derived structures (esophagus)
- Esophageal cyst
  - Spherical, unilocular cyst; within esophageal wall

- Pericardial cyst
  - Spherical or ovoid cyst; translucent thin wall
  - Watery, clear, or straw-colored fluid content
- Thymic cyst
  - Spherical, ovoid, or tubular (with neck extension), unilocular or multilocular thin-walled cyst
  - Watery, clear, or straw-colored or brown (hemorrhage) fluid content

MICROSCOPIC

- Bronchogenic cyst
  - Cartilage, mucus glands, and smooth muscle in wall
  - Lined by pseudostratified columnar ciliated (respiratory) epithelium
- Esophageal cyst
  - Lamina propria, esophageal glands, and muscularis propria in wall
  - Lined by squamous or ciliated columnar epithelium; may contain ectopic gastric mucosa
- Pericardial cyst
  - Connective tissue wall
  - Lined by single layer of flat-to-cuboidal mesothelial cells
- Thymic cyst
  - Identification of thymic tissue within cyst wall required for diagnosis
  - Variable epithelial lining

Clinical Findings

Patients with bronchogenic cyst are typically young children and adults under the age of 40 years. Many are symptomatic and present because of chest pain and/or respiratory complaints related to mass effect on the airways. Patients with esophageal cysts are often asymptomatic adults and children, but some present with symptoms of esophageal and/or mediastinal mass effect or with local pain related to ectopic gastric mucosa in the cyst. Patients with pericardial cysts are invariably asymptomatic and are diagnosed incidentally. Patients with thymic cysts are often asymptomatic children and young adults.

Imaging Findings

RADIOGRAPHY

- Bronchogenic cyst
  - Well-defined spherical or ovoid middle mediastinal mass (subcarinal, paratracheal) (**Figs. 172A** and **172B**)
  - May attain large sizes and produce mass effect on adjacent structures (**Fig. 172A**)
- Esophageal cyst
  - Spherical or ovoid middle or posterior mediastinal mass
- Pericardial cyst
  - Spherical or ovoid cardiophrenic angle mass; right sided in 75% of cases
- Thymic cyst
  - Well-defined, unilateral anterior mediastinal mass

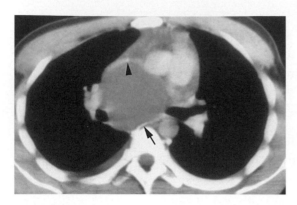

Figure 172E Contrast-enhanced chest CT (mediastinal window) of a young man with a bronchogenic cyst demonstrates a large subcarinal mass of water attenuation with a thin peripheral enhancing wall (arrow) and punctate mural calcification (arrowhead). Note the small right pleural effusion.

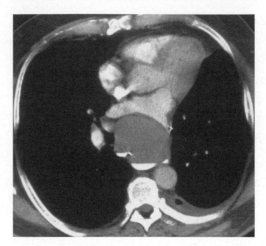

Figure 172F Contrast-enhanced chest CT (mediastinal window) of a 60-year-old man with cough, dyspnea on exertion, and a bronchogenic cyst shows a subcarinal cyst of lobular contours with internal fluid–milk of calcium levels and mass effect on the contrast-filled esophagus and the left atrium. Note left pleural thickening or fluid.

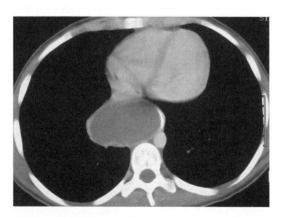

Figure 172G Contrast-enhanced chest CT (mediastinal window) of a 14-year-old girl with dysphagia and an esophageal cyst demonstrates a large ovoid cyst with water attenuation contents. Note the enhancing thin wall, thin peripheral soft tissue septa, and the elongate contour of the contrast-filled esophageal lumen consistent with the mural location of the cyst.

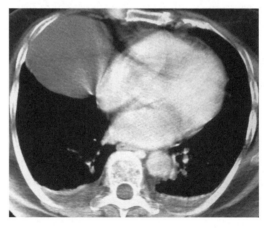

Figure 172H Contrast-enhanced chest CT (mediastinal window) of an 82-year-old woman with heart failure and an incidentally discovered pericardial cyst demonstrates a large spherical cardiophrenic angle mass of water attenuation. Note absence of enhancement, imperceptible cyst wall, and bilateral pleural effusions.

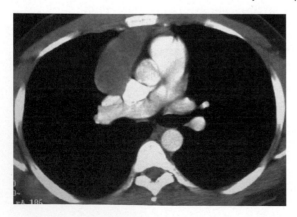

Figure 172I Contrast-enhanced chest CT (mediastinal window) of an asymptomatic 23-year-old man with a thymic cyst demonstrates a multilocular cystic right anterior mediastinal mass in the anatomic location of the thymus. Note the thin internal enhancing soft tissue septa.

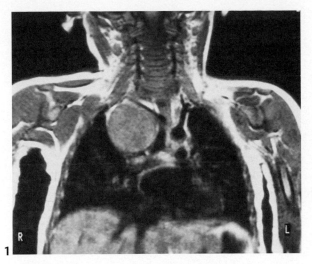
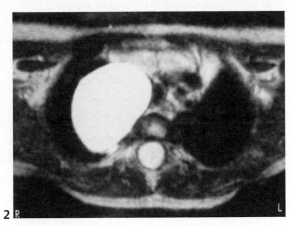

Figure 172J (1,2) Coronal T1-weighted MR **(1)** and axial T2-weighted MR **(2)** images of a 2-year-old boy with cough and a bronchogenic cyst demonstrate a spherical right middle mediastinal mass of intermediate signal intensity on the T1-weighted image **(1).** The lesion exhibits a thin, low signal intensity peripheral wall and high signal intensity contents (isointense with the adjacent cerebrospinal fluid) on the T2-weighted image **(2).**

CT

- Bronchogenic cyst
  - Well-defined spherical middle mediastinal mass (subcarinal, paratracheal) (**Figs. 172C, 172D, 172E,** and **172F**); may affect other mediastinal compartments, lung, diaphragm
  - Homogeneous internal attenuation: soft tissue (43%) (**Figs. 172C** and **172D**), water (40%) (**Figs. 172E** and **172F**); no internal enhancement (**Figs. 172C, 172D, 172E,** and **172F**)
  - Thin, smooth wall best seen on contrast-enhanced studies or because of punctate, discontinuous mural calcification (**Fig. 172E**)
  - Rarely: fluid-fluid levels, milk of calcium (**Fig. 172F**)
- Esophageal cyst
  - Relationship to esophagus and/or esophageal wall (**Fig. 172G**)
  - Otherwise indistinguishable from bronchogenic cyst
- Pericardial cyst
  - Smooth, spherical or ovoid water attenuation mass at cardiophrenic angle (**Fig. 172H**)
  - Imperceptible nonenhancing wall (**Fig. 172H**)
- Thymic cyst
  - Variable size, unilocular or multilocular cystic mass with water attenuation contents (**Fig. 172I**)
  - Thin-walled, internal soft tissue septa (**Fig. 172I**), soft tissue components, mural and/or septal calcifications

MR

- Intermediate-to-high signal intensity on T1-weighted images (**Fig. 172J1**)
- Markedly increased signal intensity on T2-weighted images (**Fig. 172J2**)
- Isointensity with cerebrospinal fluid (**Fig. 172J2**)
- Hemorrhage or infection: high signal on both T1- and T2-weighted images
- Visualization of thin wall (**Fig. 172J**) and internal soft tissue septa

SCINTIGRAPHY

- Uptake of technetium-99m (Tc-99m) sodium pertechnetate in ectopic gastric mucosa within esophageal cysts

Therapy

- Bronchogenic and esophageal cysts
  - Excision
  - Aspiration, instillation of sclerosing agents, marsupialization
  - Observation of patients who are not surgical candidates
- Pericardial cysts
  - Observation
- Thymic cysts
  - Excision for exclusion of cystic neoplasia
  - Observation in selected asymptomatic patients

Prognosis

- Excellent
- Fluid reaccumulation in aspirated cysts; recurrence of symptoms

PEARLS_____

- The diagnosis of bronchogenic cyst should be suggested based on location, morphology, and absence of internal enhancement, as attenuation and signal intensity may vary. Visualization of a thin peripheral wall (best seen after intravenous contrast administration) and/or fluid–fluid levels strongly supports the diagnosis. MR is helpful in the evaluation of high attenuation bronchogenic cysts through demonstration of isointensity to cerebrospinal fluid. Bronchogenic cyst is indistinguishable from other foregut cysts; differentiation requires histologic evaluation of the cyst wall.
- Thymic cysts are rare anterior mediastinal masses (**Fig. 172I**). Thus, cystic neoplasia should always be excluded, particularly in the presence of mural nodules or lymphadenopathy.
- Neuroenteric cysts are rare congenital foregut cysts characterized by their fibrous connection to the vertebrae. They are typically diagnosed in symptomatic infants and manifest as spherical paravertebral soft tissue masses associated with spinal dysraphism, butterfly or hemivertebrae, and/or scoliosis.

Suggested Readings

Choi YW, McAdams HP, Jeon SC, et al. Idiopathic multilocular thymic cyst: CT features with clinical and histopathologic correlation. AJR Am J Roentgenol 2001;177:881–885

Fraser RS, Müller NL, Colman N, Paré PD. Masses situated predominantly in the middle-posterior mediastinal compartment. In: Fraser RS, Müller NL, Colman N, Paré PD, eds. Fraser and Paré's Diagnosis of Diseases of the Chest, 4th ed. Philadelphia: Saunders, 1999:2938–2973

Jeung M-Y, Gasser B, Gangi A, et al. Imaging of cystic masses of the mediastinum. Radiographics 2002; 22:S79–S93

McAdams HP, Kirejczyk WM, Rosado-de-Christenson ML, Matsumoto S. Bronchogenic cyst: imaging features with clinical and histopathologic correlation. Radiology 2000;217:441–446

Shimosato Y, Mukai K. Tumors of the mediastinum excluding the thymus, heart and great vessels. In: Shimosato Y, Mukai K, eds. Atlas of Tumor Pathology: Tumors of the Mediastinum, fascicle 21, series 3. Washington, DC: Armed Forces Institute of Pathology, 1997:249–273

CASE 173 Neurogenic Neoplasms

Clinical Presentation

A 40-year-old woman with chest discomfort

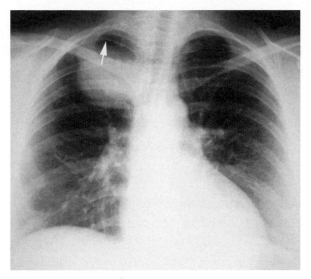

Figure 173A

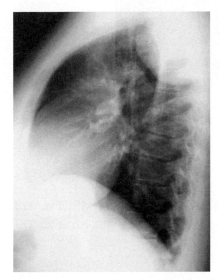

Figure 173B

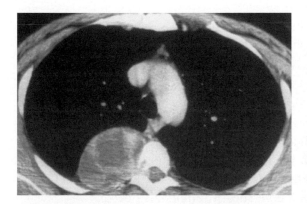

Figure 173C

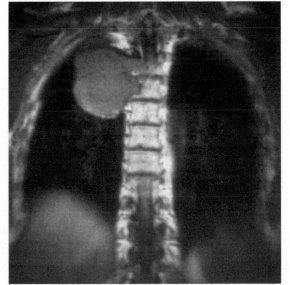

Figure 173D

Radiologic Findings

PA (**Fig. 173A**) and lateral (**Fig. 173B**) chest radiographs demonstrate a well-defined lobular mediastinal soft tissue mass situated predominantly in the right paravertebral region and extending into the middle mediastinum (**Fig. 173B**). Note the associated displacement, pressure erosion, and sclerosis of the adjacent right posterior third rib (arrow) (**Fig. 173A**). Contrast-enhanced chest CT (mediastinal window) (**Fig. 173C**) demonstrates a heterogeneously enhancing soft tissue mass, which extends through the neuroforamen into the spinal canal. Unenhanced coronal T1-weighted (**Fig. 173D**)

669

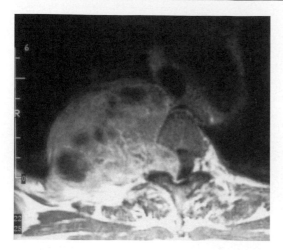

Figure 173E

and gadolinium-enhanced axial T1-weighted MR (**Fig. 173E**) images demonstrate heterogeneous enhancement of the mass and intraspinal growth (**Fig. 173E**) through at least two neuroforamina (**Fig. 173D**).

Diagnosis

Schwannoma

Differential Diagnosis

- Other neurogenic neoplasms: neurofibroma, ganglioneuroma
- Thoracic meningocele
- Extramedullary hematopoiesis

Discussion

Background

Neurogenic neoplasms represent approximately 20% of mediastinal masses in adults and approximately 35% in children. They are the most common neoplasms of the paravertebral region but may arise in other locations. Neoplasms of peripheral nerve origin are typically benign (schwannoma, neurofibroma, plexiform neurofibroma), but malignant peripheral nerve sheath tumors also occur. Schwannoma is the most frequent neurogenic neoplasm followed by neurofibroma. Neoplasms that arise from sympathetic (or parasympathetic) ganglia may be benign (ganglioneuroma) or malignant (ganglioneuroblastoma, neuroblastoma). Malignant sympathetic neurogenic neoplasms typically affect symptomatic neonates and infants, carry a poor prognosis, and will not be discussed further.

Etiology

The etiology of neurogenic neoplasms is unknown, and most lesions arise spontaneously. Neurofibromatosis type I is associated with multifocal neurogenic neoplasms and a high risk of malignant transformation.

Clinical Findings

The majority of patients with benign neurogenic neoplasms are asymptomatic. Large lesions may produce symptoms related to mass effect: cough, pain, dyspnea, and/or hoarseness. Approximately 10% exhibit intraspinal growth and may produce symptoms of spinal cord compression. Patients with peripheral nerve neoplasms (schwannoma, neurofibroma, malignant nerve sheath tumor) are typically young adults in the third and fourth decades of life. Patients with sympathetic ganglia neoplasms (ganglioneuroma) are usually older children (over the age of 4 years), adolescents, and young adults. Neurofibromatosis type I, the most common neurocutaneous disorder, is an autosomal-dominant disease (although approximately 50% of cases occur spontaneously) that manifests with multifocal cutaneous and plexiform neurofibromas, other neurogenic and nonneurogenic neoplasms, skin pigmentation, skeletal defects, and pulmonary fibrosis. Affected patients often exhibit solitary or multiple neurogenic neoplasms of the posterior mediastinum and other thoracic locations. Patients with neurofibromatosis type I have a higher risk of malignant transformation of a neurogenic neoplasm.

Pathology

GROSS

- Schwannoma
  - Encapsulated spherical, ovoid, or fusiform soft tissue mass attached to a peripheral nerve
  - Soft consistency; pink or yellow cut surface
  - Occasional calcification and cystic change
- Neurofibroma
  - Unencapsulated well-circumscribed fusiform soft tissue mass; enlarges nerve of origin
  - White-gray cut surface
- Neurofibromatosis
  - Multiple schwannomas, neurofibromas
  - Plexiform neurofibroma: long, thick, soft, and tortuous nerve enlargement (so-called "bag of worms" appearance)
- Malignant peripheral nerve sheath tumor
  - Large round, ovoid, or fusiform mass
  - Extensive necrosis, hemorrhage, or cystic change
- Ganglioneuroma
  - Well-defined encapsulated firm gray-to-yellow soft tissue mass
  - May exhibit a trabeculated cut surface

MICROSCOPIC

- Schwannoma
  - Spindle cells with elongated nuclei and indistinct cell membranes
  - Characteristic cellular Antoni A and hypocellular Antoni B areas, the latter characterized by scant cells and loose edematous myxoid stroma
- Neurofibroma
  - Schwann cells in loose edematous myxomatous stroma, fibroblasts, collagen strands, and neural fibers; less cellular than schwannomas
- Neurofibromatosis
  - Plexiform neurofibroma: neuronal axons with intermixed tangle of disorganized Schwann cells and matrix

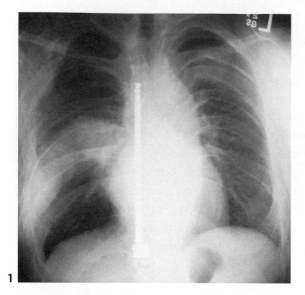

Figure 173F (1–3) PA chest radiograph **(1)** of a young woman with neurofibromatosis type I who was surgically treated for thoracic scoliosis demonstrates multifocal mediastinal and chest wall masses with numerous associated skeletal abnormalities characterized by rib deformities and benign pressure erosion along the inferior aspects of multiple ribs. T2-weighted coronal MR **(2,3)** demonstrates multifocal bilateral mediastinal (paravertebral) and chest wall masses of heterogeneous high signal intensity. Note the classic "target sign" appearance exhibited by some of the lesions **(2)**.

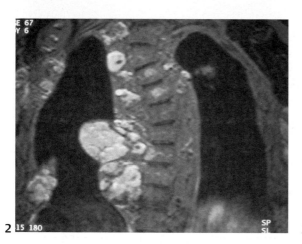

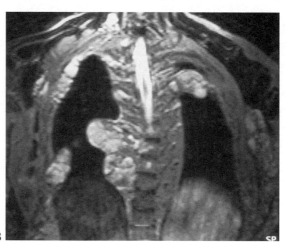

- Malignant peripheral nerve sheath tumor
  - Solid sheets of pleomorphic spindle cells, numerous mitoses, necrosis; may be indistinguishable from other sarcomas
- Ganglioneuroma
  - Mature ganglion cells, Schwann cells, and nerve fibers

Imaging Findings

RADIOGRAPHY

- Schwannoma/neurofibroma
  - Well-defined spherical or ovoid, smooth or lobular paravertebral soft tissue mass (**Figs. 173A** and **173B**)
  - Osseous abnormalities in 50% of cases: expansion of neuroforamen, pressure erosion of adjacent vertebrae and ribs, rib deformity (**Fig. 173A**)
- Neurofibromatosis
  - Focal or multifocal soft tissue masses typically adjacent to ribs, in paravertebral regions and in mediastinum (**Fig. 173F1**)
  - Rib erosion, separation of adjacent ribs, dysplastic changes ("ribbon rib" deformity) (**Fig. 173F1**); posterior scalloping of vertebral bodies, enlarged neuroforamina

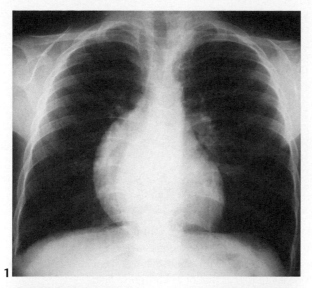
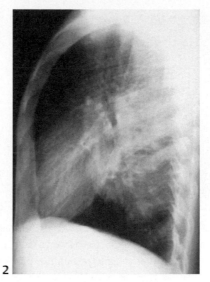
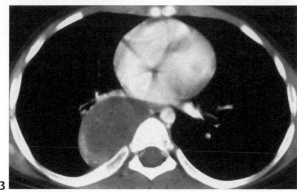

Figure 173G (1–3) PA **(1)** and lateral **(2)** chest radiographs of an asymptomatic 7-year-old boy with a ganglioneuroma demonstrate a large elongated right paraspinal soft tissue mass that produces mild displacement and sclerosis of the inferior aspects of the posteromedial right eighth and ninth ribs **(1).** Contrast-enhanced chest CT (mediastinal window) **(3)** demonstrates a heterogeneously enhancing ovoid right paraspinal mass of predominant low attenuation with multifocal internal punctate calcifications. Note the mass effect on adjacent vessels and bronchi.

- - Short-segment acute angulation scoliosis
  - Lateral meningocele, right-sided predominance
- Malignant peripheral nerve sheath tumor
  - Large, rapidly growing spherical posterior mediastinal mass
- Ganglioneuroma
  - Well-defined elongated mass along anterolateral spine (see Case 163 and **Fig. 173G**)
  - Vertical orientation, tapered appearance (see Case 163 and **Fig. 173G1,2**)
  - Associated benign skeletal erosion/sclerosis (see Case 163 and **Fig. 173G1**)

CT

- Osseous erosion/deformity, intraspinal extension (**Fig. 173C**)
- Schwannoma/neurofibroma
  - Homogeneous or heterogeneous attenuation, typically lower than that of skeletal muscle
  - Heterogeneous enhancement (**Fig. 173C**)
  - Punctate calcification in 10%
- Neurofibromatosis
  - Focal mass or multifocal masses affecting multiple thoracic nerves
  - Low attenuation, calcification
  - Pressure erosion, enlarged neuroforamina
  - Lateral thoracic meningocele: homogeneous spherical, well-defined paraspinal mass of water attenuation with adjacent osseous erosion or sclerosis and/or neuroforamen enlargement (**Fig. 173H1**)

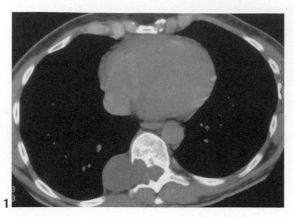 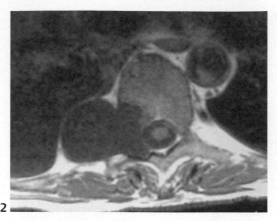

Figure 173H (1,2) Unenhanced chest CT (mediastinal window) **(1)** of a 45-year-old man with neurofibromatosis type I and a lateral thoracic meningocele demonstrates a low attenuation spherical right paraspinal mass that extends through the neuroforamen with resultant expansion and adjacent osseous sclerosis and scalloping. Axial T1-weighted MR **(2)** shows that the mass exhibits the same signal intensity as that of cerebrospinal fluid.

- Malignant peripheral nerve sheath tumor
  - Large round mass (> 5 cm in diameter)
  - Large areas of low attenuation, multifocal calcifications
  - Mass effect
  - Pleural effusion, pleural nodules
  - Pulmonary metastases
- Ganglioneuroma
  - Homogeneous or heterogeneous attenuation (**Fig. 173G3**)
  - Low-to-intermediate attenuation (**Fig. 173G3**)
  - Punctate-to-coarse calcification (**Fig. 173G3**)

MR

- Exclusion of neuroforaminal or intraspinal growth; dumbbell-shaped tumors (**Figs. 173D** and **173E**)
- Schwannoma/neurofibroma
  - Low-to-intermediate signal intensity on T1-weighted images (**Fig. 173D**)
  - Intermediate-to-high signal intensity on T2-weighted images
- Neurofibromatosis
  - Focal or multifocal neurogenic neoplasms (**Fig. 173F2,3**)
  - Variable signal intensity on T1-weighted images; peripheral hyperintensity and central hypointensity on T2-weighted images (target sign) (**Fig. 173F2**)
  - Lateral thoracic meningocele: low signal intensity on T1-weighted images (**Fig. 173H2**), high signal intensity on T2-weighted images, parallels cerebrospinal fluid signal; no contrast enhancement
- Ganglioneuroma
  - Low signal intensity on T1-weighted images
  - High signal intensity on T2-weighted images
  - Whorled heterogeneous appearance (see Case 163)
  - Gradually increasing enhancement on dynamic MR imaging

Treatment

- Surgical excision

Prognosis

- Excellent prognosis for patients with excised benign neurogenic neoplasms
- Excised solitary malignant peripheral nerve sheath tumor: 75% 5-year survival
- Patients with neurofibromatosis and malignant peripheral nerve sheath tumor: 15 to 30% 5-year survival

PEARL_____

- Thoracic meningocele (intrathoracic extrusion of meningeal membranes and their fluid content) typically affects patients with neurofibromatosis and manifests on radiography as a well-defined spherical paravertebral mass that may mimic a neurogenic neoplasm. Associated findings include enlargement of an adjacent neuroforamen and pressure erosion or sclerosis of adjacent vertebrae. CT demonstrates osseous "scalloping" and sclerosis and fluid attenuation (**Fig. 173H1**). MR establishes the diagnosis by demonstrating signal intensity that parallels that of cerebrospinal fluid (**Fig. 173H2**).

Suggested Readings

Armstrong P. Mediastinal and hilar disorders. In: Armstrong P, Wilson AG, Dee P, Hansell DM, eds. Imaging of Diseases of the Chest, 3rd ed. London: Mosby, 2000:789–892

Fraser RS, Müller NL, Colman N, Paré PD. Masses situated predominantly in the paravertebral region. In: Fraser RS, Müller NL, Colman N, Paré PD, eds. Fraser and Paré's Diagnosis of Diseases of the Chest, 4th ed. Philadelphia: Saunders, 1999:2974–2983

Ichikawa T, Ohtomo K, Araki T, et al. Ganglioneuroma: computed tomography and magnetic resonance features. Br J Radiol 1996;69:114–121

Marchevsky AM. Mediastinal tumors of peripheral nervous system origin. Semin Diagn Pathol 1999; 16:65–78

Moon WK, Im J-G, Han MC. Malignant schwannomas of the thorax: CT findings. J Comput Assist Tomogr 1993;17:274–276

Rossi SE, Erasmus JJ, McAdams HP, Donnelly LF. Thoracic manifestations of neurofibromatosis-I. AJR Am J Roentgenol 1999;173:1631–1638

CASE 174 Mediastinal Goiter

Clinical Presentation

An elderly woman with respiratory distress and a chronic left neck mass

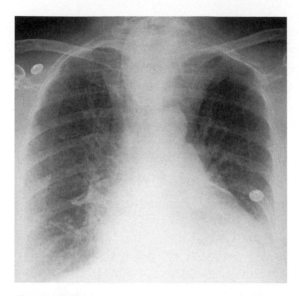

Figure 174A

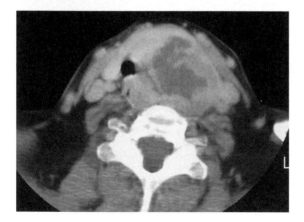

Figure 174B

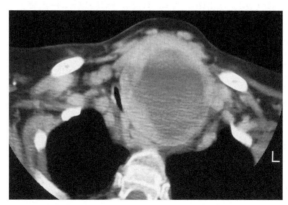

Figure 174C

Radiologic Findings

PA chest radiograph (**Fig. 174A**) demonstrates a large, well-defined left-sided mediastinal soft tissue mass and an associated ipsilateral neck mass. Note the marked mass effect on the cervical and intrathoracic portions of the trachea. Contrast-enhanced chest CT (mediastinal window) (**Figs. 174B** and **174C**) demonstrates a large heterogeneously enhancing soft tissue mass that arises from the left lobe of the thyroid gland (**Fig. 174B**) and extends into the mediastinum (**Fig. 174C**). Note the large area of central low attenuation surrounded by irregular enhancing soft tissue and significant mass effect on the trachea, esophagus, and mediastinal great vessels.

Diagnosis

Mediastinal goiter

Differential Diagnosis

- Thyroid carcinoma
- Lymphadenopathy, lymphoma
- Neurogenic neoplasm

Discussion

Background

Mediastinal (intrathoracic, substernal, retrosternal) goiter refers to abnormal thyroid tissue within the mediastinum. Mediastinal goiter affects approximately 5% of the world's population. The term *substernal goiter* is sometimes used to refer to mediastinal goiters in which over 50% of the mass resides below the thoracic inlet. Approximately 80% of mediastinal goiters arise from the inferior aspect of a thyroid lobe or from the thyroid isthmus and extend into the anterior and/or middle mediastinum. The rest arise from the posterior aspect of the thyroid, extend into the posterior mediastinum (so-called posterior descending goiters), and are predominantly right sided.

Etiology

Most mediastinal goiters result from intrathoracic growth of a thyroid goiter, and up to 17% of cervical goiters extend into the thorax. Primary intrathoracic (aberrant or ectopic) goiters are rare (accounting for less than 1% of excised lesions) and are thought to result from abnormal embryologic migration of the thyroid cells.

Clinical Findings

Most affected patients are women in the fifth decade of life. Patients with mediastinal goiter are usually asymptomatic adults with a long history of a thyroid mass. Symptoms of tracheal, esophageal, vascular, or recurrent laryngeal nerve compression may occur, typically dyspnea, wheezing, stridor, dysphagia, and hoarseness.

Pathology

GROSS

- Well-defined, encapsulated lobular soft tissue masses of variable size (6–10 cm)
- Cut section: nodular soft tissue with frequent hemorrhage, calcification, and cystic change

MICROSCOPIC

- Multinodular goiter
- Rarely carcinoma or thyroiditis

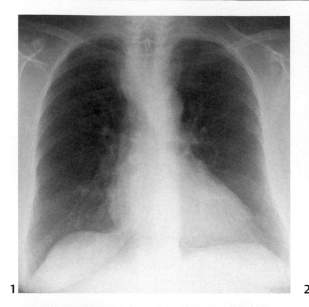

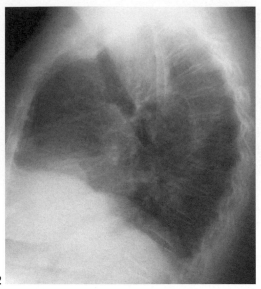

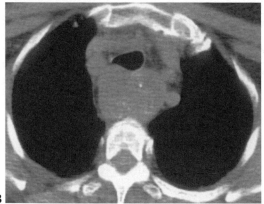

Figure 174D (1–3) PA **(1)** and lateral **(2)** chest radiographs of an asymptomatic middle-aged woman with a posterior descending goiter demonstrate a middle mediastinal mass, which produces mass effect on the posterior trachea. Unenhanced chest CT (mediastinal window) **(3)** demonstrates a soft tissue mass with subtle multifocal punctate calcifications that produces mass effect on the posterior aspect of the trachea and the mediastinal great vessels.

Imaging Findings

RADIOGRAPHY

- Well-defined smooth or lobular mediastinal soft tissue mass with frequent mass effect on the airway (**Figs. 174A, 174D1, and 174D2**)
  - Associated cervical or thoracic inlet mass with contralateral airway displacement (**Fig. 174A**)
  - Isolated mediastinal mass (**Figs. 174D1 and 174D2**)
- Focal or multifocal calcification
- Right-sided mediastinal mass in most posterior mediastinal goiters, even when originating from the left thyroid lobe

CT

- Well-defined high attenuation soft tissue mass on unenhanced CT
- Heterogeneous attenuation from focal or multifocal punctate or coarse calcification (**Fig. 174D3**) or hemorrhage or cystic change (**Figs. 174B and 174C**)
- Early intense and sustained contrast enhancement; frequent foci of low attenuation (**Figs. 174B and 174C**)
- Continuity with cervical thyroid (**Figs. 174B and 174C**)

MR

- Demonstration of continuity with cervical thyroid on sagittal and coronal imaging
- Heterogeneous signal intensity on T1- and T2-weighted images

SCINTIGRAPHY

- Uptake of technetium-99m (Tc-99m)
- Uptake of I-123 and I-131; false-positives reported

Treatment

- Recognition and observation in asymptomatic patients
- Surgical excision in symptomatic patients (tracheal, esophageal, vascular, nerve compression) and in those with malignant transformation

Prognosis

- Favorable prognosis in patients with multinodular goiter
- Guarded prognosis in patients with thyroiditis or malignancy

PEARLS

- The presumptive diagnosis of mediastinal goiter can be made in most asymptomatic patients with a known chronic cervical goiter based on clinical presentation and imaging features.
- CT is the imaging modality of choice for the evaluation of mediastinal goiter. While scintigraphy is useful, it may fail to demonstrate features of malignancy, and false-positive studies are reported.
- Local invasion and lymphadenopathy suggest thyroid carcinoma.
- The diagnosis of ectopic mediastinal goiter should be considered in asymptomatic patients with isolated high attenuation anterior mediastinal masses that exhibit intense and sustained contrast enhancement. The diagnosis may be confirmed with scintigraphy.

Suggested Readings

Buckley JA, Stark P. Intrathoracic mediastinal thyroid goiter: imaging manifestations. AJR Am J Roentgenol 1999;173:471–475

Fraser RS, Müller NL, Colman N, Paré PD. Masses situated predominantly in the anterior mediastinal compartment. In: Fraser RS, Müller NL, Colman N, Paré PD, eds. Fraser and Paré's Diagnosis of Diseases of the Chest, 4th ed. Philadelphia: Saunders, 1999:2875–2937

Hopkins CR, Reading CC. Thyroid and parathyroid imaging. Semin Ultrasound CT MR 1995;16: 279–295

CASE 175 Lymphangioma

Clinical Presentation

A 24-year-old woman with a palpable neck mass

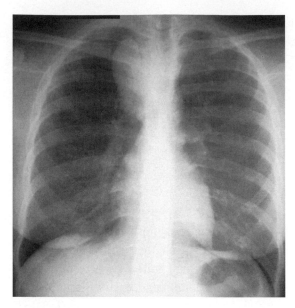

Figure 175A

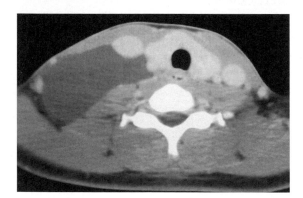

Figure 175B

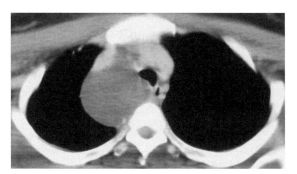

Figure 175C

Radiologic Findings

PA chest radiograph (**Fig. 175A**) demonstrates a well-defined right middle mediastinal (paratracheal) mass that produces mass effect on the cervical and intrathoracic portions of the trachea. Contrast-enhanced chest CT (mediastinal window) (**Figs. 175B** and **175C**) demonstrates a multilocular cystic right neck mass of water attenuation contents with thin internal soft tissue septa (**Fig. 175B**) that extends into the mediastinum, protrudes between adjacent vascular structures (**Fig. 175C**), and produces mass effect on the trachea (**Fig. 175C**).

Diagnosis

Lymphangioma

Differential Diagnosis

- Congenital or acquired cyst: bronchogenic, thyroglossal, branchial cleft, thymic
- Mature teratoma

Discussion

Background

The majority of lymphangiomas affect infants, who typically present with a soft, palpable cystic mass in the neck, head, and/or axilla. Approximately 10% of lymphangiomas extend into the mediastinum, and primary mediastinal lymphangiomas are rare. Mediastinal lymphangioma represents up to 4.5% of all mediastinal masses in adults. Rarely, mediastinal lymphangiomas result from recurrence of previously excised lymphangiomas. Hemangioma is a related vascular lesion and may coexist with lymphangioma or may occur as an isolated mass.

Etiology

The etiology of lymphangioma is poorly understood. Developmental, hamartomatous, and neoplastic origins have been postulated.

Clinical Findings

Approximately 90% of patients with lymphangioma are diagnosed in infancy (under the age of 2 years) because of a palpable mass in the neck, chest wall, and/or axilla. Affected patients may present with symptoms related to mass effect, including cough, wheezing, and pain. Isolated mediastinal lymphangiomas are rare (less than 1%), typically affect asymptomatic adults, and may be more common in men.

Pathology

GROSS

- Soft, thin-walled, multilocular cystic mass
- Chylous fluid content
- Variable size

MICROSCOPIC

- Intercommunicating lymphatic vessels of variable sizes; capillary, cavernous, and cystic (cystic hygroma) varieties described based on size of vascular structures
- Endothelial cell lining of vascular spaces
- Mural connective tissue, smooth muscle, adipose tissue, lymphoid tissue
- Identification of coexistent hemangioma

Imaging Findings

RADIOGRAPHY

- Well-defined mediastinal mass (**Fig. 175A**)
  - Mediastinal mass with cervical and/or chest wall component (**Fig. 175A**)
  - Isolated mediastinal mass

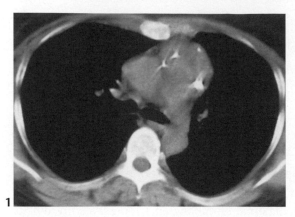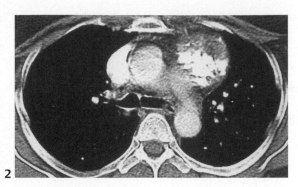

Figure 175D (1,2) Unenhanced **(1)** and contrast-enhanced chest CT **(2)** (mediastinal window) of an asymptomatic middle-aged woman with a mediastinal hemangioma demonstrates a well-defined heterogeneous mediastinal mass with multifocal punctate calcifications **(1)**. Note the intense heterogeneous enhancement of the lesion after contrast administration that parallels the attenuation of the pulmonary and mediastinal vascular structures **(2)**.

- Anterior-superior mediastinum; other compartments also affected
- May produce mass effect on mediastinal structures and/or cervical trachea (**Fig. 175A**)

CT

- Well-defined mediastinal mass (may exhibit continuity with ipsilateral cervical mass) (**Figs. 175B** and **175C**)
- Unilocular or multilocular (heterogeneous) cystic mass with water attenuation contents and enhancing soft tissue elements (thin septa, larger soft tissue components) (**Figs. 175B** and **175C**)
- Nonenhancing low (water or soft tissue) attenuation mass (**Fig. 175C**)
- May conform to or insinuate around normal structures; may produce mass effect (**Fig. 175C**)
- Rarely calcification, soft tissue attenuation, spiculated borders

MR

- Intermediate-to-high signal intensity on T1-weighted images
- Heterogeneous high signal intensity on T2-weighted images; low signal intensity on T2-weighted images with hemorrhage or fibrosis
- Enhancing thin tissue septa surrounding intermediate signal intensity cystic spaces

Treatment

- Surgical excision

Prognosis

- Excellent
- Reports of local recurrence

PEARLS

- Lymphangioma should be included in the differential diagnosis of multilocular cystic mediastinal masses affecting young patients, particularly when the lesion exhibits extension into the neck, chest wall, and/or axilla.
- Mediastinal hemangioma is a rare benign vascular mediastinal tumor that is typically diagnosed in asymptomatic young adults and is composed of interconnecting blood-filled endothelial-lined

vascular channels with foci of organized thrombus and phleboliths. Radiography demonstrates a well-defined mediastinal soft tissue mass. CT demonstrates multifocal punctate calcifications in 28% of cases (**Fig. 175D1**), heterogeneous attenuation on unenhanced studies (**Fig. 175D1**), and intense heterogeneous enhancement that parallels vascular enhancement following contrast administration (**Fig. 175D2**).

Suggested Readings

Charruau L, Parrens M, Jougon J, et al. Mediastinal lymphangioma in adults: CT and MR imaging features. Eur Radiol 2000;10:1310–1314

McAdams HP, Rosado-de-Christenson ML, Moran CA. Mediastinal hemangioma: radiographic and CT features in 14 patients. Radiology 1994;193:399–402

Miyake H, Shiga M, Takaki H, Hata H, Osini R, Mori H. Mediastinal lymphangiomas in adults: CT findings. J Thorac Imaging 1996;11:83–85

Shaffer K, Rosado-de-Christenson ML, Patz EF Jr, Young S, Farver CF. Thoracic lymphangioma in adults: CT and MR imaging features. AJR Am J Roentgenol 1994;162:283–289

Shimosato Y, Mukai K. Tumors of the mediastinum excluding the thymus, heart and great vessels. In: Rosai J, ed. Atlas of Tumor Pathology: Tumors of the Mediastinum, fascicle 21, series 3. Washington, DC: American Registry of Pathology and Armed Forces Institute of Pathology, 1997:249–273

CASE 176 Paraesophageal Varices

Clinical Presentation

An asymptomatic elderly man with known cirrhosis and portal hypertension

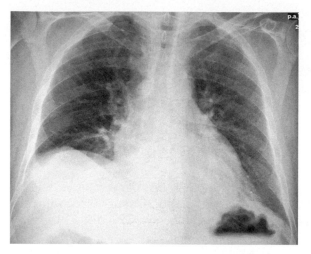

Figure 176A

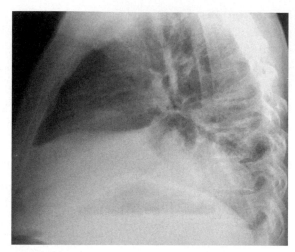

Figure 176B

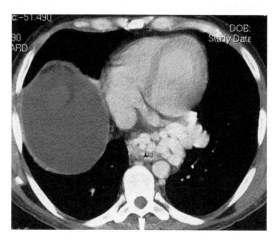

Figure 176C

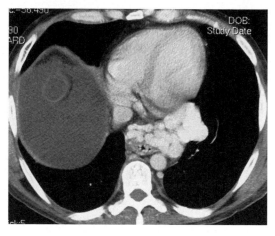

Figure 176D

(Figs. 176A, 176B, 176C, and 176D courtesy of H. Page McAdams, M.D., Duke University Medical Center, Durham, North Carolina.)

Radiologic Findings

PA (**Fig. 176A**) and lateral (**Fig. 176B**) chest radiographs demonstrate a large retrocardiac middle and posterior mediastinal mass, abnormal interstitial lung markings, and elevation of the right hemidiaphragm. Contrast-enhanced chest CT (mediastinal window) (**Figs. 176C** and **176D**) demonstrates a complex middle mediastinal mass composed of numerous enhancing tortuous serpiginous structures. The degree of contrast enhancement within the lesion parallels that of the adjacent aorta and hemiazygos vein. Note the thickened nodular esophageal wall with minute intensely enhancing foci adjacent to the esophageal lumen and abdominal ascites.

684

Diagnosis

Paraesophageal and esophageal varices

Differential Diagnosis

None

Discussion

Background

Paraesophageal and esophageal varices represent dilated extrinsic and intrinsic esophageal veins, respectively. They are supplied by the left gastric vein, which arises at the portal venous confluence and courses through the gastric fundus to drain into the lower esophageal plexus veins, serving as a portosystemic collateral pathway in patients with portal hypertension. The posterior branch of the left gastric vein supplies the paraesophageal varices, and the anterior branch supplies the gastroesophageal varices. Paraesophageal varices are located outside the esophageal wall, communicate with esophageal varices, and typically drain into the azygos and/or hemiazygos system, the subclavian and/or brachiocephalic system, and/or the inferior vena cava. Esophageal varices are located within the wall of the inferior esophagus.

Etiology

Paraesophageal varices result from severe liver disease and portal hypertension (portal venous pressure greater than 10 mm Hg). Two hypotheses are proposed in their pathogenesis: (1) increased sinusoidal pressure (and increased resistance to flow) resulting from collagen deposition in the spaces of Disse and hepatocyte swelling, and (2) endogenous hepatic vasoconstrictors and mesenteric vasodilators that produce increased blood flow and pressure in the portal venous system. It is probable that both mechanisms play a role. Portal venous hypertension results in reversal of flow (away from the liver, or hepatofugal) through intrahepatic arterioportal communications, through the vasa vasorum that supply the walls of the portal veins, or at the portal triad through direct blood shunting from the hepatic arteries to the capillaries to the portal vein. The end result is enlargement of portosystemic collateral vessels and the formation of varices.

Clinical Findings

Patients with paraesophageal varices are typically adults with portal hypertension secondary to hepatic cirrhosis and characteristically have a history of alcohol abuse. They may present with fatigue, weight loss, abdominal pain, jaundice, and/or upper gastrointestinal hemorrhage. Physical examination may reveal gynecomastia, digital clubbing, peripheral edema, abdominal ascites, hepatosplenomegaly, and/or enlarged abdominal wall veins. Children may develop portal hypertension secondary to extrahepatic portal venous obstruction.

Pathology

- Paraesophageal varices
  - Serpiginous network of dilated veins that surround the esophagus and aorta

- Esophageal varices
  - Dilated veins within the esophageal wall that may protrude into the esophageal lumen

Imaging Findings

RADIOGRAPHY

- Middle and/or posterior mediastinal, paraaortic/paravertebral lobular soft tissue masses (**Figs. 176A** and **176B**)
  - Visible in less than 10% of cases
  - Also known as mediastinal pseudotumor
- Obliteration or nodularity of descending thoracic aortic interface
- Lateral displacement of inferior paraspinal interfaces (**Fig. 176A**)
- Lateral displacement or obliteration of inferior azygoesophageal recess
- Mass in the region of the pulmonary ligament (**Fig. 176A**)
- Splenomegaly

CT

- Dilated serpiginous soft tissue masses closely related to the outer wall of the esophagus; may reach large sizes (**Figs. 176C** and **176D**)
- Intense contrast enhancement that parallels aortic enhancement (**Figs. 176C** and **176D**)
- Visualization of vascular communications with the systemic venous circulation (precaval draining vein, preaortic esophageal veins)
- Associated esophageal varices:
  - Thickened esophageal wall with lobular outer contour (**Figs. 176C** and **176D**)
  - Scalloped esophageal lumen with nodular intraluminal protrusions (**Figs. 176C** and **176D**)
  - Focal or circumferential mural (nodular) enhancement (similar to that of the thoracic aorta) with associated esophageal wall thickening
- Use of CT angiography with two-dimensional and three-dimensional rendering for anatomic visualization of collateral pathways; evaluation of patients with known cirrhosis, esophageal varices and a mediastinal mass
- Abdominal findings of hepatic cirrhosis: dilated left gastric vein (5–6 mm in diameter) or multiple dilated veins (4–6 mm in diameter) located between the stomach and the posterior left hepatic lobe, abdominal ascites (**Figs. 176C** and **176D**)

MR

- Use of axial three-dimensional gradient-echo MR imaging for depiction of abnormal upper abdominal vascular anatomy
- Use of gadolinium-enhanced three-dimensional MR portal venography

Treatment

- Sclerotherapy or banding for bleeding esophageal varices

Prognosis

- Poor prognosis in patients with bleeding esophageal varices and paraesophageal varices on CT; prolonged and more frequent sclerotherapy

Suggested Readings

Henseler KP, Pozniak MA, Lee FT Jr, Winter TC III. Three-dimensional CT angiography of spontaneous portosystemic shunts. Radiographics 2001;21:691–704

Ibukuro K, Tsukiyama T, Mori K, Inoue Y. Precaval draining vein from paraesophageal varices: radiologic-anatomic correlation. AJR Am J Roentgenol 1999;172:651–654

Ibukuro K, Tsukiyama T, Mori K, Inoue Y. Preaortic esophageal veins: CT appearance. AJR Am J Roentgenol 1998;170:1535–1538

Kim M-J, Mitchell DG, Ito K. Portosystemic collaterals of the upper abdomen: review of anatomy and demonstration on MR imaging. Abdom Imaging 2000;25:462–470

Lee SJ, Lee KS, Kim SA, Kim TS, Hwang JH, Lim JH. Computed radiography of the chest in patients with paraesophageal varices: diagnostic accuracy and characteristic findings. AJR Am J Roentgenol 1998;170:1527–1531

CASE 177 Hiatus Hernia

Clinical Presentation

A middle-aged woman with recurrent epigastric pain

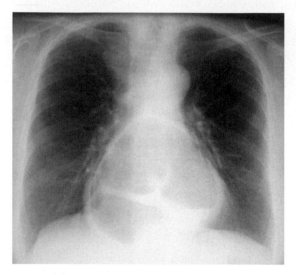

Figure 177A

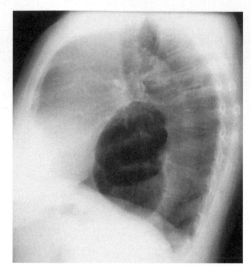

Figure 177B

Radiologic Findings

PA (**Fig. 177A**) and lateral (**Fig. 177B**) chest radiographs demonstrate a large middle mediastinal (retrocardiac) mass. The mass contains the air-filled stomach, possibly bowel, and at least one air–fluid level (**Fig. 177A**).

Diagnosis

Hiatus hernia

Differential Diagnosis

None

Discussion

Background

Hiatus hernia results from intrathoracic gastric herniation through an enlarged esophageal hiatus. Herniation of omentum and other portions of the gastrointestinal tract (hollow viscera and solid organs) occasionally occurs. Abdominal fluid may also herniate through the esophageal hiatus in patients with ascites.

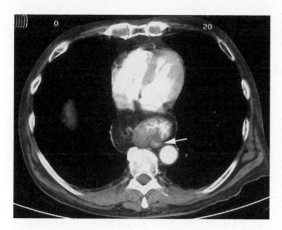

Figure 177C Contrast-enhanced chest CT (mediastinal window) of an elderly man with a hiatus hernia demonstrates herniation of the stomach and omental fat through the esophageal hiatus. Note the location of the distal esophagus (arrow).

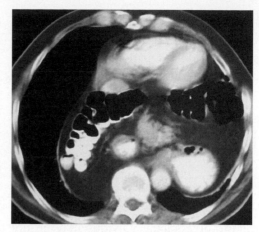

Figure 177D Contrast-enhanced chest CT (mediastinal window) of an asymptomatic 67-year-old man with a large hiatus hernia demonstrates mediastinal herniation of the transverse colon, omentum, and stomach.

Etiology

Hiatus hernia results from acquired widening of the esophageal hiatus related to increased intraabdominal pressure associated with obesity and/or pregnancy. Congenital weakness of the esophageal hiatus may play a role in some cases.

Clinical Findings

The prevalence of hiatus hernia increases with age, and most affected patients are older than 60 years. Patients with hiatus hernia are typically asymptomatic middle-aged or elderly individuals who are diagnosed incidentally because of an abnormal chest radiograph. Symptomatic patients complain of abdominal burning pain that is worse after meals and in the supine position and is typically alleviated by antacids. Upper gastrointestinal bleeding may also occur and may manifest with anemiae, frank hematemesis, or melena.

Imaging Findings

RADIOGRAPHY

- Retrocardiac middle mediastinal mass
  - Homogeneous soft tissue mass
  - Air-filled mass (**Figs. 177A** and **177B**)
  - Mass with one or more air–fluid levels (**Fig. 177A**)
- Organoaxial volvulus in cases of significant gastric herniation; large air-filled mass; may exhibit two air-fluid levels

CT

- Visualization of gastric herniation through esophageal hiatus (**Figs. 177C** and **177D**)
- Visualization of other herniated abdominal organs and/or structures (**Fig. 177D**)

Treatment

- Recognition and observation
- Antacids in symptomatic patients
- Immediate surgical intervention in cases of strangulation or symptomatic gastric volvulus

Prognosis

- Good

PEARLS_____

- Asymptomatic organoaxial volvulus may be present in patients with completely intrathoracic stomachs due to large hiatus hernias.
- Acute upper gastrointestinal symptoms in a patient with a known hiatus hernia should prompt exclusion of strangulation or symptomatic gastric volvulus.

PITFALL_____

- Large hiatus hernias may lateralize to one side of the hemithorax and may mimic a lung mass or abscess on radiography.

Suggested Readings

Armstrong P. Mediastinal and hilar disorders. In: Armstrong P, Wilson AG, Dee P, Hansell DM, eds. Imaging of Diseases of the Chest, 3rd ed. London: Mosby, 2000:789–892

Fraser RS, Müller NL, Colman N, Paré PD. The diaphragm. In: Fraser RS, Müller NL, Colman N, Paré PD, eds. Fraser and Paré's Diagnosis of Diseases of the Chest, 4th ed. Philadelphia: Saunders, 1999:2987–3010

CASE 178 Achalasia

Clinical Presentation

An elderly woman with dysphagia, weight loss, and halitosis

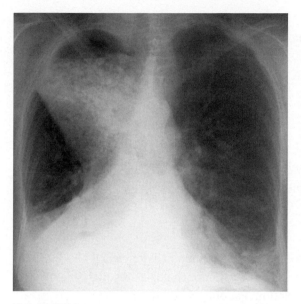

Figure 178A

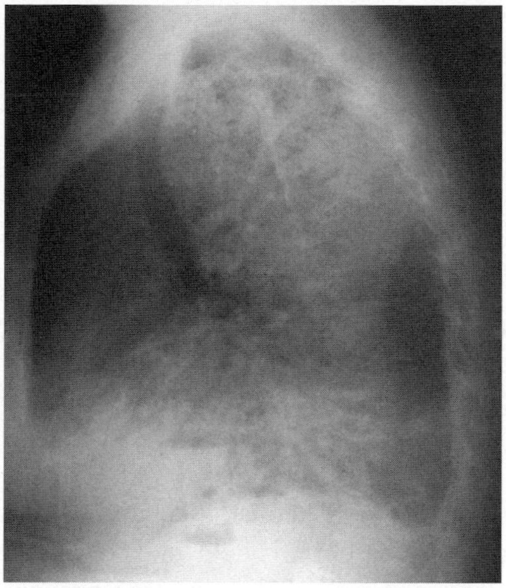

Figure 178B

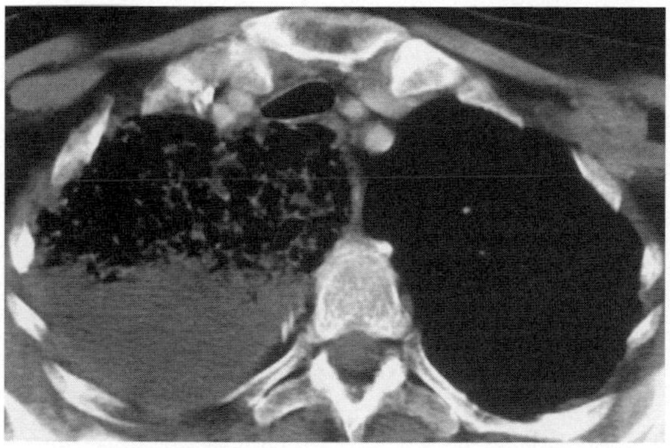

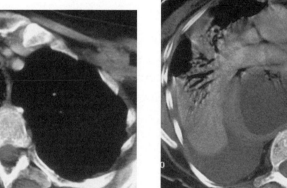

Figure 178C

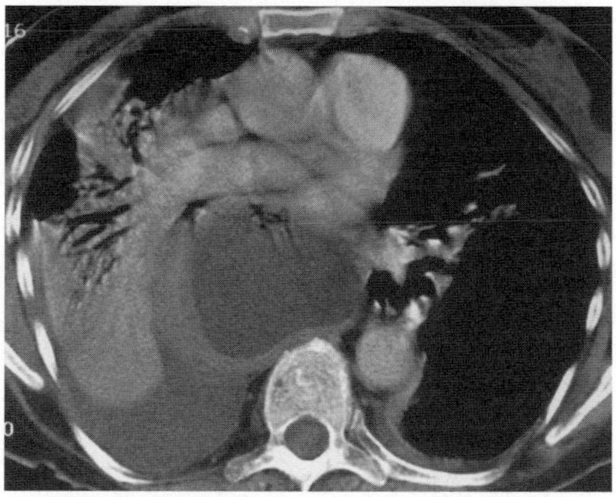

Figure 178D

Radiologic Findings

PA (**Fig. 178A**) and lateral (**Fig. 178B**) chest radiographs demonstrate a large elongated middle-posterior mediastinal mass that extends to the paravertebral region, projects to the right of the midline, and contains heterogeneous debris admixed with air and a large air–debris level (**Fig. 178A**). The mass produces right middle and right lower lobe atelectasis, and there is a small right pleural effusion. Contrast-enhanced chest CT (mediastinal window) (**Figs. 178C** and **178D**) demonstrates a massively dilated esophagus with heterogeneous contents that produces mass effect on the mediastinum and bronchus intermedius (**Fig. 178D**), with resultant right middle and right lower lobe atelectasis. Note the right pleural effusion.

691

Diagnosis

Achalasia

Differential Diagnosis

- Esophageal dilatation from progressive systemic sclerosis
- Esophageal dilatation from acquired focal obstruction: carcinoma, metastatic disease, nonneoplastic stenosis

Discussion

Background

Achalasia is characterized by absent peristalsis and incomplete relaxation of the lower esophageal sphincter, resulting in marked esophageal dilatation and poor esophageal emptying.

Etiology

In most cases, achalasia is a primary or idiopathic condition that correlates with ganglion cell deficiency in the esophageal myenteric smooth muscle plexus. Secondary achalasia (or pseudoachalasia) results from Chagas disease or from malignancy at the gastroesophageal junction. Esophageal dilatation may also result from progressive systemic sclerosis, reflux esophagitis, and mediastinal fibrosis.

Clinical Findings

Patients with primary achalasia usually experience an insidious onset of symptoms and typically present between the ages of 30 and 50 years. Symptomatic patients complain of dysphagia, foul breath, regurgitation, and symptoms related to aspiration and recurrent pulmonary infection. Patients with secondary achalasia (from malignancy) are usually older (over 60 years) and have a recent onset of dysphagia and substantial weight loss.

Pathology

- Diffuse deficiency of esophageal myenteric plexus ganglion cells
- Neoplastic cells, fibrosis, or esophagitis in cases of secondary achalasia

Imaging Findings

RADIOGRAPHY

- Elongated middle mediastinal mass (dilated esophagus) (**Figs. 178B** and **178E1**); commonly exhibits an air–fluid level (**Fig. 178A**)
- Marked esophageal dilatation with esophageal displacement to the right of midline (**Figs. 178A** and **178E1**)
- Anterior tracheal displacement on lateral chest radiography (**Fig. 178B**)
- Associated pulmonary consolidation/atelectasis from recurrent aspiration (**Figs. 178A** and **178B**)
- Esophagram
  - Esophageal dilatation (typically > 4 cm in diameter) (**Fig. 178E2**)
  - Absent peristalsis

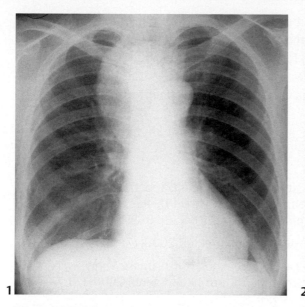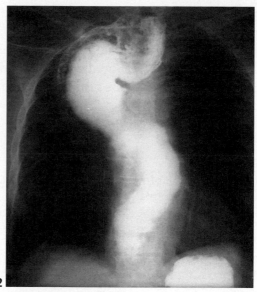

Figure 178E (1) PA chest radiograph of a 45-year-old woman with dysphagia and mild weight loss secondary to primary achalasia demonstrates a large, elongated right middle mediastinal mass that represented a dilated esophagus. **(2)** Barium esophagram demonstrates marked dilatation and tortuosity of the entire esophagus. Decreased-to-absent peristalsis was noted at fluoroscopy.

- Smooth narrowing of distal esophagus under 3.5 cm in length (in primary achalasia)
- Failure of lower esophageal sphincter to relax with swallowing (**Fig. 178E2**)

CT

- Dilated esophagus with air–fluid level (**Figs. 178C** and **178D**)
- Normal esophageal wall thickness (**Figs. 178C** and **178D**)
- Poor visualization of gastric cardia due to poor esophageal emptying
- Associated pulmonary consolidation, atelectasis (**Figs. 178C** and **178D**), and/or bronchiectasis from mass effect and recurrent aspiration

Treatment

- Laparoscopic esophagogastric myotomy with fundoplication
- Endoscopic injection of botulinum toxin into the lower esophageal sphincter
- Progressive balloon dilation of distal esophagus under fluoroscopic guidance; may require repeated treatments; may be complicated by esophageal perforation

Prognosis

- Good

PEARLS

- Approximately 75% of patients with secondary achalasia have carcinoma of the gastric cardia or metastatic neoplasm to this area. These patients may exhibit asymmetric thickening of the distal esophageal wall, a soft tissue mass at the cardia, and mediastinal lymphadenopathy.
- Eccentricity, nodularity, angulation, straightening, and proximal shouldering of the narrowed esophageal segment and a length of narrowing greater than 3.5 cm on barium esophagram suggest secondary achalasia; malignancy must be excluded.

- Chagas disease is a parasitic infection caused by *Trypanosoma cruzi* that occurs only on the American continents anywhere from Mexico to the south of Argentina. Approximately 18 million persons are affected each year. An acute stage is followed by a symptom-free (silent) period that may last for many years. Chronic disease causes irreversible damage to the heart, esophagus, colon, and peripheral nervous system. Approximately 6% of affected individuals develop megaviscera.

Suggested Readings

Fraser RS, Müller NL, Colman N, Paré PD. Masses situated predominantly in the middle-posterior mediastinal compartment. In: Fraser RS, Müller NL, Colman N, Paré PD, eds. Fraser and Paré's Diagnosis of Diseases of the Chest, 4th ed. Philadelphia: Saunders, 1999:2938–2973

Mueller CF, Klecker RJ, King MA. Case 3. Achalasia. AJR Am J Roentgenol 2000;175:867;870–871

Woodfield CA, Levine MS, Rubesin SE, Langlotz CP, Laufer I. Diagnosis of primary versus secondary achalasia: reassessment of clinical and radiographic criteria. AJR Am J Roentgenol 2000;175:727–731

CASE 179 Extramedullary Hematopoiesis

Clinical Presentation

A 25-year-old man with thalassemia major and profound hemolytic anemia

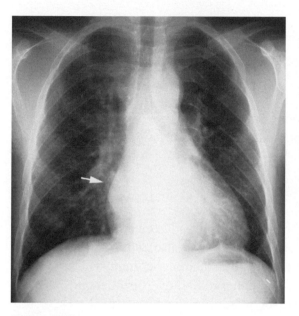

Figure 179A

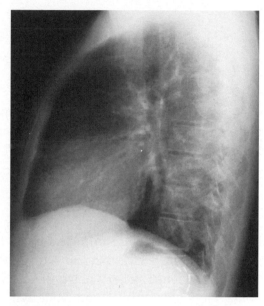

Figure 179B

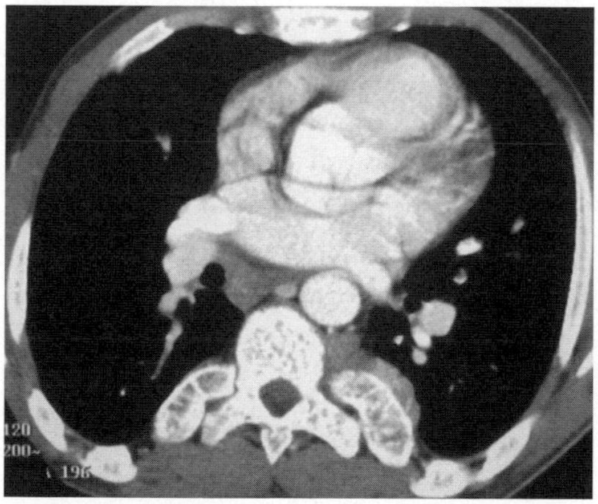

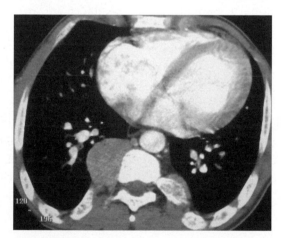

Figure 179C

Figure 179D

Radiologic Findings

PA (**Fig. 179A**) and lateral (**Fig. 179B**) chest radiographs demonstrate a well-defined right paravertebral soft tissue mass (arrow) and expansion of all osseous medullary spaces. Note the left upper quadrant metallic surgical clips from a prior splenectomy. Contrast-enhanced chest CT (mediastinal window) (**Figs. 179C** and **179D**) demonstrates an ovoid, well-defined right paraspinal soft tissue mass (**Fig. 179D**) and a smaller left paraspinal mass (**Fig. 179C**). Note the expansion of the marrow spaces and the increased trabeculation of the adjacent ribs.

695

Diagnosis

Extramedullary hematopoiesis

Differential Diagnosis

- Neurogenic neoplasm
- Lymphadenopathy

Discussion

Background

Extramedullary hematopoiesis represents the compensatory formation of blood elements outside the osseous medulla, most commonly in the liver, spleen, and lymph nodes but also in the posterior mediastinum (paravertebral region).

Etiology

The etiology of extramedullary hematopoiesis is incompletely understood. It usually occurs as a response to inadequate erythrocyte production or excessive hemolysis but may also represent an abnormal cellular proliferation. It is associated with severe congenital hemolytic anemias (hereditary spherocytosis, thalassemia major), polycythemia vera, lymphoproliferative disorders (myelofibrosis, lymphoma, chronic leukemia), and sickle cell disease. It has also been described in association with hyperparathyroidism and chronic pneumonia. It has been postulated that mediastinal extramedullary hematopoiesis results from paravertebral extrusion of marrow elements through the abnormally thinned cortex of adjacent ribs and vertebrae. An embolic mechanism has also been suggested.

Clinical Findings

Mediastinal extramedullary hematopoiesis does not usually produce symptoms, and affected patients are diagnosed incidentally because of an abnormal chest radiograph. There are rare reports of associated spontaneous hemothorax and spinal cord compression. Patients may also present with symptoms related to one of the associated disease processes described above.

Pathology

GROSS

- Reddish soft nodule(s) or mass(es)
- Cut surface may resemble a hematoma.

MICROSCOPIC

- All marrow elements represented: erythroid hyperplasia, lymphocytes, adipose tissue

Imaging Findings

RADIOGRAPHY

- Focal or multifocal smooth or lobular paravertebral soft tissue mass(es)
  - Unilateral or bilateral (**Figs. 179A** and **179E1**)

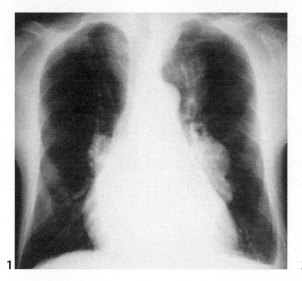 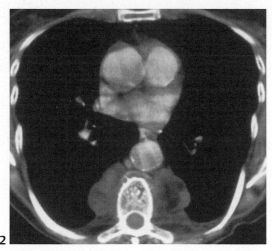

Figure 179E (1) PA chest radiograph of an elderly woman with chronic anemia and extramedullary hematopoiesis demonstrates bilateral lobular paravertebral masses that span the length of the thorax. **(2)** Contrast-enhanced chest CT (mediastinal window) demonstrates bilateral lobular paraspinal soft tissue masses with central areas of fat attenuation.

- Typically in the inferior hemithorax between the 6th and 12th vertebral bodies (**Fig. 179A**)
- May affect entire length of the thoracic paravertebral region (**Fig. 179E1**)
- Expansion of osseous erythroid bone marrow spaces (**Fig. 179A**) with coarse trabeculation

CT

- Well-defined lobular homogeneous soft tissue masses (**Figs. 179C** and **179D**)
- May exhibit internal fat attenuation (particularly following splenectomy) (**Fig. 179E2**)
- Marrow expansion of adjacent skeletal structures with lacy appearance of ribs and vertebrae (**Figs. 179C** and **179D**)
- Rarely abnormal interstitial and ground-glass pulmonary opacities; pleural effusion

MR

- Extramedullary mass with slightly higher signal intensity than that of adjacent marrow on T1- and T2-weighted images
- Evaluation of the epidural space for exclusion of involvement

SCINTIGRAPHY

- Uptake of Tc-99m–labeled monoclonal antibody
  - High sensitivity
  - Binds to hematopoietic cells beyond promyelocytes
- Uptake of In-111-chloride–labeled and Tc-99m–labeled colloids

Treatment

- Recognition and observation in asymptomatic patients
- Radiation therapy for epidural involvement with spinal cord compression

Prognosis

- Variable prognosis based on underlying condition
- Durable control of spinal cord compression in affected patients treated with radiation

Suggested Readings

Dunnick NR. Image interpretation session: 1999. Extramedullary hematopoiesis in a patient with beta thalassemia. Radiographics 2000;20:266–268

Fraser RS, Müller NL, Colman N, Paré PD. Masses situated predominantly in the paravertebral region. In: Fraser RS, Müller NL, Colman N, Paré PD, eds. Fraser and Paré's Diagnosis of Diseases of the Chest, 4th ed. Philadelphia: Saunders, 1999:2974–2983

Gilkeson RC, Basile V, Sands MJ, Hsu JT. Chest case of the day: extramedullary hematopoiesis (EMH). AJR Am J Roentgenol 1997;169:267,270–273

Moellers MO, Bader JB, Alexander C, Samnick S, Kirsch C-M. Localization of extramedullary hematopoiesis with Tc-99m-labeled monoclonal antibodies (BW 250/183). Clin Nucl Med 2002;27: 354–357

CASE 180 Acute Mediastinitis

Clinical Presentation

A 70-year-old woman status post–left lower lobectomy for adenocarcinoma complicated by pharyngeal perforation

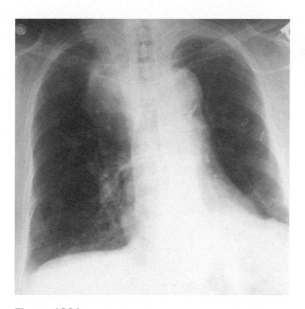

Figure 180A

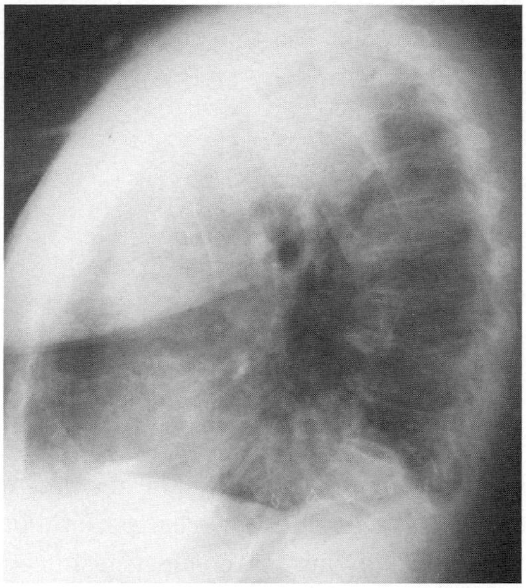

Figure 180B

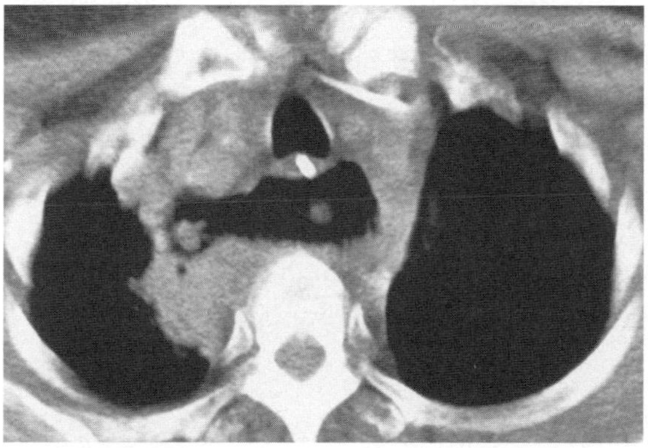

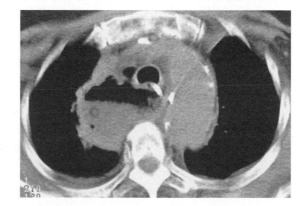

Figure 180C

Figure 180D

(Figs. 180A, 180B, 180C, and 180D courtesy of Diane C. Strollo, M.D., University of Pittsburgh Medical Center, Pittsburgh, Pennsylvania)

Radiologic Findings

PA (**Fig. 180A**) and lateral (**Fig. 180B**) chest radiographs demonstrate a large heterogeneous air-containing middle mediastinal mass, findings of prior left lower lobectomy, and bilateral pleural effusions. Unenhanced chest CT (mediastinal window) (**Figs. 180C** and **180D**) demonstrates a complex middle mediastinal mass with a large air–fluid level, irregular borders, and extension behind the trachea and esophagus. Note the obliteration of normal mediastinal tissue planes.

699

Diagnosis

Mediastinal abscess

Differential Diagnosis

- Tuberculous mediastinitis
- Status post–mediastinal biopsy or instrumentation
- Mediastinal neoplasm with necrosis or fistulous communication with aerodigestive tract

Discussion

Background

Acute mediastinal infection is an uncommon but potentially life-threatening inflammatory condition.

Etiology

The majority of cases of acute mediastinitis (acute mediastinal infection) result from surgery or iatrogenic instrumentation. Iatrogenic esophageal perforation during surgery or endoscopy and accidental perforation from swallowing sharp objects or forceful vomiting are important etiologies. Postoperative mediastinitis occurs in up to 1% of patients who undergo sternotomy for cardiac surgery. Acute mediastinitis may also result from contiguous or remote spread of infection from an infected organ or site. Other associated conditions are empyema and subphrenic abscess. Pyogenic and tuberculous vertebral infections may also result in the development of paravertebral abscesses.

Clinical Findings

Patients with acute mediastinal infection are typically quite ill, present with chest pain, high fever, and chills, and may progress to septic shock. Patients with esophageal perforation may complain of dysphagia.

Imaging Findings

RADIOGRAPHY

- Focal or diffuse mediastinal widening (**Fig. 180A**)
- Air in the soft tissues of the neck
- Pneumomediastinum (**Fig. 180A**)
- Associated pleural effusion and pulmonary consolidation (**Figs. 180A** and **180B**); pneumothorax, hydropneumothorax
- Extravasation of ingested contrast material

CT

- Esophageal thickening
- Mediastinal air (bubbly or streaky patterns) in cases of esophageal perforation (**Figs. 180C** and **180D**)
- Obliteration of mediastinal tissue planes (**Figs. 180C, 180D,** and **180E**)

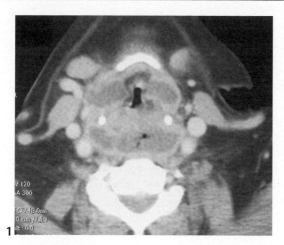
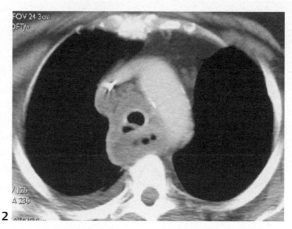

Figure 180E (1,2) Contrast-enhanced chest CT (mediastinal window) of a 70-year-old woman with mediastinal extension of a retropharyngeal abscess demonstrates a complex peripharyngeal fluid collection **(1)** with enhancing borders and internal air bubbles. The process extends into the middle mediastinum **(2)** and surrounds the trachea and esophagus. Note a small right pleural effusion. (Courtesy of Diane C. Strollo, M.D., University of Pittsburgh Medical Center, Pittsburgh, Pennsylvania.)

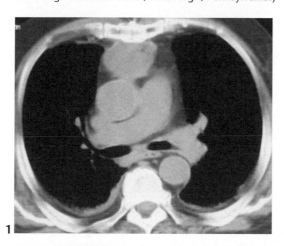
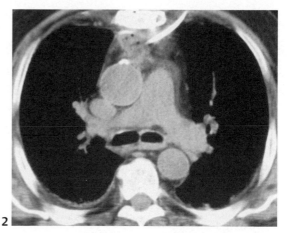

Figure 180F (1,2) Unenhanced chest CT (mediastinal window) of an 81-year-old man who developed a post-sternotomy mediastinal abscess demonstrates a retrosternal (anterior mediastinal) rounded lobular soft tissue mass **(1). (2)** Unenhanced chest CT (mediastinal window) following placement of a mediastinal drainage catheter demonstrates a smaller retrosternal collection with internal iatrogenic air bubbles. (Courtesy of Diane C. Strollo, M.D., University of Pittsburgh Medical Center, Pittsburgh, Pennsylvania.)

- Focal or multifocal abscesses
  - Low-attenuation fluid collections (**Figs. 180C, 180D,** and **180E**)
  - Internal air, air–fluid levels (**Figs. 180C, 180D, 180E,** and **180F2**)
- Extraluminal contrast material
- Associated empyema, abscess; adjacent osseous (spinal) involvement

MR

- Intermediate signal intensity on T1-weighted images
- High signal intensity on T2-weighted images

Treatment

- Percutaneous or open drainage (**Fig. 180F**)
- Antibiotics

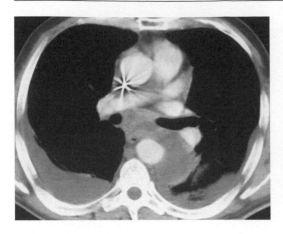

Figure 180G Contrast-enhanced chest CT (mediastinal window) of a 50-year-old man with a pancreatic pseudocyst with extension into the mediastinum demonstrates a heterogeneous mediastinal mass with enhancing borders affecting the subcarinal region, partially encasing the descending thoracic aorta, and extending posteriorly to the left paravertebral region. Note the bilateral pleural effusions and bilateral dependent atelectasis. (Courtesy of Diane C. Strollo, M.D., University of Pittsburgh Medical Center, Pittsburgh, Pennsylvania.)

Prognosis

- Poor when mediastinitis results from esophageal perforation
- High fatality rate in the presence of sepsis

PEARLS

- Substernal fluid collections and mediastinal air are normal findings in the 2-week period that follows median sternotomy. However, persistence of these findings after the 14th postoperative day is highly suggestive of mediastinitis (**Fig. 180F**).
- Mediastinal pancreatic pseudocysts are rare lesions that affect patients with a history of recurrent pancreatitis, alcohol abuse, and abdominal trauma or surgery. The pseudocyst is a peripancreatic fluid collection surrounded by a fibrous wall that lacks a true epithelial lining. An abdominal pseudocyst may communicate with the thorax via the esophageal hiatus or the aortic hiatus and may manifest as a mediastinal mass (**Fig. 180G**) with associated left or bilateral pleural effusions (**Fig. 180G**). CT demonstrates a thin-walled cyst of low-attenuation content, which is typically located in the posterior mediastinum and usually produces mass effect (**Fig. 180G**). There is typically an associated pancreatic pseudocyst or peripancreatic fluid collection.

Suggested Readings

Armstrong P. Mediastinal and hilar disorders. In: Armstrong P, Wilson AG, Dee P, Hansell DM, eds. Imaging of Diseases of the Chest, 3rd ed. London: Mosby, 2000:789–892

Fraser RS, Müller NL, Colman N, Paré PD. Masses situated predominantly in the middle-posterior mediastinal compartment. In: Fraser RS, Müller NL, Colman N, Paré PD, eds. Fraser and Paré's Diagnosis of Diseases of the Chest, 4th ed. Philadelphia: Saunders, 1999:2938–2973

Fraser RS, Müller NL, Colman N, Paré PD. Mediastinitis, pneumomediastinum and mediastinal hemorrhage. In: Fraser RS, Müller NL, Colman N, Paré PD, eds. Fraser and Paré's Diagnosis of Diseases of the Chest, 4th ed. Philadelphia: Saunders, 1999:2851–2874

Jeung M-Y, Gasser B, Gangi A, et al. Imaging of cystic masses of the mediastinum. Radiographics 2002; 22:S79–S93

SECTION XIII

Pleura, Chest Wall, and Diaphragm

CASE 181 Pleural Effusion: Heart Failure

Clinical Presentation

A 54-year-old man with increasing dyspnea

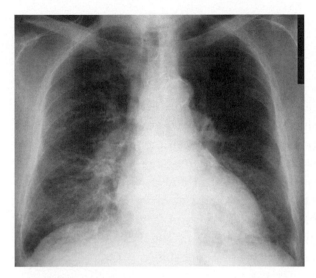

Figure 181A

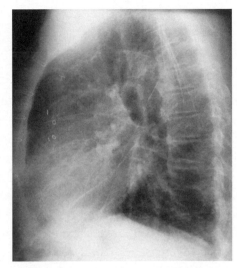

Figure 181B

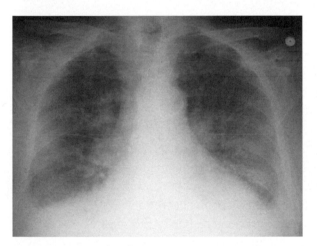

Figure 181C

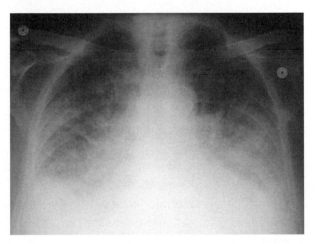

Figure 181D

Radiologic Findings

PA (**Fig. 181A**) and lateral (**Fig. 181B**) chest radiographs demonstrate cardiomegaly, increased interstitial opacities, thickening of the interlobar fissures, and findings of prior median sternotomy for coronary artery revascularization. AP portable chest radiograph obtained 1 day later (**Fig. 181C**) demonstrates mild widening of the vascular pedicle, indistinct bronchovascular margins, smooth thickening of the minor fissure, and bilateral pleural effusions. AP portable chest radiograph obtained the following day (**Fig. 181D**) shows further widening of the vascular pedicle, increasing bilateral pleural effusions, and bilateral central airspace opacities consistent with pulmonary edema.

Diagnosis

Heart failure with bilateral pleural effusions

Differential Diagnosis

None

Discussion

Background

Pleural effusion is a common manifestation of local and systemic diseases that involve the thorax, affecting an estimated 1.3 million individuals each year. A small amount of fluid (5–15 mL) is normally present within the pleural space and provides a frictionless surface between the visceral and parietal pleura as lung volume changes during respiration. Under normal circumstances, pleural fluid forms and flows from capillaries in the parietal pleura into the pleural space and is absorbed through the parietal lymphatics. The parietal pleura vasculature drains to the right side of the heart, whereas the visceral pleura vasculature drains to the left side of the heart. A variety of factors may cause an imbalance in the formation and absorption of pleural fluid: increased hydrostatic pressure, decreased oncotic pressure, decreased pleural space pressure, increased permeability of the microvascular circulation, and impaired lymphatic drainage. Fluid may also move from the peritoneal space into the pleural space through diaphragmatic lymphatics or through anatomic defects.

Etiology

Thoracentesis is usually performed to evaluate pleural effusions of unknown etiology. The fluid is examined grossly and submitted for biochemical analysis, white blood cell and red blood cell counts, Gram and acid-fast stains, and cytologic evaluation. Invasive diagnostic procedures, including closed, open, or thoracoscopic biopsy, are sometimes necessary to establish a diagnosis. Most pleural effusions are categorized as transudates or exudates using the criteria established by Light. Exudates exhibit one or more of the following characteristics: fluid-to-serum protein ratio > 0.5; pleural fluid lactate dehydrogenase (LDH) > 200 IU; fluid-to-serum LDH ratio > 0.6. Transudative pleural effusions are characteristically caused by systemic factors that alter pleural fluid formation or absorption, most commonly heart failure, cirrhosis, and pulmonary embolism. Exudative effusions result from diseases that alter the pleural surface and its permeability to protein. The most common causes are pneumonia, malignant neoplasia, and pulmonary embolism. If pleural fluid analysis reveals a transudate, the systemic disorder can be treated, and no further investigation is required. When an exudate is found, further investigation is warranted to determine its etiology. Bilateral pleural effusions may sometimes have different etiologies (Contarini's condition), for example, an exudative pleural effusion (empyema) on one side, and a transudative pleural effusion (secondary to fluid overload or heart failure) on the other side.

Clinical Findings

Patients with pleural effusion may be asymptomatic (15%) or may present with dull aching chest pain, cough, and/or dyspnea. Large pleural effusions may displace the mediastinum and cause respiratory distress. Dullness to percussion and decreased or absent breath sounds are characteristic features. Other physical findings may suggest the etiology (e.g., distended neck veins and peripheral edema in heart failure).

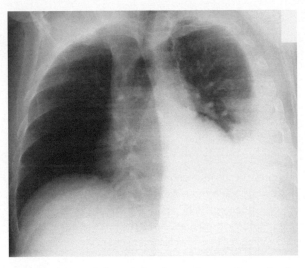

Figure 181E Left lateral decubitus chest radiograph of a 43-year-old man with a parapneumonic pleural effusion shows dependent layering of a free left pleural effusion. The left lower lobe is obscured by the pleural effusion and underlying consolidation.

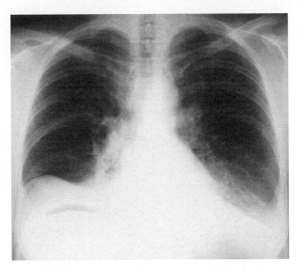

Figure 181F PA chest radiograph of a 34-year-old woman who had recent abdominal surgery demonstrates a right subpulmonic effusion that mimics elevation of the right hemidiaphragm ("pseudodiaphragm") and lateral displacement of its superior border. Pneumoperitoneum outlines the undersurface of the right hemidiaphragm and reveals the extent of the subpulmonic fluid accumulation. Note the left pleural effusion.

Pathology

- Fibrinous exudates, organizing granulation tissue, or fibrous tissue in fibrinous pleuritis (e.g., pneumonia, pericarditis, hepatitis, peritonitis, pancreatitis, collagen-vascular disease, drug reaction, and cancer)
- Granulomatous inflammation or well-formed granulomas with or without central necrosis (e.g., tuberculosis, fungal infection, sarcoidosis, Wegener granulomatosis)
- Eosinophilic infiltrates, reactive mesothelial cells, histiocytes, lymphocytes, and giant cells (e.g., eosinophilic pleuritis)

Imaging Findings

RADIOGRAPHY

- Hazy increase in radiopacity (i.e., ground-glass veil) that does not obscure bronchovascular markings on supine radiography
- Radiopacity involving posterior or lateral costophrenic sulcus with meniscus-shaped upper border (i.e., blunting) on upright radiography (**Figs. 181C** and **181D**)
- Smooth meniscus-shaped upper border that curves gently downward from its lateral aspect to the mid-cardiac region in small to moderate pleural effusions (**Figs. 181C** and **181D**)
- Posterior costodiaphragmatic sulcus blunting on lateral radiography: 25 to 50 mL
- Lateral costodiaphragmatic sulcus blunting on frontal radiography: 200 mL (**Figs. 181C** and **181D**)
- Obscuration of ipsilateral hemidiaphragm on frontal radiography: more than 500 mL (**Figs. 181C** and **181D**)
- Pleural thickening (layering) on lateral decubitus radiography: more than 5 mL (**Fig. 181E**)

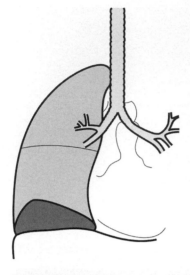

Figure 181G Diagram illustrates the location and morphology of a subpulmonic pleural effusion. The fluid accumulates in the pleural space between the visceral pleura lining the undersurface of the lower lobe and the parietal pleura covering the ipsilateral hemidiaphragm. Note the preservation of a sharp costophrenic angle and mass effect on the hemidiaphragm. There is a characteristic lateral displacement of the apex of the pleural fluid collection (pseudodiaphragm).

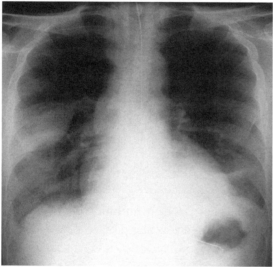
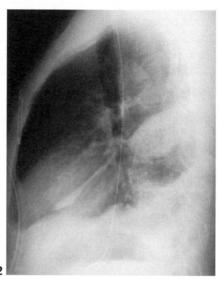

Figure 181H (1,2) PA **(1)** and lateral **(2)** chest radiographs demonstrate localized fluid collections (i.e., pseudotumors) in the right major fissure manifesting as elliptical opacities with incomplete borders **(1)** that taper toward the fissure **(2)**.

- Subpulmonic (subpulmonary) effusion
  - Lateral displacement of apex of apparent diaphragm (i.e., pseudodiaphragm) on frontal radiography (**Figs. 181F** and **181G**)
  - Left-sided effusion may be characterized by downward displacement of gastric air bubble from pseudodiaphragm contour by 2.0 cm or more.
  - Small amount of fluid may be seen in inferior aspect of major fissure on lateral radiography.
  - Convex upper margin of fluid flattens as it contacts major fissure and descends abruptly to anterior costophrenic sulcus on lateral radiography (i.e., Rock of Gibraltar sign).
- Pseudotumor
  - Elliptical opacity within interlobar fissure ("pseudotumor") (**Fig. 181H**)
- Loculated effusion
  - Nonmobile mass-like peripheral opacity

CT

- Thickening of posterior pleural space with concave or meniscoid anterior margin (**Fig. 181I**)

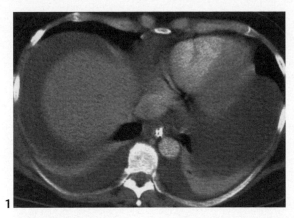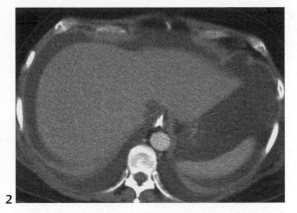

Figure 181I (1,2) Contrast-enhanced abdominal CT (soft tissue window) demonstrates bilateral pleural effusions and abdominal ascites. The pleural effusions are peripheral or lateral to the respective hemidiaphragms. Ascites is located central (medial) to the hemidiaphragms and forms a sharp interface with the anterolateral hepatic surface, but it is anatomically prevented from extending along the posterior hepatic surface because this region of the right hepatic lobe lacks a peritoneal covering and is directly apposed to the posterior abdominal wall (bare area).

- CT attenuation values between those of water [0 Hounsfield units (HU)] and soft tissue (100 HU) (**Fig. 181I**)
- Pleural thickening with anterior and cephalad tracking and extension into interlobar fissures

Treatment

- Treatment of underlying cause

Prognosis

- Good; resolution with treatment of underlying cause

PEARLS_____

- Heart failure is the most common cause of transudative pleural effusion encountered in clinical practice.
- Pleural effusion caused by heart failure is typically bilateral and associated with cardiomegaly and variable degrees of pulmonary venous hypertension (**Figs. 181C** and **181D**).
- Malignancy is the most common cause of an exudative pleural effusion, followed by infection and pulmonary thromboembolic disease. Pleural biopsy may be required for definitive diagnosis.
- Subpulmonic pleural effusions simulate hypoventilation when bilateral, and elevation of the ipsilateral hemidiaphragm ("pseudodiaphragm") when unilateral. Unilateral subpulmonic effusions may manifest on upright radiography with lateral displacement of the apex of the "pseudodiaphragm" (**Figs. 181F** and **181G**).
- Interlobar accumulations of pleural fluid (pseudotumor, vanishing tumor, phantom tumor) (**Fig. 181H**) are most commonly associated with cardiac decompensation and typically resolve spontaneously when heart failure has been relieved.
- Large pleural effusions may invert the ipsilateral hemidiaphragm (**Fig. 181G**). Inversion of the left hemidiaphragm may manifest with medial and inferior displacement of the gastric air bubble and/or deformity of the superolateral margin of the air bubble. The inverted hemidiaphragm may also move paradoxically and may impair ventilation.

Suggested Readings

Blackmore CC, Black WC, Dallas RV, Crow HC. Pleural fluid volume estimation: a chest radiograph prediction rule. Acad Radiol 1996;3:103–109

Fraser RS, Müller NL, Colman N, Paré PD. Pleural abnormalities. In: Fraser RS, Müller NL, Colman N, Paré PD, eds. Fraser and Paré's Diagnosis of Diseases of the Chest, 4th ed. Philadelphia: Saunders, 1999:563–594.

Fraser RS, Müller NL, Colman N, Paré PD. Pleural effusion. In: Fraser RS, Müller NL, Colman N, Paré PD, eds. Fraser and Paré's Diagnosis of Diseases of the Chest, 4th ed. Philadelphia: Saunders, 1999: 2739–2779

Light RW. Clinical practice: pleural effusion. N Engl J Med 2002;346:1971–1977

Travis WD, Colby TV, Koss MN, Rosado-de-Christenson ML, Müller NL, King TE Jr. Pleural disorders. In: King DW, ed. Atlas of Nontumor Pathology: Non-Neoplastic Disorders of the Lower Respiratory Tract, first series, fascicle 2. Washington, DC: American Registry of Pathology; 2002:901–921

CASE 182 Empyema: Bronchopleural Fistula

Clinical Presentation

A 40-year-old woman with cough and fever

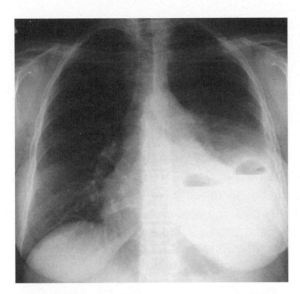

Figure 182A

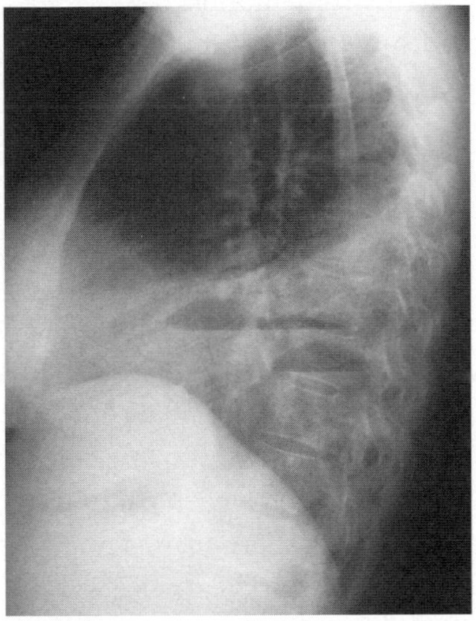

Figure 182B

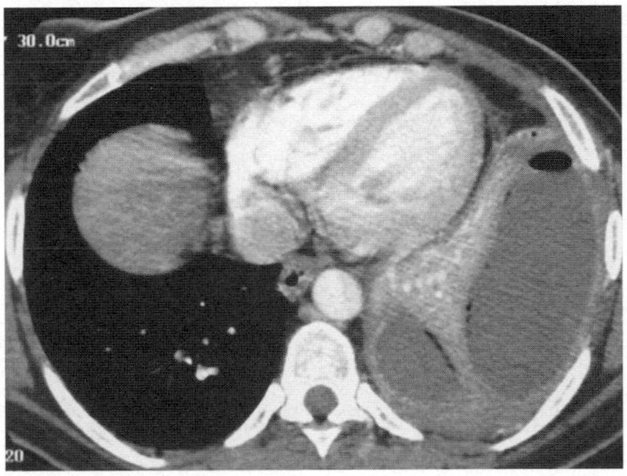

Figure 182C

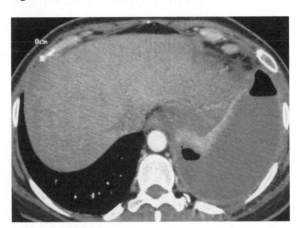

Figure 182D

Radiologic Findings

PA (**Fig. 182A**) and lateral (**Fig. 182B**) chest radiographs demonstrate a large left pleural effusion with two air–fluid levels. Note the difference in length of the superior air–fluid level on the two orthogonal radiographs (**Figs. 182A** and **182B**). Contrast-enhanced chest CT (mediastinal window) (**Figs. 182C** and **182D**) demonstrates a loculated left pleural effusion with two air–fluid levels (**Fig. 182D**) and smooth, mildly thickened enhancing visceral and parietal pleural surfaces (i.e., "split pleura sign") that surround the intervening low-attenuation fluid (**Fig. 182D**). Note the mass effect on the adjacent atelectatic left lower lobe (**Fig. 182C**).

Diagnosis

Empyema; bronchopleural fistula

Differential Diagnosis

- Loculated pleural effusion postinstrumentation
- Malignant pleural effusion with bronchopleural fistula

Discussion

Background

Pleural effusions caused by infection are generally exudative and are classified into three groups, based on pleural fluid analysis. *Simple parapneumonic effusions* are culture- and gram-negative. *Complicated parapneumonic effusions* are culture- and gram-negative but have high lactate dehydrogenase (LDH) levels, low pH ($<$ 7.2), or low glucose levels ($<$ 40 mg/dL). *Empyema* is characteristically purulent on gross inspection, has high neutrophil counts and low pH, and may be culture- or gram-positive. Differentiation between parapneumonic pleural effusions and empyemas is based on pleural fluid analysis rather than on imaging features. Empyema may be associated with bronchopleural fistula when a communication is established between the infected pleural fluid and adjacent airways. Bronchopleural fistula is the most frequent cause of abnormal air collections and air–fluid levels within empyemas. Pleural infection may result in progressive pleural thickening with formation of an inelastic fibrous membrane that may encase the lung and restrict function (pleural peel).

Etiology

Empyema is most commonly due to pleural extension of infection from adjacent pneumonia, typically caused by gram-negative bacteria, anaerobic bacteria, *Staphylococcus aureus*, *Streptococcus pneumoniae*, or *Mycobacterium tuberculosis*. Other causes include lung abscess, septic emboli, and subphrenic infection.

Clinical Findings

Affected patients present with fever, chills, cough, and pleuritic chest pain. Physical examination may reveal chest wall erythema and edema. Absence of fever or leukocytosis does not exclude the possibility of empyema. Detection of grossly purulent pleural fluid by thoracentesis is diagnostic.

Pathology

GROSS

- Purulent pleural fluid
- Fibrin deposition on visceral and parietal pleural surfaces
- Loculated pleural effusion
- Pleural thickening that may progress to formation of a pleural peel

MICROSCOPIC

- Demonstration of microorganisms in pleural fluid
- Gram-negative anaerobes in most culture-positive parapneumonic pleural effusions

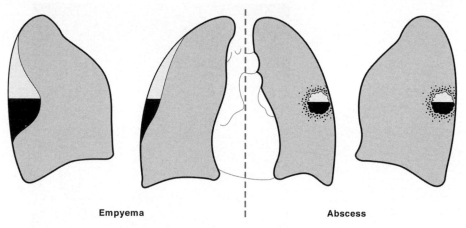

Empyema   **Abscess**

Figure 182E The morphology of empyema with bronchopleural fistula, contrasted with that of lung abscess. An empyema is an elongated or lenticular pleural fluid collection and, when associated with a bronchopleural fistula, may exhibit discrepant lengths of intrinsic air–fluid levels on orthogonal radiographs. A lung abscess is a spherical lung lesion that exhibits no discrepancy in the length of an associated air–fluid level on orthogonal radiographs.

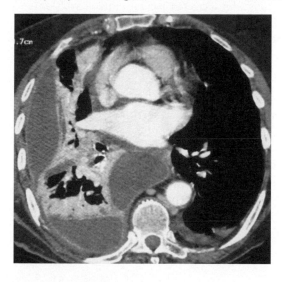

Figure 182F Contrast-enhanced chest CT (mediastinal window) of an 80-year-old woman with empyema demonstrates a multi-locular right pleural effusion that produces mass effect on the adjacent consolidated/atelectatic lung. The "split pleura" sign is demonstrated in the three areas of loculation.

Imaging Findings

RADIOGRAPHY

- Findings of uncomplicated pleural effusion (see Case 181)
- Ovoid, lenticular, or rounded pleural mass; loculated pleural effusion (**Figs. 182A** and **182B**)
- Lesion margins often better defined in one of two orthogonal radiographs, discrepant margin visualization ("incomplete border" sign)
- Bronchopleural fistula
  - Air–fluid level(s) within a pleural mass (loculated empyema) or pleural effusion (**Figs. 182A** and **182B**)
  - Disparity in length of an air–fluid level on paired orthogonal radiographs (**Figs. 182A, 182B,** and **182E**)

CT

- Pleural effusion (**Figs. 182C, 182D,** and **182F**)
- Focal or multifocal loculated pleural effusion (**Figs. 182C, 182D,** and **182F**)
- Loculated pleural fluid forms obtuse angles with adjacent pleura, exhibits a lenticular shape (**Figs. 182C, 182D,** and **182F**) and produces mass effect on the adjacent lung (**Figs. 182C** and **182F**)

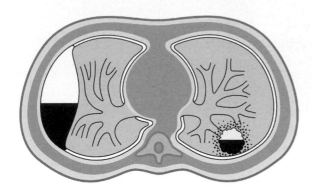

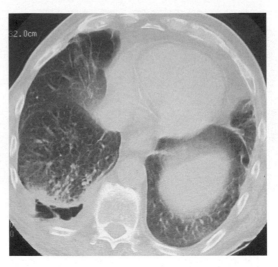

Figure 182G The CT features of empyema, contrasted with those of lung abscess. An empyema is an elongated pleural collection with tapered borders toward the adjacent pleura and smooth, uniformly thickened walls formed by the visceral and parietal pleural surfaces. The pleural collection displaces adjacent parenchymal structures. A lung abscess is spherical in morphology, has thick walls, forms acute borders in relation to the adjacent pleural surface, and does not displace parenchymal structures.

Figure 182H Unenhanced chest CT (lung window) of a 57-year-old HIV-positive man with bronchopleural fistula and empyema necessitatis demonstrates a right posterior loculated pleural effusion with an air–fluid level. Note the thin soft tissue septa that compartmentalize the loculated hydropneumothorax and that the pleural process extends into the soft tissues of the adjacent chest wall.

- Uniformly thickened visceral and parietal pleura; exhibits contrast enhancement and surrounds pleural fluid collection, the so-called "split pleura" sign (**Figs. 182D** and **182F**)
- Air–fluid level within pleural fluid collection (bronchopleural fistula) (**Figs. 182C, 182D,** and **182G**)

Treatment

- Prompt closed chest tube drainage
- Antibiotics, empiric initially followed by specific antibiotics based on culture results
- Early administration of fibrinolytic agents (streptokinase, urokinase) through the drainage tube
- Thoracotomy or thoracoscopic lysis of adhesions for patients who fail to respond to antibiotics and closed drainage; open drainage required in up to 30% of affected patients
- Surgical decortication in late-stage empyema with significantly thickened pleura
- Open thoracotomy and thoracoplasty with muscle flap transposition procedures for drainage of chronic empyema with or without complicating bronchopleural fistula

Prognosis

- Good; frequent response to antibiotics and closed chest tube therapy
- Slower recovery for patients requiring open drainage
- Adequate drainage of bronchopleural fistulas imperative to avoid back-spillage into lung and resultant diffuse pneumonia
- Variable prognosis depending on age, underlying disease, and organism; increased morbidity/mortality when drainage is inadequate
- Pleural squamous cell carcinoma and malignant lymphoma, may complicate untreated or chronic empyema.

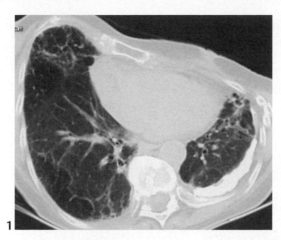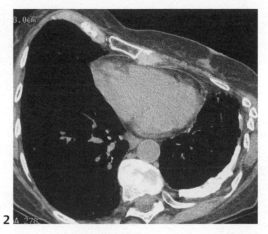

Figure 182I (1,2) Unenhanced chest CT [lung **(1)** and mediastinal **(2)** window] of an 83-year-old woman with fibrothorax related to childhood tuberculosis demonstrates volume loss in the left hemithorax and ipsilateral pleural thickening and calcification (e.g., calcific pleuritis). The patient had decreased left respiratory excursions.

PEARLS

- Radiographic evaluation of internal air–fluid levels in thoracic disorders may allow distinction of empyema with bronchopleural fistula from lung abscess. Empyemas exhibit lenticular shapes, disparate lengths of air–fluid levels, and tapering smooth borders (**Figs. 182A, 182B,** and **182E**). Lung abscesses exhibit spherical shapes, air–fluid levels of equal lengths on orthogonal views, and irregular borders. On cross-sectional imaging, empyemas exhibit loculation, lenticular shapes, and displace adjacent lung (**Figs. 182C, 182D, 182F,** and **182G**), whereas lung abscesses do not.

- Postsurgical bronchopleural fistula develops in 2.5 to 3% of patients who undergo lobectomy or pneumonectomy, and typically manifest within the first 2 weeks after surgery. They are usually caused by necrosis of the bronchial stump or dehiscence of the suture line and most commonly occur following surgery for infectious disease, especially tuberculosis.

- Ultrasonography often reveals septations within empyemas. CT does not reveal such septations directly, but often shows indirect evidence of their presence by demonstrating small air and fluid collections trapped within multiple spaces (**Figs. 182C, 182D, 182F,** and **182H**).

- Untreated and inappropriately treated empyemas may drain spontaneously into the subcutaneous tissues of the adjacent chest wall (e.g., empyema necessitatis) (**Fig. 182H**). This complication is most commonly associated with tuberculosis, actinomycosis, aspergillosis, blastomycosis, and nocardiosis, and may result in a palpable mass with associated erythema. Prior to the advent of antibiotics, empyema necessitatis was most commonly associated with tuberculosis. Today, it is most often encountered in immunocompromised individuals.

- Tuberculosis is also associated with chronic changes of healed tuberculosis that characteristically manifest as parenchymal scarring and associated pleural thickening, which may be extensive (fibrothorax) and frequently calcifies (e.g., calcific pleuritis) (**Fig. 182I**).

Suggested Readings

Fraser RS, Müller NL, Colman N, Paré PD. Pleural abnormalities. In: Fraser RS, Müller NL, Colman N, Paré PD, eds. Fraser and Paré's Diagnosis of Diseases of the Chest, 4th ed. Philadelphia: Saunders, 1999:563–594

Fraser RS, Müller NL, Colman N, Paré PD. Pleural effusion. In: Fraser RS, Müller NL, Colman N, Paré PD, eds. Fraser and Paré's Diagnosis of Diseases of the Chest, 4th ed. Philadelphia: Saunders, 1999:2739–2779

Travis WD, Colby TV, Koss MN, Rosado-de-Christenson ML, Müller NL, King TE Jr. Pleural disorders. In: King DW, ed. Atlas of Nontumor Pathology: Non-Neoplastic Disorders of the Lower Respiratory Tract, first series, fascicle 2. Washington, DC: American Registry of Pathology; 2002:901–921

CASE 183 Asbestos-Related Pleural Disease

Clinical Presentation

A 78-year-old man with a history of colon cancer

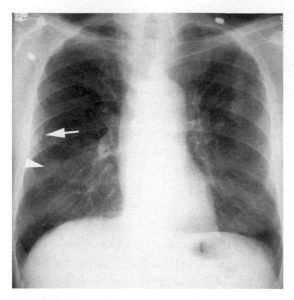

Figure 183A

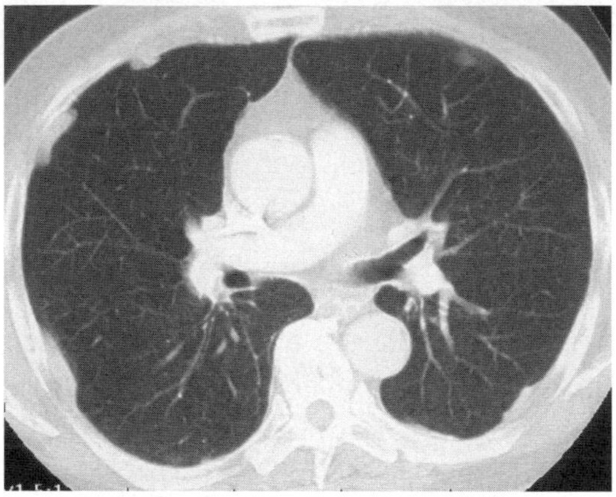

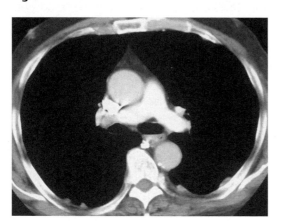

Figure 183C

Figure 183B

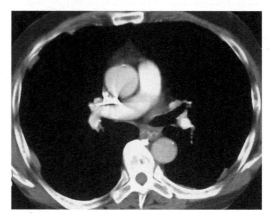

Figure 183D

Radiologic Findings

PA chest radiograph (**Fig. 183A**) demonstrates multifocal bilateral nodular opacities. Note discrepant visualization of the lesion borders [some ill-defined lesion borders (arrowhead) and sharp margination (arrow) of others] consistent with an extrapulmonary location. Contrast-enhanced chest CT [lung (**Fig. 183B**) and mediastinal (**Figs. 183C** and **183D**) window] demonstrates multifocal discontinuous areas of pleural thickening, many of which are adjacent to ribs.

Diagnosis

Pleural plaques

Differential Diagnosis

None

Discussion

Background

Benign asbestos-related pleural diseases include noncalcified and calcified pleural plaques, benign asbestos pleural effusion, diffuse pleural fibrosis or thickening, and parenchymal rounded atelectasis as a sequela of an asbestos pleural effusion (see Section IV, Case 49). Pleural plaques are the macroscopic and radiologic hallmarks of past asbestos exposure and typically develop 15 to 20 years after the initial exposure. Pleural plaques tend to occur on the parietal pleural surface adjacent to relatively rigid structures such as the ribs, vertebrae, and the tendinous portion of the diaphragms. Subsequent calcium deposition often occurs in pleural plaques, beginning as fine, punctate flecks that may coalesce over time to form dense streaks or plate-like deposits.

Benign asbestos pleural effusions are dose-related manifestations of asbestos exposure that may develop within a shorter latency period than that of other asbestos-related pleural diseases (1 to 20 years). The effusions are usually small (i.e., less than 500 mL), unilateral, sometimes hemorrhagic, and are typically exudates. Benign asbestos pleural effusions may persist from 2 weeks to 6 months and are recurrent in 15 to 30% of cases. The diagnosis is established based on a history of exposure and through exclusion of other etiologies, particularly malignancy. Diffuse pleural thickening and diffuse pleural fibrosis are thought to develop after a previous asbestos-related pleural effusion, involve the visceral pleura, and affect the pleural surface adjacent to the costophrenic angle, a distinguishing feature from pleural plaques. Rounded atelectasis is an unusual form of atelectasis that most commonly occurs in asbestos-exposed individuals but is also associated with other etiologies (see Case 49).

Etiology

The pathogenesis of pleural plaques is unclear. It has been hypothesized that plaques result from mechanical irritation of the parietal pleura by asbestos fibers. Recent studies suggest that short asbestos fibers (chrysotile) reach the parietal pleura by passage through lymphatic channels, where they cause an inflammatory reaction, whereas larger fibers (amphiboles) are retained in the lung.

Clinical Findings

Patients with pleural plaques are typically asymptomatic and have a history of asbestos exposure. Pleural plaques are invariably found more frequently in men than in women and exhibit increasing incidence and extent with advancing age.

Pathology

GROSS

- Multifocal, discontinuous bilateral parietal pleural thickening
- White, irregular nodules or masses along the parietal pleura lining the inner surface of ribs, extending across intercostal muscles and along the parietal pleura over the central tendinous portion of the diaphragm

MICROSCOPIC

- Acellular bundles of collagen in undulating "basket weave" pattern

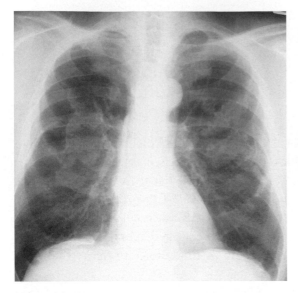

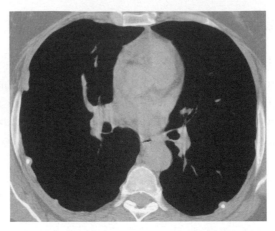

Figure 183E PA chest radiograph of a 75-year-old man with pleural plaques demonstrates the "holly-leaf" appearance of partially calcified plaques when radiographed *en face*. Note the densely calcified pleural plaques over the central tendinous portion of the hemidiaphragms.

Figure 183F Unenhanced chest CT (mediastinal window) of a 60-year-old man with pleural plaques demonstrates small bilateral, multifocal, discontinuous pleural nodules, some of which exhibit central calcification.

Imaging Findings

RADIOGRAPHY

- Bilateral, discontinuous multifocal areas of pleural thickening characteristically distributed on the posterolateral chest wall (7th to 10th ribs), the lateral chest wall (6th to 9th ribs), the domes of the diaphragms, and the mediastinal pleura (**Figs. 183A** and **183E**)
- Characteristic sparing of the pleural surfaces adjacent to the lung apices and costophrenic angles (**Figs. 183A** and **183E**)
- Variable calcification (**Figs. 183A** and **183E**)
- Characteristic serpentine marginal calcification (so-called "holly-leaf" pattern of calcification) in peripherally calcified plaques imaged *en face* (**Fig. 183E**)

CT

- Multifocal discontinuous bilateral pleural nodules; most profuse along costovertebral pleural surfaces and posterolateral chest wall (**Figs. 183B, 183C, 183D, 183F, 183G,** and **183H**)
- Pleural plaques along the anterior aspects of the upper ribs on CT, an area poorly visualized on radiography (**Figs. 183B, 183D,** and **183G**)
- More conspicuous calcification of plaques than on radiography (**Figs. 183F, 183G,** and **183H**)

Treatment

- None

Prognosis

- Good; no proven long-term sequelae
- Conflicting reports regarding likelihood of development of malignant pleural mesothelioma in patients with pleural plaques

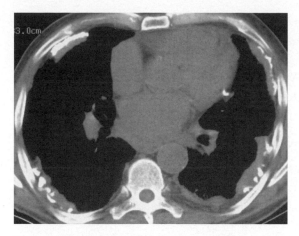

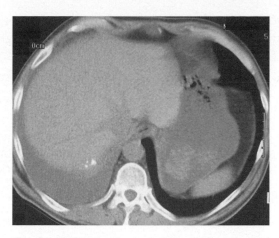

Figure 183G Unenhanced chest CT (mediastinal window) of a 68-year-old man with pleural plaques demonstrates bilateral large, thick discontinuous foci of pleural thickening with dense calcification extending along multiple ribs.

Figure 183H Unenhanced chest CT (mediastinal window) of a 63-year-old man with an asbestos-related pleural effusion demonstrates a right-sided pleural effusion and a calcified pleural plaque over the tendinous portion of the right hemidiaphragm.

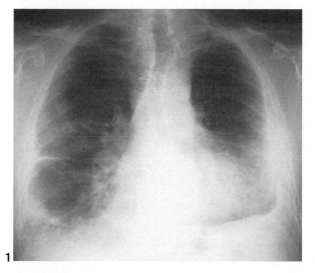

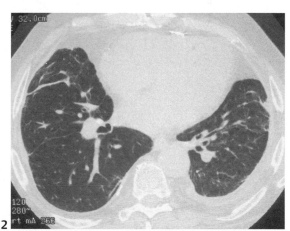

Figure 183I (1,2) PA chest radiograph **(1)** of a 72-year-old man with dyspnea and asbestosis demonstrates diffuse bilateral smooth pleural thickening that produces blunting of the costophrenic angles. **(2)** High-resolution chest CT (lung window) demonstrates diffuse continuous bilateral pleural thickening more pronounced on the left. Note interstitial peripheral parenchymal bands, nonseptal juxtapleural linear opacities, and architectural distortion.

PEARLS_____

- Asbestos-related pleural effusion (**Fig. 183H**) is a diagnosis of exclusion and can only be attributed to asbestos when there is a history of asbestos exposure and all other etiologies have been excluded, particularly malignancy.

- Diffuse pleural fibrosis typically manifests as diffuse pleural thickening that results in blunting of the costophrenic angles (**Figs. 183I1 and 183I2**), and may mimic malignant pleural mesothelioma on histologic evaluation.

- Asbestosis (**Figs. 183I1 and 183I2**) (see Case 136) should not be confused with asbestos-related pleural disease. The former refers to interstitial lung disease characterized by pulmonary fibrosis resulting from occupational exposure to asbestos. The latter does not affect the lung and typically occurs in asymptomatic individuals.

Suggested Readings

Chapman SJ, Cookson WO, Musk AW, Lee YC. Benign asbestos pleural diseases. Curr Opin Pulm Med 2003;9:266–271

Cugell DW, Kamp DW. Asbestos and the pleura: a review. Chest 2004;125:1103–1117

Peacock C, Copley SJ, Hansell DM. Asbestos-related benign pleural disease. Clin Radiol 2000;55: 422–432

Travis WD, Colby TV, Koss MN, Rosado-de-Christenson ML, Müller NL, King TE Jr. Pleural disorders. In: King DW, ed. Atlas of Nontumor Pathology: Non-Neoplastic Disorders of the Lower Respiratory Tract, first series, fascicle 2. Washington, DC: American Registry of Pathology; 2002:901–921

CASE 184 Pneumothorax

Clinical Presentation

A 47-year-old man with sudden onset of dyspnea

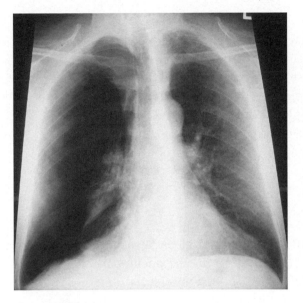

Figure 184A

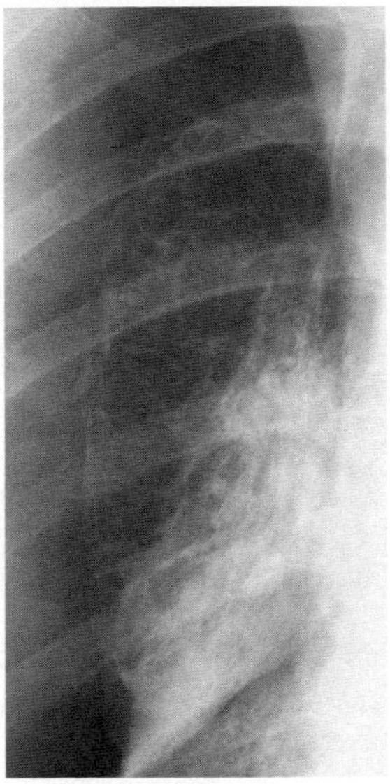

Figure 184B

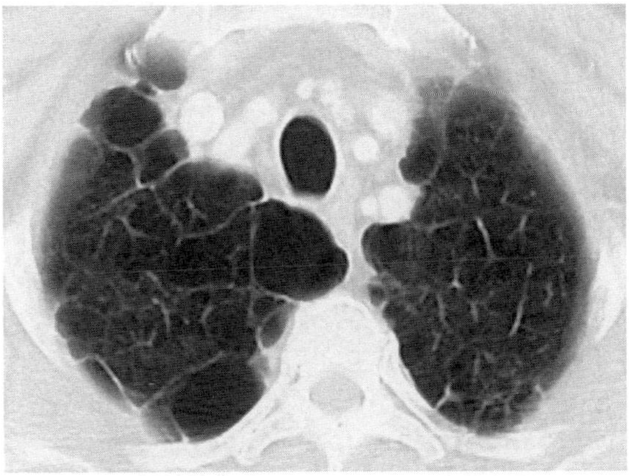

Figure 184C

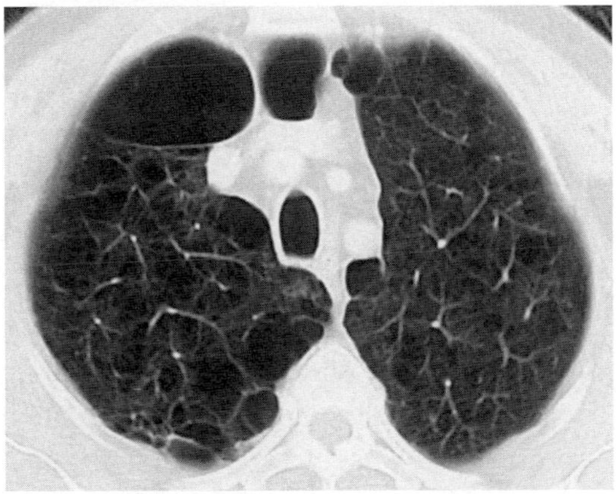

Figure 184D

Radiologic Findings

PA chest radiograph (**Fig. 184A**) demonstrates a large right pneumothorax with severe right lung volume loss. Coned-down PA chest radiograph (**Fig. 184B**) shows right upper lobe bullae and the visceral pleural (pleural line) of the atelectatic right lung. Note complete absence of bronchovascular markings lateral to the pleural line. Unenhanced chest CT (lung window) (**Figs. 184C** and **184D**) after chest tube placement and evacuation of the pneumothorax demonstrates bilateral upper lobe emphysema and right upper lobe bullae.

Diagnosis

Pneumothorax with bullous emphysema

Differential Diagnosis

None

Discussion

Background

Pneumothorax is defined as air within the pleural space and may be classified as spontaneous or traumatic (the latter includes iatrogenic pneumothorax). Spontaneous pneumothorax may be further classified as primary (in patients without coexisting lung disease) or secondary (in patients with known lung disease). The incidence of spontaneous pneumothorax is approximately 9 cases per 100,000 persons/year. *Tension pneumothorax* may occur following blunt or penetrating lung trauma when air enters the pleural space and is unable to escape, resulting in increased intrapleural pressure. With sufficient increased intrapleural pressure, venous return to the heart may be compromised, with resultant cardiovascular collapse.

Etiology

Most primary spontaneous pneumothoraces result from rupture of apical bullae or blebs. Secondary spontaneous pneumothorax may result from cavitary infections (*Pneumocystis jiroveci* pneumonia, tuberculosis, necrotizing pneumonia), primary or secondary malignancy, diffuse interstitial lung diseases (sarcoidosis, Langerhans' cell histiocytosis, lymphangioleiomyomatosis), and miscellaneous conditions (asthma, cystic fibrosis, pleural endometriosis). Tension pneumothorax usually results from traumatic lung injury that produces a one-way valve in which air enters the pleural space with each inspiration but does not escape during expiration.

Clinical Findings

Most patients with pneumothorax present with sudden onset of chest pain and dyspnea, often with associated tachypnea and tachycardia. Physical examination reveals diminished or absent breath sounds and hyperresonance of the affected hemithorax. Spontaneous pneumothorax typically affects young individuals who are tall and thin, and most frequently male (male-to-female-ratio of 6:1). Mass effect on the lung and mediastinum in patients with tension pneumothorax may compromise vascular return to the heart, eventually leading to cyanosis, hypotension, shock, and death.

Pathologic Features

- Emphysema with bulla formation (80% of cases)
- Pleural fibrosis
- Eosinophilic pleuritis

Imaging Findings

RADIOGRAPHY

- Visible thin, white visceral pleural line (**Figs. 184A, 184B, 184E, 184F, 184G, 184H,** and **184I1**)
- Peripheral radiolucency and absent bronchovascular markings beyond visceral pleural line (**Figs. 184A, 184B, 184E, 184F, 184G, 184H,** and **184I1**)

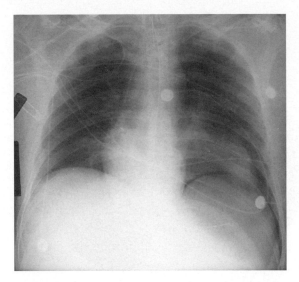

Figure 184E Portable AP supine chest radiograph of a 32-year-old man with pneumothorax demonstrates hyperlucency over the left hemidiaphragm that extends caudally into the costophrenic sulcus ("deep sulcus" sign). Note visible pleural line surrounding the left lower lobe.

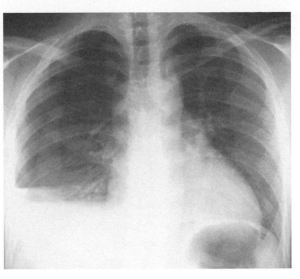

Figure 184F PA chest radiograph of a 20-year-old man with a hydropneumothorax following penetrating thoracic injury demonstrates an air–fluid level in the right pleural space consistent with a hemopneumothorax.

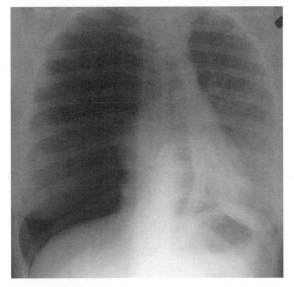

Figure 184G Portable AP chest radiograph of a young woman who sustained a penetrating injury to the chest demonstrates a right tension pneumothorax displacing the mediastinum and anterior junction line toward the contralateral hemithorax.

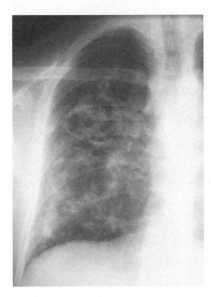

Figure 184H Coned-down PA chest radiograph of a 47-year-old woman with stage IV sarcoidosis demonstrates reticulonodular opacities and cystic changes in the right upper lung and a spontaneous right pneumothorax.

- Increased conspicuity of pneumothorax on expiratory radiography
- Radiolucency extending inferiorly within lateral costophrenic sulcus in supine patients: "deep sulcus" sign (**Fig. 184E**)
- Air–fluid level in the pleural space in hydropneumothorax or hemopneumothorax (**Fig. 184F**)
- Contralateral tracheal and/or mediastinal shift (**Figs. 184E** and **184G**) and/or ipsilateral diaphragmatic inversion in tension pneumothorax

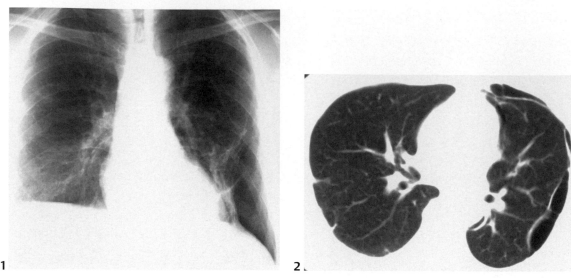

Figure 184I (1,2) PA chest radiograph **(1)** and unenhanced chest CT (lung window) **(2)** of a 52-year-old man with a loculated left pneumothorax demonstrate the localized pleural air collection. The location and configuration of the pneumothorax did not change on supine CT imaging. Note the pleural adhesions that resulted in loculation **(2)**.

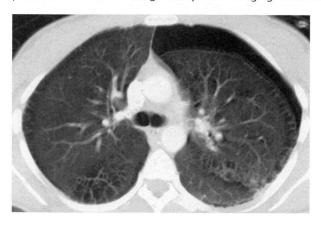

Figure 184J Contrast-enhanced chest CT (lung window) of a 21-year-old woman smoker demonstrates a small to moderate left pneumothorax and bilateral severe proximal and distal acinar emphysema.

- Cavitary, cystic, or infiltrative lung disease in cases of secondary spontaneous pneumothorax (**Fig. 184H**)
- Loculation of pneumothorax in patients with pleural adhesions (**Fig. 184I1**)

CT

- Direct visualization of air within the pleural space; high sensitivity for small pneumothorax (**Figs. 184I2** and **184J**)
- Assessment and characterization of pneumothorax (**Figs. 184I2** and **184J**)
- Evaluation of adjacent lung in cases of spontaneous pneumothorax (**Figs. 184C, 184D, 184I2, and 184J**); demonstration of emphysema in up to 80% of patients with spontaneous pneumothorax (**Figs. 184C, 184D,** and **184J**)

Treatment

- Observation for small (< 20%) pneumothorax
- Supplemental oxygen; accelerates rate of pleural air resorption by a factor of 4
- Removal of air by simple aspiration (16-gauge needle), chest tube drainage, pleurodesis for patients with moderate to large pneumothorax (> 20%); emergent chest tube evacuation of tension pneumothorax

Prognosis

- Recurrence of primary spontaneous pneumothorax in up to 25% of patients within 2 years, most frequently involving the ipsilateral hemithorax (75%)
- Hypotension, shock, and death in untreated tension pneumothorax

PEARLS_____

- Decubitus or cross-table lateral chest radiographs may be useful in patients who cannot be imaged in the upright position. Supine radiographs are used in the settings of trauma and intensive care facilities and demonstrate abnormal radiolucency in the lower hemithorax that often extends into the lateral costophrenic sulcus ("deep sulcus" sign) (**Figs. 184E** and **184G**).
- Catamenial pneumothorax affects women and occurs at or around the time of menstruation. It has been attributed to air migrating to the pleural space through the vagina, uterus, fallopian tubes, and/or diaphragmatic fenestrations as well as to pleural endometriosis.
- Reexpansion pulmonary edema may occur following rapid evacuation of a pneumothorax and reexpansion of previously atelectatic lung. Reexpansion pulmonary edema typically occurs acutely, but its appearance may be delayed for up to 24 hours.

PITFALLS_____

- Pneumothorax is optimally demonstrated on upright inspiratory and/or expiratory PA or AP chest radiography. Perception of the visceral pleural line may be difficult since volume loss associated with pneumothorax does not always result in an increase in lung opacity. Concomitant pleural effusion or parenchymal disease may obscure the visceral pleural line. Radiographic detection of pneumothorax may be difficult in patients with bullous or cystic lung disease.
- Skinfolds, chest tube tracks, the scapular edge, and rib companion shadows are frequent mimics of pneumothorax.

Suggested Readings

Fraser RS, Müller NL, Colman N, Paré PD. Pneumothorax. In: Fraser RS, Müller NL, Colman N, Paré PD, eds. Fraser and Paré's Diagnosis of Diseases of the Chest, 4th ed. Philadelphia: Saunders, 1999: 2781–2794

Kong A. The deep sulcus sign. Radiology 2003;228:415–416

Maeder M, Ullmer E. Pneumomediastinum and bilateral pneumothorax as a complication of cocaine smoking. Respiration 2003;70:407

Travis WD, Colby TV, Koss MN, Rosado-de-Christenson ML, Müller NL, King TE Jr. Pleural disorders. In: King DW, ed. Atlas of Nontumor Pathology: Non-Neoplastic Disorders of the Lower Respiratory Tract, first series, fascicle 2. Washington, DC: American Registry of Pathology; 2002:901–921

Trotman-Dickenson B. Radiology in the intensive care unit (part I). J Intensive Care Med 2003;18: 198–210

CASE 185 Malignant Pleural Mesothelioma

Clinical Presentation

A 73-year-old woman with malaise and left-sided pleuritic chest pain

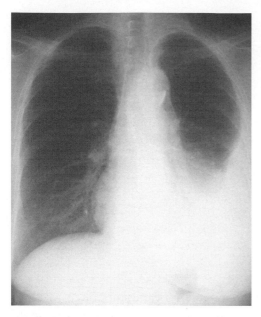

Figure 185A

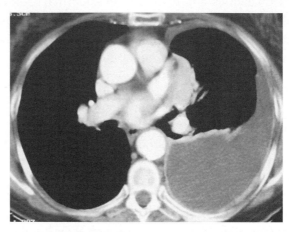

Figure 185B

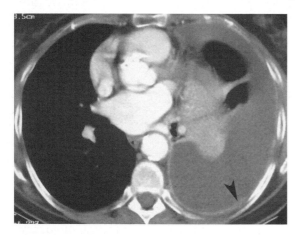

Figure 185C

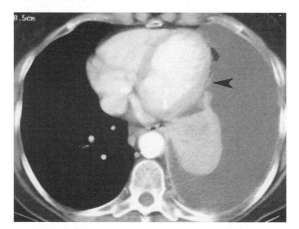

Figure 185D

Radiologic Findings

PA (**Fig. 185A**) chest radiograph demonstrates a moderate left pleural effusion. Note mild pleural thickening along the superolateral left pleural surface. Contrast-enhanced chest CT (mediastinal window) (**Figs. 185B, 185C,** and **185D**) demonstrates the left pleural effusion and subtle nodular pleural thickening (arrowheads).

Diagnosis

Malignant pleural mesothelioma

Differential Diagnosis

- Pleural effusion of nonneoplastic etiology
- Malignant pleural effusion; pleural metastases (adenocarcinoma, carcinoma of other cell type, lymphoma)

Discussion

Background

Malignant pleural mesothelioma is a relatively rare pleural malignancy, but it is the most common primary pleural neoplasm.

Etiology

The majority of cases of malignant pleural mesothelioma (80–90%) are related to the carcinogenic effects of asbestos, and most lesions occur in individuals with documented occupational or environmental asbestos exposure. Approximately 6% of asbestos workers develop mesothelioma. Although a higher incidence of mesothelioma is observed in patients with continuous exposure to asbestos, intermittent, brief, and indirect exposures have also been implicated in the development of this neoplasm. Occupations with increased exposure to asbestos include construction, shipyard, and insulation work. The latency period between onset of exposure and the development of mesothelioma is between 20 and 40 years. Both amphibole and chrysotile asbestos fibers are associated with the development of mesothelioma. Amphiboles are long, needle-like fibers that penetrate deeply in the lung, resist clearance, and are considered more tumorigenic than the serpiginous chrysotile asbestos fibers.

Clinical Findings

Patients with malignant pleural mesothelioma often have an insidious onset of symptoms—commonly dyspnea and chest pain. Affected patients may also present with cough and constitutional symptoms such as weight loss and fatigue. Most (approximately 75%) of affected patients are men, typically between the ages of 40 and 60 years. A history of asbestos exposure can be documented in 40 to 80% of patients with mesothelioma.

Pathology

GROSS

- Multiple pleural nodules (affecting the parietal pleura more extensively than visceral pleura); frequent coalescence into larger tumor masses
- Bulk of tumor in inferior hemithorax; involvement of interlobar fissures; encasement of ipsilateral lung
- Direct invasion of lung, mediastinum, pericardium, chest wall, contralateral pleura, diaphragm, peritoneal cavity, and abdominal organs

MICROSCOPIC

- Epithelioid (> 50%), sarcomatoid, mixed or biphasic and undifferentiated cell types
- Epithelioid is most frequent; uniform cuboidal or polyhedral cells, moderate cytoplasm, central nuclei, distinct nucleoli
- Difficult distinction of mesothelioma from adenocarcinoma and mesothelial hyperplasia; requires immunohistochemical techniques

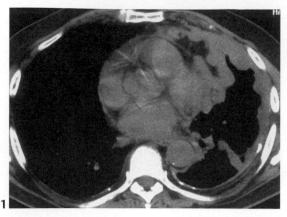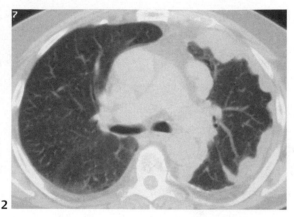

Figure 185E (1,2) Unenhanced chest CT [mediastinal **(1)** and lung **(2)** window] of a 62-year-old man with malignant pleural mesothelioma demonstrates circumferential nodular left pleural thickening with involvement of the major fissure and direct mediastinal invasion (T4; stage IV by imaging). Note decreased size and encasement of the left lung and bilateral calcified pleural plaques. The patient worked in the shipbuilding industry for 35 years and had documented asbestos exposure.

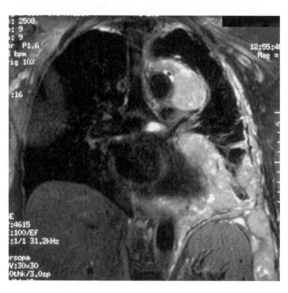

Figure 185F Coronal T2-weighted MR image of an elderly man with malignant pleural mesothelioma demonstrates circumferential left pleural thickening by high-signal nodular masses. Note extension into the inferior left costodiaphragmatic recess, involvement of the mediastinal pleura, and invasion of the diaphragm and mediastinum (T4; stage IV by imaging). (Courtesy of Jeremy J. Erasmus M.D., M.D. Anderson Cancer Center, Houston, Texas.)

Imaging Findings

RADIOGRAPHY

- Unilateral pleural effusion (40%) (**Fig. 185A**)
- Unilateral pleural thickening (**Fig. 185A**); diffuse, nodular, circumferential, fissural
- Decrease in size of affected hemithorax

CT

- Pleural effusion (**Figs. 185B, 185C,** and **185D**)
- Plaque-like (**Figs. 185B, 185C,** and **185D**) or nodular (**Fig. 185E**) pleural thickening
- Smooth or lobulated pleural thickening of greater than 1 cm (**Fig. 185E**)
- Mediastinal pleural involvement (**Figs. 185D** and **185E**)
- Lung encasement, extension into interlobar fissures (**Fig. 185E**)
- Invasion of chest wall, mediastinum (**Fig. 185E**), diaphragm, or pericardium
- Concomitant pleural plaques in 25% of cases (**Fig. 185E1**)

Table 185-1 International TNM Staging System for Diffuse Malignant Pleural Mesothelioma

T (Tumor)	
T1a	Limited to ipsilateral parietal pleura
	No visceral pleura involvement
T1b	Involves ipsilateral parietal pleura
	Scattered foci involving visceral pleura
T2	Involves each ipsilateral pleural surface and at least one of the following:
	Diaphragmatic muscle
	Confluent visceral tumor (including fissures) or extension into underlying lung
T3*	Involving all of the ipsilateral pleural surfaces and at least one of the following:
	Involves endothoracic fascia
	Extension into mediastinal fat
	Solitary focus extending into soft tissues of chest wall
	Nontransmural pericardial involvement
T4†	Involving all of the ipsilateral pleural surfaces and at least one of the following:
	Diffuse extension into chest wall with or without rib destruction
	Direct transdiaphragmatic spread into peritoneum
	Direct extension to contralateral pleura
	Direct extension to one or more mediastinal organs
	Direct extension to spine
	Extends through to internal pericardial surface, with or without pericardial effusion, or myocardial involvement
N (Lymph nodes)	
NX	Regional lymph nodes cannot be assessed
N0	No regional lymph nodes
N1	Ipsilateral bronchopulmonary or hilar nodes
N2	Subcarinal or ipsilateral mediastinal nodes
N3	Contralateral mediastinal, contralateral internal thoracic, ipsilateral or contralateral supraclavicular nodes
M (Metastases)	
MX	Cannot assess for distant metastases
M0	No distant metastases
M1	Distant metastases present

*Locally advanced but potentially resectable disease
†Locally advanced but technically unresectable disease
Adapted from Rusch VW, Venkatraman E. The importance of surgical staging in the treatment of malignant pleural mesothelioma. J Thorac Cardiovasc Surg 1996; 111:815

MR

- Minimally increased signal relative to chest wall muscles on T1-weighted images
- Moderately increased signal relative to muscle on T2-weighted images (**Fig. 185F**)
- Improved detection of local invasion of chest wall, diaphragm, and mediastinum (**Fig. 185F**)

Treatment

- Surgery: pleurectomy (stripping of the parietal pleura), extrapleural pneumonectomy (en bloc removal of the affected lung, parietal pleura, pericardium, and a portion of the ipsilateral hemidiaphragm)
- Radiation therapy
- Chemotherapy; systemic, intrapleural

Table 185-2 International TNM Staging System for Diffuse Malignant Pleural Mesothelioma

Stage	TNM
Ia	T1aN0M0
Ib	T1bN0M0
II	T2N0M0
III	Any T3 M0
	Any N1M0
	Any N2M0
IV	Any T4
	Any N3
	Any M1

Adapted from Rusch VW, Venkatraman E. The importance of surgical staging in the treatment of malignant pleural mesothelioma. J Thorac Cardiovasc Surg 1996; 111:815

- Immunotherapy
- Photodynamic therapy, gene therapy, multimodality therapy

Prognosis

- Poor; 12-month median survival after diagnosis
- Better with early diagnosis and extrapleural pneumonectomy
- Reports of median survival of 18 to 19 months with radical pleurectomy-decortication and aggressive radiation therapy with or without chemotherapy

PEARLS_____

- The imaging features of malignant mesothelioma cannot be reliably distinguished from those of pleural metastases (adenocarcinoma, metastatic lymphoma, invasive thymoma).
- The clinical staging of mesothelioma (see **Tables 185-1** and **185-2**) relies primarily on CT, but MR and positron emission tomography (PET) imaging may add important additional diagnostic and prognostic information.
- The diagnosis is often established through open lung or video assisted thoracoscopic (VATS) biopsy, whereas fine-needle biopsies are usually inadequate.
- Because of the reported predilection of malignant pleural mesothelioma to seed biopsy needle tracts, thoracostomy tube tracts, and thoracoscopy ports, localized radiation therapy is often advocated for these specific sites following instrumentation.

Suggested Readings

Antman KH, Pass HI, Schiff PB. Malignant mesothelioma. In: DeVita VT, Hellman S, Rosenberg SA, eds. Cancer: Principles and Practice of Oncology. New York: Lippincott Williams & Wilkins, 2001: 1943–1969

Fraser RS, Müller NL, Colman N, Paré PD. Pleural neoplasms. In: Fraser RS, Müller NL, Colman N, Paré PD, eds. Fraser and Paré's Diagnosis of Diseases of the Chest, 4th ed. Philadelphia: Saunders, 1999:2807–2847

Miller BH, Rosado-de-Christenson ML, Mason AC, Fleming MV, White CC, Krasna MJ. Malignant pleural mesothelioma: radiologic-pathologic correlation. Radiographics 1996;16:613–644

Sharma A, Fidias P, Hayman LA, Loomis SL, Taber KH, Aquino SL. Patterns of lymphadenopathy in thoracic malignancies. Radiographics 2004;24:419–434

Stewart DJ, Edwards JG, Smythe WR, Waller DA, O'Byrne KJ. Malignant pleural mesothelioma—an update. Int J Occup Environ Health 2004;10:26–39

Wang ZJ, Reddy GP, Gotway MB, et al. Malignant pleura mesothelioma: evaluation with CT, MR Imaging, and PET. Radiographics 2004;24:105–119

CASE 186 Pleural Metastases

Clinical Presentation

A 48-year-old woman with recently diagnosed lung cancer

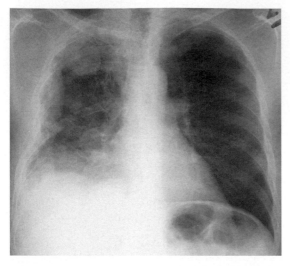

Figure 186A

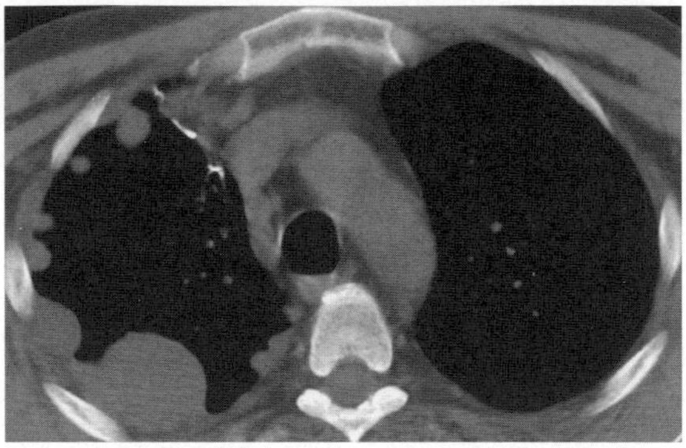

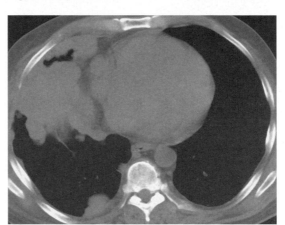

Figure 186B

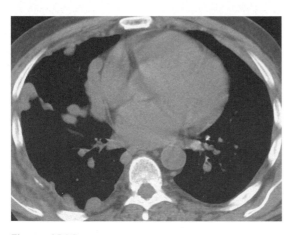

Figure 186C

Figure 186D

Radiologic Findings

PA chest radiograph (**Fig. 186A**) demonstrates circumferential nodular right pleural thickening with encasement and loss of volume of the right lung. Note the right upper lobe surgical sutures. Unenhanced chest CT (mediastinal window) (**Figs. 186B, 186C,** and **186D**) demonstrates circumferential nodular pleural thickening that involves the major fissure (**Fig. 186C**) and multifocal pleural masses of various sizes along the lateral chest wall, ipsilateral mediastinal pleural reflection, and pericardium (**Figs. 186B, 186C,** and **186D**). Many pleural nodules and masses measure over 1 cm in thickness. Right upper lobe surgical chain sutures (**Fig. 186B**) are from prior wedge resection of a primary lung adenocarcinoma.

Diagnosis

Pleural metastases from recurrent adenocarcinoma of the lung

Differential Diagnosis

- Pleural metastases from extrapulmonary primary malignancy
- Malignant pleural mesothelioma
- Lymphoma
- Invasive thymoma

Discussion

Background

Pleural metastases are the most common pleural malignancy and typically result from primary cancers of the lung, breast, pancreas, stomach, and ovary. However, pleural metastases can originate from primary neoplasms in almost any organ. Malignant pleural effusion is the most common manifestation of metastatic pleural disease and occurs in approximately 60% of patients with pleural metastases. The majority of malignant pleural effusions (75%) occur as a result of lung and breast cancers and lymphoma. Pleural metastases may also manifest as soft tissue nodules or masses.

Etiology

Metastases may disseminate to the pleura via hematogenous and lymphatic routes. Pleural metastases may also develop from direct pleural invasion by an adjacent peripheral lung cancer. "Drop" metastases may produce circumferential pleural involvement and may develop in patients with invasive thymoma.

Clinical Findings

Patients with pleural metastases typically have a known primary malignancy. Most patients present with dyspnea on exertion. Chest pain is relatively uncommon ($< 25\%$), in contradistinction to its frequent occurrence in patients with malignant pleural mesothelioma.

Pathology

GROSS

- Pleural effusion
- Focal or multifocal plaque-like and nodular pleural masses
- Circumferential pleural thickening with frequent fissural involvement

MICROSCOPIC

- Histologic and immunohistochemical features identical to those of the primary tumor
- Most frequently adenocarcinoma

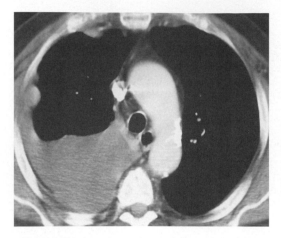

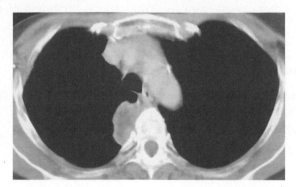

Figure 186E Contrast-enhanced chest CT (mediastinal window) of a 79-year-old man with metastatic melanoma demonstrates a large right pleural effusion. Note multifocal enhancing soft tissue nodules along the anterior and lateral pleural surfaces and band-like enhancing soft tissue measuring 1 cm in thickness along the right mediastinal pleural surface.

Figure 186F Contrast-enhanced chest CT (mediastinal window) of a 60-year-old woman with metastatic breast cancer demonstrates a focal mass along the right posterior mediastinal pleura. The lesion is heterogeneous and exhibits well-defined lobular contours without invasion of adjacent osseous structures. There was no associated pleural effusion.

Imaging Findings

RADIOGRAPHY

- Unilateral or bilateral pleural effusion
- Focal or diffuse pleural thickening (**Fig. 186A**)
  - Nodular
  - Circumferential
- Pleural effusion and nodular pleural thickening

CT/ HRCT

- Pleural effusion (**Fig. 186E**)
- Pleural effusion and nodular pleural thickening and/or pleural masses (**Fig. 186E**)
- Nodular pleural thickening
  - Circumferential (**Figs. 186B, 186C,** and **186D**)
  - Fissural (**Fig. 186C**)
  - Mediastinal (**Figs. 186B, 186C, 186D, 186E,** and **186F**)
  - Thickening greater than 1 cm (**Figs. 186B, 186C, 186D, 186E,** and **186F**)

Treatment

- Pleurodesis for control of malignant pleural effusions
- Pleural and systemic chemotherapy
- Radiation therapy

Prognosis

- Poor
- Mean survival for patients with lung cancer and malignant pleural effusion of 2 to 3 months
- Mean survival for patients with breast cancer and malignant pleural effusion of 7 to 15 months

- Pleural metastases, invasive thymoma, and lymphoma may be radiologically indistinguishable from malignant pleural mesothelioma.
- The presence of a pleural effusion in the setting of lung cancer does not necessarily imply malignancy, as affected patients may develop parapneumonic pleural effusions and pleural effusions unrelated to the primary neoplasm.

Suggested Readings

Aquino SL, Chen MY, Kuo WT, Chiles C. The CT appearance of pleural and extrapleural disease in lymphoma. Clin Radiol 1999;54:647–650

Fraser RS, Müller NL, Colman N, Paré PD. Pleural neoplasms. In: Fraser RS, Müller NL, Colman N, Paré PD, eds. Fraser and Paré's Diagnosis of Diseases of the Chest, 4th ed. Philadelphia: Saunders, 1999:2807–2847

Laucirica R. Pleural metastases. In: Cagle PT, ed. Color Atlas and Text of Pulmonary Pathology. Philadelphia: Lippincott Williams & Willkins, 2005:163–164

Leung AN, Müller NL, Miller RR. CT in differential diagnosis of diffuse pleural disease. AJR Am J Roentgenol 1990;154:487–492

CASE 187 Localized Fibrous Tumor

Clinical Presentation

An asymptomatic 62-year-old man

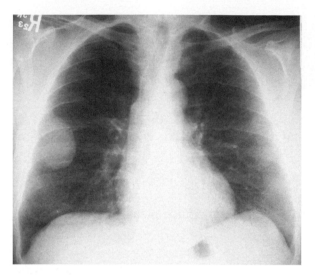

Figure 187A

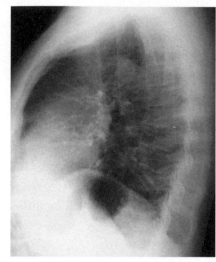

Figure 187B

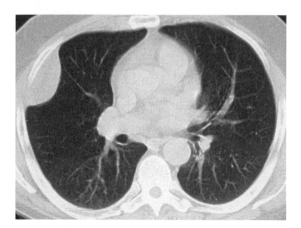

Figure 187C

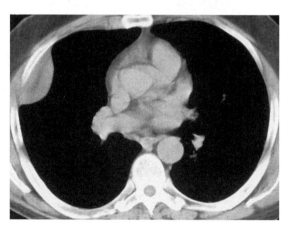

Figure 187D

Radiologic Findings

PA (**Fig. 187A**) and lateral (**Fig. 187B**) chest radiographs demonstrate an ovoid mass in the peripheral right mid-thorax. The mass has a well-defined medial border and an indistinct lateral border (**Fig. 187A**) and is not readily visible on the lateral radiograph. The lesion's obtuse angles with the adjacent pleura result in nonvisualization on the lateral radiograph ("incomplete border" sign). Unenhanced chest CT [lung (**Fig. 187C**) and mediastinal (**Fig. 187D**) window] shows a well-defined homogeneous soft tissue mass that forms obtuse angles with the adjacent pleura. There is no evidence of chest wall involvement.

Diagnosis

Localized fibrous tumor of the pleura

Differential Diagnosis

- Other mesenchymal pleural neoplasm
- Chest wall neoplasm (schwannoma, neurofibroma)
- Pleural metastasis

Discussion

Background

Localized or solitary fibrous tumors of the pleura are rare but represent the second most common primary pleural neoplasm after malignant mesothelioma. They probably arise from submesothelial mesenchymal cells that undergo fibroblastic differentiation. While most are related to the pleura, they have also been described in other intra- and extrathoracic locations. Localized fibrous tumors are not related to mesothelioma or to asbestos exposure.

Etiology

Localized fibrous tumors are neoplasms of unknown etiology.

Clinical Findings

Localized fibrous tumors typically occur in adult men and women in the fifth through eighth decades of life. Many patients (particularly those with small tumors) are asymptomatic and diagnosed incidentally because of an abnormal chest radiograph. Symptoms typically relate to tumor size and include cough, chest pain, and dyspnea. Hypertrophic pulmonary osteoarthropathy is observed in 20 to 35% of patients. The association of hypertrophic pulmonary osteoarthropathy with localized fibrous tumor of the pleura is much stronger than with primary lung cancer, and its presence in a patient with a large intrathoracic mass should suggest this diagnosis. Symptomatic hypoglycemia (Doege-Potter syndrome) occurs in less than 5% of patients with localized fibrous tumors of the pleura, and is somewhat more common with malignant lesions.

Pathology

GROSS

- Most originate from visceral pleural surface; approximately 50% are pedunculated
- Well-defined lobular masses; wide size range
- Whorled fibrous appearance on cut section; necrosis, hemorrhage, and cystic change in large lesions

MICROSCOPIC

- Ovoid or spindle-shaped cells, eosinophilic cytoplasm, and indistinct cell borders
- Frequent collagen surrounding tumor cells or occupying hypocellular areas
- Numerous histologic patterns including a hemangiopericytoma-like appearance
- Malignant localized fibrous tumor: high cellularity, pleomorphism, more than four mitoses per 10 high-power fields

Imaging Findings

RADIOGRAPHY

- Well-defined lobular nodules or masses (**Fig. 187A**) typically abut the pleura
- Variable size; approximately one third occupy half a hemithorax

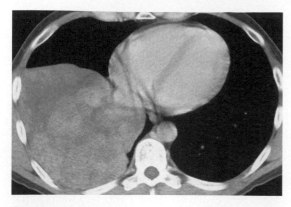

Figure 187E Contrast-enhanced chest CT (mediastinal window) of a 49-year-old man with a localized fibrous tumor of the pleura demonstrates a large mass in the right inferior hemithorax. The mass exhibits well-defined borders, acute angles with the adjacent pleura, and heterogeneous contrast enhancement with nodular areas of high attenuation surrounded by irregular low-attenuation areas.

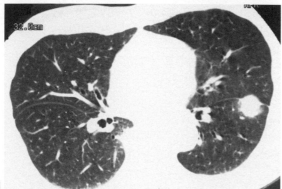
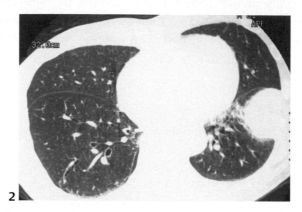

Figure 187F (1,2) Unenhanced chest CT (lung window) of a 58-year-old man with an asymptomatic localized fibrous tumor of the pleura demonstrates a peripheral soft tissue mass in the left hemithorax that forms acute angles with the adjacent pleural surface **(2)** and extends into the left major fissure **(1)**.

- May exhibit the "incomplete border" sign (discrepant border visualization on orthogonal radiographs) (**Figs. 187A** and **187B**)
- Approximately 80% extend to or occupy the inferior hemithorax; may mimic diaphragmatic elevation
- Ipsilateral pleural effusion in 20%

CT

- Noninvasive lobular soft tissue mass of variable size that abuts at least one pleural surface (**Figs. 187C, 187D, 187E, 187F,** and **187G**)
- Typically exhibit acute angles against adjacent pleura (**Figs. 187E, 187F2,** and **187G**); approximately one third exhibit at least one obtuse angle (**Figs. 187C** and **187D**)
- Contrast enhancement is typical (**Figs. 187E** and **187G**)
- Homogeneous attenuation in small lesions; heterogeneous attenuation/enhancement in large lesions (**Figs. 187E** and **187G**): low-attenuation areas (**Figs. 187E** and **187G**), calcification, and enhancing vessels within lesion
- Ipsilateral pleural effusion in approximately one third of cases (**Fig. 187G**)
- May exhibit fissural location (**Fig. 187F**)
- Rare direct visualization of pedicle

MR

- Well-defined, noninvasive mass of heterogeneous signal
- Low or intermediate signal intensity on both T1- and T2-weighted images; high signal intensity on T2-weighted images
- Multiplanar imaging helpful in excluding local invasion and establishing intrathoracic location

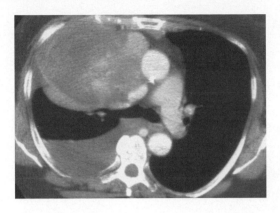

Figure 187G Contrast-enhanced chest CT (mediastinal window) of a 50-year-old man with a malignant localized fibrous tumor of the pleura demonstrates a large heterogeneous soft tissue mass in the anterior aspect of the right hemithorax that produces mass effect on the mediastinum and exhibits extensive low attenuation with central foci of enhancement. Note the large right-sided pleural effusion.

Treatment

- Complete surgical excision

Prognosis

- Favorable prognosis with benign course in up to 90% of patients
- Infrequent local recurrence and distant metastases

PEARLS_____

- The radiographic "incomplete border" sign refers to discrepancy of margin visualization of thoracic lesions and typically implies an extrapulmonary location. It is typically exhibited by lesions that form obtuse borders with the adjacent pleura (**Figs. 187A** and **187B**). Although most thoracic localized fibrous tumors arise from the pleura, they infrequently exhibit the "incomplete border" sign, as most of these tumors form acute angles with the adjacent pleura (**Figs. 187E, 187F2,** and **187G**).
- Localized fibrous tumors of the pleura are not related to mesothelioma, asbestos exposure, or tobacco abuse. Benign and malignant variants are described. Prognosis relates more to resectability than to histologic features.
- Pedunculated lesions may move or change position in the thorax with changes in patient position. Some authorities regard such changes in lesion position as a pathognomic feature of localized fibrous tumors of the pleura. Interestingly, a small percentage of patients with pedunculated lesions complain of a "rolling" sensation in their chest when they change position.

Suggested Readings

Magdeleinat P, Alifano M, Petino A, et al. Solitary fibrous tumors of the pleura: clinical characteristics, surgical treatment and outcome. Eur J Cardiothorac Surg 2002;21:1087–1093

Rosado-de-Christenson ML, Abbott GF, McAdams HP, Franks TJ, Galvin JR. Localized fibrous tumors of the pleura. Radiographics 2003;23:759–783

CASE 188 Chest Wall Infection

Clinical Presentation

A 23-year old man with chest pain and a palpable chest wall mass

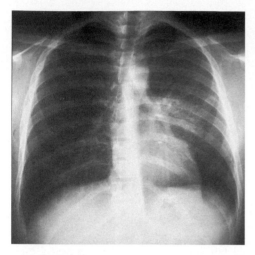

Figure 188A

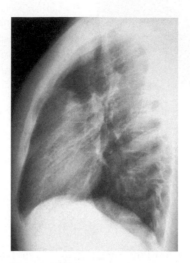

Figure 188B

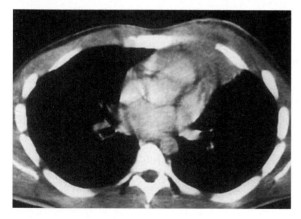

Figure 188C

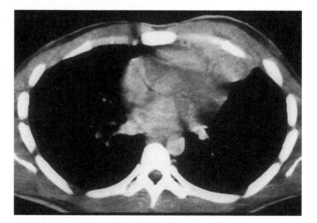

Figure 188D

Radiologic Findings

PA (**Fig. 188A**) and lateral (**Fig. 188B**) chest radiographs demonstrate a left upper lobe mass-like consolidation. Contrast-enhanced chest CT (mediastinal window) (**Figs. 188C** and **188D**) demonstrates a left anterior mediastinal soft tissue mass with contiguous chest wall involvement. The chest wall lesion exhibits heterogeneous attenuation (**Fig. 188C**) but no evidence of osseous destruction. (Courtesy of Aletta A. Frazier, M.D., Armed Forces Institute of Pathology, Washington, District of Columbia).

Diagnosis

Actinomycosis; pulmonary, mediastinal, and chest wall involvement

Differential Diagnosis

- Lung cancer with adjacent mediastinal and chest wall involvement
- Pulmonary, mediastinal, and chest wall involvement by other malignancy
- Other thoracic infections (aspergillosis, nocardiosis, blastomycosis, tuberculosis, pyogenic infection)

Discussion

Background

Actinomycosis is a rare bacterial pneumonia that often extends across anatomic barriers to involve the pleura and chest wall. Pulmonary actinomycosis typically occurs as a chronic suppurative and granulomatous infection. Spread of infection is related to proteolytic enzymes and fistula formation between involved lung and adjacent tissues. Thoracic infection most commonly occurs through aspiration of contaminated oral secretions.

Etiology

Actinomycosis is caused by infection with organisms in the genus *Actinomyces*. The most common pathogen is *Actinomyces israelii*. Less common pathogens include *A. naeslundii*, *A. viscosus*, and *A. propionica*.

Clinical Findings

Patients with actinomycosis may present with cough, sputum production, fever, and weight loss. Hemoptysis and chest pain occur less frequently. Affected patients often have poor dental hygiene that promotes growth of actinomyces organisms normally present in the oropharynx. The cervicofacial region is most commonly affected. Abdominal infection is usually related to surgery or intestinal trauma, and pelvic disease may be associated with intrauterine contraceptive devices in women. Cerebral actinomycosis may also occur.

Pathology

GROSS

- Parenchymal mass-like consolidation; often mimics a neoplasm
- "Sulfur granules" (yellow-orange macroscopic masses of filamentous bacterial cells resembling sunbursts) within abscesses or airways
- Pleural effusion and empyema with or without chest wall involvement

MICROSCOPIC

- Acute suppurative inflammation
- Gram-positive, beaded, branching, filamentous bacteria
- Acute bronchopneumonia with abscess formation
- Histiocytic reaction
- Sulfur granules characterized by Splendore-Hoeppli phenomenon (an eosinophilic proteinaceous deposit encasing the filamentous bacteria)

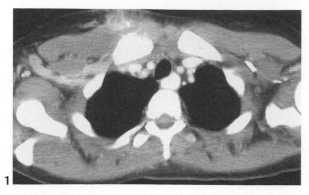 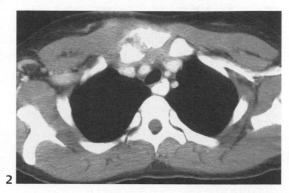

Figure 188E (1,2) Contrast-enhanced chest CT (mediastinal window) of an intravenous drug user with chest wall *Staphylococcus aureus* osteomyelitis demonstrates enhancing soft tissue infiltration of the subcutaneous fat of the right anterior chest wall, thickening of adjacent muscles **(1)**, and involvement of the ipsilateral sternoclavicular joint **(2)**.

Imaging Features

RADIOGRAPHY

- Peripheral, unilateral patchy consolidation (may be chronic)
- Mass-like consolidation; may mimic lung cancer (**Figs. 188A** and **188B**)
- Multifocal nodules/masses
- Soft tissue thickening or mass of adjacent chest wall
- Wavy periostitis; rarely rib destruction

CT

- Mass-like consolidation; homogeneous or heterogeneous with peripheral enhancement and central low attenuation/cavitation (**Fig. 188C**)
- Pleural thickening, pleural effusion
- Hilar/mediastinal lymphadenopathy
- Mediastinal involvement (**Figs. 188C** and **188D**)
- Chest wall soft tissue mass or thickening, (**Figs. 188C** and **188D**)
- Wavy periostitis of adjacent osseous structures

Treatment

- Prolonged therapy with penicillin; 4 to 6 weeks of intravenous penicillin followed by 6 to 12 months of an oral regimen
- Improved oral hygiene

Prognosis

- Good with antibiotic treatment but slow response; prolonged indolent disease reported
- Cure in 90% of patients treated with penicillin
- Morbidity from central nervous system involvement (i.e., brain abscess, meningitis)

PEARLS

- Thoracic actinomycosis is often difficult to diagnose and can mimic lung cancer and tuberculosis in its clinical presentation and imaging features. The majority of patients undergo surgery for definitive diagnosis.

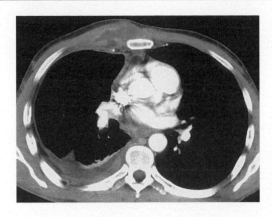

Figure 188F Contrast-enhanced CT (mediastinal window) of a 41-year-old man with tuberculosis demonstrates a heterogeneous irregular mass in the soft tissues of the right anterior chest wall. Note subtle peripheral enhancement and central low attenuation consistent with tissue necrosis. There is right pleural thickening, a small right pleural effusion, and lymphadenopathy in the azygoesophageal recess.

- Heroin addicts have a striking tendency to develop septic arthritis of the sternoclavicular and sternochondral joints, typically caused by *Staphylococcus aureus* (**Fig. 188E**) and *Pseudomonas aeruginosa*.
- Tuberculous chest wall abscesses are most frequently found at the margins of the sternum and along rib shafts (**Fig. 188F**).

Suggested Readings

Colmegna I, Rodriguez-Barradas M, Rauch R, Clarridge J, Young EJ. Disseminated *Actinomyces meyeri* infection resembling lung cancer with brain metastases. Am J Med Sci 2003;326:152–155

Fraser RS, Müller NL, Colman N, Paré PD. Fungi and actinomyces. In: Fraser RS, Müller NL, Colman N, Paré PD, eds. Fraser and Paré's Diagnosis of Diseases of the Chest, 4th ed. Philadelphia: Saunders, 1999:875–978

Mabeza GF, Macfarlane J. Pulmonary actinomycosis. Eur Respir J 2003;21:545–551

Morris BS, Maheshwari M, Chalwa A. Chest wall tuberculosis: a review of CT appearances. Br J Radiol 2004;77:449–457

CASE 189 Chest Wall Lipoma

Clinical Presentation

An asymptomatic 91-year-old woman

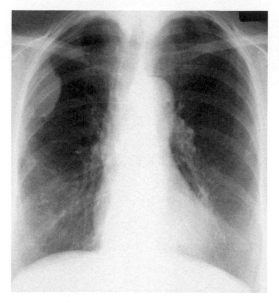

Figure 189A

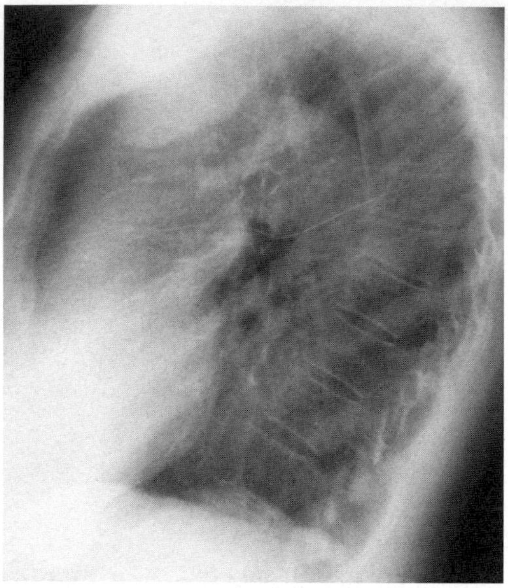

Figure 189B

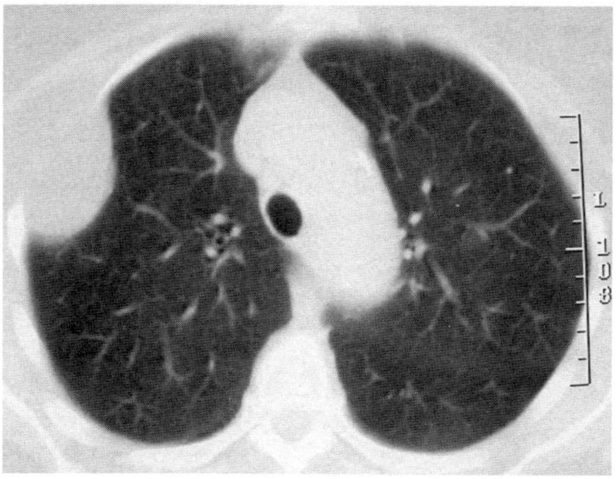

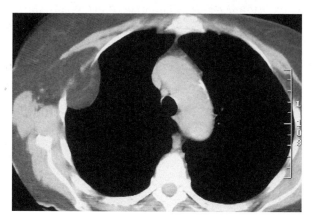

Figure 189C

Figure 189D

Radiologic Findings

PA (**Fig. 189A**) and lateral (**Fig. 189B**) chest radiographs demonstrate a peripheral opacity in the right superior hemithorax that forms obtuse angles with the adjacent chest wall (**Fig. 189A**). There is a discrepancy in margin visualization consistent with an extrapulmonary location. Contrast-enhanced chest CT [lung (**Fig. 189C**) and mediastinal window (**Fig. 189D**)] demonstrates a peripheral mass that forms at least one obtuse angle with the adjacent chest wall (**Figs. 189C** and **189D**) and exhibits fat attenuation with scant thin linear and punctate soft tissue elements (**Fig. 189D**). The mass is contiguous with subcutaneous fat attenuation tissue. There is no appreciable rib destruction.

744

Diagnosis

Chest wall lipoma

Differential Diagnosis

None

Discussion

Background

Benign chest wall tumors may originate from blood vessels, nerves, bone, cartilage, or fat. The imaging manifestations of benign and malignant chest wall lesions overlap, but some entities have characteristic imaging features that allow a confident diagnosis. Lipomas represent the most common soft tissue chest wall tumors. They are well-circumscribed, encapsulated masses of adipose tissue that may lie deep within the chest wall or protrude into the thorax and displace the pleura, mimicking other benign or malignant pleural lesions. Most lipomas that arise between the ribs have a dumbbell or hourglass configuration (part projecting inside and part projecting outside of the thorax) (**Fig. 189D**).

Etiology

The etiology of chest wall lipomas is unknown.

Clinical Findings

Chest wall lipomas are typically incidental findings in asymptomatic patients. They occur most frequently in patients who are 50 to 70 years of age and are more common in obese individuals.

Pathology

GROSS

- Soft, well-circumscribed, encapsulated fatty mass

MICROSCOPIC

- Encapsulated mature adipose tissue

Imaging Findings

RADIOGRAPHY

- Well-marginated ovoid or lens-shaped chest wall mass (**Figs. 189A** and **189B**)
- Lesions may exhibit the "incomplete border" sign (**Figs. 189A** and **189B**).
- Lesions may change shape with respiration.

CT

- Chest wall mass with intrathoracic extension and well-defined borders (**Figs. 189C** and **189D**)
- Fat attenuation mass (**Fig. 189D**); may contain scant thin linear and punctate soft tissue elements (**Fig. 189D**)

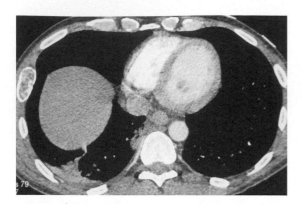

Figure 189E Contrast-enhanced chest CT (mediastinal window) of a 42-year-old man with monostotic fibrous dysplasia demonstrates a right rib expansile lesion with intact cortical margins.

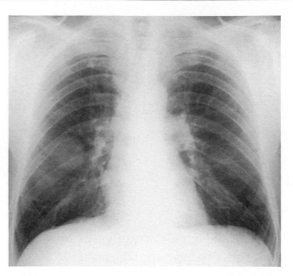

Figure 189F PA chest radiograph of a 29-year-old man with neurofibromatosis demonstrates smooth notching and sclerosis of the undersurface of the right eighth posterior rib that conforms to the superior contour of an adjacent nodular opacity with "incomplete" and ill-defined borders.

- Occasional punctate calcification in areas of fat necrosis
- Completely intrathoracic, subcutaneous, or both (**Figs. 189C** and **189D**)

MR

- High signal intensity on T1-weighted images
- Intermediate signal intensity on T2-weighted images
- Low signal intensity on fat-saturation images

Treatment

- None
- Surgical excision in selected patients with large lesions

Prognosis

- Excellent

PEARLS_____

- Predominance of soft tissue elements in a fatty chest wall lesion should suggest the possibility of liposarcoma or lipoblastoma. Large lesion size should also prompt exclusion of malignancy.
- Fibrous dysplasia is a developmental skeletal anomaly that commonly affects the ribs and may be monostotic (70–80%) or polyostotic. The lesion is related to failure of mesenchymal osteoblasts to achieve normal morphologic differentiation and maturation. Imaging studies typically demonstrate unilateral fusiform rib enlargement and deformity with cortical thickening and increased trabeculation (**Fig. 189E**).
- Neurofibromas are peripheral nerve neoplasms that most commonly affect young adults between the ages of 20 and 30 years. The majority of patients (60–90%) have type 1 neurofibromatosis

(NF1). Neurofibromas may develop along the thoracic spine roots, the paraspinal ganglia of the sympathetic chain, the intercostal nerves, or the peripheral nerves of the chest wall. Those arising from intercostal nerves may produce rib erosion, notching, and/or sclerosis (**Fig. 189F**).

• CT is more cost-effective than radiography for establishing the diagnosis of chest wall lipoma and for demonstrating small calcifications and subtle bone destruction. MR imaging is the preferred modality for delineating intramuscular neurofibromas, for demonstrating soft tissue, intraspinal, and marrow involvement by neurogenic tumors, and for surgical planning.

Suggested Readings

Fraser RS, Müller NL, Colman N, Paré PD. The chest wall. In: Fraser RS, Müller NL, Colman N, Paré PD, eds. Fraser and Paré's Diagnosis of Diseases of the Chest, 4th ed. Philadelphia: Saunders, 1999: 3011–3042

Kuhlman JE, Bouchardy L, Fishman EK, Zerhouni EA. CT and MR imaging evaluation of chest wall disorders. Radiographics 1994;14:571–595

Tateishi U, Gladish GW, Kusumoto M, et al. Chest wall tumors: radiologic findings and pathologic correlation. Part 1. Benign tumors. Radiographics 2003;23:1477–1490

CASE 190 Chondrosarcoma

Clinical Presentation

A 57-year-old man with chest pain and a palpable right anterior chest wall mass

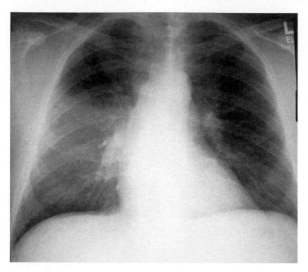

Figure 190A

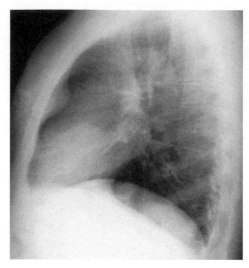

Figure 190B

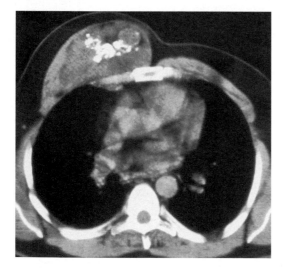

Figure 190C

Radiologic Findings

PA (**Fig. 190A**) and lateral (**Fig. 190B**) chest radiographs demonstrate a right anterior chest wall mass. The lesion exhibits a well-defined border with obtuse angles against the adjacent chest wall on the lateral radiograph (**Fig. 190B**) and manifests as a right midthoracic opacity with poorly defined margins on the frontal radiograph (**Fig. 190A**). Note the flocculent calcifications within the subcutaneous portion of the right anterior chest wall mass on the lateral radiograph (**Fig. 190B**). Unenhanced chest CT (mediastinal window) (**Fig. 190C**) demonstrates a heterogeneous right anterior chest wall mass arising near the chondral cartilage with multifocal dense, amorphous calcifications.

748

Diagnosis

Chondrosarcoma

Differential Diagnosis

- Metastasis from primary chondrosarcoma or other primary malignant neoplasm
- Primitive neuroectodermal tumor (PNET)
- Malignant fibrous histiocytoma (MFH)
- Fibrosarcoma; neurofibrosarcoma

Discussion

Background

Chondrosarcomas are malignant neoplasms with cartilaginous differentiation. They represent the most common primary malignant tumor of the chest wall. They typically arise in the anterior chest wall and involve the sternum or costochondral arches. Less frequently chondrosarcomas arise in the ribs (17%) and scapulae.

Clinical Findings

Chondrosarcomas occur across a wide age range but typically affect patients between the ages of 30 and 60 years. Most tumors manifest as palpable chest wall masses that may be painful. The lesions may grow rapidly and cause chest pain. Males are affected slightly more frequently than females (male to female ratio of 1.3:1.0).

Pathology

GROSS

- Lobular glistening mass with frequent disruption of the osseous cortex; nodules of white to bluish white cartilaginous tissue
- Size range from 1.5 to 3.0 cm
- Local invasion

MICROSCOPIC

- Round to stellate cells with eosinophilic cytoplasm and dark chromatin arranged in rows and in a chain-like pattern
- Calcification in 60 to 75%

Imaging Findings

RADIOGRAPHY

- Large chest wall mass (**Figs. 190A** and **190B**); bone destruction; typically affects sternum, costochondral junction or ribs
- Incomplete border sign as in other extrapulmonary masses (see Case 187) (**Figs. 190A** and **190B**)
- Variable intratumoral calcification (rings, arches, flocculent, or stippled) (**Fig. 190B**)

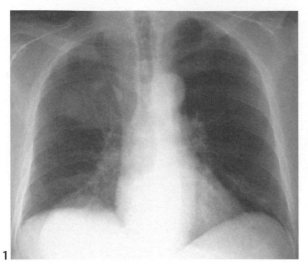
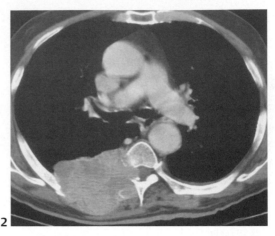

Figure 190D (1,2) PA chest radiograph **(1)** of a 69-year-old man with metastatic hepatocellular carcinoma demonstrates an ill-defined opacity projecting over the right superior hemithorax with associated destruction of the posterior right fifth rib. Contrast-enhanced chest CT (mediastinal window) **(2)** demonstrates a large soft tissue mass of the right posterior chest wall that exhibits rib destruction and invasion of the adjacent soft tissue. Note partial destruction of the adjacent vertebral body and intraspinal tumor growth **(2).**

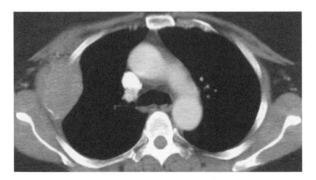
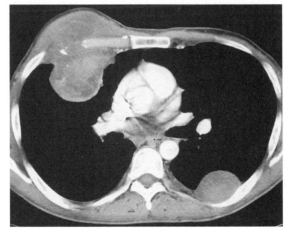

Figure 190E Contrast-enhanced chest CT of a 53-year old woman with multiple myeloma demonstrates a homogeneous soft tissue mass in the right lateral chest wall with associated rib destruction, involvement of the chest wall soft tissues, and smooth effacement of the adjacent pleura.

Figure 190F Contrast-enhanced chest CT of a 46-year-old man with neurofibromatosis type 1 (NF1) demonstrates a benign neurofibroma manifesting as a well-defined homogeneous soft tissue mass of the left posterior chest wall that manifests with benign pressure erosion on an adjacent rib and a malignant right anterior chest wall neurofibrosarcoma. The neurofibrosarcoma exhibits heterogeneous enhancement, amorphous calcification, extension into the right chest cavity, and involvement of the anterior chest wall soft tissues and osseous structures.

CT

- Well-defined soft tissue mass (**Fig. 190C**)
- Osseous destruction
- Higher sensitivity for detection of tumor calcification, which may be amorphous, popcorn-like, or curvilinear (**Fig. 190C**)

MR

- Lobular chest wall mass
- Heterogeneous signal intensity on T1- and T2-weighted images
- Heterogeneous contrast enhancement, especially at the periphery

Treatment

- Surgical resection
- Chemotherapy and radiation in selected cases

Prognosis

- Five-year survival more than 60% (greater than 80% in patients without metastases)
- Poor prognosis associated with incomplete resection, metastases, local recurrence, and patient age over 50 years

PEARLS

- Chest wall metastases represent the most common malignant chest wall neoplasm (**Fig. 190D**).
- Chest wall neoplasms that exhibit imaging features of osseous destruction in adults include chest wall metastases (**Fig. 190D**), multiple myeloma (**Fig. 190E**), and neurofibrosarcoma (**Fig. 190F**).
- CT and MR imaging have complementary roles in evaluating chest wall lesions. CT more readily shows calcifications (**Figs. 190C** and **190F**) and bone destruction (**Figs. 190D2, 190E,** and **190F**), and is faster and less expensive. MR may better delineate the extent of tumor invasion and is superior for depicting bone marrow infiltration and the extent of soft tissue involvement.

Suggested Readings

Fraser RS, Müller NL, Colman N, Paré PD. The chest wall. In: Fraser RS, Müller NL, Colman N, Paré PD, eds. Fraser and Paré's Diagnosis of Diseases of the Chest, 4th ed. Philadelphia: Saunders, 1999: 3011–3042

Gladish GW, Sabloff BM, Munden RF, Truong MT, Erasmus JJ, Chasen MH. Primary thoracic sarcomas. Radiographics 2002;22:621–637

Kuhlman JE, Bouchardy L, Fishman EK, Zerhouni EA. CT and MR imaging evaluation of chest wall disorders. Radiographics 1994;14:571–595

Tateishi U, Gladish GW, Kusumoto M, et al. Chest wall tumors: radiologic findings and pathologic correlation. Part 2. Malignant tumors. Radiographics 2003;23:1491–1508

Clinical Presentation

An asymptomatic 65-year-old woman

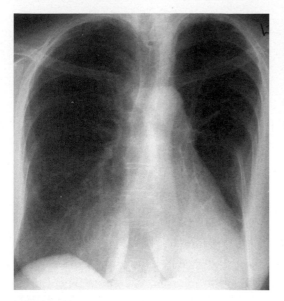

Figure 191A

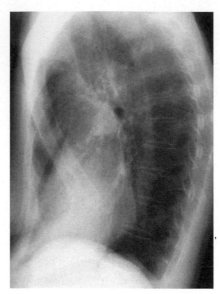

Figure 191B

Radiologic Findings

PA (**Fig. 191A**) and lateral (**Fig. 191B**) chest radiographs demonstrate a severe pectus excavatum deformity. Note vertical orientation of the anterior ribs and obscuration of the right cardiac border in the absence of right middle lobe consolidation.

Diagnosis

Pectus excavatum

Differential Diagnosis

None

Discussion

Background

Pectus deformities (pectus excavatum and pectus carinatum) are among the most common chest wall anomalies in the general population. There is great variability in the anatomy and morphology of the anterior chest wall of asymptomatic children. Thus, mild asymmetry and mild degrees of pectus deformity are sometimes considered normal variants. Pectus excavatum is also referred to as "funnel chest."

Etiology

Pectus excavatum is thought to result from abnormal growth of the costal cartilages that produces depression of the sternum (typically its inferior portion) often associated with sternal rotation to the right. Typically, there is associated rotation and displacement of the heart and mediastinum to the left. Pectus carinatum and localized pectus excavatum probably result from sternal growth disturbances with or without associated costal cartilage abnormalities.

Pathology

- Overgrowth of the costal cartilages
- Sternal depression and rotation

Clinical Findings

Pectus excavatum is found in about 0.13 to 0.4% of the general population and affects males three to four times more frequently than females. While it is usually a sporadic condition, there are reports of an increased familial incidence. Associated conditions include Marfan syndrome, congenital heart disease (2%), and mitral valve prolapse. Most patients with pectus excavatum are asymptomatic. Symptomatic patients complain of dyspnea, chest pain, and palpitations. Severe pectus excavatum deformity may result in exercise-induced cardiopulmonary dysfunction. There is an increased incidence of mild scoliosis (15–22% of cases). There may also be large airway compression, malacia, and a predisposition to atelectasis. Physical examination may reveal a heart murmur that may relate to flow abnormalities from mediastinal distortion. Impaired cardiac function is primarily exercise-induced with decreased stroke volume and respiratory reserve.

Imaging Findings

RADIOGRAPHY

- Mediastinal shift to the left, upturned configuration of the cardiac apex, and straightening of the left heart border (from mediastinal rotation) on frontal radiographs (**Fig. 191A**)
- Posterior depression of the inferior sternum with narrow anteroposterior diameter on lateral radiographs (**Fig. 191B**)
- Prominent right pulmonary vasculature and poor visualization of the right cardiac border suggesting right middle lobe consolidation and/or volume loss on frontal radiographs (**Fig. 191A**)
- Increased downward sloping of anterior ribs on frontal radiographs (**Fig. 191A**)

CT

- Visualization of location and degree of pectus deformity and its effect on intrathoracic structures
- Evaluation of mediastinum and airways and exclusion of pulmonary disease
- Calculation of "pectus index," the ratio of the transverse thoracic diameter to the AP diameter at the deepest point of the pectus deformity

Treatment

- Surgical correction for patients with cardiorespiratory symptoms or for cosmetic reasons
- Resection of costal cartilage with placement of a transverse metallic strut

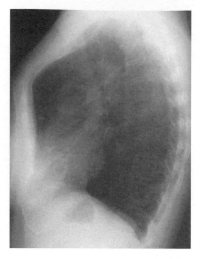

Figure 191C Lateral chest radiograph of an asymptomatic woman with pectus carinatum demonstrates focal sternal deformity with increased anteroposterior thoracic diameter.

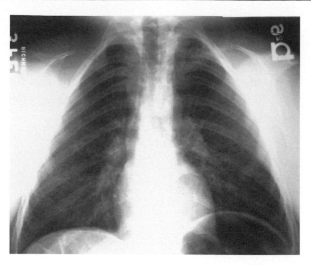

Figure 191D PA chest radiograph of an asymptomatic young man with cleidocranial dysostosis demonstrates small rudimentary clavicles bilaterally and a bell-shaped thorax.

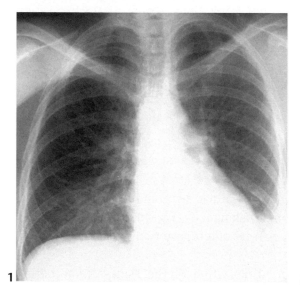

1

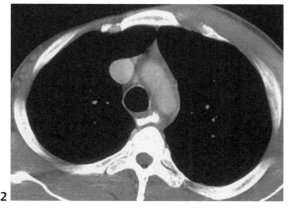

2

Figure 191E (1,2) PA chest radiograph **(1)** of an asymptomatic patient with Poland syndrome demonstrates hyperlucency of the right hemithorax secondary to asymmetry of the chest wall soft tissues and absence of the right breast. Contrast-enhanced chest CT (mediastinal window) **(2)** demonstrates absence of the right pectoralis muscles.

Prognosis

- Excellent for asymptomatic patients with mild pectus deformity
- Excellent for surgically treated patients; best results when surgery is performed between ages 4 and 10 years, but successful surgery reported in adolescents and adults

PEARLS

- A "pectus index" over 3.25 is one of the parameters used to select candidates for surgical correction of the pectus excavatum deformity.

- Pectus carinatum or "pigeon breast" is less common than pectus excavatum. It may result from abnormal growth of the costal cartilage or abnormal fusion of the sternal segments and manubrium sternum with resultant sternal protrusion (**Fig. 191C**).
- Cleidocranial dysostosis is an autosomal-dominant disorder of membranous bone in which the outer portions of the clavicles are typically absent. The scapula may be hypoplastic, and the glenoid is often small. The thorax may be bell-shaped (**Fig. 191D**)
- Poland syndrome refers to congenital absence or hypoplasia of the pectoralis major muscle. Associated anomalies include malformations of ipsilateral ribs (typically 2 through 5) and clavicle and congenital absence of ipsilateral breast tissue (**Fig. 191E**).

Suggested Readings

Grissom LE, Harcke HT. Thoracic deformities and the growing lung. Semin Roentgenol 1998;33: 199–208

Lancaster L, McIlhenny J, Rodgers B, Alford B. Radiographic findings after pectus excavatum repair. Pediatr Radiol 1995;25:452–454

Takahashi K, Sugimoto H, Ohsawa T. Obliteration of the descending aortic interface in pectus excavatum: correlation with clockwise rotation of the heart. Radiology 1992;182:825–828

CASE 192 Bochdalek Hernia

Clinical Presentation

An asymptomatic 74-year-old man with slowly enlarging mass on serial chest radiography

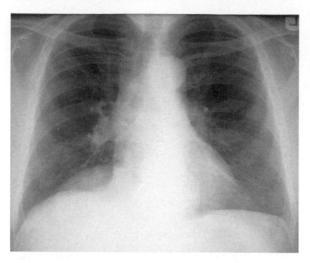

Figure 192A

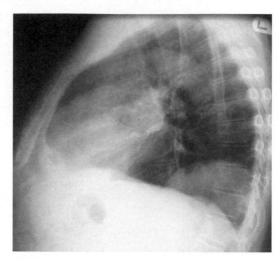

Figure 192B

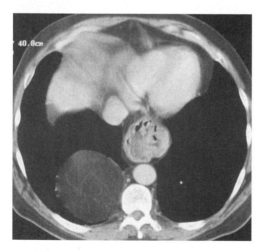

Figure 192C

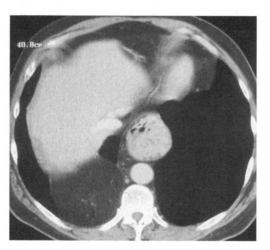

Figure 192D

Radiologic Findings

PA (**Fig. 192A**) and lateral (**Fig. 192B**) chest radiographs demonstrate a well-defined mass in the posteromedial right inferior hemithorax that appears to abut the adjacent hemidiaphragm. Contrast-enhanced chest CT (mediastinal window) (**Figs. 192C** and **192D**) demonstrates a well-defined mass that abuts the right hemidiaphragm and exhibits predominant fat attenuation with thin linear and small nodular soft tissue foci representing vascular structures (**Figs. 192C** and **192D**). Note the moderate hiatus hernia.

Diagnosis

Bochdalek hernia

Differential Diagnosis

None

Discussion

Background

Abdominal contents may herniate into the thorax through congenital or acquired diaphragmatic weak areas or through rents caused by trauma. Nontraumatic diaphragmatic herniation occurs most frequently through the esophageal hiatus and is usually related to obesity or pregnancy. Less commonly, herniation occurs through the pleuroperitoneal hiatus (Bochdalek hernia) or the parasternal hiatus (Morgagni hernia). Bochdalek hernias have been reported to occur more commonly on the left side, although a recent small series described a right-sided predominance (68%) with bilateral involvement in 14% of affected patients. Bochdalek hernias are associated with protrusion of omental or retroperitoneal fat that may be accompanied by abdominal organs, most often the kidney. Morgagni hernias are less common and represent 3% of diaphragmatic hernias. They are frequently located lateral to the xiphoid but may be directly posterior to it. The foramina of Morgagni are small triangular diaphragmatic clefts bounded medially by muscle fibers originating from the sternum and laterally by the seventh costal cartilages. Morgagni hernias are typically unilateral and occur more commonly on the right (90%), as the left foramen is protected by the pericardium.

Etiology

Bochdalek hernias are typically acquired lesions of adults and relate to focal weaknesses or defects in the diaphragm near the pleuroperitoneal hiatus.

Clinical Findings

The incidence of Bochdalek hernias in the adult population is approximately 1%, and women are more commonly affected than men. The incidence of Bochdalek hernias increases with age, suggesting that they are acquired lesions. Affected patients are often asymptomatic but may complain of vague symptoms including chest pain, abdominal pain, and rarely bowel obstruction. Large hernias may produce mass effect and pulmonary insufficiency.

Pathology

- Omental fat, bowel or abdominal viscera contained in hernia sac

Imaging Findings

RADIOGRAPHY

- Focal bulge in hemidiaphragm or mass in posteromedial inferior hemithorax (**Figs. 192A** and **192B**)
- Lesion density may appear lower than soft tissue (**Fig. 192B**).
- Visualization of internal air-containing bowel loops

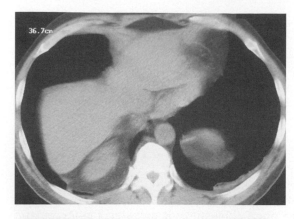

Figure 192E Unenhanced chest CT (mediastinal window) of a 49-year-old man with a Bochdalek hernia demonstrates herniation of the right kidney and retroperitoneal fat into the right inferior hemithorax. Note right diaphragmatic discontinuity posterolateral to the kidney.

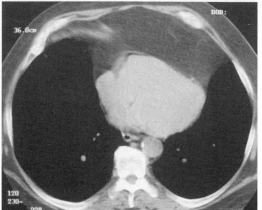
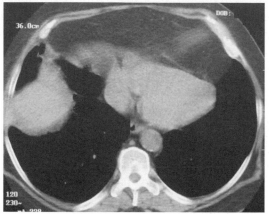

Figure 192F (1,2) Unenhanced chest CT (mediastinal window) of a 58-year-old man with bilateral Morgagni hernias demonstrates protrusion of omental fat into the anterior thorax.

CT

- Continuity with diaphragm and abdomen (**Figs. 192D** and **192E**)
- Demonstration of fat attenuation with intrinsic punctate or thin, linear soft tissue foci representing omental vessels (**Figs. 192C** and **192D**)
- Herniated viscera, most often a kidney (**Fig. 192E**)

Treatment

- Surgical repair in symptomatic patients

Prognosis

- Good; most patients remain asymptomatic.
- Large hernias may contain viscera or bowel that may experience vascular compromise or obstruction.

PEARLS

- Morgagni hernia manifests as a well-defined mass located in the right costophrenic angle in asymptomatic patients (**Figs. 192F** and **192G**). In contrast to Bochdalek hernias, a hernia sac is

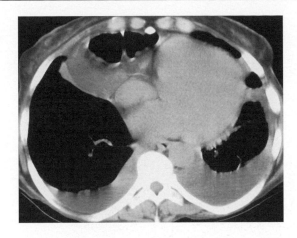

Figure 192G Unenhanced chest CT (mediastinal window) of a 50-year-old woman with a Morgagni hernia demonstrates a right costophrenic angle hernia sac that contains air-filled bowel surrounded by abdominal ascites. Note bilateral pleural effusions.

usually present and contains omentum (**Fig. 192F**) or bowel (**Fig. 192G**), typically transverse colon. In some cases, the hernia sac may extend into the pericardium.

• Congenital Bochdalek hernias relate to anomalies of the pleuroperitoneal canal, often secondary to partial agenesis of the hemidiaphragm. These lesions are typically left-sided and, when large, are associated with neonatal respiratory distress. Large congenital Bochdalek hernias may contain large amounts of bowel and abdominal viscera and may result in pulmonary hypoplasia.

Suggested Readings

Caskey CI, Zerhouni EA, Fishman EK, Rahmouni AD. Aging of the diaphragm: a CT study. Radiology 1989;171:385–389

Fraser RS, Müller NL, Colman N, Paré PD. The Diaphragm. In: Fraser RS, Müller NL, Colman N, Paré PD, eds. Fraser and Paré's Diagnosis of Diseases of the Chest, 4th ed. Philadelphia: Saunders, 1999:2987–3010

Gaerte SC, Meyer CA, Winer-Muram HT, Tarver RD, Conces DJ Jr. Fat-containing lesions of the chest. Radiographics 2002;22:S61–S78

Mullins ME, Stein J, Saini SS, Mueller PR. Prevalence of incidental Bochdalek's hernia in a large adult population. AJR Am J Roentgenol 2001;177:363–366

INDEX

Page numbers followed by f or t indicate figures and tables respectively.